Bancroft's Theory and Practice of Histological Techniques

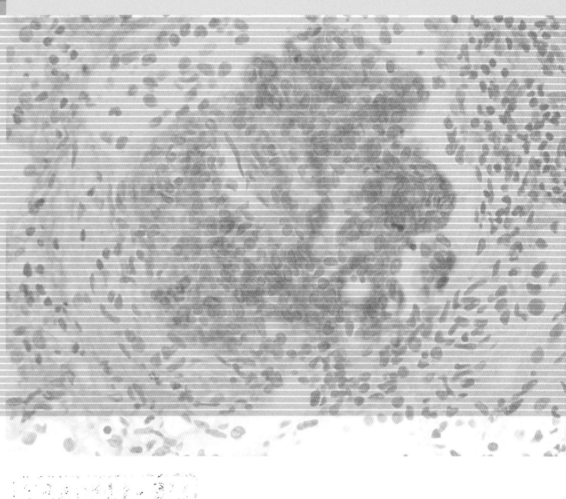

Content Strategist: Michael Houston
Content Development Specialists: Michael Parkinson and Alexandra Mortimer
Project Manager: Caroline Jones
Design: Stewart Larking
Marketing Manager: Abby Swartz

Bancroft's
THEORY and PRACTICE of HISTOLOGICAL TECHNIQUES

SEVENTH EDITION

S. Kim Suvarna
Consultant Pathologist
Histopathology Department,
Northern General Hospital
Sheffield, UK

Christopher Layton
Specialist Section Lead in Specimen Dissection
Histopathology Department,
Northern General Hospital
Sheffield, UK

John D. Bancroft
Formerly Pathology Directorate Manager and Business Manager,
Queen's Medical Centre,
Nottingham, UK

CHURCHILL LIVINGSTONE

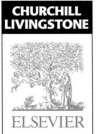

ELSEVIER

CHURCHILL
LIVINGSTONE
ELSEVIER

is an imprint of Elsevier Limited
© 2013, Elsevier Limited. All rights reserved.

First edition 1977
Second edition 1982
Third edition 1990
Fourth edition 1996
Fifth edition 2002
Sixth edition 2008

Notices
Knowledge and best practice in this field are constantly changing. As new research and experience broaden our understanding, changes in research methods, professional practices, or medical treatment may become necessary.

Practitioners and researchers must always rely on their own experience and knowledge in evaluating and using any information, methods, compounds, or experiments described herein. In using such information or methods they should be mindful of their own safety and the safety of others, including parties for whom they have a professional responsibility.

With respect to any drug or pharmaceutical products identified, readers are advised to check the most current information provided (i) on procedures featured or (ii) by the manufacturer of each product to be administered, to verify the recommended dose or formula, the method and duration of administration, and contraindications. It is the responsibility of practitioners, relying on their own experience and knowledge of their patients, to make diagnoses, to determine dosages and the best treatment for each individual patient, and to take all appropriate safety precautions.

To the fullest extent of the law, neither the Publisher nor the authors, contributors, or editors, assume any liability for any injury and/or damage to persons or property as a matter of products liability, negligence or otherwise, or from any use or operation of any methods, products, instructions, or ideas contained in the material herein.

Churchill Livingstone

British Library Cataloguing in Publication Data
Bancroft's theory and practice of histological techniques.
 – 7th ed.
 1. Histology, Pathological – Technique.
 I. Theory and practice of histological techniques
 II. Suvarna, Kim.   III. Layton, Christopher.   IV. Bancroft,
 John D.
 616'.07583 – dc23

ISBN-13: 9780702042263
ISBN: 978-0-7020-4226-3
Ebook ISBN: 978-0-7020-5032-9

Printed in China
Last digit is the print number: 9 8 7 6 5 4 3 2 1

Contents

Foreword   *vii*

Preface to the seventh edition   *ix*

Preface to the first edition   *xi*

List of contributors   *xiii*

Acknowledgments   *xv*

1. Managing the laboratory   1
   Louise Dunk

2. Safety and ergonomics in the laboratory   11
   John D. Bancroft

3. Light microscopy   37
   John D. Bancroft and Alton D. Floyd

4. Fixation of tissues   69
   Anthony Rhodes

5. The gross room/surgical cut-up   95
   S. Kim Suvarna and Christopher Layton

6. Tissue processing and microarray   105
   Lena T. Spencer, John D. Bancroft and Wanda Grace Jones

7. Microtomy: Paraffin and frozen   125
   Lena T. Spencer and John D. Bancroft

8. Plastic embedding for light microscopy   139
   Neil M. Hand

9. How histological stains work   157
   Richard W. Horobin

10. The hematoxylins and eosin   173
    John D. Bancroft and Christopher Layton

11. Connective and mesenchymal tissues with their stains   187
    John D. Bancroft and Christopher Layton

12. Carbohydrates   215
    Christopher Layton and John D. Bancroft

13. Pigments and minerals   239
    Guy E. Orchard

14. Amyloid   271
    Janet A. Gilbertson and Toby Hunt

15. Microorganisms   291
    Jeanine H. Bartlett

16. Bone   317
    Diane L. Sterchi

17. Techniques in neuropathology   353
    J. Robin Highley and Nicky Sullivan

18. Immunohistochemical techniques   381
    Peter Jackson and David Blythe

19. Immunofluorescent techniques   427
    Graeme Wild

20. Immunohistochemistry quality control   435
    Tracy Sanderson and Gregory Zardin

21. Molecular pathology   455
    Diane L. Sterchi and Caroline Astbury

22. Transmission electron microscopy   493
    Anthony E. Woods and John W. Stirling

23. Quantitative data from microscopic specimens   539
    Alton D. Floyd

Appendices
    Diagnostic appendices   561
        Appendix I: Classical histochemical methods   563
        John D. Bancroft and Jennifer H. Stonard

        Appendix II: Applications of immunohistochemistry   577
        Laura J. Keeling and Sherin Jos Payyappilly

    Technical appendices   585
        Appendix III: Measurement units   587
        Jennifer H. Stonard

        Appendix IV: Preparation of solutions   589
        Danielle Maddocks

        Appendix V: Buffer solutions   593
        Paul Samuel

        Appendix VI: Solubility of some common reagents and dyes   597
        Stuart Inglut

        Appendix VII: Mounting media and slide coatings   601
        Ann Michelle Moon

        Appendix VIII: Molecular pathology reagents   603
        Diane L. Sterchi

Staining methods index   605
Subject index   609

Foreword

You are familiar with earlier editions of *Theory and Practice of Histological Techniques*. So, you may be wondering 'What's all this about? Why the name change?' As the only author contributing to this new edition who also contributed to the first edition, and as someone originally recruited by the eponymous John Bancroft and his then co-editor Alan Stevens, it falls to me to offer an explanation. It is simple enough. John has now pulled back into a more hands-off editorial role. Yet his energy and persistence over many years are the key to this publishing epic – seven editions of a technical manual, continuously in print for 35 years, wow! So Churchill Livingstone Elsevier, the publishers, wish to celebrate John's part in the success of this world-renowned text from its origins to this new edition, both as editor and contributor. Moreover, the successive editions of this remarkable book were, for much of the time, produced in parallel with and enriched by John's contributions to research and teaching in our field, and of course whilst managing a histopathology department in a large teaching hospital. So let us salute *Bancroft's Theory and Practice of Histological Techniques*!

Richard Horobin
2012

Preface to the seventh edition

In the 35 years since the first edition of this book, the histological laboratory has changed dramatically. Whilst some techniques of tissue selection, fixation and section production have remained relatively static, there have been great advances in terms of immunological and molecular diagnostic methodology. Immunohistochemistry and immunofluorescence now have well-defined roles with quality assurance realities, and are to be found throughout the world with pivotal interactions with tissue diagnosis and patient management. In the last 20 years, the progressive development of molecular techniques revolving around DNA and *in situ* hybridization has permitted the creation of new genetic tests and diagnostic opportunities for the laboratory. These are currently at the forefront of guiding treatment choices for patients. At the same time, these have permitted review of some classic histological tests resulting in a reduced histochemical repertoire in many laboratories. Knowledge of both the old and new is required by trained, as well as trainee, histotechnologists working alongside the pathologist. A thorough grounding in all these aspects of diagnostic methodology is still required.

In producing this edition we were faced with choices about classical and rarely used methodologies, and concluded that many needed to be removed from the text or reduced in volume into the appendices. These include the chapters on lipids, proteins and nucleic acids, neuroendocrine system and cytoplasmic granules and enzyme histochemistry. This has allowed for expansion and update in some areas, particularly the newer diagnostic methodologies. We recognized that some sections on classic stains have not changed dramatically, and have simply reviewed these to ensure that modern relevance has been achieved. Other chapters have been amalgamated, such as the *in situ* hybridization and genetic testing sections.

There are a number of new contributors for this edition. They include Louise Dunk, who contributed the management chapter and Anthony Rhodes, who updated fixation of tissues. The gross room/surgical cut-up chapter has been rewritten by Kim Suvarna and Christopher Layton. The pigment and minerals chapter has been revamped by Guy Orchard and the amyloid chapter by Janet Gilbertson and Tony Hunt. Neuropathology has been rewritten by Robin Highly and Nicky Sullivan. Some immunohistochemistry and immunofluorescent techniques have required a rewrite reflecting current modalities, and this has been accomplished by Tracy Sanderson, Greg Zardin and Graeme Wild.

Having said this, we are conscious that we are all part of the lineage of previous authors that have contributed to the first six editions of the book. We salute and thank them for their previous work. Indeed, their contribution to the success of this ongoing text cannot be underestimated. We would not wish to single out any one person, or group of individuals, but rather express great thanks to all the previous contributors over the decades that this book has been in existence.

Ultimately, we hope that we have produced a modern and relevant histotechnology text that will be of use to those in training as well as established practitioners across the world. As always, we recognize that this edition is but one step of the ongoing story and hope that colleagues across the world will enjoy and approve of the changes that have taken place.

S. Kim Suvarna, Christopher Layton
and John D. Bancroft
February 2012

Preface to the first edition

In recent years histological techniques have become increasingly sophisticated, incorporating a whole variety of specialties, and there has been a corresponding dramatic rise in the level and breadth of knowledge demanded by the examiner of trainees in histology and histopathology technology.

We believe that the time has arrived when no single author can produce a comprehensive book on histology technique sufficiently authoritative in the many differing fields of knowledge with which the technologist must be familiar. Many books exist which are solely devoted to one particular facet such as electron microscopy or autoradiography, and the dedicated technologist will, of course, read these in the process of self-education. Nevertheless the need has arisen for a book which covers the entire spectrum of histology technology, from the principles of tissue fixation and the production of paraffin sections to the more esoteric level of the principles of scanning electron microscopy. It has been our aim then, to produce a book which the trainee technologist can purchase at the beginning of his career and which will remain valuable to him as he rises on the ladder of experience and seniority.

The book has been designed as a comprehensive reference work for those preparing for examinations in histopathology, both in Britain and elsewhere.

Although the content is particularly suitable for students working towards the Special Examination in Histopathology of the Institute of Medical Laboratory Sciences, the level is such that more advanced students, along with research workers, histologists, and pathologists, will find the book beneficial. To achieve this we have gathered a team of expert contributors, many of whom have written specialized books or articles on their own subject; most are intimately involved in the teaching of histology and some are examiners in the HNC and Special Examination in Histopathology. The medically qualified contributors are also involved in technician education.

All contributors have taken care to give, where applicable, the theoretical basis of the techniques, for we believe that the standard of their education has risen so remarkably in recent years that the time is surely coming when medical laboratory technicians will be renamed 'medical laboratory scientists'; we hope that the increase in 'scientific' content in parts of this book will assist in this essential transformation.

John D. Bancroft
Alan Stevens
Nottingham, 1977

List of contributors

Caroline Astbury PhD FACMG
Department of Pathology and
Laboratory Medicine
Nationwide Children's Hospital
Columbus, OH, USA

John D. Bancroft
Formerly Pathology Directorate
Manager and Business Manager
Queen's Medical Centre
Nottingham, UK

**Jeanine H. Bartlett BS HT
(ASCP), QIHC**
Biologist
Centers for Disease Control and
Prevention
Infectious Diseases Pathology
Branch
Division of High-Consequence
Pathogens and Pathology
National Center for Emerging
and Zoonotic Infectious Diseases
Atlanta, GA, USA

David Blythe FIBMS
Chief Biomedical Scientist
HMDS Laboratory
Leeds Teaching Hospitals NHS
Trust
Leeds, UK

Louise Dunk MSc FIBMS
Lead Laboratory Manager
Histopathology
Sheffield Teaching Hospitals
Sheffield, UK

Alton D. Floyd PhD
ImagePath Systems Inc.
Edwardsburg, MI, USA

**Janet A. Gilbertson CSci
FIBMS**
National Amyloidosis Centre
Royal Free and University
College Medical School
London, UK

**Neil M. Hand MPhil C.Sci
FIBMS**
Operational Manager
Immunocytochemistry
Histopathology Department
Nottingham University Hospitals
NHS Trust
Nottingham, UK

**J. Robin Highley DPhil
FRCPath**
Clinical Fellow in
Neuropathology
Sheffield Institute for
Translational Neuroscience
Department of Neuroscience
Sheffield University Medical
School

Richard W. Horobin BSc PhD
School of Life Sciences
College of Medical, Veterinary
and Life Sciences
University of Glasgow
Glasgow, UK

Toby Hunt MSc BSc FIBMS
Laboratory and Mortuary
Manager
Department of Histopathology
Great Ormond Street Hospital

Stuart Inglut BSc (Hons)
Histopathology Department
Sheffield Teaching Hospitals
Sheffield, UK

**Peter Jackson MPhil CSi
FIBMS**
Formerly Department of
Histopathology and Molecular
Pathology
Leeds Teaching Hospitals
NHS Trust Leeds
Leeds, UK

**Wanda Grace Jones
Ht(ASCP)**
Immunohistochemistry Specialist
Department of Pathology
Emory University Hospital
Atlanta, GA, USA

Laura J. Keeling
Histopathology Department
Sheffield Teaching Hospitals
Sheffield, UK

Christopher Layton PhD
Specialist Section Lead in
Specimen Dissection
Histopathology Department
Sheffield Teaching Hospitals
Sheffield, UK

**Danielle Maddocks BSc
(Hons)**
Histopathology Department
Sheffield Teaching Hospitals
Sheffield, UK

**Ann Michelle Moon MSc
MIBMS**
Histopathology Department
Sheffield Teaching Hospitals
Sheffield, UK

**Guy E. Orchard PhD C.Sci
MSc FIBMS**
Laboratory Manager
Histopathology Department
St. John's Institute of
Dermatology
St. Thomas' Hospital
London, UK

**Sherin Jos Payyappilly
FRCPath**
Department of Histopathology
Birmingham Heartlands Hospital
Birmingham, UK

Anthony Rhodes BSc MSc PhD CSi FIBMS
Professor
Centre for Research in Biosciences
Faculty of Health and Life Sciences
University of the West of England
Bristol, UK

Paul Samuel BSc DMLT MIBMS
Histopathology Department
Sheffield Teaching Hospitals
Sheffield, UK

Tracy Sanderson FIBMS
Immunohistology Lead
Histopathology Department
Sheffield Teaching Hospitals
Sheffield, UK

Lena T. Spencer MA HTL(ASCP)QIHC
Senior Histotechnologist
Norton Healthcare
Louisville, KY, USA

Diane L. Sterchi MS HTL(ASCP)
Senior Research Associate
Histomorphometry Lead
Department of Pathology
Covance Laboratories Inc.
Greenfield, IN, USA

John W. Stirling BSc (Hons), MLett, AFRCPA, MAIMS, FRMS
Head of Unit
The Centre for Ultrastructural Pathology
Surgical Pathology – SA Pathology
Adelaide, Australia

Jennifer H. Stonard BSc (Hons), LIBMS
Histopathology Department
Sheffield Teaching Hospitals
Sheffield, UK

Nicky Sullivan CSci FIBMS
Department of Neuropathology and Ocular Pathology
John Radcliffe Hospital
Oxford, UK

S. Kim Suvarna MBBS BSc FRCP FRCPath
Consultant Pathologist
Histopathology Department
Sheffield Teaching Hospitals
Sheffield, UK

Graeme Wild
Immunology Department
Sheffield Teaching Hospitals
Sheffield, UK

Anthony E. Woods BA BSc (Hons) PhD MAIMS FFSc(RCPA)
School of Pharmacy and Medical Sciences
University of South Australia
Adelaide, Australia

Gregory Zardin BSc (Hons) MSc MIBMS
Histopathology Department
Sheffield Teaching Hospitals
Sheffield, UK

Acknowledgments

General acknowledgments

Many Laboratory Scientists and Pathologists have contributed in different ways to the seven editions of this text and to acknowledge their individual advice and assistance is impossible. We express our thanks to everyone who has contributed since 1977. We owe Harry Cook special thanks for his advice and contributions to the earlier editions. Our thanks are also due to the colleagues we worked with in Nottingham and Sheffield during the production of this book.

We would like to thank all of our current authors, and those contributors whose previous work remains in some of the chapters in this new edition. Special thanks go to Richard Horobin who has contributed to all of the editions and to Marilyn Gamble for her work on the previous edition. Our thanks go to those who assisted in the preparation of the manuscripts and the production of the illustrations. We are grateful to Carol Bancroft for her considerable help with the editing and proof-reading.

Finally, we wish to thank the staff of our publishers for their unfailing help and courtesy.

John D. Bancroft, Kim Suvarna and
Christopher Layton
Nottingham and Sheffield, UK
2012

Acknowledgment to Alan Stevens

I have known Alan since he joined the Pathology Department at the University of Nottingham some 30 years ago. We had many discussions in those early years over whether the time had arrived for a multi-authored text on histological technique. It was apparent at that time that the subject was becoming too diverse for any single or two authors to cover in the depth that was required in the laboratories or the colleges where histotechnologists received their academic education.

In 1977 the first edition of this text was published and was due in no small part to Alan's vision and diligent work in editing and even rewriting some of the chapters. His contributions to the succeeding editions were just as important and his medical knowledge was a significant factor in the development of the book. It has been a great pleasure working with him and I have greatly missed his contribution to the editing of this new edition, although much of his writing in the various chapters remains. The success over the years of Bancroft and Stevens owes a great deal to Alan Stevens. I wish to thank him and wish him well in his current and future medical education publications.

John D. Bancroft
Nottingham, UK
2001

Managing the laboratory 1

Louise Dunk

Introduction

Management is an integral aspect of the day-to-day life of the histopathology laboratory and is a major requirement of the accreditation process required by legislation in some countries. The accreditation standards include management as part of the evaluation and it is necessary that the laboratory worker is familiar with all of the processes involved. There are excellent books available which cover management issues in depth, and it is not the objective of this chapter to be a comprehensive guide to the subject. Rather, it discusses and concentrates on specific areas which have an impact on the operation of the laboratory; namely:

- Governance
- Risk management
- Quality management and establishing a quality system
- Personnel management

Other areas would include the management of estate, assets, equipment and supplies, business and budget management, and management of the scientific aspect and test repertoire of the service.

A pathology service may include a histology laboratory, an autopsy service, general cytology and a cervical screening/testing service. These areas will have many common management requirements but there will be some areas such as risk management where the issues will be individual to that section.

The surgical biopsy is sent for histopathological assessment to corroborate or dispute a clinical diagnosis by providing confirmation of data provided from other diagnostic tests. It should provide the clinician with valuable information on how to proceed with the treatment of the disease. Some resection specimens are taken as part of the treatment process, being referred to confirm the diagnosis, ensure adequate resection margins, to determine the extent of lymphatic/vascular involvement, staging, likely outcome and prognosis. Aside from simply determining a cause of death, autopsies may provide definitive data for a medical audit. They may be used to determine where medical procedures have been ineffective, or may give additional data for the future treatment of other patients. They can also provide a much needed final diagnosis and resolution for relatives.

Cytology samples are used as a screening process (e.g. cervical smears) and may assist in the early diagnosis of disease prior to the development of symptoms and thereby enable effective treatment. Cytology tests can also be used to monitor the stage of disease before/after treatment. This is accomplished by using non-invasive or minimally invasive techniques, which have a low risk of complications to the patient.

Governance

Risk management

Risk management is an essential and central part of all laboratory work. Organizations such as the Health and Safety Executive (HSE) and the Health Protection Agency (HPA) exist to ensure the safety of employees, patients and the general public in the United Kingdom. In the USA the Occupational Safety and Health Administration's mission is to prevent work-related injuries, illnesses, and occupational fatality by issuing and enforcing standards for workplace safety and health, and most countries will have equivalent bodies and standards.

Regulations made under the Health and Safety at Work Act 1974 apply to all work situations, for example the Control of Substances Hazardous to Health (COSHH) Regulations and the Workplace (Health, Safety and Welfare) Regulations. The HSE enforces this act along with others, including the Health and Safety Offences Act 2008. The overall message is that that employees are entitled to work in environments where risks to their health and safety are properly controlled (i.e. minimized). Under health and safety law, the primary responsibility is owed by employers, with employees expected to ensure their own safety, and that of their colleagues and/or patient's by adhering to policies and procedures.

To comply with legislation and maintain accreditation, a laboratory must have an effective risk management policy. Any chance of something going wrong should be either negated or minimized, and therefore a laboratory's risk management process should have procedures in place for:

- Identifying all risks that exist within the environment
- Assessing those risks for likelihood and severity
- Eliminating those risks that can be removed
- Reducing the effect of risks that cannot be eliminated

The pathology laboratory should have close links with, and feed into, the host organization's risk management process. In most hospital laboratories, the laboratory manager will be accountable for risk management and the health and safety of the staff in their department, and often will be supported by a Risk Lead who will be responsible for the operational aspects of the system.

To function effectively and safely, all of a laboratory's procedures and activities must be subjected to the risk management process. The risks in the laboratory are similar worldwide, albeit with a variation due to local circumstances. Health and safety and quality assurance incorporate a major aspect of risk management. All aspects of our working life incorporate a degree of risk and the risk management process allows us to prioritize, evaluate, and handle the risk appropriately. It is not possible to avoid or eliminate all risks, and in reality this may not be practical. It is important to identify and understand the risks that are involved in a laboratory's working practices. An individual's responsibility for risk management is dependent upon that individual's role within the organization. The Chief Executive, for example, will be concerned mainly with risks associated with strategic issues affecting the organization as a whole and would only include histopathology within the risk assessment if it had a direct impact on these issues. Matters concerning the day-to-day running of the laboratory would not be of direct interest unless, of course, there was a significant reason for involvement such as major clinical or financial concerns or unmanaged risks or incidents, especially those likely to cause harm to patients, cause the organization to fail to achieve agreed targets or might attract adverse media publicity. A laboratory manager would be concerned with all risks associated with the department that they manage, but also how these might impact on other areas of the organization such as porters transporting samples or chemicals to the laboratory. They would also be required to alert the organization to the presence of risks which cannot be adequately controlled within or by the department.

The laboratory management team will deal with any laboratory-associated risk by ensuring that adequate resources are available to deliver the service, and by guaranteeing that the laboratory provides a service that is safe both for staff and patients. Staffing levels and competence, timeliness and quality of results, budgetary management, consumable and equipment supplies, and maintenance are some of the areas of concern. The laboratory management team must also ensure risk management procedures are in place for every aspect of a laboratory's processes and environment.

The laboratory manager must ensure that day-to-day errors do not arise as a result of inadequacies in laboratory procedures and that quality control checks are in place to minimize the possibility of human errors: for example, a transcription error or mislabeling. Standard operating procedures (SOPs) should include COSHH data, risk assessments or equivalent, and also to include other health and safety information relevant to the procedure. This should include national legislation and guidance where available.

Scientific and support staff at the bench may be exposed to risks involving equipment malfunction due to poor maintenance or design. Poor-quality reagents may produce poor processing of tissues or inaccurate staining results. One of the most common accidents in the histopathology laboratory is the injury to fingers or hands from microtome blades or laboratory knives. It is the responsibility of each laboratory worker to reduce the risks associated with their day-to-day work by working in accordance with SOPs and associated risk and COSHH assessments. This will help ensure that everyone is working to the same standard and understands what is required to minimize risk to themselves, their colleagues and/or patients. It is importance that where risks are identified, the risk management measures which are put in place are regularly audited to assess whether they are being followed and are still appropriate and effective.

Risk identification

The risks within each laboratory section are best identified by the section lead and members of that team, working in conjunction with the laboratory's health and safety lead. This ensures that the broadest possible spectrum of viewpoints is considered. During this process it is also useful to divide the risks into different categories, such as clinical, physical, chemical, infectious, etc., and even organizational, financial and political, depending on the area being risk assessed. For example a support worker unpacking the samples delivered to the laboratory might have noticed that more samples than usual have leaked. This could put both themselves and the porter at risk from infection and exposure to fixative, and if any of the contents has leaked beyond the specimen bag there could be a risk to other health workers and patients/visitors using the same route. This could just be a problem with one batch of specimen pots, but could also be a training issue for staff putting the samples in the pots. In raising the issue with their supervisor and giving them the opportunity to investigate the root cause, the support worker may have prevented harm to others and potential damage to the sample.

Risk analysis/evaluation

Analysis and evaluation of potential risks is an essential part of the process, and one that is used to identify both the likelihood and severity of these risks. By scoring the risks for likelihood and severity, it is then possible to use a matrix such as the one described below as a tool that will put a value on specific risks. This will then help prioritize them for further action.

The risk manager should put a system in place whereby all incidents and accidents are reported no matter how small. It is only by recording data that the full picture can be obtained and analysed and areas possibly overlooked initially be risk assessed and managed.

Severity and likelihood values

The following is an example of a severity scoring scale for incidents:

1. **Low**
   - Minor injury or harm
   - Minor loss of non-critical service
   - Minor non-compliance with standards
   - Minor out-of-court settlement
   - Publicity mostly contained within organization. Local press coverage of no more than one day

2. **Slight**
   - Injury or harm requiring less than 3 days absence from work or less than 2 days hospital stay
   - Loss of service for less than 2 hours in a number of non-critical areas or less than 6 hours in one area

- Single failure to meet internal standards
- Civil action with or without defense, improvement notice
- Regulatory concern
- Local media coverage of less than 7 days

3. **Moderate**
   - Medical treatment required and more than 3 days' absence from work or more than 2 days' extended hospital stay
   - Loss of services in any critical area
   - Repeated failures to meet internal standards or follow protocols
   - Class action, criminal prosecution or prohibition notice served

4. **Severe**
   - Fatality, permanent disability or multiple injuries
   - Extended loss of essential service in more than one critical area
   - Failure to meet national standards
   - Executive officer fined or imprisoned, criminal prosecution – no defense
   - Political concern, questions in parliament, national media coverage greater than 3 days

5. **Catastrophic**
   - Multiple fatalities
   - Loss of multiple essential services in critical areas
   - Failure to meet professional standards
   - Imprisonment of executive from organization
   - Full public enquiry

   Incidents may also be scored 1–5 for likelihood:

1. Incident unlikely to occur.
2. Incident likely to occur once in a 5-year period.
3. Incident likely to occur yearly.
4. Incident likely to occur once in a 6-month period.
5. Incident likely to occur once every 4 weeks or more frequently.

   The risk factor is the severity multiplied by the likelihood of occurrence:

Very Low Risk – The majority of control measures in place or harm/severity small. Action may be long term.

Low Risk – Moderate probability of major harm or high probability of minor harm if control measures are not implemented. Action in the medium term.

Moderate Risk – Urgent action to remove or reduce the risk.

High Risk – Immediate action to remove/reduce the risk.

Risk management

The objective of the whole risk management process is to either remove or avoid risks, or manage them where removal is not an option. Removal would be possible, for example, by looking for alternatives to high-risk, harmful chemicals used in the laboratory. For example, prior to the 1970s, it was common practice to use mercuric chloride as a constituent of fixatives and, although this gave excellent quality fixation, it was extremely harmful to the environment and also to laboratory staff. Its use was subsequently stopped and alternative fixatives replaced it. Where risks remain, efforts should be made to reduce the effect or the possibility of the risk happening. The ways of controlling risk are numerous, but frequently there will be expert guidance or regulations issued by professional bodies or government agencies that the Risk Lead should ensure are implemented. Informal networking with professionals in similar laboratories can also provide valuable information and ideas as to how others have overcome the challenges of managing certain risks.

Audit is an essential tool in risk management. Regular audits of the effectiveness of the risk management measures put in place and the frequency and nature of incidents will allow the laboratory's risk management team to assess them and amend and improve if required. Audit will also identify areas or tasks that may need more regular monitoring and may highlight training gaps for individuals or groups of staff. In addition, regular and targeted audits will provide evidence to assist with driving change should the risk be due to lack of funding for certain tasks or process or to processes outside the control of the laboratory management (e.g. labeling of samples in the operating theater).

Risk funding

Risk management should also consider insurance (individual or laboratory), although this is an important option. All medical staff carry medical liability insurance, which covers them in the event of any negligence claims. Similarly, professional indemnity insurance is commonly available today for non-medical laboratory staff who are much more at risk in today's litigation-conscious society. The decision regarding whether or not to insure should be based on the risk assessment and the severity and likelihood of the risk. Some risks will not be appropriate for insurance cover for whatever reason, and in these instances the risk must be accepted by the organization.

Quality management

A quality management system is essential in order to provide the best possible service for the patient and clinicians. Quality is defined as a measure of how well a product or service does the job for which it is designed (i.e. conformity to specification).

Internal quality control of work processes is an important part of quality management, and has been the traditional way that bench work has been checked for many years. External quality assurance (EQA) schemes provide benchmarking against other laboratories and often provide access to best practice methods and expert advice on improving techniques/specific tests. However, a full quality management system should also encompass systems to ensure consistency, quality of service, confidence, standardization and continual improvement of all laboratory processes.

Quality management of a laboratory should ensure there are systems in place to monitor and improve areas such as organization and quality management systems. This will involve liaison with users, human resources, premises, the local environment, equipment management, information systems and materials. It will address the pre-examination process, the examination process, the post-examination phase as well as evaluation and quality assurance. Regular audit of the various components of the system will provide evidence of compliance with standards for accreditation. It should identify any trends and issues for concern, and confirm quality systems are working. Overall, all these measures should identify areas for quality improvement and show whether any improvements are working.

Accreditation

Accreditation is an important and long-established part of quality management in pathology laboratories. Accreditation allows confirmation that a department meets specific requirements for the users and clients, and fulfills appropriate legal requirements. The process will normally reduce risks from areas such as product failure, health risks, and company reputation. Many countries have their own long-established accreditation bodies and systems, but the International Organization for Standardization or ISO standards are being adopted by many countries as the standards they wish to work to and be accredited by. ISO is the world's largest developer and publisher of international standards. There are ISO standards that cover many areas of activity, with the ones that affect medical laboratories being:

ISO 15189 – *Medical laboratories – Particular requirements for quality and competence.* This is the main standard that affects medical laboratories and that the majority will seek to become accredited to.

ISO 17043 – *Conformity assessment – General requirements for proficiency testing.* This standard specifies general requirements for the competence of providers of proficiency testing schemes, which would include external quality assurance schemes.

ISO 17011 – *Conformity assessment – General requirements for accreditation bodies accrediting conformity assessment bodies.* In order to assess and accredit laboratories according to ISO standards within their own country, national accreditation bodies such as CPA in the UK must themselves be accredited under this standard.

Laboratories wishing to be accredited must demonstrate a robust quality management system and consistent application of the standards, usually by undergoing assessment and surveillance visits from the accrediting body, plus providing annual reviews of the quality management system.

Quality control (QC)

This system checks that the work process is functioning properly. It includes processes utilized in the laboratory to recognize and eliminate errors. It ensures that the quality of work produced by the laboratory conforms to specified requirements prior to its release for diagnosis. Errors and/or deviations from expected results must be documented and include the corrective action taken, if required. In the laboratory, quality control has long been a component of accreditation requirements and should be ingrained in scientists as a daily practice.

Most laboratories have experienced scientists and support staff who have the responsibility of performing routine quality control checks prior to the release of slides for diagnosis. This QC evaluation will include, but is not limited to: accurate patient identification, fixation, adequate processing, appropriate embedding techniques, acceptable microtomy, unacceptable artifacts, and inspection of controls to determine quality and specificity of special staining and immunohistochemistry methods. Criteria should be established that would trigger a repeat if the QC findings were qualitatively or quantitatively unacceptable. Despite having a conscientious QC system in the laboratory, pathologists (having a higher level of expertise) perform the final QC examination as they assess/report the slide. It is their responsibility to determine that this is adequate for diagnostic interpretation. However, all personnel are responsible, such that errors and incidents should be recorded and audited regularly to identify trends. This will highlight any training needs and gaps.

External quality assurance (EQA)

In addition to local data collection and monitoring for internal quality control, external mechanisms provide valuable information regarding quality and peer comparisons and as an educational tool. In the UK, quality assurance of laboratory techniques is organized on a national basis. It is a system of peer review and registration with appropriate (approved) schemes. The non-profit-making NEQAS (National External Quality Assurance Scheme) organizes programs for histochemistry and immunohistochemistry.

In the USA, the National Society of Histotechnology (NSH) in partnership with the College of American Pathologists (CAP) (2006), created the Histology Quality Improvement Program (Histo-QIP). Their system scores each slide, assessing the fixation, processing, embedding, microtomy, staining and coverslipping. Additionally, CAP establishes national surveys for immunohistochemistry.

The UK quality assurance schemes were started by members of the profession to establish quality standards within histopathology. Registration with the schemes is now a requirement for accreditation. The quality assurance process is based on peer review of the stained sections submitted by participating laboratories. There are also medical quality assurance schemes for pathologists that cover many of the sub-specialties of histopathology.

The quality assurance schemes currently used in the UK are coordinated under the auspices of UK NEQAS and within this organization there are two individual schemes for histopathology, the NEQAS for immunohistochemistry and the NEQAS for cellular pathology techniques. The immunohistochemistry scheme gives participants the option to be assessed on general antibody panels, or more specialist laboratories may choose to participate only in the lymphoma or breast specialist areas. The cellular pathology scheme is subdivided into general, veterinary and neuropathology.

Accreditation standards require action be taken by poor performers to improve the quality of their preparations. Most schemes offer expert assistance and advice to laboratories that fall below the defined acceptable score.

Organization and liaison with users

An appropriate management structure for the department should exist so that the main functions can be adequately delivered. Staff at all levels should be qualified and trained for the work that they do and hold appropriate registration, if required. Competencies for the tasks performed should be regularly assessed, checked and recorded.

Many departments publish a mission statement outlining their business and aims. The quality objectives need to be documented so that all have clear objectives outlining who is responsible for achieving them and when they should be achieved by.

A laboratory will have many users, including patients, clinicians and those purchasing its services. It is essential when planning and developing a laboratory service that all users are consulted. In short, the department must know about the service it is providing/will provide. Likewise when monitoring the effectiveness and quality of a service, user feedback should be sought so that the service can be properly evaluated. Any complaints/praise should be followed up immediately, and should feed into the quality management system.

Premises, equipment and materials

The laboratory environment and equipment must be fit for all laboratory processes. Managers should ensure that there are adequate basic facilities for staff to do their jobs, such as rest and toilet facilities, adequate lighting, IT provision and space. There should also be enough space for equipment and storage. Equipment should be functional and be regularly maintained for safe use.

Staff must be trained and competent (in their own areas) to use all of the equipment and materials in a safe and effective way. Materials and equipment must be managed with regard to stock control and servicing. Procurement policies should ensure that quality stock is purchased, being fit for purpose and value for money.

Examination procedures

Any laboratory's testing procedures may be multiple and complex, and in many laboratories its staff are required to rotate between sections. Also, it is essential that the methodology for all procedures and tests are documented in standard operating procedures (SOPs) to permit all staff to operate in a standardized and appropriate way. SOPs should cover all aspects of the testing process, from delivery of samples or reagents to the issuing of the final laboratory report. The SOPs therefore include not only the laboratory procedures but also those carried out by pathologist and clerical staff. It is important that SOPs that impact on areas or staff outside of the laboratory (e.g. porters delivering samples from operating theaters) are shared with the other departments responsible for managing that part of the process.

Accreditation standards require that SOPs and other policies are controlled within a document control system. This is usually a central database that holds authorized copies of documents, with controls on who can modify the data. The document control system must also ensure that only authorized and up-to-date copies of SOPs and policies are being used by staff performing the tasks. Any changes to a procedure must be captured within a further updated SOP. This must then be issued and any old SOPs removed from circulation.

Continuous quality improvement (CQI)

This is the system that is used proactively, to approach and identify opportunities to improve quality, before problems occur. It operates through evaluation and audit of all systems and processes in the laboratory. The goal is to improve care and safety for patients and staff through recognition of potential problems and errors – before they can occur. Good managers now realize that often failures, errors, and problems are usually due to the system processes and not necessarily the fault of the employee(s).

Regular and thorough audit of the many components of the laboratory's quality management system and performance should be mapped against accreditation standards. This will help highlight any problem areas. Feedback from users provides useful information when evaluating the effectiveness and quality of the service. Any criticism received may well prompt an unscheduled audit of that particular part of the system.

CQI should include auditing of the laboratory's procedures against not only accreditation standards but also those of the host organization/other services. Any audit findings that show that the laboratory's processes are not adequate should result in corrective actions. These audit findings might also highlight improvements for processes, documentation, staff training or monitoring aspects of competency. Any corrective actions required should be completed as soon as possible in order that the service required by the users can be improved and brought up to standard quickly. CQI is a continuous cycle of audit and assessment of the service. If not monitored regularly, quality standards can slip as staff, equipment and reagents change. It is useful for the manager to establish an audit calendar to ensure that all areas are audited regularly with particular attention to 'problem areas'.

Personnel management

One of the most important assets for a histology laboratory is its staff or personnel. More than any other pathology specialty, the laboratory process in histology is a very manual procedure, from sample receipt, through dissection (grossing), embedding, sectioning and staining. Many techniques are still reliant on skilled personnel rather than automation, and the laboratory manager must ensure that the department is staffed by an appropriate number of staff with the right level of skills to ensure that the process is robust, safe and cost-effective.

The role of the laboratory manager in staff management

The laboratory manager is accountable for the service provided by the laboratory, and should have the appropriate qualifications experience to undertake this task. As well as being the lead scientist for the department, laboratory managers are usually responsible for recruiting the appropriate staff, and also managing the human resource needs and professional direction of their staff. All staff should have comprehensive job descriptions so that they and their manager and supervisor know what is expected from them and to whom they are accountable. They should also have contracts that specify the terms and conditions that they are employed under.

Staff should have access to basic facilities such as handwashing, toilets and rest rooms. The manager should ensure that adequate breaks are allowed, especially in areas where staff cannot easily break off from what they are doing due to the high levels of concentration required, or because they work in areas where personal protective equipment is needed due to chemical or biological hazards. The European Working Time Directive and United States Department of Labor give guidance on how long staff can work without a break and maximum working hours per week.

The manager must ensure that there are appropriate numbers of staff with the required education, qualifications, training and competence to provide the service required. Managers must also ensure that staff have access to further education as required in order to continue to keep up with the latest knowledge and techniques related to the service being provided. The competency of staff to do the tasks within their job description needs to be assessed at regular intervals, and this together with regular formal appraisals should ensure staff are supported and provided with what they require to fulfill their roles. The manager must also address any issues with discipline or excessive absence from work to ensure that the workforce team functions optimally.

Regular staff meetings should be held that involve all levels of staff, in order that any new information can be passed on, such as new procedures or updates related to the risk and quality management systems. Regular meetings also allow staff to feed back any information they have or raise queries, and gives them access to supervisors or managers that they may not easily get during their routine day. Management techniques such as 'Lean' encourage short staff meetings at the start of each day so that any issues related to the days work can be raised and planned for, e.g. staff absence, workload, or other factors that might interrupt or disrupt the workflow.

Staffing the laboratory

Ensuring the right number and level of staff depends on the manager having a good understanding of the volume and complexity of work received. Good information systems are essential for recording and analyzing the work performed in a laboratory every year, and for understanding trends in workflow and complexity.

Guidelines such as those issued by the Royal College of Pathologists and the Institute of Biomedical Science in the UK advise what level of laboratory duties may be undertaken by which grade of staff, and have their own training and examination systems to enable consultant and postgraduate scientist staff to gain the qualifications they require. Scientific staff working in accredited laboratories in the UK should be registered by the Health Professions Council.

In the USA the National Accrediting Agency for Clinical Laboratory Sciences (NAACLS) fully accredits about 479 programs for medical and clinical laboratory technologists, medical and clinical laboratory technicians, and related professions. Other nationally recognized agencies that accredit specific areas for clinical laboratory workers include the Commission on Accreditation of Allied Health Education Programs and the Accrediting Bureau of Health Education Schools. Some States require laboratory personnel to be licensed or registered. Licensure of technologists often requires a bachelor's degree and the passing of an exam, but requirements vary by State and specialty. Scientists may also gain certification by a recognized professional association, including the Board of Registry of the American Society for Clinical Pathology, the American Medical Technologists, the National Credentialing Agency for Laboratory Personnel, and the Board of Registry of the American Association of Bioanalysts.

Once the level and complexity of the workload is known, the workforce can be profiled to match its requirements, remembering that to be cost-effective, tasks not requiring registered or licensed scientists should be performed by support staff where possible.

Acknowledgments

With thanks to Sheffield Teaching Hospitals NHSFT for their kind permission to adapt and use the risk severity and likelihood values from the Trust risk policy.

Further reading

Accrediting Bureau of Health Education Schools (ABHES), website www.abhes.org

American Medical Technologists (AMT), website www.amt1.com

American Society for Clinical Pathology (ASCP) – Board of Registry, website www.ascp.org

Board of Registry of the American Association of Bioanalysts (ABB), website www.aab.org

Clinical and Laboratory Standards Institute, 2006. Press release: From NCCLS to CLSI: One year. Online. Available at www.clsi.org

Clinical Pathology Accreditation (UK) Ltd Standards for the Medical Laboratory. Document name: PD-LAB-Standards v2.02 Nov 2010

College of American Pathologists (CAP)HistoQIP programme. Available at www.cap.org

Commission on Accreditation of Allied Health Education Programs (CAAHEP), website www.caahep.org

DOH, 1994. Risk management in the NHS: D026/RISK/3M. Department of Health, London.

Health and Safety at Work etc Act 1974. Available at www.legislation.gov.uk

Health and Safety Offences Act 2008, http://news.hse.gov.uk

Health Professions Council (HPC), website www.hpc-uk.org

Institute of Biomedical Science (IBMS): Managing staffing and workload in UK clinical diagnostic laboratories. Available at www.ibms.org

ISO 15189, 2007. Medical laboratories – particular requirements for quality and competence. International Organization for Standardization, Geneva, Switzerland.

ISO 17011, 2004. Conformity assessment – General requirements for accreditation bodies accrediting conformity assessment bodies. International Organization for Standardization, Geneva, Switzerland.

ISO 17043, 2010. Conformity assessment –General requirements for proficiency testing. International Organization for Standardization, Geneva, Switzerland.

National Accrediting Agency for Clinical Laboratory Sciences (NAACLS), website www.naacls.org

National Association of Histotechnology (NSH), website www.nsh.org

National Credentialing Agency for Laboratory Personnel (NCA), website www.nca-info.org

Royal College of Pathologist (RCPath), 2005. Guidelines on staffing and workload in histopathology and cytopathology departments, second ed. Available at www.rcpath.org

UK National External Quality Assessment Service (UKNEQAS), website www.ukneqas.org.uk

Working with substances hazardous to health: what you need to know about COSHH, HSE leaflet INDG136(rev4), revised 06/09. Available at www.hse.gov.uk

Workplace (Health, Safety and Welfare) Regulations, HSE leaflet INDG244(rev2). Available at www.hse.gov.uk

Safety and ergonomics in the laboratory

2

John D. Bancroft

There are numerous workplace hazards in histology laboratories, and most countries have now passed regulations designed to improve this. These vary from country to country but the underlying theme is universal.

Risk management pertains not just to personal health and safety, but also to environmental health and safety. Hospital laboratories and research facilities have seen significant improvements in workplace conditions, but they remain contributors to environmental pollution.

The goal of this chapter is to lay out a risk management plan that is applicable worldwide. While general in scope to encompass a variety of regulations, it is specific regarding the hazards unique to histology. Most of the information is from Dapson and Dapson (2005). Other references which should be in every laboratory include Montgomery (1995), the Prudent Practices Series (National Research Council 1989, 1995), aids for preparing chemical hygiene plans (Stricoff & Walters 1990), as well as guidelines from the Clinical and Laboratory Standards Institute concerning laboratory safety (2004), biohazards (2005) and waste management (2002). Indispensable publications from the Centers for Disease Control (USA) include guidelines for safety (1988), HIV and tuberculosis (1990, 1994).

Risk management

Identify and evaluate hazards

The first step in risk management is to identify hazards in and emanating from the workplace. If this has never been done, it may be a formidable task, especially if there are old reagents or chemicals in poorly labeled containers. Anything that is unidentifiable or questionable should be set aside for disposal. Identification of hazards goes beyond making a chemical inventory, although that is a significant part of the effort. Electrical, mechanical and biological hazards are also included. In this initial identification stage, include the nature of the hazard(s) with the name, its location and the procedure(s) involved with its use. If no current use is found, then dispose of the item.

For hazardous chemicals, data sheets are available in most countries, and available from databases on the Internet. A file of data sheets should be kept in a secure location, and employees must be given reasonable access to it. It is also advisable to keep a duplicate file readily accessible in the laboratory in case of emergencies. Some reagents found in storage areas may be obsolete; sheets will be impossible to find for these. This creates a problem with no simple solution, because legitimate disposal may require having a data sheet, yet keeping the chemical also dictates that a sheet be on file. You will have to create one, or hire a qualified firm to do that for you.

Evaluate the severity of each of the hazards. What is the volume or magnitude of the hazardous item? How much is used per day (or some other meaningful unit of time)? Now put that information together with the data sheet. These are written for industrial-scale exposures, and you must weigh that against the scale of use in your laboratory. This evaluation must include risks associated with spillage and disposal as well as normal use. The hazards of a bulk container of formalin emptying onto the floor of a laboratory are quite different from spilling a

30 ml specimen container in a dermatologist's office. Likewise, emptying hundreds of small formalin-filled specimen containers into a disposal drum or sink might present far greater exposure risk than handling each one during grossing. Do not underestimate risk, but keep the assessment proportional to scale and scope of operations.

Plan to minimize risk

Once the hazards have been listed and evaluated, decide how to reduce risk. Each item should be scrutinized, not just those offering the greatest dangers. Prioritize later. The goal is to reduce risks to acceptable levels, preferably through a cascading series of options that become progressively more burdensome and expensive. Work practice controls are the best way to tackle the problem; when pursued aggressively and with commitment at all levels of the institution, they usually are the only changes needed. Work practice controls involve eliminating, reducing and recycling everything possible. If they do not succeed, engineering controls should be implemented. These involve ventilation systems, fire protection devices and other expensive alterations to the facility. If all of these measures fail or are impossible to accomplish, personal protective equipment (PPE) must be used as a last resort. PPE should never be the first choice, although it may seem the most obvious way to protect workers.

There are several ways to reduce risk, the first of which should be to eliminate the hazard altogether. The list of obsolete chemicals in some of our labs is growing rapidly; how many does your laboratory still use? Remember using benzene and dioxane? No? Then do not be surprised in another few years to have histologists and biomedical scientists who never used xylene, toluene, chloroform, methacrylate, picric acid, uranyl nitrate and formaldehyde. A surprising number of laboratories are free of one or more of these highly dangerous substances and a few have eliminated all of them

Practically every hazardous chemical can be replaced today with a safer and technically superior substitute. The question is not whether it can be done, but if it might be done. The obstacle is rarely technical feasibility; most likely, it is human obstinacy. The notion that substitutes are not as good has been debased so often in everyday life that it is a wonder that it persists so strongly in the medical profession. Antifreeze, correction fluid, nail polish, hard surface cleaners, cosmetics, contact lens solutions and gasoline are just a few of the thousands of common materials in our lives that have undergone radical reformulation. In all cases, the products are safer, many work better, and some are less expensive.

If elimination of a hazard is out of the question, consider reduction. This will involve procedural changes, so be sure to weigh all implications before pushing ahead. A common idea for reduction is to use smaller specimen containers for fixation. Recycling is a final option for risk minimization. The volume in use at any given time might not be reduced, but the amount involved in storage and disposal will be cut drastically.

The plan must include justification to managers. Rationale for change should not rely solely upon improving safety. Financial considerations weigh heavily in any business, and could be your strongest argument for change. While many changes will cost more money initially, the long-term benefits are usually easy to calculate. For example, formalin substitutes are more expensive than formalin, but their use creates significant savings later. Workplaces and personnel do not need to be monitored for hazardous vapors, and disposal costs are usually reduced to zero. Less tangible but nonetheless real are the cost benefits of a healthier work force.

Implement the plan

Having a plan will do no good unless it is implemented. Prioritize the changes described in the plan. While easy changes should be tackled immediately, do not put off the challenging items that carry high health or environmental risk. Achieving financial gain quickly will help your cause, so be sure to include something at the outset with immediate positive economic impact.

Design standard operating procedures for working with hazards

Nearly all laboratories operate under a set of written, standard operating procedures (SOPs) mandated by a variety of accrediting or regulatory agencies. Detailed procedures for handling hazardous substances certainly should be central in these procedures, but other topics ought to be addressed as well. Personal hygiene practices should be a subconscious part of every workers' behavior, but must be spelled out in the SOPs. Define the criteria for invoking the use of specific control measures, such as the use of protective equipment. Describe how to assure that fume hoods and other pieces of protective equipment are functioning properly. Make provisions for employee training, medical consultations and medical examinations. Detail spill procedures; define the kinds of spills that should be handled by laboratory workers and those too serious for anyone except trained HazMat responders. Establish a qualified officer or committee of qualified people to develop and administer these safety procedures.

Train personnel

Safety training is mandated by a variety of governmental regulations in several countries, and should be part of every department's personnel practices. Trained people work more safely, efficiently and economically. In addition, the threat of employee litigation against the department is reduced. Regulations rarely address the issue of who should provide the training. In the past, it was common for one of the technical staff (usually the supervisor) to do this, that person obtaining the information as best he/she could. It is preferable, however, to have the trainer who is specially educated and experienced in health and safety matters.

Training must include general practices and may deal with very specific topics such as respirator use, handling select carcinogens, and working with formaldehyde. Each employee should sign a form verifying that training was received, a copy of which becomes part of the employee's permanent record.

The employee's name, date and subject of training should be included on the certification form. Yearly retraining should be mandatory and documented. New employees, or employee's assigned new hazardous tasks, must be adequately trained before beginning work.

Periodic reviews

On at least a yearly basis, all SOPs, risk assessments and training programs should be reviewed and updated as needed. Each written document should bear the date of creation and latest revision. Continue to minimize risks. Address any new risks that occur when different hazardous materials are brought into the workplace. Revise risk assessments and protocols to accommodate increased use of hazardous substances, especially as workloads increase.

Record keeping

Regulations often prescribe what records must be kept and for how long. It is prudent to record everything that pertains to regulatory compliance, risk assessment, causes and prevention of occupational illness or injury, employee health and safety training, exposure monitoring, occupational medical records, personal protective equipment and hazardous waste disposal practices. Records should be kept indefinitely, although 30 years past the duration of a worker's employment is the term often prescribed by regulatory agencies. If in doubt, consider this: for how long would you want your estate to have access to health and safety records relating to your employment?

Occupational exposure limits

Most chemicals are hazardous to some degree; the question really is how hazardous are they? In other words, what would a safe level of exposure be? From many years of actual industrial experience, various agencies have developed standards for exposure to widely used chemicals. Generically, these are called occupational exposure limits, but each agency refers to its own values by unique names. OSHA's Permissible Exposure Limits (PELs) are based upon scientifically based recommendations from the National Institute of Occupational Safety and Health, or NIOSH (2003), but are also influenced by special interest groups and Congressional actions. OSHA limits therefore typically are more lenient. Another source of exposure limits, called Threshold Limit Values (TLVs®) is ACGIH®, the American Conference of Governmental Industrial Hygienists (2004). These limits are more widely used around the world for occupational standards.

An exposure limit is the maximum allowable airborne concentration of a chemical (vapor, fume or dust) to which a worker may be exposed. Presumably, it represents the concentration at or below which it is safe for most people to work; there will be individuals who react adversely below the limits because of hypersensitivity.

It is important to realize that exposure limits are properties of the worker and the workplace combined. They are not simply the maximum limits of vapor, fume or dust in the workplace; they are the maximum limits of exposure. This is especially important to consider when monitoring exposure levels. Monitor employees, not the workplace. Monitoring devices should be positioned as close as possible to the worker's face in order to capture actual breathable quantities of hazardous material. For example, airborne levels of formaldehyde vapor a few inches above a grossing station's cutting board may be much higher than concentrations at nose level, especially with well-designed ventilation.

Kinds of exposure limits based upon the duration of exposure

TWA (or TWAEV). The time-weighted average (time-weighted average exposure value) is the employee's average exposure over 8 hours. Shorter exposures may exceed this value as long as the average exposure does not. There may be some short exposure that is too high for safety; that is covered below. When additional exposure is likely through the skin, that may be noted after the TWA. This is especially true for

chemicals like phenol and methanol that pass quickly through skin.

STEL (or STEV). The short-term exposure limit (or value) is the highest permissible time-weighted average exposure for any 15-minute period during the work shift. It should be measured during the worst 15-minute period. The STEL is always higher than the TWA.

CL (or CEV). The Ceiling Limit (Ceiling Exposure Value) is the maximum permissible instantaneous exposure during any part of the work shift. Few chemicals are given both a STEL and a CL; the CL is usually reserved for highly dangerous substances.

For chemicals lacking either a STEL or CL, prudent values may be determined by multiplying the TWA by 3 for the STEL or by 5 for the CL, as is suggested by the Ontario (Canada) Ministry of Labor (1991). When more than one harmful substance is present, complex formulas must be used to determine combined occupational exposure limits. These formulas are prescribed by various governments and vary from country to country.

IDLH. This airborne concentration is immediately dangerous to life and health. Chemicals with low IDLH should be considered very dangerous when spilled or when significant volumes are being dispensed. A single inhalation at or above this limit could have serious, if not lethal consequences.

Biological exposure indices

Can a worker determine if significant exposure has occurred? Can the chemical in question be detected in the worker by a clinical test? In a few instances, the answer is 'yes'. ACGIH® has established Biological Exposure Indices (BEIs®) as maximum values of analytes determined from clinical tests on exhaled air, urine or blood for a variety of hazardous chemicals, but only four are pertinent to histology: N, N-dimethylformamide, methanol, phenol and xylenes. Consult the latest booklet issued yearly by ACGIH® for details on the first three chemicals.

Because xylene is used so pervasively in histology, and so many histologists are concerned with its effects, further information is presented here on this chemical. The isomers of xylene are metabolized to methylhippuric acids, which can be measured in exposed workers' urine. The BEI® for xylenes is 1.5 g methylhippuric acids per g creatinine. Samples are collected immediately at the end of a work shift.

BEIs® are not intended to be used in diagnosing occupational illness. They are not maximum safe permissible values. Rather, they are to be used as indicators that workers may be exposed to significant concentrations of harmful substances, particularly if a worker or a group of co-workers repeatedly show values of the analyte at or above the BEI®. For xylene in a well-ventilated histology lab, high methylhippuric acids in urine would probably indicate significant skin exposure.

Types of hazard

Systems of classifying the hazardous nature of chemicals range from simple pictographs with numerical ratings to comprehensive lists of formally defined terms. Even within a single country, government agencies may differ in how hazards are defined. While no single system will suffice worldwide, the following terms do have nearly universal meaning and should serve on a practical basis for describing the hazards encountered in histology. For convenience, hazards are first divided into two broad categories, health and physical. The latter certainly have ramifications for health, but present more immediate problems for storage, handling and building codes.

Biohazards can be infectious agents themselves or items (solutions, specimens or objects) contaminated with them. Anything that can cause disease in humans, regardless of its source, is considered biohazardous, even if the disease primarily occurs in animals. In many countries, biohazardous materials are specially labeled and disposal is generally strictly controlled.

Irritants are chemicals that cause reversible inflammatory effects at the site of contact with living tissue. Most often, eyes, skin and respiratory passages are affected. Nearly all chemicals can be irritating given sufficient exposure to tissue, so general hygiene practices dictate that direct contact be avoided as much as possible.

Corrosive chemicals present both physical and health hazards. When exposed to living tissue, destruction or irreversible alteration occurs. In contact with certain inanimate surfaces (generally metal), corrosives destroy the material. A chemical may be corrosive to tissue but not to steel, or vice versa; few are corrosive to both.

Sensitizers cause allergic reactions in a substantial proportion of exposed subjects. Nearly any chemical may cause an allergic reaction in hypersensitive individuals, so the key here is the prevalence of the reaction in the exposed population. True sensitizers are serious hazards, because sensitization lasts for life and only gets worse with subsequent exposure. It may occur at work because of the high exposure level, but chances are the chemicals will also be found outside the workplace in lower concentrations that aggravate the allergy. Formaldehyde is a prime example. Its vapors come off permanent press clothing, draperies, upholstery, wall coverings, plywood and many other building materials.

Carcinogens: While many substances induce tumors in experimental animals exposed to unrealistically high dosages, officially recognized carcinogens must present a special risk to humans. Criteria for the carcinogenic designation differ slightly among agencies, but in the end, any carcinogenic chemical used in histology is universally recognized as such. Examples include chloroform, chromic acid, dioxane, formaldehyde, nickel chloride, and potassium dichromate. Additionally, a number of dyes are carcinogens: auramine O (CI 41000), basic fuchsin (pararosaniline hydrochloride, CI 42500), ponceau 2R (ponceau de xylidine, CI 16150) and any dye derived from benzidine (including Congo red, CI 22120; diaminobenzidine and Chlorazol black E, CI 30235).

Toxic materials are capable of causing death by ingestion, skin contact or inhalation at certain specified concentrations. These concentrations vary slightly according to the agency making the designation, but differences are insignificant to the histologist. Some countries use the term *poison* when referring to this category. Toxic chemicals pose an immediate risk greater than the previously covered hazards, and some are so dangerous that they are given the designation *highly toxic*. Methanol is toxic; chromic acid, osmium tetroxide and uranyl nitrate are highly toxic. Use extreme caution when handling toxic substances; avoid highly toxic ones if possible.

Chemicals causing specific harm to select anatomical or physiological systems are said to have *target organ effects*. These are particularly dangerous substances because their effects are not immediately evident but are cumulative and frequently irreversible. There are numerous histological relevant examples: xylene and toluene are neurotoxins and benzene affects the blood. Reproductive toxins are especially prevalent (chloroform, methanol, methyl methacrylate, mercuric chloride, xylene and toluene, to name a few) and may warrant special consideration under occupational safety regulations of some countries.

The remaining hazard classes pertain to physical risks. *Combustibles* have flash points at or above a specified temperature. Flash point is the temperature at which vapors will ignite in the presence of an ignition source under carefully defined conditions using specified test equipment. It is a guide to the likelihood vapors might ignite under real workplace conditions. Flash point is not the temperature at which a substance will ignite spontaneously. Different countries and various agencies within those countries have their own unique values for the specified temperature. In the USA, OSHA defines it as 38°C, while the Department of Transportation uses 60.5 °C. Combustible liquids pose little risk of fire under routine laboratory conditions, but they will burn readily during a fire. It is better to choose a combustible product over a flammable one if all other considerations are equal. Clearing agents offer this choice.

Flammable materials have flash points below the specified temperature discussed above, and thus

are of greater concern. Vapors should be controlled carefully to prevent buildup around electrical devices that spark. Special provisions for storage are usually mandated by national regulations, but local codes may impose even stricter measures. Storage rooms, cabinets and containers may have to be specially designed for flammable liquids; volumes stored therein may also be limited. Original manufacturers' containers should be used whenever possible, and preferably should not exceed 1 gallon (4–5 liters).

Explosive chemicals are rare in histology, the primary example being picric acid. Certain silver solutions may become explosive upon aging; they should never be stored after use. In both cases, explosions may occur by shaking. Picric acid also forms dangerous salts with certain metals, which, unlike the parent compound, are potentially explosive even when wet. The best defense against explosive reagents is to avoid them altogether; this is certainly feasible today with picric acid.

Oxidizers initiate or promote combustion in other materials. Harmless by themselves, they may present a serious fire risk when in contact with suitable substances. Sodium iodate is a mild oxidizer that poses little risk under routine laboratory conditions. Mercuric oxide and chromic acid are oxidants that are more serious. *Organic peroxides* are particularly dangerous oxidizers sometimes used to polymerize plastic resins. Limit their volume on hand to extremely small quantities. *Pyrophoric, unstable (reactive)* and *water-reactive* substances are not generally found in histology. All involve fire or excessive heat.

Control of chemicals hazardous to health and the environment

Personal hygiene practices

There must be no eating, drinking or smoking in the lab. Application of cosmetics other than hand lotion likewise has no place within the laboratory setting. Wash hands frequently, but keep skin supple and hydrated with a good lotion. If hazardous powders have been handled, wash around your nose and mouth so that adherent particles are not ingested or inhaled. Solutions must never be pipetted by mouth.

Labeling

Every chemical should be labeled with certain basic information; proper labeling of all containers of chemicals is mandated in some countries. Most reagents purchased recently will have most of the following already on the label, but older inventories may lack certain critical hazard warnings. Remember that solutions created in your laboratory must be fully labeled. Minimum information includes:

- chemical name and, if a mixture, names of all ingredients;
- manufacturer's name and address if purchased commercially, or person making the reagent;
- date purchased or made;
- expiration date, if known;
- hazard warnings and safety precautions.

When putting a reagent's name (or names of ingredients) on the label, use terminology that will be useful to those needing the information. In histology, we have many reagent names that are unfamiliar to chemically knowledgeable people who might be involved in an emergency. This is why it is so important to list ingredients, using names with widespread acceptance in the general field of chemistry; for example, use formaldehyde for formalin, acid fuchsin and picric acid for Van Gieson's, and mercuric chloride, sodium acetate and formaldehyde for B-5.

Commercial products in their original containers will have the name and address of the manufacturer or supplier. If you put the material into another container, even 'temporarily', include this information on the new label. Chemicals in 'temporary' storage conditions have a bad habit of remaining there for years after laboratory personnel have moved on.

If the reagent is made in the laboratory, indicate who made it and when. Traceability could be critical if other information is lacking, as in the case of a Coplin jar of 'silver stain' left in a refrigerator. Is the solution one of those that is potentially explosive? Does anyone know which silver solution it is?

Many laboratories use small self-adhesive labels that say 'Received: ____'. These are dated and affixed to each incoming container. Similarly, an expiration date should also be included for those chemicals that do not have an indefinite shelf life. Most inorganic compounds and many non-perishable organic chemicals are good for many years, but mixtures frequently deteriorate in a shorter time. Information on shelf life is hard to come by, and the best source is your own experience since each laboratory has different conditions and perhaps slightly varied formulations. Kiernan (1999) has included shelf-life data from his own extensive experience, which should serve as a good first approximation for your use.

Hazard warnings at a minimum should include the designations listed in the preceding section. This is the simplest and least ambiguous system. Pictographs (flames, corroding objects, etc.) are not universally recognized; some are obscure as to their meaning. Hazard diamonds are popular but carry risks of misinterpretation, especially since there are several systems in use. When there is an emergency, people may not think clearly or have time to figure something out. They need immediate access to the nature of the danger, and nothing provides that so effectively as the printed word. Briefly worded safety precautions may be appended to the hazard warning: for example, irritant, avoid contact with skin and eyes.

A multicultural workforce, not all of who may have the same native language, staff many labs. It is prudent to accommodate their needs by providing multilingual hazard warnings. Again, in an emergency you want no impediments to prompt and correct action.

Warning signs

Various countries have established different guidelines or mandatory regulations involving signage, so specific recommendations cannot be given here.

Protective equipment

There are certain general guidelines for clothing suitable for laboratory work that should be considered before protective equipment. Secure, close-toed footwear should be mandated; open-toed shoes and sandals offer no protection against spills or dropped items. While nearly all fabric today is resistant to destruction by histological solvents, such was not always the case. Certain early acrylic and acetate fibers dissolved almost instantly when in contact with xylene or toluene, creating a great deal of embarrassment when tiny drops of solvent hit the cloth. The possibility that such fabric still exists is real enough to take heed.

Aprons, goggles, gloves and respirators are the personal protective equipment (PPE) most likely to be used in the histology laboratory. In some countries, law for certain hazardous situations requires specified PPE. The following set of recommendations should be a routine part of general laboratory hygiene and will satisfy the most stringent regulations. When specific requirements exist for certain chemicals, such information will be included below in the section detailing common histological reagents. Aprons should be made of material impervious to the chemicals being used. Simple disposable plastic aprons are usually quite satisfactory, although heavy rubber aprons may be warranted when handling concentrated acids. Cloth laboratory coats are suitable only for protection against powders or very small quantities of hazardous liquids. Do not use them for protection against formaldehyde.

Goggles should be chosen specifically for each worker to accommodate the diversity of facial shapes and prescription glasses. Goggles not only come in a variety of sizes and shapes but also they are made for different functions. Choose only vented splashproof goggles for routine work in histology. These allow for ventilation, which reduces bothersome fogging of the lenses, but the vent holes are baffled so that splashing liquids are not likely to

reach the eyes. Never cut holes in goggles to improve ventilation, as this defeats the protective function of the equipment. For severe conditions of exposure, wear a faceshield over splashproof goggles; never use a faceshield without the goggles. Finally, safety glasses are no substitute for goggles when handling hazardous liquids.

The issue of contact lenses arises frequently in discussions about eye protection (American College of Occupational and Environmental Medicine 2003). If liquids with no irritating fumes are being handled, contact lenses may be used safely in conjunction with appropriate goggles. Conventional goggles offer no protection against harmful vapors, which can become trapped beneath the lenses, causing corneal damage. If your eyes sting or water, your inhalation exposure is almost certainly beyond permissible or prudent limits. Regardless of whether you wear contact lenses, do not work under those conditions, even for brief periods.

Gloves are the most controversial PPE, and misinformation abounds. It is important to understand how gloves work, so that informed decisions can be made about glove selection. Glove material is rarely completely impermeable; it delays penetration of harmful material for a time sufficient to provide adequate protection. Chemical resistance refers to how well material holds up in the presence of solvents, but says nothing about how readily substances move through the material. In most cases, liquids rarely penetrate intact glove material. The vapors are the problem, both because they penetrate more efficiently through gloves and skin, and because the worker usually cannot detect them. Reputable manufacturers of gloves evaluate their products in standardized tests, measuring the time it takes for detectable amounts of a particular chemical to appear on the far side of the material. This is called the breakthrough time, and it increases nonlinearly with glove thickness. A glove twice as thick as another made from the same material will not have a breakthrough time that is double that of the thinner glove. Schwope et al. (1987) present the most comprehensive listing of data on this subject.

Latex is one of the most permeable of all glove materials. Thick (8 mil) rubber gloves have a breakthrough time of 12 minutes with formaldehyde solutions. Latex surgical gloves are so thin (1.0–1.5 mil) that they offer *no* effective protection against formaldehyde or histological solvents. These gloves are suitable only for protection from biohazards. Keep in mind the startling increase in the incidence of latex sensitization, which has accompanied the widespread use of these gloves since the beginning of the AIDS epidemic.

Nitrile gloves are the best option for histological use. They are available in surgical-type thinness for brief intermittent exposures where fine dexterity is necessary. Exposures that are more serious can be safely tolerated with 8 mil nitrile gloves. Remember, however, that no glove material is effective against all classes of chemicals, and nitrile is no exception. Some chemicals in wide histological usage (xylene, toluene, chloroform) will permeate nitrile in seconds.

Respiratory protection against chemical vapors should rarely if ever be needed except in emergencies. Regulatory agencies stress that respirators are the protective equipment of last resort. No one in histology should be in a workplace whose vapor levels are even transiently higher than the PELs. Wearing respirators is uncomfortable, expensive and fraught with compliance hassles. Leave them to the people specially trained not only in respiratory use but also in dealing with such dangerous environments.

In the following discussion, the word 'should' is used, but substitute 'must' in countries having stringent respiratory protection standards. Workers should receive special training for wearing respirators because of the complexities of proper usage. Each worker needing this level of protection should be individually fitted with a respirator that exactly fits the contours of the face. The efficacy of the fit is then assured through a series of complicated tests that should be documented and repeated on a periodic basis. Workers should undergo medical evaluations and respiratory function tests to determine if they are physically qualified to wear respirators. Cartridges for respirators must be chosen carefully for the chemical environment. Both the type of chemical and the vapor concentration are vitally important considerations. Respiratory protection

from airborne infectious materials is another matter altogether. Surgical masks are unacceptable because they fit poorly and have too large a pore size to filter out aerosols. HEPA (high efficiency particulate air) filters are suitable. Workers wearing HEPA masks may have to comply with applicable provisions of respiratory protection standards.

Ventilation

Ventilation is the foremost engineering control; ensuring proper airflow through a laboratory is the first critical step in improving working conditions. Every laboratory scientist should be aware of the following basic principles. For further details on hood design and placement, see Dapson and Dapson (2005) and Saunders (1993). Laboratories should have two separate systems of ventilation, one for general air circulation (often combined with heating and air conditioning and called HVAC), and the other for local removal of hazardous fumes. They must work in concert to be effective, and must not merely shift the noxious vapors to another part of the facility.

General ventilation is for the physical comfort of the occupants of the room. Each hour, the entire volume of room air should be exchanged 4–12 times. That air should not contain significant quantities of hazardous vapors. If such vapors are originating somewhere in the room (from a grossing area, for instance), they should be dealt with at their source with an independent system of local ventilation.

Properly designed chemical fume hoods enclose the emission area, isolating it structurally and functionally from the rest of the room. A motor somewhere in the ductwork (preferably far from the hood) moves air directly to the outside. A sliding door (sash) usually fronts the system, and is an integral part of the way it works by controlling the face velocity of air entering the enclosure. It is a common misconception that high face velocities are good. In fact, strong airflow may create such turbulence inside the hood that contaminated air spills back out into the room. For vapor levels usually encountered in histology labs, a face velocity of 80–120 linear feet per minute is ideal. Control this by adjusting the height of the sash. As lifting the sash enlarges the opening, face velocity declines. Either a vaneometer built into the hood or obtained as an inexpensive handheld device measures face velocity. Always keep the sash at least partially open (unless the hood is designed to admit room air from another port) to prevent overtaxing the motor.

Improperly designed hoods will not be able to achieve optimal face velocity with the sash opened to a comfortable working height. Avoid these literally at all costs, for your facility's money will only be wasted, giving you a false sense of security. There are important dimensional considerations that determine a hood's effectiveness: the hood will develop dangerous eddies if too shallow and may not be able to move the full volume of air if too expansive.

There are other, external factors that influence how a hood works, and all center on the air supplied to the face of the hood. It should be obvious that a device removing air from a workplace must have a supply to draw upon. This is in addition to the amount required by the general ventilating system to exchange 4–12 room air changes per hour. Heating and air conditioning must also be balanced to account for the removal of air through the hood. Location of a hood is critical. Airflow into the face should be smooth and unimpeded. Surprisingly strong crosscurrents are generated by doors opening and closing, or by people walking by. Even the draft from general HVAC ducts can adversely affect hood performance. Any of these disturbances can draw harmful vapors out of the enclosure into the room, even against a net inward flow of air. Locate the hood, and by inference the hazardous work area, out of main traffic patterns and away from HVAC ducts.

Do not use fume hoods as storage or disposal devices. Objects within a hood disrupt airflow, and may block important air passages. Containers that emit vapors should not be placed within a hood except as a temporary safety measure. Remove the offending substance as soon as possible and put it into a secure container. Finally, do not put a waste chemical into a hood for evaporating it away unless there is no alternative in an emergency. Doing so is probably a violation of environmental regulations,

and it may exceed the capacity of the hood to carry fumes away safely.

Ventilation devices other than fume hoods are used in histology labs; few are suitable unless vapor levels are already low. A non-enclosed system, such as a duct located above or behind the work area, may be powerful enough to draw contaminated air away from the worker as long as no crosscurrents are generated, but that is an unrealistic assumption. Workers must move about, and that usually destroys the effectiveness of unenclosed devices. Hoods that return air to the room after passing it through a filter may be suitable for localized workstations generating modest vapor emissions. Filters must be chosen with care. Vapor levels will dictate the size needed. Formaldehyde is not effectively captured by the filtration media used for solvent vapors. Filters become loaded and must be replaced, but how often this occurs is usually a mystery until odors are noticed out in the room. Since most workers in histology labs have impaired senses of smell, dangerous vapor levels may accumulate before anyone detects them. If filtration devices must be used, figure out how to determine effective life of the filters and establish a strict replacement regimen.

Air purification systems based upon ozone should not be used. They generate a chemical that is more hazardous than most of the fumes found in histology labs: ozone has a Ceiling Limit of 0.1 ppm according to ACGIH®. Further, ozone from these purifiers does not seem to be effective in destroying formaldehyde vapors (Esswein & Boeniger 1994).

First aid

With laboratory chemicals, the most common accidents requiring first aid are ingestion, eye contact and extensive skin contact. All health care professionals should have basic training in dealing with these situations at least and preferably with all aspects of first aid. Yearly safety training should include preparedness exercises on the most likely chemical accidents. Ingestion is encountered with patients and other non-laboratory staff, and frequently involves formalin. This is a tragic consequence of administrative neglect of basic safety issues. Laboratory chemicals should never be accessible to unattended patients, particularly those who because of age or illness are unable to think clearly about their actions. Improperly labeled containers are another cause of accidental ingestion. Patients should not be allowed to take fixed surgical specimens home; they present such a large risk from poisoning that no argument to the contrary is sufficient. If a body part needs to be specially cared for as part of a religious need, it should be given only to a responsible adult who can assure that it will never be accessible to unattended children.

First aid for ingestion of hazardous chemicals is not a simple matter. Some reagents will cause more damage if vomited and subsequently aspirated into respiratory passages; others are so toxic that the risk of aspiration is outweighed by the necessity to get the offending substance out of the body quickly. To solve this dilemma, some countries have established sophisticated networks of emergency response teams, which are admirably qualified to provide the best advice. If you have access to a Poison Control Center, or something similar, post the telephone number on each telephone in your laboratory. Time is of the essence in such emergencies, and preparedness may save a life. If enough people are available, get the victim to the emergency room while someone else contacts a Poison Control Center. If outside help is not possible, give a conscious victim a large quantity of water.

Splashing of dangerous chemicals into eyes is a common accident among those who fail to wear suitable goggles. Except for concentrated mineral acids, routine histological chemicals, including formaldehyde, are not likely to cause serious harm to eyes as long as proper treatment immediately follows an accident. All labs should be equipped with emergency eyewash stations, as either freestanding devices or small appliances affixed to sink faucets (the latter must be tested frequently to assure free flow of water). Current recommendations are to have such devices no more than 10 seconds or 30 meters from hazardous work areas. Ideally, the water temperature should be controlled to a range of 15–35°C.

Portable eyewash bottles are not recommended and may be deemed unacceptable by regulatory agencies. These containers hold little liquid and may become contaminated with microorganisms.

Rinse the affected eye for 15–30 minutes, pulling the lids away from the eyeball. This is a seemingly interminable period, but do not shorten it. Emergency health care should be sought only after this treatment.

Treatment of skin contact with hazardous chemicals is simple: wash with water for 15–30 minutes. A quick rinse will not be sufficient for the more dangerous chemicals. Emergency showers should be as accessible as eyewash stations. If the substance is not readily water-soluble, use soap with the water wash. Immediately remove contaminated clothing, including wet shoes. Launder before wearing again, or discard the article. Formaldehyde-soaked leather will be difficult to salvage.

Radiation

The advantages of using radioactive chemicals are rarely sufficient to justify their risks to health and the environment. Exceptions may pertain to therapeutic radioisotopes used as tracers. These emit very low levels of poorly penetrating radiation, and have half-lives measured in hours.

If radioactive substances are handled, a qualified radiation safety officer must oversee all aspects of the project, including waste disposal. Participating staff must be specially trained in radiation safety. This will allay fears as much as create a responsible work force. The work area should be monitored periodically with a radiation detector. Workers should wear dosimeters.

Storage of hazardous chemicals

Most laboratory chemicals can be safely stored in conventional cupboards. Dangerous liquids are best stored below countertop height to minimize the risk of bodily exposure in case a bottle is dropped and broken. Buy dangerous reagents in plastic or plastic-coated glass bottles whenever possible. Special storage provisions are warranted for acids, flammables, radioactive isotopes, controlled substances and hazardous chemicals in bulk containers.

Specialized acid cabinets are designed to contain the fumes emanating from most containers of strong mineral acids. They should be vented to the outside, using acid-resistant ductwork. Curiously, many of these storage devices contain some mild steel parts, which soon rust. Choose this equipment carefully for that reason. Paper labels on acid bottles should be checked periodically for corrosion that could lead to illegibility. Other special storage cabinets are usually mandated for all but the smallest quantities of flammable materials. These are designed to contain a fire within the cabinet. If they are vented, provisions must be made in the ductwork to prevent the spread of fire from the cabinet.

Certain flammable liquids present unusual fire and explosion risks because of their highly volatile nature and very low flash point. Isopentane and diethyl ether ('ether') are common examples. Opened containers cannot be resealed reliably. Never store these in a refrigerator or freezer unless these appliances are certified as suitable for an explosive atmosphere (mistakenly referred to as 'explosion-proof'). The best advice is to avoid using these chemicals altogether. If that is not possible, buy only the quantity immediately needed, use it up if possible and do not try to store any leftovers.

Radioactive chemicals and controlled substances must be stored separately from other reagents. Cabinets should be locked. Access should be limited to a few specially qualified people.

Large containers present other risks. Even 5-gallon (20-liter) quantities can be too heavy for people to handle, especially for pouring operations. Equip these containers with spigots and keep the spigot above fluid level when not in use. Larger drums more than 200 liters require special handling equipment for moving and dispensing. Be sure any pumping device is completely compatible with the chemical. Avoid mild steel parts for fixatives and most plastics for xylene and toluene.

Transporting hazardous materials from storage to work areas can be risky. Carry glass containers with both hands, one hand beneath the jar or bottle. Rubber buckets should be used to carry highly dangerous materials like glass containers of mineral acids.

Spills and containment

Preparedness for spills begins with laboratory design. The goal is to prevent hazardous materials from reaching the outside environment. There should be no open floor drains unless they lead to special containment equipment that can be pumped out or drained by a hazardous waste hauler. Floor drains for showers can be built with a low dyke that prevents liquids on the floor from entering and keeps most of the water from the shower from getting out onto the floor.

How laboratory personnel respond to a spill will depend upon the nature of the hazard, the volume of the spill and the qualifications of the staff. Each chemical should be evaluated with these factors in mind. A gallon of alcohol spilled onto the floor presents a risk of fire but little health hazard, while the same quantity of formalin could be life threatening (20 ppm is imminently hazardous to life). Small spills are defined as those that can be safely handled by the immediate staff. Large spills present risks that surpass the qualifications of the same people to deal safely with the emergency and require specially trained HazMat or emergency response teams.

Develop plans for dealing with each family of hazardous material (acids, bases, flammables, etc.). Detail exactly what protective equipment is needed, and how each type of spill will be handled. Establish who will be called in the event the spill requires outside help, then contact them so they will be prepared. They may want an on-site visit to familiarize themselves with your facility's layout, and certainly will want to discuss the types and magnitudes of hazards. Finally, train the laboratory staff on spill procedures and practice doing it with harmless material. Not having had the time to do this will prove to be a sorry excuse when the accident occurs.

If the amount of spilled material is limited to a few grams or milliliters, simply wipe it up with towel or sponge, protecting your hands with suitable gloves.

Dispose of the towel or sponge appropriately; do not put it into the general trash, and protect the room from its vapors by sealing it within an impermeable plastic bag or other container.

In contrast to such very small incidents, an entirely different approach should be used for any other spills of dangerous materials. All personnel should evacuate the room or immediate vicinity of the problem. Assemble in a designated spot, and be certain everyone is there. On your way out, watch for your co-workers and assist anyone needing help getting out. Provide first aid if anyone has been splashed or is feeling the effects of vapors. Calmly discuss the magnitude of the spill and determine if it is large or small. There should be no mention of cause or blame here: it is immaterial to the immediate problem. If the spill is large, call an emergency response team and seal off the area. If small, decide how to handle the spill based on prearranged plans.

Spill neutralizing and containment kits should be available immediately outside the hazardous work area. These may be commercially purchased or assembled from common materials, and should include protective equipment and cleanup aids. Nitrile gloves similar in thickness to dishwashing gloves are adequate for most spills likely in histology; several sizes are available. Splashproof goggles and a faceshield are important. Provide disposable plastic aprons for chemical spills and disposable gowns for biohazards. If the staff is qualified and trained, equip the kit with respirators appropriate for the type of spill (a HEPA respirator for biohazards).

A good basic kit would also include cleanup items such as a dustpan and brush for powders, sponges, towels and mops for liquids, adsorbent material (vermiculite, kitty litter or a commercial sorbent), bleach (sodium hypochlorite) for biohazards, baking soda for acids, vinegar (5% acetic acid) for alkalis, and a commercial formalin neutralizing product. Have a sealable plastic bucket and heavy plastic bags for containment of the salvaged waste. Kits that are more sophisticated would contain instantaneous vapor monitoring devices so that the contaminated area can be checked before cleanup operations begin. Remember: the level of expertise of the staff will dictate how far to go with this.

Recycling

One effective way to control hazardous chemicals is through recycling, as this reduces the quantities purchased, stored and discarded. Many clearing agents, alcohol and formalin can be recycled satisfactorily with proper equipment. Because these are the highest-volume chemicals in histology, the cost savings can be impressive, despite an initial outlay of capital funds.

Formalin is a mixture of volatile formaldehyde and nonvolatile salts in a solvent of water or water and alcohol (the small amount of stabilizing methanol can be ignored). Used solutions also contain solubilized and particulate components from the specimens. Through the process of simple distillation, water and formaldehyde are separated from all the other constituents. While that leaves the undesirable parts behind, the recycled product now lacks its salts and may not be at the proper concentration. Formaldehyde content can be assayed with a simple kit and adjusted as necessary. Fresh salts are readily restored to the solution.

Solvents should be fractionally distilled, as some of the contaminants in the waste are also volatile. Simple distillation will not separate these, and the resultant product may contain unacceptable amounts of water.

The most common problem with good distillation equipment is a foul amine odor detectable in the recycled product. It comes from deamination of protein in the waste during the distillation process. The freed amines evaporate readily and pass over with the other volatile components. Keeping the distillation chamber scrupulously clean is usually the key to avoiding the problem altogether. Formalin that has been heavily enriched with blood protein (as from fixing placentas) may require diluting with less bloody waste formalin. Pre-filter solutions contain many tissue fragments or coagulated protein.

Hazardous chemical waste disposal

Health care facilities are to prevent and treat illness, yet they are significant contributors to environmental harm especially in countries that have seen significant improvements in industrial pollution. On the other hand, if an effective pollution prevention program has been put into effect, there should be little waste to deal with. Reducing toxics use by substitution and minimization, coupled with recycling, could lead to amazingly low quantities of waste to be hauled away. The three highest-volume reagents, formalin, alcohol and clearant, can all be recycled. Formalin can be replaced with an effective glyoxal-based fixative that is drain-disposable in nearly all communities because of its ready biodegradability and low aquatic toxicity.

Options for disposal of hazardous chemical waste depend heavily upon national and local regulations, but the following recommendations should be valid anywhere. First, keep waste streams separated; do not mix different chemicals together unless told to do so by a qualified waste official. Second, know the hazard(s) of the waste. Is it flammable? Water-soluble? Toxic? Each of these factors affects the choice of disposal method. The best option for disposal is to pour the waste down the sanitary drain, from which it can be treated before entering the environment. Such waste, however, must not harm the biological processes that waste treatment facilities depend upon; nor must it pass through the system untreated. An example of the former would be formaldehyde in sufficient strength and quantity to kill off the bacteria driving the treatment process. Xylene typifies the latter, because its rate of biodegradation is too slow to be affected by the 1–3 day residence time in the wastewater treatment plant.

Formaldehyde is readily biodegradable. Nearly all organisms have an enzyme, formaldehyde dehydrogenase, which decomposes this chemical. The trick is to feed it into the system slowly enough so that it is diluted below toxic concentrations by the normal flow of water. Never dilute toxic material before pouring it down the drain, or follow disposal by 'flushing with copious amounts of water'; this practice increases the volume passing through the treatment plant, which shortens the residence time and may impair biodegradation.

Work with your wastewater authorities, inform them of the nature of the waste (chemical composition and hazardous characteristics), and offer material safety data sheets. Propose a plan for disposal which includes the volume of waste, the time period over which it will be dumped, and the frequency of disposal. For example, you may wish to dispose of large quantities of waste formalin containing 3.7% or 37,000 ppm formaldehyde over a 1-hour period each working day. This could be accomplished by trickling the waste into a sink from a carboy equipped with bottom spigot adjusted so that it takes an hour to become empty. There would be no risk to the treatment plant at this flow rate of 2 ml/second. Dumping a large volume of waste all at once is not good because it tends to travel in a slug and may fail to become sufficiently diluted to protect the treatment plant.

Some waste can be rendered more acceptable for drain disposal. Acids and bases can be neutralized and formalin can be detoxified with commercial products. Be sure the pretreatment process is safe, effective and acceptable. Never attempt to detoxify formalin by mixing with bleach (sodium hypochlorite) or ammonia. Both reactions are exothermic and could quickly get out of control, spewing vapors and hot fluid all over the lab. Know what the reaction products are, and be certain that they are indeed suitably low in toxicity. Water-insoluble solvents are never drain disposable, even if purportedly biodegradable. If they are combustible with sufficiently high caloric value, they may be eligible to be mixed with the fuel in an oil-fired heating system in certain countries. Good candidates for this option are any of the clearing agents except the halogenated solvents chloroform, trichloroethane and their relatives. Note that this method is not burning the waste in an incinerator. The difference is subtle but important. An incinerator exists for the sole purpose of destroying waste, while a furnace provides heat.

If you cannot get rid of a waste by drain disposal or combustion in a furnace, you must resort to a waste hauler. In some countries, the waste generator (your facility) bears the ultimate responsibility and liability for the waste that someone else takes away and supposedly deals with properly. If you are generating waste that must be removed from the premises for burial or incineration, you should do everything possible to eliminate that chemical from your lab. There is no better advice; however, you want to view it, whether from a financial, health or environmental perspective.

Control of biological substances hazardous to health and the environment

Preparation

An Exposure Control Plan for biohazards should be written. It may be part of the Chemical Hygiene Plan or an independent document, but definitely should be part of your SOPs. As with chemical hazards, workers should be trained initially, refreshed at least yearly and immediately introduced to any new procedures that present additional risks.

Handling

People who work in histology laboratories may not be exposed to quite the level of risk that many health care workers are, but they face hazards that may be more subtle. There are three potential routes of exposure: inhalation of aerosols, contact with non-intact skin and contact with mucous membranes (eyes, nose and mouth). Knowing how infectious agents can reach you is the foundation of protecting yourself and your co-workers. Practice universal precautions: handle every specimen as if it were infectious.

Fresh specimens of human origin must always be considered potentially infectious. Most animal tissue does not carry that risk, but there are important exceptions. Species known to be capable of transmitting disease to humans, and animals intentionally infected or known to be naturally infected with transmissible diseases, must be handled with the same precautions as would be used for human tissue.

The first and most obvious source of biological risk is with fresh tissue and body fluids; grossing carries the highest risk of all histological activities.

Fixed specimens have a much-reduced risk because nearly all infectious agents are readily deactivated by fixation. Specimens must be thoroughly fixed for this to happen. Certain tissues like liver, spleen, placenta and lung do not fix well unless grossed thinly, and may remain raw (unfixed) in the center after days of exposure to the fixative. Those centers are potentially infectious. Some fixatives require more time than that available in rushed pathology labs, so tissues in the first several stations of a tissue processor may remain biohazardous. Complete penetration by alcohol will kill all infectious agents except prions, so it is safe that properly processed specimens are free from microbial risk and can be handled without special precautions.

Prions, the agents of spongiform encephalopathies like Creutzfeldt-Jakob disease, scrapie, chronic wasting disease and mad cow disease, present a more difficult challenge. Even normal steam sterilization fails to inactivate these particles, and common effective chemical treatments like sodium hypochlorite and phenol create artifacts in tissue. Histological specimens can be decontaminated by immersion in formalin for 48 hours, followed by treatment for 1 hour in concentrated formic acid and additional formalin fixation for another 48 hours. Rank (1999) reviewed the risks and decontamination protocols for histology labs.

Cryotomy presents special risks because tissue is usually fresh. Small dust-like particles generated from sectioning may become airborne, a risk vastly magnified with the use of cryogenic sprays. Do not clean the cabinet with a vacuum unless the device is equipped with a HEPA filter. Sterilize surfaces with chlorine bleach or a suitable commercial disinfectant; avoid formaldehyde solutions as these present a chemical risk to the person doing the cleaning. Good-quality latex or nitrile surgical gloves are perfectly acceptable protective devices for biohazards. Goggles should be worn during grossing anyway to protect against chemical splashes, and will do double duty against infectious agents. A faceshield may be warranted in some cases. Aprons or laboratory coats will keep clothes clean, but do not wear these used protective articles outside the laboratory (especially to the cafeteria!).

Disposal of biohazardous waste

Biohazardous waste should be incinerated on-site or hauled away. Either way, potentially infectious waste ought to be segregated from chemical and non-regulated waste, which may be barred from incinerators designed for biohazardous materials. Fixed wet specimens and their fluid are chemically hazardous and may be infectious. Together they pose a difficult problem.

Control of physical hazards

From equipment

Equipment may present risks from electrical and mechanical factors, which can be minimized by proper installation, care and personnel training. Keep a log for each piece of equipment, listing its installation date, the person and firm performing the installation, and the initial diagnostic test results that assure the item is working properly. Include a schedule for preventive maintenance and a complete service record is good laboratory practice.

Electrical shock most often arises from improperly grounded devices. Have a qualified person verify that all outlets are properly polarized and grounded. Plug equipment into outlets, not into extension cords.

Electrical equipment poses a risk of igniting flammable vapors. Nearly all switches may spark, including those associated with doors. Devices sold as 'explosion-proof' have their switches sealed to prevent contact with flammable vapors. Refrigerators and freezers must never be used to store highly flammable chemicals like ether and isopentane unless they are rated as suitable for flammable environments. Likewise, household microwave ovens should not be used to heat flammables because the door interlock switch may spark (this switch stops the magnetron when the door is opened). Some laboratory microwave appliances vent the chamber sufficiently to prevent potentially explosive vapor concentrations from building.

Today, mechanical dangers from histological equipment are generally confined to burns from hot surfaces. Most modern devices have adequate safety features that have eliminated some of the more common hazards encountered decades ago. If you use older equipment, be aware of its shortcomings. Many centrifuges have lockout devices that prevent the lid from being opened while the rotor is moving. Distillation equipment should be purchased only if it has safety features that include high temperature and low liquid volume cutoff switches. Specialized apparatus for electron microscopy should be used only by people specially trained in the inherent risks.

Devices that emit an open flame (such as Bunsen burners or alcohol lamps) must never be used in an environment where flammable solvents are present. Electrical appliances for heating or sterilizing are far safer and more convenient than a gas-fired or alcohol-fueled implement.

Broken glass and disposable microtome blades present risks, particularly if they are contaminated with chemical or biological material. Special 'sharps' containers are used for the disposal of such items. Microtomes and cryostats are particularly dangerous; be sure to remove blades before cleaning such equipment.

Hazards and handling of common histological chemicals

Extracting succinct information from data sheets and reference books is a time-consuming task that has served as a major impediment to designing proper training programs and labels. The following compilation includes most of the chemicals commonly used in histology laboratories on a routine basis. Permissible exposure values are from OSHA unless otherwise indicated as being taken from ACGIH® (2004) or NIOSH (2003). All IDLH values are from NIOSH and Biological Exposure Indices (BEIs) are from ACGIH®. Many PELs have been revised downward since 2002. The listed hazards are applicable to the quantities normally handled on a laboratory scale and may be inappropriate for bulk quantities. Recommendations for glove material are from Schwope et al. (1987). In reality, selection of glove material may have to balance chemical resistance against practicality for the tasks likely to be encountered. Some chemicals have been deemed essentially non-hazardous under normal laboratory conditions of use.

The intent of this section, and indeed this entire chapter, is to provide guidelines for a safe workplace. Most hazardous chemicals can be handled safely with a minimum of effort and equipment, but a few cannot. These have been identified clearly and should be eliminated or at least reduced to the smallest quantity possible. Suitable substitutes have been identified. The toxicology of most chemicals is not well known, and new information, usually damaging, continues to become available.

Acetic acid. TWA = 10 ppm; STEL = 15 ppm (ACGIH®); IDHL = 50 ppm. Irritating to respiratory system (target organ effects); concentrated solutions are severe skin and eye irritants, corrosive to most metals and combustible (flash point = 43°C). Avoid skin, eye and respiratory contact. Use a chemical fume hood, nitrile gloves, goggles and impermeable apron when dispensing concentrated acid. Do not use rubber (latex) gloves. Always add acid to water, never water to acid, to avoid severe splattering. Do not mix concentrated (glacial) acetic acid with chromic acid, nitric acid or sodium/potassium hydroxide. Dilute (1–10%) aqueous solutions are relatively benign.

Acetone. TWA = 1000 ppm (500 ppm ACGIH®, 250 ppm NIOSH); STEL 750 ppm; BEI = 50 mg acetone/liter of urine at the end of the shift. Highly flammable (flash point = −16°C) and very volatile. Great risk of fire from heavy vapors traveling along counters or floors to a distant ignition source. Not a serious health hazard under most conditions of use but be aware that acetone can be narcotic in high concentration. Inhalation may cause dizziness, headache and irritation to respiratory passages. Skin contact can cause excessive drying and dermatitis.

Moderately toxic by ingestion. Protect skin with Neoprene gloves.

Aliphatic hydrocarbon clearing agents. TWA = 196 ppm (manufacturer's recommendation). Very low toxicity: non-irritating and non-sensitizing to normal human skin. Combustible (40°C) or flammable (flash point = 24°C). Limit skin exposure to minimize de-fatting effects. Neoprene or nitrile gloves are satisfactory. Recycle by fractional distillation, burn as a fuel supplement or use a licensed waste hauler for disposal.

Aluminum ammonium sulfate, aluminum potassium sulfate and aluminum sulfate. Not dangerous in laboratory quantities except as eye irritants.

Ammonium hydroxide. TWA = 50 ppm OSHA (25 ppm ACGIH®); STEL = 35 ppm as ammonia gas; IDLH = 300 ppm. Severe irritant to skin, eyes and respiratory tract. Target organ effects on respiratory system (fibrosis and edema). Wear rubber or nitrile gloves. Store away from acids. Do not mix with formaldehyde as this generates heat and toxic vapors. Spills of 500 ml or more may warrant evacuation of the room.

Aniline. TWA = 5 ppm (2 ppm ACGIH®) with additional exposure likely through the skin; IDLH = 100 ppm. A very dangerous reagent, which should not be used if possible. Moderate skin and severe eye irritant, sensitizer, toxic by skin absorption, carcinogen. Excessive exposure may cause drowsiness, headache, nausea and blue discoloration of extremities.

Celloidin (stabilized nitrocellulose). Harmless as a health hazard but dangerously flammable as a solid. May deteriorate into a crumbly, potentially explosive substance requiring professional assistance for removal. Solutions usually contain highly flammable ether and alcohol.

Chloroform. CL = 50 ppm; STEL = 2 ppm (NIOSH); IDLH = 500 ppm. Toxic by ingestion and inhalation. Overexposure to vapors can cause disorientation, unconsciousness and death. Target organ effects on liver, reproductive, fetal, and central nervous, blood and gastrointestinal systems. Carcinogenic. Practical glove materials are not available. This is one of the most dangerous and difficult chemicals in histology because workers in most laboratories simply cannot receive adequate protection from vapors and skin contact. Legitimate disposal may be very challenging. Do not burn. Do not evaporate solvent to the atmosphere. Avoid all use.

Chromic acid (chromium trioxide). TWA = 0.5 mg chromium/cubic meter (ACGIH®); CL = 0.1 (0.05 ACGIH®) mg chromium/cubic meter; IDLH = 15 mg chromium/cubic meter. Highly toxic with target organ effects on kidneys; corrosive to skin and mucous membranes; carcinogenic. Strong oxidizer. Avoid all skin contact. Nitrile, latex and Neoprene gloves are not suitable except for limited contact; suitable protective material not readily available or practical for laboratory use. Chromium is a serious environmental toxin. Drain disposal is not a legitimate option for any solution containing chromium, including subsequent processing fluids following fixation or rinses after staining procedures involving chromium. Give this chemical high priority for complete elimination from your lab.

Diaminobenzidine (DAB). Human carcinogen. Solutions pose little health risk under normal conditions of use. Disposal of DAB and subsequent rinse solutions down the drain creates environmental problems. These wastes can be detoxified with acidified potassium permanganate according to the methods of Lunn and Sansone (1990); see Dapson and Dapson (2005) for a simplified procedure. Do not use chlorine bleach, as the reaction products remain mutagenic (Lunn & Sansone 1991).

Dimethylformamide (DMF). TWA = 10 ppm; additional exposure likely through skin contact; IDLH = 500 ppm. Eye, nose and skin irritant. May cause nausea. May be a reproductive toxin. Facilitates transport of other harmful materials through skin and mucous membranes. Combustible liquid (flash point = 136°F). Avoid all skin and respiratory contact. Use DMF only in a fume hood with suitable gloves (butyl rubber). Common glove materials do not provide adequate protection. Dispose of DMF only through a licensed waste hauler.

Dioxane (1,4-dioxane). TWA = 100 pm (20 ppm ACGIH®); additional exposure likely through skin contact; CL 1 ppm (NIOSH); IDLH = 500 ppm. Skin and eye irritant: overexposure may cause corneal damage. Readily absorbed through skin and mucous membranes. Delayed target organ effects in central nervous system, liver and kidneys. Only butyl or Teflon gloves are suitable. Flammable liquid, which develops explosive properties (peroxides) after a year. Do not recycle, as the risk of creating explosive peroxides increases greatly. Avoid all use of this chemical.

Dyes. There are thousands of dyes and many have been implicated in causing cancers in rats under highly unrealistic circumstances. All should be handled with due caution when in the powder state, but liquids pose little risks except through skin contact and ingestion. Dyes containing the benzidine nucleus are now considered known human carcinogens and must be treated accordingly in both handling and disposal. See the section on carcinogens earlier in this chapter for examples.

Ethanol. TWA = 1000 ppm. Skin and eye irritant. Toxic properties are not likely to be significant under intended conditions of use in a laboratory. Use butyl or nitrile gloves, not rubber or Neoprene. Flammable liquid. Recycle via distillation.

Ether (diethyl ether). TWA = 400 ppm. Mild to moderate skin and eye irritant. Overexposure to vapors can produce disorientation, unconsciousness or death. Target organ effects on nervous system following inhalation or skin absorption. Dangerously flammable liquid that forms explosive peroxides. It is extremely volatile and difficult to contain. Do not store in a refrigerator or freezer unless the appliance is rated for an explosive atmosphere. Use a licensed waste hauler. Because of the uncontrollable physical hazard, avoid use of this substance if possible.

Ethidium bromide. May be harmful by ingestion, inhalation or absorption through the skin. Irritating to skin, eyes, mucous membranes and upper respiratory tract. Chronic exposure may cause alteration of genetic material. Dispense powder under a fume hood and wear any type of gloves.

Ethylene glycol ethers (ethylene glycol monomethyl or monoethyl ether, Cellosolves). TWA = 200 ppm (5 ppm (ACGIH®); additional exposure likely through skin. Toxic by inhalation, skin contact and ingestion, with target organ effects involving reproductive, fetal, urinary and blood systems. Combustible liquids (flash point = 43–49°C). Avoid all use, substituting propylene-based glycol ethers. If substitution is not possible, wear butyl gloves and use a fume hood for all tasks involving these reagents.

Formaldehyde and paraformaldehyde. TWA = 0.75 ppm (0.016 ppm NIOSH); STEL = 2 ppm; CL = 0.3 ppm for 15 minutes ACGIH® (0.1 ppm NIOSH); IDLH = 20 ppm. Severe eye and skin irritant. Sensitizer by skin and respiratory contact (this is the most serious hazard for most laboratory workers). Toxic by ingestion and inhalation. Target organ effects on respiratory system. Carcinogen. Corrosive to most metals. All workers exposed to formaldehyde should be monitored for exposure levels on a periodic basis. Exposure of the skin during grossing is the greatest risk in a well-ventilated lab. Latex surgical gloves are nearly worthless as protective devices. Thin nitrile gloves are better but cannot be used safely for extended periods. Recycle as much waste as possible by distillation and have the remainder taken away by a licensed waste hauler or detoxified by a commercial product. Drain disposal of limited quantities of formaldehyde may be permitted in some communities. Satisfactory substitutes are now available worldwide and offer substantial technical advantages.

Formic acid. TWA = 5 ppm; STEL = 10 ppm (ACGIH®); IDLH = 30 ppm. Mild skin and severe eye irritant. Corrosive to metal. Avoid skin, eye and respiratory contact; use a chemical fume hood. All common glove materials except latex are suitable. Always add acid to water, never water to acid, to avoid severe splattering.

Glutaraldehyde. CL = 0.2 ppm NIOSH (0.05 ppm ACGIH®). Severe skin and eye irritant; toxic by ingestion. Wear butyl or Neoprene gloves and use a hood.

Glycol methacrylate monomer. No established PELs. Sensitizer. Flammable liquid. Avoid all skin, eye and respiratory contact. Common glove materials are probably not suitable, based on information concerning other methacrylates. To avoid a dangerous exothermic reaction, do not polymerize large quantities of this monomer. Polymerize small quantities for disposal.

Glyoxal. No established PELs. Glyoxal solutions have no vapor pressure (do not give off fumes) and thus pose no inhalation risk. Irritant to skin and eyes. Ingestion may produce adverse fixative effects on the gastrointestinal tract. Wear nitrile gloves and goggles. Favorable ecotoxicity profile. An excellent substitute for formaldehyde-based fixatives.

Hydrochloric acid. CL = 5 ppm (2 ppm ACGIH®); IDLH = 50 ppm. Strong irritant to skin, eyes and respiratory system. Target organ effects via inhalation on respiratory, reproductive and fetal systems. Corrosive to most metals. Concentrated acid is particularly dangerous because it fumes. Use a fume hood, goggles, apron and gloves made of any common material except butyl rubber. Always add acid to water, never water to acid, to avoid severe splattering.

Hydrogen peroxide. TWA = 1 ppm; IDLH = 75 ppm. Solutions less than 5% are essentially harmless. Concentrated solutions are very hazardous and should not be used.

Hydroquinone. TWA = 2 mg/cubic meter; CL = 2 mg/cubic meter for 15 minutes (NIOSH). Irritant capable of causing dermatitis and corneal ulceration. Toxic by ingestion and inhalation. May cause dizziness, sense of suffocation, vomiting, headache, cyanosis, delirium and collapse. Urine may become green or brownish green. Lethal adult dose is 2 grams. All common glove materials are suitable except latex. Avoid contact with sodium hydroxide.

Iodine. CL = 0.1 ppm; IDLH = 2 ppm. Strong irritant and possibly corrosive to eyes, skin and respiratory system. Dermal sensitizer. Toxic by ingestion and inhalation. Wear nitrile gloves and use a hood when handling iodine crystals. Histological solutions are essentially harmless except if ingested.

Isopentane. TWA = 1000 ppm (600 ppm ACGIH®, 120 ppm NIOSH); CL = 610 ppm for 15 minutes; IDLH = 1500 ppm. Excessive exposure to vapors causes irritation of respiratory tract, cough, mild depression and irregular heartbeat. Ingestion causes vomiting, swelling of abdomen, headache and depression. Chilled isopentane may freeze the skin but otherwise is harmless to it. Extremely flammable (flash point = −57°C) and highly volatile, making this a very dangerous chemical. Never store it in a refrigerator or freezer unless the appliance is rated for an explosive atmosphere. Protect hands from frostbite.

Isopropanol. TWA = 400 ppm (200 ppm ACGIH®); STEL = 400 ppm; IDLH = 2000 ppm. Mild skin and moderate eye irritant. Toxic by ingestion. Flammable liquid (flash point = 12°C). Practically harmless except for flammability under normal conditions of use. Recycle by fractional distillation.

Limonene. No PELs established. Generally regarded as safe as a food additive in minute quantities, but a dangerous sensitizer when handled as in histology. May cause respiratory distress if inhaled. Use a hood and gloves (butyl, Neoprene or nitrile). Clearing agents containing limonene usually cannot be recycled back to the original product because they also include non-volatile antioxidants and diluents.

Mercuric chloride. TWA = 0.01 mg mercury/cubic meter; additional exposure likely through skin contact; IDLH = 10 mg mercury/cubic meter. Severe skin and eye irritant; target organ effects on reproductive, urogenital, respiratory, gastrointestinal and fetal systems following ingestion and inhalation. Severe environmental hazard. Corrosive to metals. Avoid all use if possible because of the impossibility of preventing environmental contamination. Most processing solutions will become contaminated with mercury if any specimens have been fixed in B-5, Helly's, Zenker's or similar fixatives. Reagents used to 'de-Zenkerize' sections release mercury. None of these must be allowed to go down the drain. Legitimate disposal of mercury-containing waste is difficult and very expensive, if not impossible, in some areas of the world. Replace mercuric fixatives with zinc formalin or glyoxal solutions.

Mercuric oxide. Strong oxidizer. See mercuric chloride for other information.

Methanol. TWA = 200 ppm, STEL = 250 ppm (ACGIH®); additional exposure likely through the skin; IDLH = 6000 ppm. Moderate skin and eye irritant. Toxic by ingestion and inhalation, with target organ effects on reproductive, fetal, respiratory, gastrointestinal and nervous systems. May cause blindness or death. Flammable (flash point = 12°C) and rather volatile. Use butyl gloves; other common glove materials are ineffective. Recyclable.

Methenamine. No PELs established. Powder may cause irritation; solutions pose little risk under normal conditions of use.

Methyl methacrylate monomer. TWA = 100 ppm (50 ppm ACGIH®); STEL 100 ppm ACGIH®; IDLH = 1000 ppm. Target organ effects from inhalation include fetal, reproductive and behavioral symptoms. Flammable liquid. May overheat dangerously if large quantities are mixed with polymerizing agents. Keep away from strong acids and bases. Common glove materials are not effective; use Teflon. Work in a hood. Polymerize small quantities for disposal.

Nickel chloride. TWA = 1.0 mg nickel/cubic meter (0.1 mg nickel/cubic meter ACGIH®, 0.015 mg nickel/cubic meter NIOSH); IDLH = 10 mg nickel/cubic meter. Carcinogenic to humans. Toxic by inhalation of dust. Solutions pose little risk to workers but are an environmental problem. Use gloves (any material) and hood when handling the powder. Do not use drain disposal for these solutions or for subsequent rinse fluids.

Nitric acid. TWA = 2 ppm; STEL = 4 ppm ACGIH®, NIOSH; IDLH = 25 ppm. Corrosive to skin, mucous membranes and most metals. Toxic by inhalation. Target organ effects on reproductive and fetal systems after ingestion. Oxidizer. Concentrated acid is very hazardous. Use Neoprene gloves for extensive use; nitrile, butyl and latex are not effective except to protect against minor splashes. Wear apron and goggles for handling any quantity. Always add acid to water, never water to acid, to avoid severe splattering. Explosive mixtures may be formed with hydrogen peroxide, diethyl ether and anion exchange resins.

Nitrogen, liquid. No PELs established. Asphyxiant gas: excessive inhalation may cause dizziness, unconsciousness or death. Use extreme caution to avoid thermal (cold) burns.

Osmium tetroxide (osmic acid). TWA = 0.0002 ppm osmium; STEL = 0.0006 ppm osmium (ACGIH®); IDLH = 0.1 ppm. Vapors are extremely dangerous. Corrosive to eyes and mucous membranes. Toxic by inhalation with target effects on reproductive, sensory and respiratory systems. Avoid all contact with vapors. Do not open containers in air. In a hood, score vial and break under water or other solvent. Information on protective glove materials is not available.

Oxalic acid. TWA = 1 mg/cubic meter; STEL = 2 mg/cubic meter; IDLH = 500 mg/cubic meter. Corrosive solid; causes severe burns of the eyes, skin and mucous membranes. Toxic by inhalation and ingestion, with target organ effects on kidneys and cardiovascular systems.

Repeated skin contact can cause dermatitis and slow-healing ulcers. Will corrode most metals. Risks are minimal with quantities usually encountered in histology.

Periodic acid. No PELs established. Mild oxidizer. Quantities used in histology pose little physical or health risk.

Phenol. TWA = 5 ppm; additional exposure likely through skin contact; CL = 15.6 ppm for 15 minutes; IDLH = 250 ppm. Toxic by ingestion, inhalation and skin absorption. Readily absorbed through skin, causing increased heart rate, convulsions and death. Will burn eyes and skin. Target organ effects on digestive, urinary and nervous systems. Combustible liquid (flash point = 172°F). Avoid all contact if possible, or use extreme caution. Purchase the smallest quantity possible. Use only butyl rubber gloves and work only under a fume hood. Mixing concentrated formaldehyde and phenol may produce an uncontrollable reaction.

Phosphomolybdic and phosphotungstic acids. TWA = 1 mg/cubic meter ACGIH®; STEL = 3 mg/cubic meter ACGIH®, NIOSH; IDLH = 1000 mg/cubic meter. All PELs are expressed as the quantity of the metal molybdenum or tungsten. Oxidants. These reagents present minor risk under normal conditions of use in histology.

Picric acid. TWA = 0.1 mg/cubic meter; additional exposure likely through skin contact. Toxic by skin absorption. Explosive when dry or when complexed with metal and metallic salts. Do not move bottles containing dry picric acid; get professional help immediately. Do not allow any picric acid solutions, including yellow rinse fluids or processing solvents, to go down the drain, as these may form explosive picrates with metal pipes. Avoid all use if possible, substituting zinc formalin or glyoxal for Bouin's or similar fixatives, and tartrazine for a yellow counterstain. If you must have it, check containers monthly to keep the salts wet. Always wipe jar and cap threads with a damp towel to prevent material from drying within them.

Potassium dichromate. See chromic acid for information on chromium toxicity.

Potassium ferricyanide and potassium ferrocyanide. Low toxicity to humans and the environment in quantities likely to be encountered in histology.

Potassium hydroxide. CL = 2 mg/cubic meter as dust (NIOSH, ACGIH®). Corrosive to eyes and skin. Use care when dissolving solids in water, as the reaction may be violently exothermic and cause splattering.

Potassium permanganate. Skin and eye irritant. Ingestion will cause severe gastrointestinal distress. Strong oxidant: do not mix with ethylene glycol, ethanol, acetic acid, formaldehyde, glycerol, hydrochloric acid, sulfuric acid, hydrogen peroxide or ammonium hydroxide. Use butyl gloves.

Propidium iodide. Mutagen, irritant and suspected carcinogen. Material is irritating to mucous membranes and upper respiratory tract. All common glove materials except latex are suitable.

Propylene glycol ethers. TWA = 100 ppm; STEL = 150 ppm (ACGIH®). Used as a less toxic substitute for ethylene-based glycol ethers.

Pyridine. TWA = 5 ppm (1 ppm ACGIH®); IDLH = 1000 ppm. Toxic by ingestion, inhalation and skin absorption. Overexposure causes nausea, headache and increased urinary frequency. Target organ effects on liver and kidneys. Irritant to skin and eyes. Highly offensive odor. Flammable liquid (flash point = 20°C). Use only under a fume hood, with butyl gloves. Do not mix with chromic acid.

Silver salts and solutions. TWA = 0.01 mg silver/cubic meter; IDLH = 10 mg silver/cubic meter. Skin and eye irritants. Ingestion will cause violent gastrointestinal discomfort. Little risk to workers when fresh, but some aged solutions become explosive. Serious environmental hazard. Do not discard solutions or rinse fluids down the drain. Silver may be recoverable in special equipment or by metal reclaimers.

Sodium azide. CL = 0.3 mg/cubic meter for the powder (NIOSH, ACGIH®). Poison, very toxic. May be fatal if swallowed or absorbed through the skin. Evolves highly toxic gas when mixed with acids. When used as a preservative in biochemical solutions there is little risk to workers except by ingestion and skin absorption. Forms explosive compounds with metals. Do not discard waste down the drain.

Sodium bisulfite. TWA = 5 mg/cubic meter (NIOSH, ACGIH®). Irritant to skin, eyes and mucous membranes. Strong reducing agent: keep from oxidants. Dilute solutions generally pose no risk.

Sodium hydroxide. See potassium hydroxide.

Sodium hypochlorite (liquid chlorine bleach). No PELs established. Eye irritant. May be toxic by ingestion unless diluted considerably. Strong oxidant, corrosive to most metals. All common glove materials provide suitable protection. Do not mix bleach with formaldehyde, aminoethylcarbazole (AEC) or diaminobenzidine (DAB).

Sodium iodate. Little risk likely with laboratory quantities. Use to replace mercuric oxide in Harris hematoxylin.

Sodium metabisulfite. See sodium bisulfite.

Sodium phosphate, monobasic and dibasic. Harmless to workers. May pose an environmental problem from eutrophication (over-enrichment of aquatic systems).

Sodium sulfite. See sodium bisulfite.

Sodium thiosulfate. Health risks are minimal under normal conditions of use in histology. Solutions used to 'de-Zenkerize' sections will contain significant amounts of mercury and are not discarded down the drain.

Sulfuric acid. TWA = 1 mg/cubic meter (0.2 mg/cubic meter ACGIH®); IDLH = 15 mg/cubic meter. Strong irritant to skin, eyes and respiratory system. Concentrated acid is especially dangerous because it fumes. Target organ effects from inhalation on respiratory, reproductive and fetal systems. Dilute solutions pose little risk. Corrosive to most materials. Use a fume hood, apron, goggles and gloves (any common material except butyl). Always add acid to water, never water to acid, to avoid severe splattering.

Tetrahydrofuran (THF). TWA = 200 ppm; STEL = 250 ppm; IDLH = 2000 ppm; BEI = 50 mg THF/liter urine at end of shift. Toxic by ingestion and inhalation. Vapors cause nausea, dizziness, headache and anesthesia. Liquid can defat the skin. Eye and skin irritant. Flammable liquid. Dangerous fire hazard because of low flash point (5°F) and high evaporation rate. Only Teflon gloves are suitable. Avoid all use, as there is no practical way to protect against skin contact.

Toluene. TWA = 200 ppm (50 ppm ACGIH®); STEL = 150 ppm; IDLH = 500 ppm; BEI = 50 mg o-cresol/liter urine at end of shift. Skin and eye irritant. Toxic by ingestion, inhalation and skin contact. Target organ effects on fetal, respiratory and central nervous system. Repeated exposure produces neurotoxic effects (impaired memory, poor coordination, mood swings and permanent nerve damage). Flammable (flash point = 5°C). Avoid all use if possible or restrict use severely. No common glove material will provide adequate protection. Substitute one of the short-chain aliphatic hydrocarbon clearing agents except as a diluent in mounting media and for removing coverslips. Exposure may be monitored by measuring the amount of methylhippuric acids in urine (see page 14)

Trichloroethane. TWA = 350 ppm, STEL = 450 ppm. Irritant to skin and eyes. Target organ effects on gastrointestinal and central nervous systems. Non-combustible. No common glove material is suitable. Chlorinated solvents pose severe environmental risks and serious disposal problems. Avoid all use.

Uranyl nitrate. TWA = 0.05 mg uranium/cubic meter; STEL = 0.6 mg/cubic meter ACGIH®; IDLH = 10 mg/cubic meter. Corrosive to tissue and most metals. Highly toxic, with target organ effects on liver, urinary, circulatory and respiratory systems. Radiation hazard from inhalation of fine particles; most substances block radioactivity, so handling solutions poses little risk. Any type of glove material except latex is satisfactory. Severe environmental toxin. Problems with transportation and disposal have made this chemical very difficult or impossible to obtain. Find alternate stains for most uses and employ immunohistochemistry for equivocal cases. This will eliminate both uranyl nitrate and silver from the lab.

Xylene. TWA = 100 ppm; STEL = 150 ppm; IDLH = 900 ppm; BEI = 1.6 g hippuric acid/g creatinine in urine at end of shift. See toluene for further information.

Zinc chloride. Corrosive to most metals, including stainless steel. All common glove materials except latex are satisfactory. Do not use zinc chloride solutions in tissue processors. Skin and eye irritant. Ingestion can cause intoxication and severe gastrointestinal upset.

Zinc formalin. A solution of zinc sulfate or zinc chloride and formaldehyde. See individual entries for those ingredients.

Zinc sulfate. Eye irritant, but otherwise not hazardous in quantities used in histology.

Ergonomics

This is the science concerned with the relationship between human beings, the machines and equipment they use and their working environment. It involves the application of physiological, anatomical and psychological data to the design of efficient working systems. In the histology laboratory, ergonomic considerations include work habits, posture, preference for right or left handedness, arrangement and use of instrumentation and tools, countertop heights, seating, lighting, noise levels, temperatures, and vibration. Following a situational analysis, preventive measures can be implemented.

A full discussion of ergonomics is beyond the realms of this text but the main areas pertaining to histopathology are briefly outlined below and in greater detail in the previous edition of this book.

Biomechanical risk factors include exposure to excessive force, repetitive movements, awkward working postures and vibration. A variety of musculoskeletal disorders including tendonitis, tenosynovitis, carpal tunnel syndrome and other nerve disorders can occur if these are not addressed.

The proper balance of work between people and machines is sometimes difficult to determine. Automation is desirable because it reduces the physical stresses imposed on workers, but having too much automation takes away the unique value of human interaction and decision making that is based on visual interpretation and cognitive experience. Automation should be considered to replace manual tasks that require standardization (processing and staining) and those that may contribute to musculoskeletal disorders (slide and cassette labeling, microtomy and coverslipping).

Good workstation design is essential in creating a healthy, comfortable, and task-efficient laboratory. Workstations should follow the workflow and be planned to accommodate all equipment and supplies. Consideration must also be given to the number of people who will use the space, their physical characteristics, whether they will sit, stand, or use a combination of positions, and if they need some type of aid to be able to see and reach all of the necessary components. Air quality, temperature, and humidity must be regulated and drafts must be avoided. Lighting must be task appropriate, not necessarily standard overhead lighting, and noise must be minimal.

Ideally, laboratory workstations are versatile, modular, and flexible so that they can be altered to accommodate new tasks, equipment or people. The work surface should be height adjustable, and seating should be individualized and task appropriate.

Suggestions for specific tasks

Computer operation
- Maintain good posture with joints in a relaxed, neutral position.
- Keep the keyboard at elbow height or tilted downward.
- Use a gentle touch on the keys.
- Do not hold your thumb or little finger in the air.
- Place the mouse by the keyboard. Be aware that the burden is on one hand and finger.
- Position the top of the monitor at eye level.
- Wear glasses (if needed) that allow you to keep your head upright or bent slightly forward.
- Do not cradle the phone on your shoulder while working.
- Eliminate sources of reflections and glare on the monitor screen.

Cassette and slide labeling
- Rest wrists on a padded surface when writing.
- Take rest breaks and vary tasks.
- Avoid excessive reaching.
- Use ergonomic writing utensils with large, padded grips.
- Do not use excessive force.
- Automate if possible.

Changing the solutions on the processor
- Use proper bending and lifting techniques.
- Carry containers using a power grip (whole or both hands).
- Use a stool with safe footing to reach above chest height.

Embedding
- Maintain good sitting posture.
- Keep as many items as possible within your reach area and use ergonomic tools if available.
- Keep joints in a neutral position. Do not lean arms on sharp or hard surfaces. Take mini-breaks and exercise wrists and fingers.
- Alternate the motion used to open cassette lids.
- Get up periodically and walk around.

Manual microtomy

- Maintain good sitting posture.
- Use a well-adjusted, ergonomic chair and a footrest, if necessary.
- Keep joints in a relaxed, neutral position.
- Do not rock the handwheel (wrist flexion and extension).
- Use a cut-out workstation or an L-shaped extension to reach the water bath without bending at the waist and reaching over.
- Take mini-breaks as often as time constraints allow.
- Automate as soon as possible.

Manual staining

- Maintain good standing posture.
- Prop one foot up or stand with one foot forward, and alternate often.
- Keep work as close to the body as possible.
- Use caution when bending, lifting, and reaching.
- Avoid repeatedly dipping slides (wrist flexion and extension).
- Use slide holders and racks rather than forceps.
- Avoid using excessive force to squeeze bottles.
- Automate as soon as possible.

Manual coverslipping

- Maintain correct posture with head upright and joints in a neutral position.
- Keep work at elbow height and within a close reach.
- Do not lean arms on sharp or hard surfaces.
- Take multiple mini-breaks and do stretching exercises.
- Use ergonomic forceps.

Pipetting

- Maintain correct posture. Work at a cut-out bench if possible.
- Keep work at elbow height and as close as possible.
- Use low-profile tubes, solution containers, and waste receptacles.

- Keep wrists in a neutral position.
- Do not twist or rotate at the waist.
- Use electronic, light-touch pipettes designed for multiple finger use.
- Hold the pipette with a relaxed grip.
- Take short breaks every 20–30 minutes if possible.

Cryotomy

- Keep hands as warm as possible to maintain feeling and sensitivity.
- Maintain good posture. Do not lean into the chamber.
- If standing, work with one foot propped up and alternate regularly.
- Keep ancillary items as close as possible (possibly on a cart).
- Use skills detailed under 'Manual microtomy'.

Microscopy

- Avoid static postures, get up and move around periodically and alternate tasks.
- Work with the head bent slightly down instead of back.
- Use a well-adjusted, ergonomic chair and sit close to the microscope.
- Use armrests with a soft, smooth surface.
- Use a microscope with ergonomically positioned controls.
- Use adjustable eyepieces or mount the microscope at a 30° angle.
- Request extenders for the microscope body if the eyepieces are still not high enough.
- Work in a place away from drafts and noise.

References

American College of Occupational and Environmental Medicine, 2003. The use of contact lenses in an industrial environment. Online at www.acoem.org/guidelines/article.asp?ID=58.

American Conference of Governmental Industrial Hygienists, 2004. Threshold limit values for chemical substances and physical agents, and Biological Exposure Indices. ACGIH®, Cincinnati.

Centers for Disease Control, 1988. Guidelines for protecting the safety and health of health care workers, CDC Publication #88–119. US Government Printing Office, Washington, DC.

Centers for Disease Control, 1990. Guidelines for preventing the transmission of tuberculosis in health-care settings, with special focus on HIV-related issues. Morbidity and Mortality Weekly Report 39, 1–29. US Government Printing Office, Washington, DC.

Centers for Disease Control, 1994. Guidelines for preventing the transmission of *Mycobacterium tuberculosis* in health-care facilities. Morbidity and Mortality Weekly Report 43, 1–132. Washington, DC: US Government Printing Office.

Clinical and Laboratory Standards Institute, 2002. Clinical laboratory waste management: approved guideline, second ed. Document GP05-A2. CLSI, Wayne, PA.

Clinical and Laboratory Standards Institute, 2004. Clinical laboratory safety: approved guideline, second ed. Document GP17-A2. CLSI, Wayne, PA.

Clinical and Laboratory Standards Institute, 2005. Protection of laboratory workers from occupationally acquired infections: approved guideline, third ed. Document M29-MA3. CLSI, Wayne, PA.

Dapson, J.C., Dapson, R.W., 2005. Hazardous materials in the histopathology laboratory: regulations, risks, handling and disposal, fourth ed. Anatech Ltd, Battle Creek, MI.

Esswein, E.J., Boeniger, M.F., 1994. Effect of an ozone-generating air-purifying device on reducing concentrations of formaldehyde in air. Applied Occupational Environmental Hygiene 9, 139–146.

Kiernan, J.A., 1999. Histological and histochemical methods: theory and practice, third ed. Butterworth Heinemann, Boston.

Lunn, G., Sansone, E.B., 1990. Destruction of hazardous chemicals in the laboratory. John Wiley, New York.

Lunn, G., Sansone, E.B., 1991. The safe disposal of diaminobenzidine. Applied Occupational and Environmental Hygiene 6, 49–53.

Montgomery, L., 1995. Health and safety guidelines for the laboratory. American Society of Clinical Pathologists Press, Chicago.

National Institute for Occupational Safety and Health, 2003. NIOSH pocket guide to chemical hazards. DHHS (NIOSH) Publication No. 97–140.

National Research Council, 1989. Prudent practices for the handling and disposal of infectious materials. National Academy Press, Washington, DC.

National Research Council, 1995. Prudent practices in the laboratory: handling and disposal. National Academy Press, Washington, DC.

Ontario (Canada) Ministry of Labor, 1991. Regulation respecting control of exposure to biological or chemical agents – made under the Occupational Health and Safety Act. Ontario Government Publications, Toronto.

Rank, J.P., 1999. How can histotechnologists protect themselves from Creutzfeldt-Jakob disease? Laboratory Medicine 30, 305–306.

Saunders, G.T., 1993. Laboratory fume hoods: a user's manual. American Conference of Governmental Industrial Hygienists, Cincinnati, Ohio.

Schwope, A.D., Costas, P.P., Jackson, J.O., et al., 1987. Guidelines for the selection of chemical protective clothing. American Conference of Governmental Industrial Hygienists, Cincinnati, Ohio.

Stricoff, R.S., Walters, B.D., 1990. Laboratory health and safety handbook: a guide for the preparation of a chemical hygiene plan. Wiley, New York.

Light microscopy 3

John D. Bancroft • Alton D. Floyd

Light and its properties

Visible light occupies a very narrow portion of the electromagnetic spectrum. The electromagnetic spectrum extends from radio and microwaves all the way to gamma rays. Electromagnetic energy is complex, having properties that are both wave-like and particle-like. A discussion of these topics is well beyond the scope of this chapter. Suffice to say, visible light is that portion of the electromagnetic spectrum that can be detected by the human eye. In physics texts, this range is generally defined as wavelengths of light ranging from approximately 400 nm (deep violet) to 800 nm (far red). Most humans cannot see light of wavelengths much beyond 700 nm (deep red).

It is common practice to illustrate the electromagnetic spectrum as a sine wave. This is a convenient representation as the distance from one sine peak to another represents the wavelength of light (Fig. 3.1). Light that has a single wavelength is monochromatic: that is, a single color. The majority of sources of light provide a complex mixture of light of different wavelengths, and when this mixture approximates the mixture of light that derives from the sun, we perceive this as 'white' light. By definition, white light is a mixture of light that contains some percentage of wavelengths from all of the visible portions of the electromagnetic spectrum. It should be understood that almost all light sources provide a mixture of wavelengths of light (exceptions being devices such as lasers, which generate monochromatic, coherent light). One measure of the mixture of light given off by a light source is *color temperature.* In practical terms, the higher the color temperature, the closer the light is to natural daylight derived from the sun. Natural daylight from the sun is generally stated to have a color temperature of approximately 5200 kelvin (K). Incandescent light, from tungsten bulbs, has a color temperature of approximately 3200K. These values will be familiar to those using color film for photography, as film type must be chosen to suit the illumination source. As a general rule, the higher the color temperature, the more 'blue' or white the light appears to the eye. Lower color temperatures appear more red to yellow, and are regarded as being 'warmer' in color.

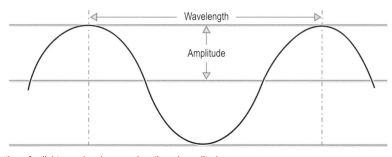

Figure 3.1 Representation of a light ray showing wavelength and amplitude.

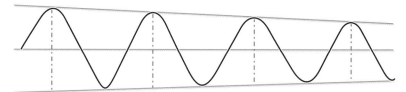

Figure 3.2 The amplitude (i.e. brightness) diminishes as light gets further from the source because of absorption into the media through which it passes.

Shorter wavelengths of light (toward the blue to violet end of the spectrum) have a higher energy content for a given brightness of light. As one goes to even shorter wavelengths of the electromagnetic spectrum, the energy content becomes even higher (X-rays and gamma rays). The energy content of light is generally expressed as an energy level, or amplitude based on the electron volts per photon (the particle representation of light). Visible light has an energy level of approximately one electron volt per photon, and the energy level increases as one moves toward the violet and ultraviolet range of the spectrum. Approaching the soft X-ray portion of the spectrum, the energy level per photon ranges from 50 to 100 electron volts (eV). It is this higher energy in the shorter wavelengths of light (the ultraviolet and blue end of the spectrum) that is exploited to elicit fluorescence in some materials.

Light sources give off light in all directions, and most light sources consist of a complex mixture of wavelengths. This mixture of wavelengths is what defines the color temperature of the light source. It should also be noted that the mixture of wavelengths is influenced by the type of material making up the source. Since the majority of light sources used in microscopy are either heated filaments or arcs of molten metal, each source will provide a specific set of wavelengths related to the material being heated. This is referred to as the *emission spectrum*. Some sources provide relatively uniform mixtures of wavelengths, although of different amplitudes or intensities, such as tungsten filament lamps and xenon lamps. Others, such as mercury lamps, provide very discrete wavelengths scattered over a broad range, but with distinct gaps of no emission between these peaks.

Although light sources are inherently non-coherent (with the exception of lasers), standard diagrams of optics always draw light rays as straight lines. This is a simplification, and it should be remembered that the actual light consists of every possible angle of light rays from the source, not just the single ray illustrated in the diagram. Another property of light that is important for an understanding of microscope optics is absorption of some of the light by the medium through which the light passes (Fig. 3.2). This is seen as a reduction in the amplitude, or energy level, of the light. The medium through which the light passes can also have an effect on the actual speed at which the light passes through the material, and this is referred to as *retardation*.

Retardation and refraction

Media through which light is able to pass will slow down or *retard* the speed of the light in proportion to the density of the medium. The higher the density, the greater the degree of *retardation*. Rays of light entering a sheet of glass at right angles are retarded in speed but their direction is unchanged (Fig. 3.3a). If the light enters the glass at any other angle, a deviation of direction will occur in addition to the retardation, and this is called *refraction* (Fig. 3.3b). A curved lens will exhibit both retardation and refraction (Fig. 3.3c), the extent of which is governed by:

(a) the angle at which the light strikes the lens – the *angle of incidence*,

(b) the density of the glass – its *refractive index*, and

(c) the curvature of the lens.

The angle by which the rays are deviated within the glass or other transparent medium is called the

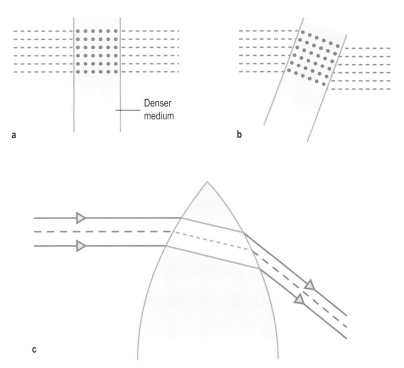

Figure 3.3 (a) Rays passing from one medium to another, perpendicular to the interface, are slowed down at the same moment. (b) Rays passing at any other angle to the interface are slowed down in the order that they cross the interface and are deviated. (c) Rays passing through a curved lens exhibit both retardation and refraction.

angle of refraction and the ratio of the sine values of the angles of incidence (i) and refraction (r) gives a figure known as the *refractive index* (RI) of the medium (Fig. 3.4a). The greater the RI, the higher the density of the medium. The RI of most transparent substances is known and is of great value in the computation and design of lenses, microscope slides and coverslips, and mounting media. Air has a refractive index of 1.00, water 1.30, and glass a range of values depending on type but averaging 1.50.

As a general rule, light passing from one medium into another of higher density is refracted towards the normal, and when passing into a less dense medium it is refracted away from the normal. The angle of incidence may increase to the point where the light emerges parallel to the surface of the lens. Beyond this angle of incidence, *total internal reflection* will occur, and no light will pass through (Fig. 3.4b).

Image formation

Parallel rays of light entering a simple lens are brought together by refraction to a single point, the 'principal focus' or *focal point*, where a clear image will be formed of an object (Fig. 3.4c). The distance between the optical center of the lens and the principal focus is the *focal length*. In addition to the principal focus, a lens also has other pairs of points, one either side of the lens, called *conjugate foci*, such that an object placed at one will form a clear image on a screen placed at the other. The conjugate foci vary in position, and as the object is moved nearer the lens the image will be formed further away, at a greater magnification, and inverted. This is the '*real image*' and is that formed by the objective lens of the microscope (Fig. 3.5).

If the object is placed yet nearer the lens, within the principal focus, the image is formed on the same side as the object, is enlarged, the right way up, and

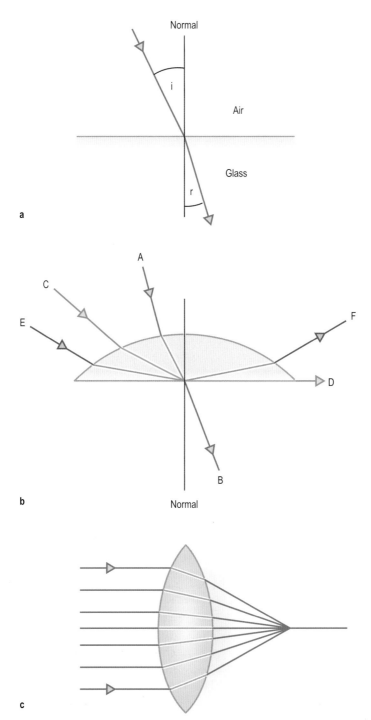

Figure 3.4 (a) Angle of incidence (i) and refraction (r). (b) Ray C–D is lost through the edge of the lens. Ray E–F shows total internal reflection. (c) Parallel rays entering a curved lens are brought to a common focus.

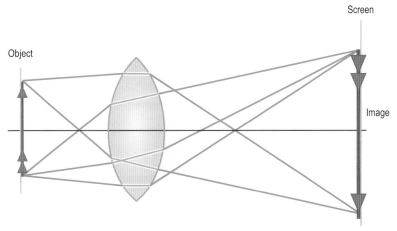

Figure 3.5 A real image is formed by rays passing through the lens from the object, and can be focused on a screen.

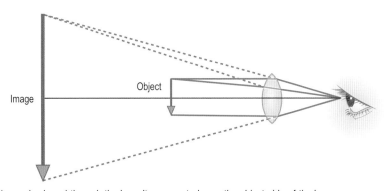

Figure 3.6 A virtual image is viewed through the lens. It appears to be on the object side of the lens.

cannot be projected onto a screen. This is the '*virtual image*' (Fig. 3.6), and is that formed by the eyepiece of the microscope of the real image projected from the objective. This appears to be at a distance of approximately 25 cm from the eye – around the object stage level. Figure 3.7 illustrates the formation of both images in the upright compound microscope, as is commonly used in histopathology.

Image quality

White light is composed of all spectral colors and, on passing through a simple lens, each wavelength will be refracted to a different extent, with blue being brought to a shorter focus than red. This lens defect is *chromatic aberration* (Fig. 3.8a) and results in an unsharp image with colored fringes. It is possible to construct compound lenses of different glass elements to correct this fault. An *achromat* is corrected for two colors, blue and red, producing a secondary spectrum of yellow/green, which in turn can be corrected by adding more lens components – the more expensive *apochromat*.

Microscope objectives of both achromatic and apochromatic types (see Fig. 3.11) are usually overcorrected for longitudinal chromatic aberration and must be combined with matched compensating eyepieces to form a good-quality image. This restriction on changing lens combinations is overcome by using chromatic, aberration-free (CF) optics, which correct for both longitudinal and lateral chromatic

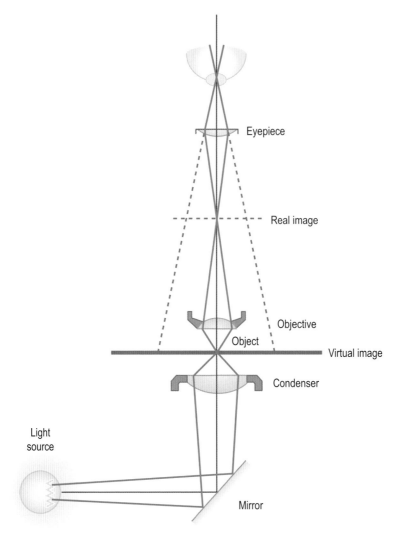

Figure 3.7 Ray path through the microscope. The eye sees the magnified virtual image of the real image, produced by the objective.

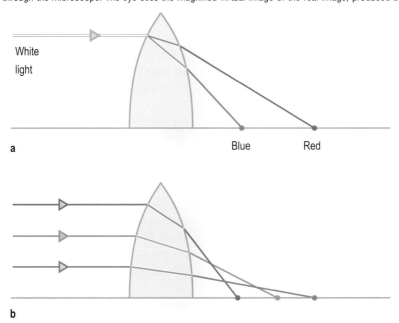

Figure 3.8 (a) Chromatic aberration. (b) Spherical aberration.

aberrations and remove all color fringes, being particularly useful for fluorescence and interference microscopes.

Other distortions in the image may be due to coma, astigmatism, curvature of field, and spherical aberration, and are due to lens shape and quality. *Spherical aberration* is caused when light rays entering a curved lens at its periphery are refracted more than those rays entering the center of the lens and are thus not brought to a common focus (Fig. 3.8b).

These faults are also corrected by making combinations of lens elements of different glass, e.g. fluorite, and of differing shapes.

The components of a microscope

Light source

Light, of course, is an essential part of the system; at one time sunlight was the usual source. A progression of light sources has developed, from oil lamps to the low-voltage electric lamps of today. These operate via a transformer and can be adjusted to the intensity required. The larger instruments have their

light sources built into them. Dispersal of heat, collection of the greatest amount of light, and direction and distance are all carefully calculated by the designer for greatest efficiency. To obtain a more balanced white light approximation, these light sources must often be operated at excessive brightness levels. The excess brightness is reduced to comfortable viewing levels through the use of *neutral density filters*.

Condensers

Light from the lamp is directed into the first major optical component, the substage condenser, either directly or by a mirror or prism. The main purpose of the condenser is to focus or concentrate the available light into the plane of the object (Fig. 3.9). Within comfortable limits, the more light at the specimen, the better is the resolution of the image.

Many microscopes have condensers capable of vertical adjustment, in order to allow for varying heights or thickness of slides. Once the correct position of the condenser has been established, there is no reason to move it, as any alteration will change the light intensity and impair the resolution. In most

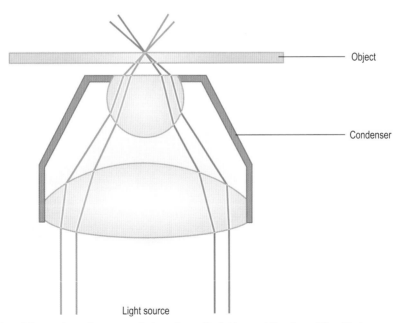

Figure 3.9 The function of the condenser is to concentrate, or focus, the light rays at the plane of the object.

cases condensers are provided with adjustment screws for centering the light path. Checking and, if necessary, adjusting the centration before using the instrument should be a routine procedure for every microscopist. All condensers have an aperture diaphragm with which the diameter of the light beam can be controlled.

Adjustment of this iris diaphragm will alter the size and volume of the cone of light focused on the object. If the diaphragm is closed too much, the image becomes too contrasty and refractile, whereas if the diaphragm is left wide open, the image will suffer from *glare* due to extraneous light interference. In both cases the resolution of the

image is poor. The correct setting for the diaphragm is when the numerical aperture of the condenser is matched to the numerical aperture of the objective in use (Fig. 3.10) and the necessary adjustment should be made when changing from one objective to another. This is achieved, approximately, by removing the eyepiece, viewing the substage iris diaphragm in the back focal plane of the objective, and closing it down to two-thirds of the field of view.

With experience the correct setting can be estimated from the image quality. Under no circumstances should the iris diaphragm be closed to reduce the intensity of the light; use filters or the rheostat of the lamp transformer. Many condensers

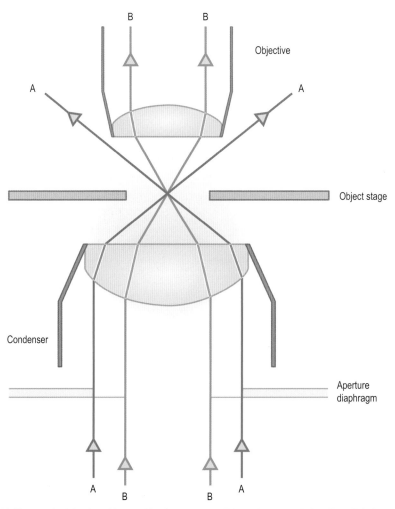

Figure 3.10 Rays A illustrate the 'glare' position resulting in extraneous light and poor resolution. Rays B indicate the correct setting of the substage iris diaphragm.

are fitted with a swing-out top lens. This is turned into the light path when the higher-power objectives are in use. It focuses the light into a field more suited to the smaller diameter of the objective front lens. Swing it out of the path with the lower power objectives, or the field of view will only be illuminated at the center. When using apochromatic or fluorite objectives the substage condenser should also be of a suitable quality, such as an aplanatic or a highly corrected achromatic condenser.

Object stage

Above the condenser is the object stage, which is a rigid platform with an aperture through which the light may pass. The stage supports the glass slide bearing the specimen, and should therefore be sturdy and perpendicular to the optical path. In order to hold the slide firmly, and to allow the operator to move it easily and smoothly, a mechanical stage is either attached or built in. This allows controlled movement in two directions, and in most cases Vernier scales are incorporated to enable the operator to return to an exact location in the specimen at a later occasion.

Objectives

The next and most important piece of the microscope's equipment is the objective, the type and quality of the objective having the greatest influence on the performance of the microscope as a whole.

Within the objective there may be from 5 to 15 lenses and elements, depending on image ratio, type and quality (Fig. 3.11). The main task of the objective is to collect the maximum amount of light possible from the object, unite it, and form a high-quality magnified real image, some distance above. Older microscopes used objectives computed for an optical tube length of 160 mm (DIN standard), or 170 mm (Leitz only), but these fixed tube length systems have now been largely replaced by *infinity corrected objectives* that can greatly extend this tube length and permit the addition of other devices into the optical path.

Magnifying powers or, more correctly, object-to-image ratios of objectives are from 1:1 to 100:1 in normal biological instruments.

The ability of an objective to resolve detail is indicated by its *numerical aperture* and not by its magnifying power. The numerical aperture or NA is expressed as a value, and will be found engraved on the body of the objective. The value expresses the product of two factors and can be calculated from the formula:

$$NA = n \times sin\ u$$

where n is the refractive index of the medium between the coverglass over the object and the front lens of the objective, for example air, water, or immersion oil, and u is the angle included between the optical axis of the lens and the outermost ray that can enter the front lens (Fig. 3.12).

In Figure 3.12 the point where the axis meets the specimen is regarded as a light source; rays radiate from this point in all directions. Some will escape to the outside, and some will be reflected back from the surface of the coverglass. Ray r is the outermost ray that can enter the front lens; the angle u between ray r and the axis gives us the *sin* value required. In theory the greatest possible angle would be if the surface of the front lens coincided with the specimen, giving a value for u of 908. In the above formula, with air (RI = 1.00) as the medium, and a value for u of 908 (*sin u* × 1), the resulting NA = 1.00. Of course this is impossible as there must always be some space between the surfaces, so a value of 908 for u is unobtainable. In practice the maximum NA attainable with a dry objective is 0.95. Similar limitations apply to water and oil immersion objectives; theoretical maximum values for NA are 1.30 and 1.50, respectively. In practice values of 1.20 and 1.40 are the highest obtainable.

Resolution does not depend entirely on the NA of a lens but also on the wavelength of light used, governed by the following relationship:

$$\frac{\lambda\ resolution}{NA} = 0.61\lambda$$

where the resolution is the smallest distance between two dots or lines that can be seen as separate entities, and λ is the wavelength of light.

The *resolving power* of the objective is its ability to resolve the detail that can be measured. In summary, as the NA of an objective increases, the resolving

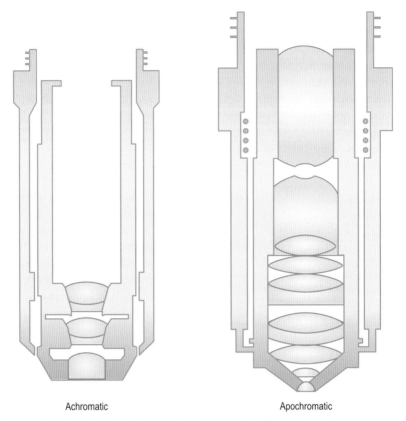

Achromatic   Apochromatic

Figure 3.11 Diagram of achromatic and apochromatic objectives. Some examples of the latter may have as many as 15 separate lens elements.

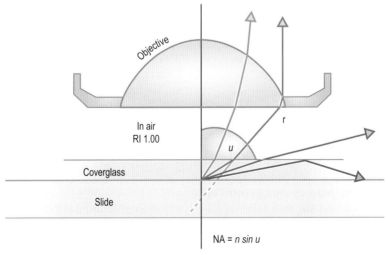

Figure 3.12 The refractive index of the medium between the coverglass and the surface of the objective's front lens (in this case air, RI = 1.00), and the sine of the angle (u) between the optical axis and the outermost accepted ray (r), gives the numerical aperture (see text).

power increases but working distance, flatness of field, and focal length decrease.

Objectives are available in varying quality and types (Fig. 3.11). The *achromatic* is the most widely used for routine purposes; the more highly corrected *apochromats*, often incorporating fluorite glass, are used for more critical work, while *plan-apochromats* (which have a field of view that is almost perfectly flat) are recommended for photomicrography. For cytology screening, flat-field objectives – often plan-achromats – are particularly useful. On modern microscopes, up to six objectives are mounted onto a revolving *nosepiece* to enable rapid change from one to another and, ideally, the focus and field location should require the minimum of adjustment. Such lenses are said to be *par-focal* and *par-central*.

Most objectives are designed for use with a cover-glass protecting the object. If so, a value giving the correct coverglass thickness should be found engraved on the objective. Usually this is 0.17 mm. Some objectives, notably apochromats between 40:1 and 63:1, require coverslip thickness to be precise. Some are mounted in a correction mount and can be adjusted to suit the actual thickness of the cover-glass used.

Body tube

Above the nosepiece is the body tube. Three main forms are available: monocular, binocular, and the combined photo-binocular. The last sometimes has a prism system allowing 100% of the light to go either to the observation eyepieces, or to the camera located on the vertical part, and sometimes has a beam-splitting prism dividing the light, 20% to the eyes and 80% to the camera. This facilitates continuous observation during photography. Provision is made in binocular tubes for the adjustment of the interpupillary distance, enabling each observer to adjust for the individual facial proportions. Alteration of this interpupillary distance may alter the mechanical tube length, and thus the length of the optical path. This can be corrected either by adjusting the individual eyepiece tubes, or by a compensating mechanism built into the body tube.

Modern design tends towards shortening the physical lengths of the components, and in consequence, the intermediate optics are sometimes included in the optical path to compensate. These lenses are mounted on a rotating turret and are designated by their magnification factor. Additionally, a tube lens may be incorporated for objectives that are *infinity corrected*, as these objectives form only a virtual image of the object, which must be converted to a real image focused at the lower focal plane of the eyepiece.

Eyepiece

Eyepieces are the final stage in the optical path of the microscope. Their function is to magnify the image formed by the objective within the body tube, and present the eye with a virtual image, apparently in the plane of the object being observed; usually this is an optical distance of 250 mm from the eye.

Early types of eyepiece, like objectives, were subject to aberrations, especially of color. Compensating eyepieces were designed to overcome these problems and can be used with all modern objectives. The eyepiece designed by Huyghens in 1690 is still available, together with periplanatic (flat-field) and wide-field types, and eyepieces for holding measuring graticules and photographic formats. High focal point eyepieces are designed for spectacle wearers. For older fixed tube length microscopes, manufacturers often placed different amounts of the various corrections in the optical train in either the objective or the eyepiece. Therefore it is important to use eyepieces from the same manufacturer with objectives from that manufacturer. Eyepieces designed for infinity objectives must be used with the newer infinity-corrected systems.

Magnification and illumination

Magnification values

Total magnification is the product of the magnification values of the objective and eyepiece, provided the system is standardized to an optical tube length

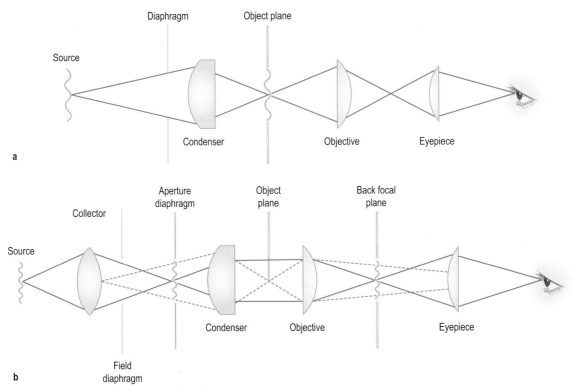

Figure 3.13 (a) Critical illumination. (b) Köhler illumination.

of 160 mm. For variations of the latter the formula is:

$$\frac{\text{Optical tube length}}{\text{Focal length of objective}} \times \text{Magnification of eyepiece}$$

Where additional tube lenses are included, simply multiply by the designated factor; for example, objective 40x, eyepiece 10x, and tube lens factor 1.25x gives a total magnification of 500x. Choosing the correct eyepiece magnification is important, as a total magnification may be reached without further resolution of the object; this is *empty magnification*. As a guide, total magnification should not exceed 1000 × NA of the objective. Therefore an objective designated 100/1.30 would allow a total magnification of 1300 (1000 × 1.3NA), so eyepieces in excess of 12.5x would serve no useful purpose. For accurate measurements, calibration of the optics with a stage micrometer is necessary.

Illumination

Critical illumination, often used with simple equipment and a separate light source, is when the light source is focused by the substage condenser in the same plane as the object, when the object is in focus (Fig. 3.13). At one time, ribbon filament lamps were available for microscope illumination. Modern filament lamps use a spring-like filament, and the image of the filament causes uneven illumination, which is unacceptable.

For photography and all the specialized forms of microscopy it is best to use *Köhler illumination*, where an image of the light source is focused by the lamp collector or field lens in the focal plane of the substage condenser (on the aperture diaphragm).

The image of the field or lamp diaphragm will now be focused in the object plane and the

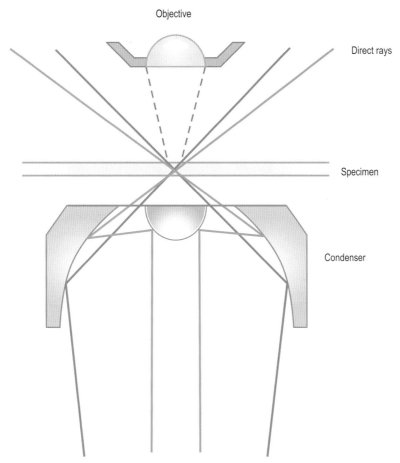

Figure 3.14 In dark-field illumination no direct rays enter the objective. Only scattered rays from the edges of structures in the specimen form the image (dashed lines).

illumination is even. The image of the light source and the aperture diaphragm will in turn be focused at the back focal plane of the objective and can be examined with the eyepiece removed. Poor resolution will result unless the illumination is centered with respect to the optical axis of the microscope. Figure 3.13 shows the main differences between critical and Köhler systems.

Dark-field illumination

So far the microscope has been shown as suitable for the examination of stained preparations. Staining aids the formation of images by absorbing part of the light (some of the wavelengths) and producing an image of amplitude differences and color. Occasions arise when it is preferable, or essential, that unstained sections or living cells are examined. Such specimens and their components have refractive indices close to that of the medium in which they are suspended and are thus difficult to see by bright-field techniques, due to their lack of contrast. Dark-field microscopy overcomes these problems by preventing direct light from entering the front of the objective and the only light gathered is that reflected or diffracted by structures within the specimen (Fig. 3.14). This causes the specimen to appear as a bright image on a dark background, the contrast being reversed and increased. Dark field permits the detection of particles smaller than the optical resolution that would be obtained in bright field, due to the high contrast of the scattered light. In the microscope, oblique light is created by using a modified or special condenser that forms a hollow cone of direct light which will pass through the specimen but outside the objective (Fig. 3.14). Dark field condensers may be for either dry, low-power objectives or for oil immersion high-power objectives. Whichever is used, the objective must have a lower numerical aperture than the condenser (in bright-field illumination, optimum efficiency is obtained when the NAs of both objective and condenser are matched). In order to obtain this condition it is sometimes necessary to use objectives with a built-in iris diaphragm or, more simply, by inserting a funnel stop into the objective. Perfect centering of the condenser is essential, and with the oil immersion systems it is necessary to put oil between the condenser and the object slide in addition to the oil between the slide and the objective. As only light diffracted by the specimen will enter the objective, a high-intensity light source is required.

Most bright-field microscopes can be converted for dark-field work by using simple patch stops, made of black paper, placed on top of the condenser lens or suspended in the filter holder. Alternatively the patch stops can be constructed from different colored filters (*Rheinberg illumination*) using a dark color for the center disc and a contrasting lighter color for the periphery. This system reduces the glare of conventional dark field and reveals the specimen in, say, red on a blue background.

Variable intensity dark field is obtained by making the Rheinberg discs from polarizing filters, the center being oriented at right angles to the periphery. This allows good photomicrography. Dark-field illumination is particularly useful for spirochetes, flagellates, cell suspensions, flow cell techniques, parasites, and autoradiographic grain counting, and was once commonly used in fluorescence microscopy. Thin slides and coverglasses should be used and the preparation must be free of hairs, dirt, and bubbles. Many small structures are more easily visualized by dark-field techniques due to increased contrast, although resolution may be inferior to bright-field microscopy.

Phase contrast microscopy

Unstained and living biological specimens have little contrast with their surrounding medium, even though small differences of refractive index (RI) exist in their structures. To see them clearly involves either:

a. closing down the iris diaphragm of the condenser, which reduces its numerical aperture (NA) producing diffraction effects and destroying the resolving power of the objective, *or*

b. using dark-field illumination, which enhances contrast by reversal, but often fails to reveal internal detail.

Phase contrast overcomes these problems by a controlled illumination using the full aperture of the condenser and improving resolution. The higher the RI of a structure, the darker it will appear against a light background, i.e. with more contrast.

Optical principle

If a diffraction grating is examined under the microscope, diffraction spectra are formed in the back focal plane (BFP) of the objective due to interference between the direct and diffracted rays of light. The grating consists of alternate strips of material with slightly different RIs, through which light acquires small phase differences, and these form the image. Unstained cells are similar to diffraction gratings as their contents also differ very slightly in RI.

Two rays of light from the same source with the same frequency are said to be coherent, and when recombined they will double in amplitude or brightness if they are in phase with each other (*constructive interference*). However, if they are out of phase with each other, *destructive interference* will occur.

Figure 3.15a represents the waveform of a light ray. In Figure 3.15b the rays are identical but one is $\frac{1}{4}\lambda$ out of phase with the other and they interfere

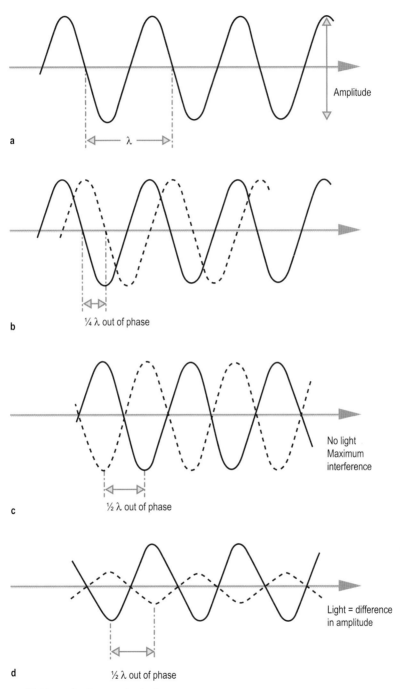

Figure 3.15 Interference of light rays in phase contrast microscopy.

but with no increase in amplitude. Figure 3.15c shows one ray now $\frac{1}{2}\lambda$ out of phase with the other, and they cancel each other out. This is maximum destructive interference and no light is seen, resulting in maximum contrast. However, if one ray is brighter than the other (increased amplitude) but is still $\frac{1}{2}\lambda$ out of phase (Fig. 3.15d) then the difference in amplitude can be seen, while maintaining maximum interference. This last position is that which occurs in the phase contrast microscope.

The phase contrast microscope

To achieve phase contrast the microscope requires modified objectives and condenser, and relies on the specimen retarding light by between $\frac{1}{8}$ and $\frac{1}{4}\lambda$. An intense light source is required to be set up for Köhler illumination.

The microscope condenser usually carries a series of annular diaphragms made of opaque glass, with a clear narrow ring, to produce a controlled hollow cone of light. Each objective requires a different size of annulus, an image of which is formed by the condenser in the back focal plane (BFP) of the objective as a bright ring of light (Fig. 3.16). The objective is modified by a phase plate which is placed at its BFP (Fig. 3.16). A positive phase plate consists of a clear glass disc with a circular trough etched in it, to half the depth of the disc. The light passing through the trough has a phase difference of $\frac{1}{4}\lambda$ compared to the rest of the plate. The trough also contains a neutral-density light-absorbing material to reduce the brightness of the direct rays, which would otherwise obscure the contrast obtained.

It is essential that the image of the bright annular ring from the condenser is centered and superimposed on the dull trough of the objective phase plate. This is achieved by using either a focusing telescope in place of the eyepiece or a Bertrand lens situated in the body tube of the microscope. Each combination of annulus and objective phase plate will require centering. When the hollow cone of direct light from the annulus enters the specimen, some will pass through unaltered while some rays will be retarded (or diffracted) by approximately $\frac{1}{4}\lambda$. The direct light

will mostly pass through the trough in the phase plate while the diffracted rays pass through the thicker clear glass and are further retarded.

The total retardation of the diffracted rays is now $\frac{1}{2}\lambda$ and interference will occur when they are recombined with the direct light. Thus an image of contrast is achieved, revealing even small details within unstained cells. This is a quick and efficient way of examining unstained paraffin, resin, and frozen sections, as well as studying living cells and their behavior.

Interference microscopy

In phase contrast microscopy, the specimen retards some light rays with respect to those which pass through the surrounding medium. The resulting interference of these rays provides image contrast but with an artifact called the 'phase halo'. In the interference microscope the retarded rays are entirely separated from the direct or reference rays, allowing improved image contrast, color graduation, and quantitative measurements of phase change (or 'optical path difference'), refractive index, dry mass of cells (optical weighing), and section thickness.

Whenever light passes across the edge of an opaque object the rays close to that edge are diffracted, or bent away from their normal path. If, instead of a single edge, the rays pass through a narrow slit, then the rays at the edge of the beam will fan out on either side to quite wide angles (Fig. 3.17a). Two slits closely side by side form two fans of rays which will cross (Fig. 3.17b) and, if coherent, will observably 'interfere'. If each ray is regarded as a wave it can be seen that phase conditions of increased amplitude and extinction are bound to occur at points where the waves cross and interfere (Figs 3.17c, d). The result of this in the microscope is a series of parallel bands, alternately bright and dark across the field of view. With white light, bands of the spectral colors are seen, because the wavelengths making up white light are diffracted at different angles. With monochromatic light, the bands are alternately dark and light, and of a single color. The same effect can be shown if separate beams of

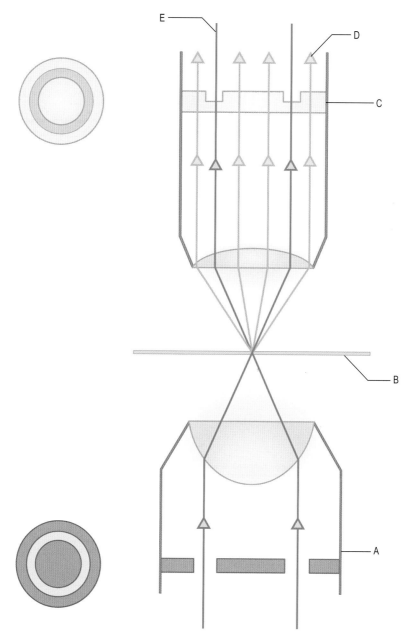

Figure 3.16 A = annulus at focal plane of condenser; B = object plane; C = phase plate at BFP of objective; D = light rays diffracted and retarded by specimen, total retardation $\frac{1}{2}\lambda$ compared with direct light; E = direct light rays unaffected by specimen.

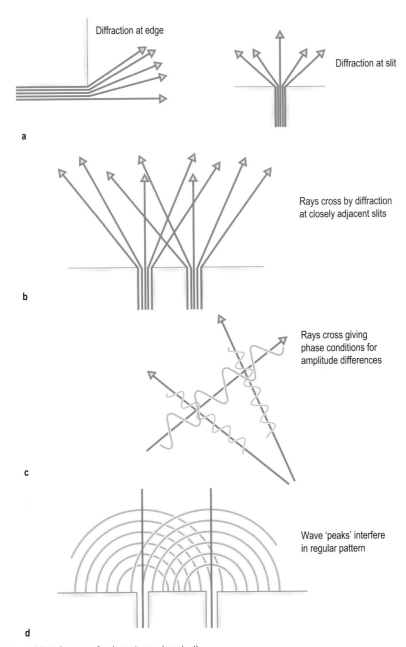

Figure 3.17 Diffraction and interference of coherent rays (see text).

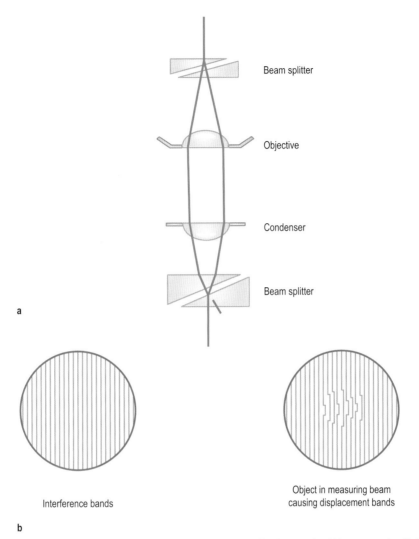

a

b

Interference bands

Object in measuring beam
causing displacement bands

Figure 3.18 (a) Ray path of an interference microscope using a single objective. The beams should be separated sufficiently for one to pass through an empty part of the preparation, otherwise the 'ghost' images formed can cause confusion. (b) Appearance of interference bands in the field of view.

coherent light are reunited. This phenomenon is known as 'interference'.

Early microscope models split a light beam into two parts, each traversing two sets of perfectly matched optics, one beam passing through the specimen (measuring beam) and the other acting as a reference beam. The beams were widely separated and suitable only for large specimens and interference fringe measurements. Later models used a double-beam system, where the separation is produced by birefringent materials and is close enough to require only one objective (Fig. 3.18a).

If the two paths are equal and in the same phase, the interference bands can be seen running straight and parallel across the field. If an object is introduced into one beam path that causes some shift in the phase, this will be seen as a displacement in the interference bands (Fig. 3.18b). When using monochromatic light, each interval comprising one dark and one light band is one wavelength wide, and

Figure 3.19 (a) A Wollaston prism is so constructed that rays passing through the center are in phase. Those passing at other points have a phase difference. The arrows and dot represent the optic axes of the prisms, being at right angles to each other. (b) Ray path in the microscope. Each ray is polarized on separation and they vibrate at right angles to each other, producing interference colors when recombined.

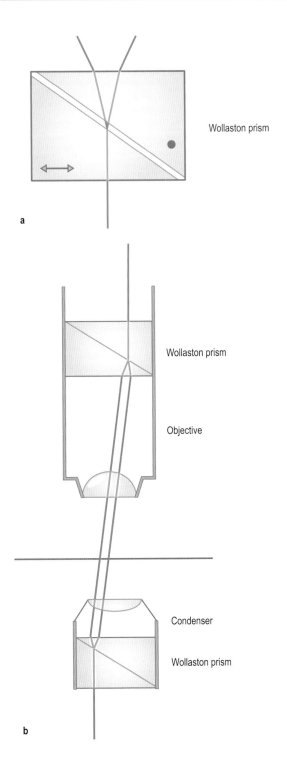

thus the distance in nanometers is known. Displacement of the bands is measured with a micrometer eyepiece and with this information, coupled with either the RI or object thickness, the measurements referred to earlier can be determined.

Two types of double-beam system have been used. One involved focusing the reference beam below the object – the 'double focus' system – and the other involved a lateral displacement of the reference beam called 'shearing', where the separation of the beams is very small. Figure 3.19a, b illustrates this latter system using polarized light and Wollaston prisms. The first birefringent prism in the condenser separates the beams and after passing through the object they are recombined by the second identical prism at the back of the objective. A different pair of prisms is required for each magnification. This produces 'interference contrast' and together with rotation of the polarizers enhances the three-dimensional (3D) effect in the image. In 1952, Nomarski modified the Wollaston prisms, so that the lateral separation is less than the resolving power of the microscope, producing excellent 3D colored images from unstained specimens. This system is referred to as *differential interference contrast* or DIC. Additionally, only one such prism is required at the objective level for all magnifications. This system permits enhanced visualization of immunohistochemical preparations.

Polarized light microscopy

The use of polarized light in microscopy has many useful and diagnostic applications. Numerous crystals, fibrous structures (both natural and artificial), pigments, lipids, proteins, bone, and amyloid deposits exhibit birefringence. Every cellular pathology laboratory should have at least a simple system of polarizing microscopy.

Earlier in this chapter, light was described as a series of pulses of energy radiating away from a source, and shown diagrammatically as a sine curve, with wavelength and amplitude defined. Light can also be described as an electromagnetic vibration, which travels outwards from the source of its propagation, much in the same way as a vibration will travel along a rope when it is jerked in a direction at right angles to its length. The vibrations in the rope will be generated in the direction of the force that caused them, and this is called the *plane of vibration*, or *vibration direction* (Fig. 3.20). Natural light vibrates in many planes or vibration directions, whereas polarized light vibrates in only one plane, as in the rope, and can be produced for microscopy purpose by passing natural light through a polarizer, which is an optical component made from a substance that will allow vibrations of only one vibration direction to pass.

Substances or crystals capable of producing plane-polarized light are called *birefringent*. Light entering

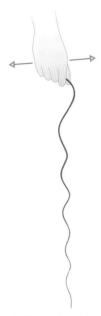

Figure 3.20 Plane of vibration produced on a rope.

a birefringent crystal such as calcite is split into two light paths, each determined by a different refractive index (RI) and each vibrating in one direction only (i.e. polarized) but at right angles to each other (Fig. 3.21). The higher the RI, the greater the retardation of the ray, so that each ray leaves the crystal at a different velocity. The high RI ray is called *slow* and the low RI ray is called *fast*. There is also a phase difference between the rays, so that, if they are recombined, interference occurs and various spectral colors are seen.

Originally, polarizers, made from calcite and known as Nicol prisms after their inventor, were cemented together with Canada balsam in such a way that the *slow* ray was reflected away from the optical path and into the mount of the prism, leaving only the polarized *fast* ray to pass through (Fig. 3.22).

There will be a direction within a birefringent crystal along which light may pass unaltered; this is called the optic axis (see Wollaston prism). Substances through which light can pass in any direction and at the same velocity are called *isotropic* and are not able to produce polarized light. A knowledge of RI and polarization measurements identifies many crystalline structures and is particularly useful to the materials scientist but is of limited use to the histologist.

Some substances and crystals can produce plane polarized light by differential absorption and give rise to the phenomenon of *dichroism*. Such crystals suspended in thin plastic films and oriented in one direction have replaced the bulky and expensive Nicol prisms. These thin films totally absorb the slow rays and are *pleochroic* (absorbing all colors equally), and are the most useful in microscopy as they occupy very little space and can be used with any microscope.

The dedicated polarizing microscope uses two polarizers (Fig. 3.23). One, always referred to as the *polarizer*, is placed beneath the substage condenser and held in a rotatable graduated mount, and can be removed from the light path when not required. The other, called the *analyzer*, is placed between the objective and the eyepiece and is also graduated for measurement to be taken. A circular rotating stage would also be present for rotation of the specimen.

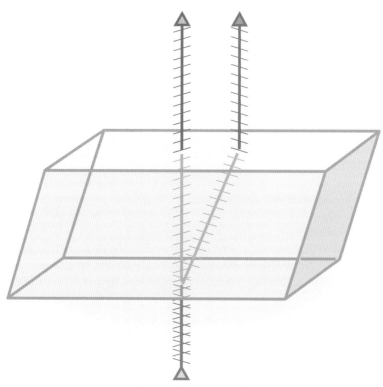

Figure 3.21 A birefringent crystal such as calcite can split a ray of light into two light paths, each vibrating at right angles to the other.

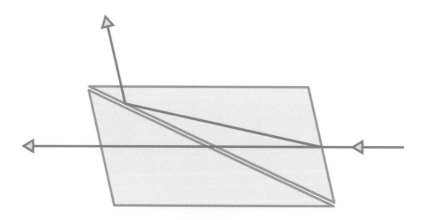

Figure 3.22 A Nicol prism is constructed so that one part of the ray is allowed to pass whilst the other is directed away from the optical path and is lost.

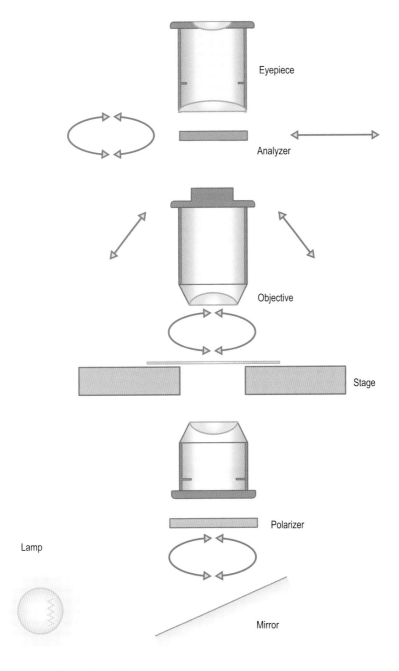

Figure 3.23 A microscope equipped for polarized light.

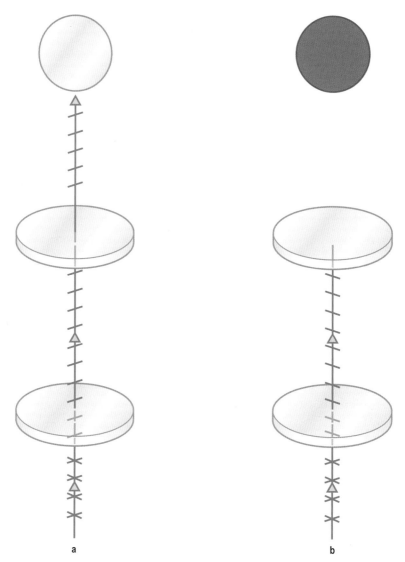

Figure 3.24 (a) When polarizer and analyzer are parallel, rays vibrating in the parallel plane are able to pass. (b) When polarizer and analyzer are crossed, rays able to pass the polarizer are blocked by the analyzer. The condition when no light reaches the observer is known as *extinction*.

The human eye is not able to distinguish any difference between polarized and natural light, although when looking through a single polarizer there is an obvious loss of intensity, some of which is due to the color of the filter, as well as the splitting and absorption of the rays. Polarizing spectacles used as sunglasses make full use of both properties, but their chief advantage is the elimination of glare and reflected light from such surfaces as water and glass, which act as polarizers, much of the reflected light being polarized at right angles to that which penetrates the surface. Looking through two polarizers, if their vibration directions are parallel, results in a further slight loss of intensity (Fig. 3.24a), due to the increase of the thickness and subsequent absorption, but as one is rotated in relation to the other, intensity decreases to extinction when the vibration directions are crossed, and at right angles (Fig. 3.24b). The first polarizer only allows the passage of rays vibrating in its own vibration direction; if parallel, the second polarizer will allow those rays to pass; if crossed, passage of the rays is blocked.

Two phenomena detected in polarized light are interesting to the histologist: birefringence and dichroism. When a birefringent substance is rotated between two crossed polarizers, the image appears and disappears alternately at each 45° of rotation. Hence, in a complete revolution of 360° the image appears four times, and likewise, it is extinguished completely four times. In a thin section of rock composed of many types of crystal this phenomenon is

very dramatic, especially when interference colors, due to varying thickness of crystal, are present. When one of the planes of vibration of the object is in a parallel plane to the polarizer, only one part ray can develop, and its further passage is blocked by the analyzer in the crossed position. At 45°, however, phase differences between the two rays which can develop are able to combine in the analyzer and form a visible image (Fig. 3.25).

Some birefringent substances are also dichroic, which is the second of the phenomena useful to the histologist. Only the polarizer is used and, if no rotating stage is available, the polarizer itself can be rotated. Changes in intensity and color are seen

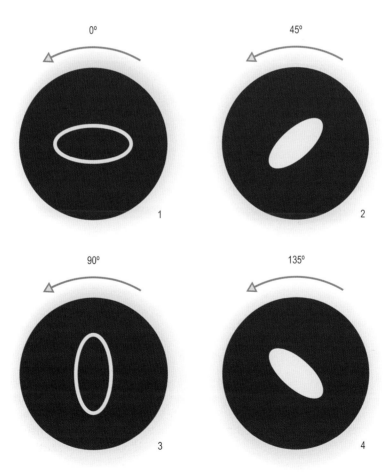

Figure 3.25 When a birefringent substance is rotated between crossed polarizers, it is visible when it is in the diagonal position (i.e. when it is halfway (45°) between the vibration planes of the polarizers). Extinction occurs when one of its planes of vibration is parallel to either polarizer. Both conditions occur four times in a complete revolution of 360°.

during rotation. The color changes in a rotation of 90°, and back to its original color in the next 90° (Fig. 3.26). This is due to differential absorption of light, depending upon the vibration direction of the two rays in a birefringent substance.

Weak birefringence in biological specimens is enhanced by the addition of dyes or impregnating metals, in an orderly linear alignment, for example along amyloid fibrils. Although only one polarizer is needed to detect the resulting dichroism, the use of the analyzer in addition can enhance the image.

Sign of birefringence

Reference was made earlier to the separated *slow* and *fast* rays in a birefringent substance. Additionally, if the *slow* ray (higher RI) is parallel to the length of the crystal or fiber, the birefringence is *positive*. If the *slow* ray is perpendicular to the long axis of the structure, the birefringence is *negative*. The *sign of birefringence* is diagnostically useful and is determined by the use of a compensator (birefringent plate of known retardation) either above the specimen or below the polarizer at 45° to the direction of polarized light. Rotate the compensator or the specimen until the *slow* direction of the compensator (indicated by arrows) is parallel to the long axis of the crystal or fiber. The field is now red and if the crystal is *blue* the birefringence is *positive*. If the crystal is *yellow*, the *slow* direction of the compensator is parallel to the *fast* direction of the crystal and the birefringence is *negative*. Quartz and collagen exhibit positive birefringence while polaroid discs, calcite, urates, and chromosomes are negative. Simple compensators can be made from mica or layers of sellotape.

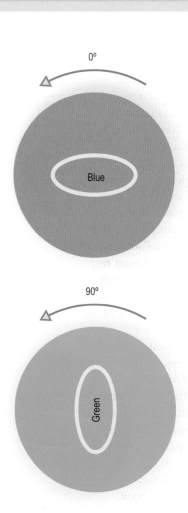

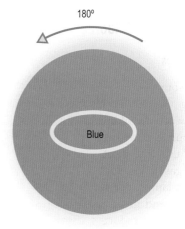

Figure 3.26 A dichroic substance rotated in polarized light (i.e. using polarizer only). Changes of color and intensity can be seen after rotating 90°. The original color returns after a further 90° rotation. This is due to the differential absorption of the two rays in some birefringent substances, depending on the direction of the polarization.

Fluorescence microscopy

Fluorescence is the property of some substances which, when illuminated by light of a certain wavelength, will re-emit the light at a longer wavelength. In fluorescence microscopy, the exciting radiation is usually in the ultraviolet wavelength (c. 360 nm) or blue region (c. 400 nm), although longer wavelengths can be used with some modern dyes.

A substance that possesses a 'fluorophore' will fluoresce naturally. This is known as *primary fluorescence* or *autofluorescence*. Ultraviolet excitation is required for optimum results with substances such as vitamin A, porphyrins, and chlorophyll. Dyes, chemicals, and antibiotics added to tissues produce *secondary fluorescence* of structures and are called 'fluorochromes'. This is the most common use of fluorescence microscopy and the majority of fluorochromes require only blue light excitation.

Induced fluorescence is a term applied to substances such as the catecholamines, which after treatment with formaldehyde vapor are converted to fluorescent quinoline compounds.

The applications of fluorescence microscopy are numerous in both qualitative and quantitative systems, and some of these are contained in other chapters of this book.

Transmitted light fluorescence

Light sources

All light sources emit a wide range of wavelengths, including the shorter ultraviolet and blue wavelengths which are of interest for fluorescence. Only a few sources emit sufficient short-wave light for practical use. The most commonly used are high-pressure gas lamps, such as the mercury vapor and xenon gas lamps. For some wavelength excitation, in the blue and green range for instance, halogen filament lamps produce enough light to be useful. The choice of a suitable source depends upon the type of work to be performed, and for routine observation purposes it is better to use the mercury vapor burners. These operate on alternating current and their starting equipment is not so costly. The xenon burners operate on direct current and require rectifiers to be included with the starter equipment if they are to be used on normal mains supply. Xenon burners on a DC supply can be stabilized and are therefore suitable for fluorimetry or the measurement of fluorescence emission. The two types of lamp differ in their emission curves: that is to say, mercury lamps reach very high amplitudes at some wavelengths, whereas at other parts of the wavelength range the emission is low, and the curve in general, has a very spiky profile. Xenon, on the other hand, has a smoother, more continuous curve. Fortunately the peaks in the mercury vapor emission coincide with the excitation wavelengths of some of the more widely used fluorochromes.

Because they contain gas at high pressure, these burners must be handled with great care, and must be housed in strong, protective lamphouses. Heat and infrared waves are filtered out before the light from the source begins its journey. At one time all fluorescence systems used the transmitted light route common to normal light microscopy. However, nowadays, the incident route is widely used. High-pressure arc lamps also have specific lifetimes, and in the case of mercury lamps this is only 200 hours. Operation for longer times than this may result in explosive destruction of the lamp, with release of mercury vapor into the immediate vicinity.

In recent years, a new type of illumination source has been introduced. This is the LED source, which is a type of solid-state, semiconductor device. These LED sources have exceptionally long lifetimes, with little change in light output over that lifetime. Another characteristic is that these sources emit light of a single wavelength, with a very narrow peak width. These advantageous features mean that these devices are finding increasing use in illuminators for microscopy. While they are not yet as bright as arc lamps, they do not require much optical filtering to select the wavelength of interest, and they do not suffer from the flicker and 'arc wandering' of the high-pressure lamps. They also do not pose the risk of explosion and they have essentially unlimited lifetimes. For different emission wavelengths, different LEDs are required, but there is no need to select a new set of emission filters as the LED itself provides a narrow band of excitation light.

Filters

Preparations for fluorescence may contain other fluorescing material in addition to that in which one is interested. It is necessary therefore to filter out all but the specific excitation wavelength to avoid confusion between the important and the unimportant fluorescence (Fig. 3.27).

A variety of filters are available for this purpose. 'Dyed in the glass' filters, with such designations as UG 1 and BG 12, are broadband filters and transmit a wide range of wavelengths, the width of the range depending upon the composition and thickness of the filter. Besides the possibility of non-specific and autofluorescence, there may also be materials that are excited at more than one excitation wavelength, so it is better to employ filters of a narrower band transmission that have their transmission peaks closer to the excitation maximum of the fluorochrome, such as FITC. Narrow band filters are often of the 'interference' filter type, and are vacuum-coated layers of metals on a glass support. They have a mirror-like surface, and must be inserted in the beam with the reflective face towards the light source. The better-quality filters are carefully selected for their transmission characteristics, and only a few

are finally judged suitable. For this reason, they are expensive; careful handling to avoid corrosive finger marks and scratches is essential. When used with high-intensity light sources, these filters may also degrade with time, and so should be checked with an accurate spectrophotometer at regular intervals.

Barrier or suppression filters are placed before the eyepiece to prevent short wavelength light from damaging the retina of the eye (Fig. 3.27). They must, however, allow the fluorescing color to pass; otherwise a negative result may be obtained. Barrier filters are colorless through yellow to dark orange and of specific wavelength transmission. For example a K.470 filter will block all wavelengths below 470 nm. Colored barrier filters may alter the final color rendering of the fluorescent specimen, and for this reason *all* filters used in the system must be recorded when reporting results.

Condensers for fluorescence microscopy

Bright-field condensers are able to illuminate the object, using all the available energy, but they also direct the rays beyond the object into the objective. Not only is this a potential hazard to the eyes of the observer but also it can set up disturbing autofluorescence in the cement and component layers in the objective itself. In consequence most systems employ a dark-field condenser which does not allow direct

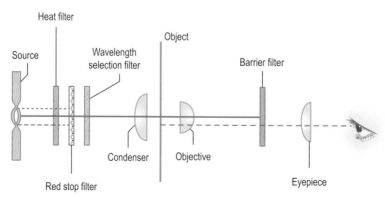

Figure 3.27 Light path for transmitted fluorescence. Light of all wavelengths passes from the source through a heat-absorbing filter, into a second filter which removes red light, and then through an exciter filter, which allows only the desired wavelength(s) to pass. On passing through the specimen, the objective collects both exciting and fluorescent wavelengths. The former is removed by a barrier filter to protect the eye of the observer.

light into the objective, and in addition is more certain to give a dark contrasting background to the fluorescence. At the same time it should be realized that only about one-tenth of the available energy is used, limited by the design of the condenser.

Fluorescent light emission is in most cases very poor in relation to the amount of energy absorbed by fluorochromes or fluorophores, with an efficiency ratio somewhere between 1:1000 and 1:100 at best, and so any system that reduces the available energy to any extent should be well considered before being put into use.

Objectives

Objectives, too, must be carefully chosen. It has already been noted that autofluorescence is a hazard with bright-field illumination, and for that system only the simpler achromat objectives are practical. With dark-ground illumination the range of objectives is considerably widened, and more elaborate lenses with higher apertures and better 'light gathering power' are possible.

Incident light fluorescence

The trend today in fluorescence techniques is in incident illumination, or lighting from above and through the objective down to the object (Fig. 3.28). A number of advantages are gained over the transmitted route.

In principle the excitation beam, after passing the selection filters, is diverted through the objective on to the preparation where fluorescence is stimulated. This fluorescence travels back to the observer

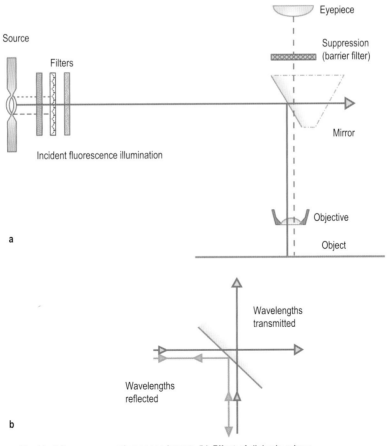

Figure 3.28 (a) Diagram of incident fluorescence microscope layout. (b) Effect of dichroic mirror.

by the normal route (Fig. 3.28a). Dichroic mirrors have been produced to divide and divert the beam. These mirrors have the property of being able to transmit light of some wavelengths and reflect other wavelengths (Fig. 3.28b). By selection of the appropriate mirror, the wavelength desired is reflected to the object; the remainder passes through to be lost. At the same time, visible fluorescent light collected by the objective in the normal way can pass to the eyepiece, and any excitation rays bouncing back (from slide and coverglass) are reflected back along their original path to the source, thus being prevented from reaching the observer. Since the objective in this system also acts as a condenser, the illumination and objective numerical apertures are one and the same, optically correct, and at their most efficient condition. Fluorescence is stimulated on the observer's side of the preparation, and is therefore more brilliant, not being masked by covering material or section thickness.

It is also possible to bring into use any type of objective, including sophisticated phase contrast and interference contrast objectives, for simultaneous transmitted illumination with normal tungsten lighting, and to demonstrate both the fluorescence and the morphology of the preparation. This is useful where normal stains cannot be used for fear of masking any fluorescent reactions.

The use of dichroic mirrors in these systems has made possible much brighter images, since up to 90% of the exciting energy can reach the preparation, and 90% of the resultant visible light can be presented to the eye. In addition, new objectives, of both oil and water immersion types, in low and high powers, have been developed. As immersion objectives they have higher numerical apertures, and can gather more light, avoiding much of the lost stray light reflected from coverslips. The use of low-magnification eyepieces is now more widely accepted, improving fluorescence techniques far beyond anything hitherto possible.

Due to the filters and light sources used in fluorescence microscopy, modern systems generally rely on digital image capture, and these images are monochrome (black and white) images. The highly colored fluorescence images which appear in publications are all the result of pseudo-coloring composite images.

The confocal microscope

In fluorescence microscopy using conventional epifluorescence microscopes, the fluorochrome present in the field of view will be excited whether it is in or out of focus. The effect is that the out-of-focus fluorescence will reduce the contrast and resolution of the image. The confocal system uses a pinhole stop to observe the specimen in such a way as to exclude the out-of-focus portion of the image. In essence the axial resolution in the confocal system is greatly improved to 0.35 mm (in reflection) with additional small but important gains in lateral resolution, and therefore the method lends itself to optical sectioning. With modern computer technology and Windows®-based software a series of optical sections can be recombined to create a 3D image of a cell or structure even with multiple labeling techniques.

Other techniques

A number of specialized techniques for use in fluorescence microscopy have appeared in recent years. One significant technique is *fluorescence resonance energy transfer* or FRET, in which the excitation of one fluorescence material is captured locally by a second material, causing fluorescence of the second material and quenching of the first. Many new techniques have been developed based on the availability of new fluorescence labels and dyes. Many of these new dyes have unique emission spectra, and may also be much more resistant to fading than earlier dyes. A promising new fluorescence label is quantum dots, a label composed on nanometer-sized particles of semiconductor metals. These quantum dots are excited over a wide range of wavelengths, and emit very narrow band light based on the size of the semiconductor particle. The advantage of quantum dots is that many different dots can be excited by the same excitation light, and each will emit a specific color based on the dot size.

The advent of powerful computers and sophisticated programs has led to many new approaches to microscopy. One specific technique that should be mentioned is *multispectral imaging*, in which a number of images are collected at narrow, specific wavelengths. Such images provide new information as individual components of the image can be easily enhanced, thus improving contrast or perceived resolution of specimen morphology.

In recent years, it has been demonstrated that images can be collected at resolutions that far exceed the resolution limits of traditional microscope lenses. These techniques require highly specialized microscopes equipped with exactingly precise scanning stages, both X and Y axis, as well as Z axis (focus) motorized functions, and in almost all cases require tiny pinholes in the optical system, similar to those used with confocal microscopy, although generally much smaller in size. These instruments are also used primarily to examine specimens that have been stained or treated with fluorescence compounds. One of the earliest demonstrations of this approach was that of Betzig et al. (1987). This early demonstration proved the concept of **Near Field Scanning Microscopy.** More recently, a variety of ancillary approaches to super resolution have been developed. A summary of current approaches to super resolution was published by Huang (2010).

Use of the microscope

The microscope itself should receive some attention before it is used. Is the illumination correctly centered? Is the condenser centered and in its proper position? Make sure that the objectives are firmly screwed home, and that the eyepieces are indeed a pair. If the microscope is set aside exclusively for your personal use, these things will probably be in order, but if the instrument is in communal use then it is likely that someone has altered or readjusted something to suit their own purpose. Above all, make sure that the optical parts are clean, and free from dust. Greasy fingerprints and dust are enemies of the optical glass.

Often when an immersion objective has been used, the next objective is swung into position, straight into the oil drop on the slide. Sometimes oil is left on the front of an immersion lens, forgotten for some time, and by the time it is used it has gathered some dust and formed a translucent film. Use oil only for an oil immersion objective. Keep it away from everything else. After a session with immersion objectives, clean them. Gross amounts of oil can be wiped off with lens tissue. The use of xylene for washing the front lens is now frowned upon. Petroleum spirit is recommended by some manufacturers. Alcohol and acetone should be avoided as they may seep into the mount and dissolve the cements.

The front lenses of some objectives are difficult to clean because of their concave shape, and many people recommend the use of swabs of cotton wool or tissue to remove the dirt from the concavity. A better method is the use of a piece of expanded polystyrene such as is used in the packing of delicate equipment and lamp bulbs. A freshly broken surface will be dust free and contain no hard crystals; it cannot scratch the glass. By pressing the polystyrene on to the lens and rotating it in the optical axis, grease, moisture, and dust are quickly removed, even from the deepest of concave lenses. Do *not* use polystyrene if the lens is wet with xylene, or it will coat the glass with a layer of dissolved plastic and make matters worse.

Eyepieces become coated with a fine film of grease from eyelashes. They should be cleaned from time to time with a lens tissue. Tissues are better than cloths as they are usually stored in small numbers in a protective packet, and are discarded after use. Cloths are liable to lie around on the bench for some time, picking up dust and other harmful substances.

Setting up the microscope

Centering the lamp

This is possible on most modern microscopes (some have pre-centered bulbs and do not require attention), either by a pair of centering screws acting against a spring, or by loosening a screw collar and orienting the lamp holder. A ground glass or plastic disc with concentric circles engraved upon it is placed in the light path, usually on the dust protection glass in the foot of the microscope. By adjusting the lamp condenser, or by moving the lamp in its mounting, the filament can be imaged on the ground-glass disc. It is then a simple matter to adjust the bulb position until the image is in the center.

Adjusting the condenser

If the microscope has an adjustable condenser, this is also a simple procedure. First, select a low-power objective (x10) and, with a suitable preparation on the stage, focus the specimen (to establish the plane of the object). Most condensers have a top lens that is normally swung into the light path for the higher-power objectives. This should be turned into position. Open the aperture diaphragm (in the condenser), close the field diaphragm (in the foot of the microscope) to a small aperture. An image of the field diaphragm should now be visible in the field of view. Adjust the height of the condenser until the image of the field diaphragm is sharply focused. This will be the correct position for slides of the same thickness. Now with the adjusting screws move the diaphragm image to the center. If the aperture is opened until it almost reaches the sides of the field of view, the centering is more accurate. When the correct position has been reached, open the field diaphragm until it just disappears from view. Adjust the aperture (or substage) iris diaphragm, by closing it down, removing an eyepiece and, while looking down the tube, open the diaphragm until it occupies one-third of the field of view. Replace the eyepiece. If the image is dark at the edge, open the aperture diaphragm a little more. This has now adjusted the numerical aperture of the condenser to approximately that of the objective in use and achieved the

optimum resolution. The illumination should now be correctly adjusted and ready for use.

Inserting the slide

When changing slides it is always good practice to lower the stage before removing the slide. The risk of damaging the objective is reduced. When a new slide is placed on the stage and the objective lowered towards the focal plane, watch from the side and gently lower the objective (or, raise the stage) until it is almost in contact, then look into the eyepieces and complete the focusing by bringing the objective away from the preparation. If you look through the eyepiece as the objective approaches the slide, you stand a great chance of missing the focus plane and of crashing the objective through the slide with the possible destruction of both the objective and the specimen.

Make sure that the slide is the right way up. With the higher-power objectives, the working distance is very short and you may never find the image.

Additional resources

Many additional resources for microscopy may be found on the internet. A site containing much information as well as graphical examples is the Molecular Expressions Microscopy Primer: http://micro.magnet.fsu.edu/primer.

References

Betzig, et al., 1987. Collection mode near-field optical scanning microscopy. Appl Phys Lett 51, 2088–2090.

Huang, B., 2010. Super-resolution optical microscopy: multiple choices. Curr Opin Chem Biol (Feb), 14.

Fixation of tissues 4

Anthony Rhodes

Introduction

Appropriate fixation of tissues for histological examination is extremely important. Without attention to this process, the range of tests performed in a modern histopathology laboratory will be rendered ineffective and practically useless. The concept of fixation of biological tissues in order to understand biological function and structure has led to the development of many types of fixatives over the last century. The mechanisms and principles by which specific fixatives act to harden and preserve tissues and prevent the loss of specific molecules fall into broad categories. These include the covalent addition of reactive groups and of cross-links, dehydration, and the effects of acids, salt formation, and heat, along with combinations of these actions. Compound fixatives may function via several of these mechanisms.

Although each fixative has advantages, they all have many disadvantages. These include molecular loss from 'fixed' tissues, swelling or shrinkage of tissues during the process, variations in the quality of histochemical and immunohistochemical staining, the ability to perform biochemical analysis accurately, and varying capabilities to maintain the structures of cellular organelles. One of the major problems with fixation using formaldehyde has been the loss of antigen immunorecognition due to that type of fixation combined with processing the tissue to paraffin wax (Eltoum et al. 2001a, 2001b). However, from a clinical perspective the advent of heat-induced epitope retrieval methods, instigated in the early 1990s, have overcome many of these limitations (Shi et al. 1991). Similarly, the analysis of mRNA and DNA from formalin-fixed,

paraffin-embedded tissue has been problematic (Grizzle et al. 2001; Jewell et al. 2002; Steg et al. 2006; Lykidis et al. 2007). All widely used fixatives are selected by compromise; their good aspects are balanced against less desirable features. This chapter discusses the basics of fixation, the advantages and disadvantages of specific fixatives, and provides some of the formulae for specific fixatives currently used in pathology, histology, and anatomy.

The major objective of fixation in pathology is to maintain clear and consistent morphological features (Eltoum et al. 2001a, 2001b; Grizzle et al. 2001). The development of specific fixatives usually has been empirical, and much of the understanding of the mechanisms of fixation has been based upon information obtained from leather tanning and vaccine production. In order to visualize the microanatomy of a tissue, its stained sections must maintain the original microscopic relationships among cells, cellular components (e.g. the cytoplasm and nuclei), and extracellular material with little disruption of the organization of the tissue, and must maintain the tissue's local chemical composition. Many tissue components are soluble in aqueous acid or other liquid environments, and a reliable view of the microanatomy and microenvironment of these tissues requires that the soluble components are not lost during fixation and tissue processing. Minimizing the loss of cellular components, including proteins, peptides, mRNA, DNA, and lipids, prevents the destruction of macromolecular structures such as cytoplasmic membranes, smooth endoplasmic reticulum, rough endoplasmic reticulum, nuclear membranes, lysosomes, and mitochondria. Each fixative, combined with the tissue processing protocol, maintains some molecular and macromolecular aspects of the tissue better than other fixative/

processing combinations. For example, if soluble components are lost from the cytoplasm of cells, the color of the cytoplasm on hematoxylin and eosin (H&E) staining will be reduced or modified and aspects of the appearance of the microanatomy of the tissue, e.g. mitochondria, will be lost or damaged. Similarly, immunohistochemical evaluations of structure and function may be reduced or lost.

Almost any method of fixation induces shrinkage/swelling, hardening of tissues and color variations in various histochemical stains (Sheehan & Hrapchak 1980; Horobin 1982; Fox et al. 1985; Carson 1990; Kiernan 1999; O'Leary & Mason 2004). Various methods of fixation always produce some artifacts in the appearance of tissue on staining; however, for diagnostic pathology it is important that such artifacts are consistent.

The fixative acts by minimizing the loss or enzymatic destruction of cellular and extracellular molecules, maintaining macromolecular structures and protecting tissues from destruction by microorganisms. This results in one view of a dynamically changing, viable tissue (Grizzle et al. 2001). A fixative should also prevent the subsequent breakdown of the tissue or molecular features by enzymatic activity and/or by microorganisms during long-term storage, because diagnostic/therapeutic tissues removed from patients are important resources which may be re-analyzed in the future.

A fixative not only interacts initially with the tissue in its aqueous environment but also, subsequently, the unreacted fixative and the chemical modifications induced by the fixative continue to react. Fixation interacts with all phases of processing and staining from dehydration to staining of tissue sections using histochemical, enzymatic or immuno-histochemical stains (Eltoum et al. 2001b; Rait et al. 2004). A stained tissue section produced after specific fixation combined with tissue processing produces a compromise in the picture that is formed of one or more features of the original living tissue. To date, a universal or ideal fixative has not been identified. Fixatives are therefore selected based on their ability to produce a final product needed to demonstrate a specific feature of a specific tissue (Grizzle et al. 2001). In diagnostic pathology, the fixative of choice for most pathologists has been 10% neutral buffered formalin (Grizzle et al. 2001).

The most important characteristic of a fixative is to support high quality and consistent staining with H&E, both initially and after storage of the paraffin blocks for at least a decade. The fixative must have the ability to prevent short- and long-term destruction of the micro-architecture of the tissue by stopping the activity of catabolic enzymes and hence autolysis, minimizing the diffusion of soluble molecules from their original locations. Another important characteristic of a good fixative, which helps maintain tissue and cellular integrity, is the inanimation of infectious agents, which helps maintain tissue and cellular integrity. It is also important to have good toxicological and flammability profiles that permit the safe use of the fixative (Grizzle & Fredenburgh 2005). The advent of new biological methods, increased understanding of the human genome, and the need to rapidly evaluate the biology of disease processes, means that fixatives should also permit the recovery of macromolecules including proteins, mRNA, and DNA without extensive biochemical modifications from fixed and paraffin-embedded tissues.

Other important characteristics of an ideal fixative include being useful for a wide variety of tissues, including fatty, lymphoid, and neural tissues. It should preserve small and large specimens and support histochemical, immunohistochemical, *in situ* hybridization and other specialized procedures. It should penetrate and fix tissues rapidly, have a shelf life of at least one year, and be compatible with modern automated tissue processors. The fixative should be readily disposable or recyclable and support long-term tissue storage giving excellent microtomy of paraffin blocks, and should be cost-effective (Dapson 1993).

Types of fixation

Fixation of tissues can be accomplished by physical and/or chemical methods. Physical methods such as heating, microwaving, and freeze-drying are independent processes and not used commonly in the routine practice of medical or veterinary pathology, anatomy, and histology, except for the use of dry heat fixation of microorganisms prior to Gram staining. Most methods of fixation used in processing of tissue for histopathological diagnoses rely on chemical fixation carried out by liquid fixatives. Reproducibility over time of the microscopic appearances of tissues after H&E staining is the prime requirement of the fixatives used for diagnostic pathology. Methods of fixation used in research protocols may be more varied, including fixation using vapors and fixation of whole animals by perfusing the animal's vascular system with a fixative (Eltoum et al. 2001a, 2001b).

Several chemicals or their combinations can act as good fixatives, and accomplish many of the stated goals of fixation. Some fixatives add covalent reactive groups which may induce cross-links between proteins, individual protein moieties, within nucleic acids, and between nucleic acids and proteins (Horobin 1982; Eltoum et al. 2001a, 2001b; Rait et al. 2004, 2005). The best examples of such 'cross-linking fixatives' are formaldehyde and glutaraldehyde. Another approach to fixation is the use of agents that remove free water from tissues and hence precipitate and coagulate proteins; examples of these dehydrants include ethanol, methanol, and acetone. These agents denature proteins by breaking the hydrophobic bonds which are responsible for the tertiary structure of proteins. Other fixatives, such as acetic acid, trichloroacetic acid, mercuric chloride, and zinc acetate, act by denaturing proteins and nucleic acids through changes in pH or via salt formation. Some fixatives are mixtures of reagents and are referred to as compound fixatives, e.g. alcoholic formalin acts to fix tissues by adding covalent hydroxymethyl groups and cross-links as well as by coagulation and dehydration.

Physical methods of fixation

Heat fixation

The simplest form of fixation is heat. Boiling or poaching an egg precipitates the proteins and, on

cutting, the yolk and egg white can be identified separately. Each component is less soluble in water after heat fixation than the same component of a fresh egg. Picking up a frozen section on a warm microscope slide both attaches the section to the slide and partially fixes it by heat and dehydration. Even though adequate morphology could be obtained by boiling tissue in normal saline, in histopathology heat is primarily used to accelerate other forms of fixation as well as the steps of tissue processing.

Microwave fixation

Microwave heating speeds fixation and can reduce times for fixation of some gross specimens and histological sections from more than 12 hours to less than 20 minutes (Anonymous 2001; Kok & Boon 2003; Leong 2005). Microwaving tissue in formalin results in the production of large amounts of dangerous vapors, so in the absence of a hood for fixation, or a microwave processing system designed to handle these vapors, this may cause safety problems. Recently, commercial glyoxal-based fixatives which do not form vapors when heated at 55°C have been introduced as an efficient method of microwave fixation.

Freeze-drying and freeze substitution

Freeze-drying is a useful technique for studying soluble materials and small molecules; tissues are cut into thin sections, immersed in liquid nitrogen, and the water is removed in a vacuum chamber at −40°C. The tissue can be post-fixed with formaldehyde vapor. In substitution, specimens are immersed in fixatives at −40°C, such as acetone or alcohol, which slowly remove water through dissolution of ice crystals, and the proteins are not denatured; bringing the temperature gradually to 4°C will complete the fixation process (Pearse 1980). These methods of fixation are used primarily in the research environment and are rarely used in the clinical laboratory setting.

Chemical fixation

Chemical fixation utilizes organic or non-organic solutions to maintain adequate morphological preservation. Chemical fixatives can be considered as members of three major categories: coagulant, cross-linking, and compound fixatives (Baker, 1958).

Coagulant fixatives

Both organic and non-organic solutions may coagulate proteins, making them insoluble. Cellular architecture is maintained primarily by lipoproteins and by fibrous proteins such as collagen; coagulating such proteins maintains tissue histomorphology at the light microscopic level. Unfortunately, because coagulant fixatives result in cytoplasmic flocculation as well as poor preservation of mitochondria and secretory granules, such fixatives are not useful in ultrastructural analysis.

Dehydrant coagulant fixatives

The most commonly used coagulating fixatives are alcohols (e.g. ethanol, methanol) and acetone. Methanol is closer to the structure of water than ethanol. Ethanol therefore competes more strongly than methanol in the interaction with hydrophobic areas of molecules; thus, coagulant fixation begins at a concentration of 50–60% for ethanol but requires a concentration of 80% or more for methanol (Lillie & Fullmer 1976). Removal and replacement of free water from tissue by any of these agents has several potential effects on proteins within the tissue. Water molecules surround hydrophobic areas of proteins and, by repulsion, force hydrophobic chemical groups into closer contact with each other and hence stabilize hydrophobic bonding. By removing water, the opposite principle weakens hydrophobic bonding. Similarly, molecules of water participate in hydrogen bonding in hydrophilic areas of proteins; so removal of water destabilizes this hydrogen bonding. Together, these changes act to disrupt the tertiary structure of proteins. In addition, with the water removed, the structure of the protein may become partially reversed, with hydrophobic groups moving to the outside surface of the protein. Once the tertiary structure of a soluble protein has been modified, the rate of reversal to a more ordered soluble state is slow and most proteins after coagulation remain insoluble even if returned to an aqueous environment.

Disruption of the tertiary structure of proteins, i.e. denaturation, changes their physical properties, potentially causing insolubility and loss of function. Even though most proteins become less soluble in organic environments, up to 13% of protein may be lost, for example with acetone fixation (Horobin 1982). Factors that influence the solubility of macromolecules include:

1. Temperature, pressure, and pH.
2. Ionic strength of the solute.
3. The salting-in constant, which expresses the contribution of the electrostatic interactions.
4. The salting-in and salting-out interactions.
5. The type(s) of denaturing reagent(s) (Herskovits et al. 1970; Horobin 1982; Papanikolau & Kokkinidis 1997; Bhakuni 1998).

Alcohol denatures protein differently, depending on the choice and concentration of alcohol, the presence of organic and non-organic substances, and the pH and temperature of fixation. For example, ethanol denatures proteins > phenols > water and polyhydric alcohols > monocarboxylic acids > dicarboxylic acids (Bhakuni 1998).

Other types of coagulant fixative

Acidic coagulants such as picric acid and trichloroacetic acid change the charges on the ionizable side chains, e.g. ($-NH_2 \rightarrow NH_3^+$) and ($COO^- \rightarrow COOH$), of proteins and disrupt electrostatic and hydrogen bonding. These acids also may insert a lipophilic anion into a hydrophilic region and hence disrupt the tertiary structures of proteins (Horobin 1982). Acetic acid coagulates nucleic acids but does not fix or precipitate proteins; it is therefore added to other fixatives to prevent the loss of nucleic acids.

Trichloroacetic acid (Cl_3CCOOH) can penetrate hydrophobic domains of proteins and the anion produced ($-C-COO^-$) reacts with charged amine groups. This interaction precipitates proteins and extracts nucleic acids. Picric acid or trinitrophenol slightly dissolves in water to form a weak acid solution (pH 2.0). In reactions, it forms salts with basic groups of proteins, causing the proteins to coagulate. If the solution is neutralized, precipitated protein may redissolve. Picric acid fixation produces brighter staining, but the low pH solutions of picric acid may cause hydrolysis and loss of nucleic acids

Non-coagulant cross-linking fixatives

Several chemicals were selected as fixatives secondary to their potential actions of forming cross-links within and between proteins and nucleic acids as well as between nucleic acids and proteins. Cross-linking may not be a major mechanism at current short times of fixation, and therefore 'covalent additive fixatives' may be a better name for this group. Examples include formaldehyde, glutaraldehyde, and other aldehydes, e.g. chloral hydrate and glyoxal, metal salts such as mercuric and zinc chloride, and other metallic compounds such as osmium tetroxide. Aldehyde groups are chemically and biologically reactive and are responsible for many histochemical reactions, e.g. free aldehyde groups may be responsible for argentaffin reactions (Papanikolau & Kokkinidis 1997).

Formaldehyde fixation

Formaldehyde in its 10% neutral buffered form (NBF) is the most common fixative used in diagnostic pathology. Pure formaldehyde is a vapor that, when completely dissolved in water, forms a solution containing 37–40% formaldehyde; this aqueous solution is known as 'formalin'. The usual '10% formalin' used in fixation of tissues is a 10% solution of formalin; i.e., it contains about 4% weight to volume of formaldehyde. The reactions of formaldehyde with macromolecules are numerous and complex. Fraenkel-Conrat and his colleagues, using simple chemistry, meticulously identified most of the reactions of formaldehyde with amino acids and proteins (French & Edsall 1945; Fraenkel-Conrat & Olcott 1948a, 1948b; Fraenkel-Conrat & Mecham 1949). In an aqueous solution formaldehyde forms methylene hydrate, a methylene glycol as the first step in fixation (Singer 1962).

$$H_2C = O + H_2O \rightarrow HOCH_2OH$$

Methylene hydrate reacts with several side chains of proteins to form reactive hydroxymethyl side groups ($-CH_2-OH$). If relatively short fixation times are used with 10% neutral buffered formalin (hours to days), the formation of hydroxymethyl side chains is probably the primary and characteristic reaction. The formation of actual cross-links may be relatively rare at the currently used relatively short times of fixation.

Formaldehyde also reacts with nuclear proteins and nucleic acids (Kok & Boon 2003; Leong 2005). It penetrates between nucleic acids and proteins and stabilizes the nucleic acid-protein shell, and it also modifies nucleotides by reacting with free amino groups, as it does with proteins. In naked and free DNA, the cross-linking reactions are believed to start at adenine-thymidine (AT)-rich regions and cross-linking increases with increasing temperature (McGhee & von Hippel 1975a, 1975b, 1977a, 1977b). Formaldehyde reacts with C=C and –SH bonds in unsaturated lipids, but does not interact with carbohydrates (French & Edsall 1945; Hayat 1981).

The side chains of peptides or proteins that are most reactive with methylene hydrate, and hence have the highest affinity for formaldehyde, include lysine, cysteine, histidine, arginine, tyrosine, and reactive hydroxyl groups of serine and threonine (see Table 4.1) (Means & Feeney 1995).

Gustavson (1956) reported that one of the most important cross-links in 'over-fixation', i.e. in tanning, is that between lysine and the amide group of the protein backbone. Due to the shorter fixation times of current diagnostic pathological and biological applications, cross-linking reactions with the protein backbone are unlikely to occur (French & Edsall 1945; Fraenkel-Conrat et al. 1945, 1947;

Table 4.1 Action of major single or combination fixatives

Category of fixative	Dehydrants	Aldehyde cross-linkers	Combination mercuric chloride with formaldehyde or acetic acid	Osmium tetroxide	Picric acid plus formalin and acetic acid	Combination alcohols plus formalin
Examples of category	Ethanol Methanol Acetone	Formaldehyde Glutaraldehyde	Zenker's B5	Post-fixation after glutaraldehyde	Bouin's	Alcoholic formalin
Effect on proteins	Precipitates without chemical addition	Cross-linkers: adds active hydroxymethyl groups to amines, amides, some reactive alcohols, and sulfydryl groups; cross-links amine/amide or sulfydryl side chains of proteins	Additive plus coagulation	Additive cross-links; some extraction some destruction	Additive and non-additive coagulant some extraction	Additive plus precipitation
mRNA/DNA	Slight	Slowly cross-links; slightly extracts	Coagulation	Slight extraction	No action	Slight
Lipids	Extensive extraction	No action	No action	Made insoluble by cross-links with double bonds	No action	Extensive extraction
Carbohydrates	No action	None on pure carbohydrates; cross-linking of glycoproteins	No action	Slight oxidation	No action	No action
Quality of H&E staining	Satisfactory	Good	Good	Poor	Good	Good

Effect on ultrastructure (organelles)	Destroys ultrastructure, including mitochondria, proteins, coagulates	Good (NBF) to excellent preservation with glutaraldehyde; adequate to good in Carson-Millonig's	Poor preservation	Used for visualization of membranes	Poor – tends to destroy membranes	Poor
Usual formulation	70–100% solution or in combination with other types of fixative	Formaldehyde (37%) – 10% V/V aqueous solution buffered with phosphates to pH 7.2–7.4. Glutaraldehyde – 2% buffered to pH 7.4	Mercuric chloride combined either with acetic acid plus dichromate or with formaldehyde plus acetate	1% solution buffered to pH 7.4	Aqueous picric acid, formalin, glacial acetic acid	10% formaldehyde (37%) with 90% ethanol
Important variables/issues	Time, specimen thickness – should be used only for small or thin specimens	Time, temperature, pH, concentration/ specimen thickness	Toxic	Extremely toxic	Mitochondria and integrity of nuclear membrane destroyed; not appropriate for some stains; mordant	Time, specimen dimensions. Note good fixative for renal tissues
Special uses	Preserves small non-lipid molecules such as glycogen; preserves enzymatic activity	General all-round fixative; best for ultrastructure if used with osmium tetroxide post-fixation	Excellent for hematopoietic tissues	Ultrastructural visualization of membranes; lipids on frozen sections	Mordant for connective tissue stains (trichrome)	Good general fixative; good for specific immunohistochemical reactions and good to detect lymph nodes in fatty tissue; removes fats from tissue

Fraenkel-Conrat & Olcott 1948a, 1948b; Fraenkel-Conrat & Mecham 1949; Gustavson 1956).

Reversibility of formaldehyde-macromolecular reactions

The reactive groups may combine with hydrogen groups or with each other, forming methylene bridges. If the formalin is washed away, reactive groups may rapidly return to their original states, but any bridging that has already occurred may remain.

Washing for 24 hours removes about half of reactive groups, and 4 weeks of washing removes up to 90% (Helander 1994). This suggests that actual cross-linking is a relatively slow process, so, in the rapid fixation used in diagnostic pathology, most 'fixation' with formaldehyde prior to tissue processing stops with the formation of reactive hydroxymethyl groups.

For long-term storage in formalin, the reactive groups may be oxidized to the more stable groups (e.g. acids –NH–COOH) which are not easily removed by washing in water or alcohol. Thus, following fixation, returning the specimen to water or alcohol further reduces the fixation of the specimen, because the reactive groups produced by the initial reaction with formalin may reverse and be removed. Although it was initially thought that cross-linking was most important in the fixation of tissue for biological uses (based on the limited number of cross-links over short periods of fixation), it is likely that formation of these hydroxymethyl groups actually denatures macromolecules and renders them insoluble. As these washing experiments have not been reproduced, the actual mechanisms and their importance to fixation by formaldehyde are uncertain. As well as simple washing under running water, over-fixation of tissue may be partially corrected by soaking the tissue in concentrated ammonia plus 20% chloral hydrate (Lhotka & Ferreira 1949). Fraenkel-Conrat and his colleagues frequently noted that the addition and condensation reactions of formaldehyde with amino acids and proteins were unstable and could be reversed easily by dilution or dialysis (Fraenkel-Conrat et al. 1945, 1947; Fraenkel-Conrat & Olcott 1948a, 1948b; Fraenkel-Conrat & Mecham 1949).

The principal type of cross-link in short-term fixation is thought to be between the hydroxymethyl group on a lysine side chain and arginine (through secondary amino groups), asparagine, glutamine (through secondary amide groups), or tyrosine (through hydroxyl group) (Tome et al. 1990). For example, a lysine methyl hydroxyl amine group can react with an arginine group to form a lysine–CH_2–arginine cross-link; similarly, a tyrosine methyl hydroxyl amine group can bind with a cysteine group to form a tyrosine–CH_2–cysteine cross-link. Each of these cross-links between macromolecules has a different degree of stability, which can be modified by the temperature, pH, and type of the environment surrounding and permeating the tissue (Eltoum et al. 2001b). The time to saturation of human and animal tissues with active groups by formalin is about 24 hours, but cross-linking may continue for many weeks (Helander 1994).

When formaldehyde dissolves in an unbuffered aqueous solution, it forms an acid solution (pH 5.0–5.5) because 5–10% of commercially available formaldehyde is formic acid. Acid formalin may react more slowly with proteins than NBF because amine groups become charged (e.g. $–N^+H_3$). In solution, this requires a much lower pH than 5.5. However, the requirement for a lower pH to produce $–N^+H_3$ groups may not be equivalent to that required in peptides. Acid formalin also preserves immuno-recognition much better than NBF (Arnold et al. 1996), and indeed the success of Taylor in the early days of immunocytochemistry to demonstrate immunoglobulins in paraffin-processed tissue sections, most probably relied on the fixation of the tissues in acid formalin (Taylor et al. 1974). The disadvantage of using acid formalin for fixation is the formation of a brown-black pigment with degraded hemoglobulin. This heme-related pigment, which forms in tissue, is usually not a great problem unless patients have a blood abnormality (e.g. sickle cell disease, malaria).

Formaldehyde primarily preserves peptide-protein bonds and the general structure of cellular organelles. It can interact with nucleic acids but has little effect on carbohydrates and preserves lipids if the solutions contain calcium (Bayliss High & Lake 1996).

Glutaraldehyde fixation

Less is known about glutaraldehyde's biological reactions and effects compared to formaldehyde, as it has not been used as widely in biological applications. Glutaraldehyde is a bifunctional aldehyde that probably combines with the same reactive groups as does formaldehyde. In aqueous solutions glutaraldehyde polymerizes, forming cyclic and oligomeric compounds (Hopwood 1985), and it is also oxidized to glutaric acid. To aid in stability, it requires storage at 4°C and at a pH of around 5 (Hopwood 1969).

Unlike formaldehyde, glutaraldehyde has an aldehyde group on both ends of the molecule. With each reaction of the first group, an unreacted aldehyde group may be introduced into the protein and these aldehyde groups can act to further cross-link the protein. Alternatively, the aldehyde groups may react with a wide range of other histochemical targets, including antibodies, enzymes, or proteins. The reaction of glutaraldehyde with an isolated protein, such as bovine serum albumin, is fastest at pH 6–7, and is faster (Habeeb 1966), and results in more cross-linking than formaldehyde (Habeeb 1966; Hopwood 1969). Cross-linking is irreversible and withstands acids, urea, semicarbazide, and heat (Hayat 1981). Like formaldehyde, reactions with lysine are the most important for forming cross-links.

Extensive cross-linking by glutaraldehyde results in better preservation of ultrastructure, but this method of fixation negatively affects immunohistochemical methods and slows the penetration by the fixative. Thus, any tissue fixed in glutaraldehyde must be small (0.5 mm maximum) and, unless the aldehyde groups are blocked, increased background staining will result if several histochemical methods are used (Grizzle 1996a). Glutaraldehyde does not react with carbohydrates or lipids unless they contain free amino groups as are found in some

phospholipids (Hayat 1981). At room temperature glutaraldehyde does not cross-link nucleic acids in the absence of nucleohistones but it may react with nucleic acids at or above 45°C (Hayat 1981).

Osmium tetroxide fixation

Osmium tetroxide (OsO_4), a toxic solid, is soluble in water as well as non-polar solvents and can react with hydrophilic and hydrophobic sites including the side chains of proteins, potentially causing cross-linking (Hopwood et al. 1990). The reactive sites include sulfydryl, disulfide, phenolic, hydroxyl, carboxyl, amide, and heterocyclic groups. Osmium tetroxide is known to interact with nucleic acids, specifically with the 2,3-glycol moiety in terminal ribose groups and the 5,6 double bonds of thymine residues. Nuclei fixed in OsO_4 and dehydrated with alcohol may show prominent clumping of DNA. This unacceptable artifact can be prevented by pre-fixation with potassium permanganate ($KMnO_4$), post-fixation with uranyl acetate, or by adding calcium ions and tryptophan during fixation (Hayat 1981). The reaction of OsO_4 with carbohydrates is uncertain (Hayat 1981). Large proportions of proteins and carbohydrates are lost from tissues during osmium fixation; some of this may be due to the superficial limited penetration of OsO_4 (i.e. <1 mm) into tissues or its slow rates of reaction. In electron microscopy, this loss is minimized by initial fixation of tissue in glutaraldehyde.

The best characterized reaction of osmium is its reaction with unsaturated bonds within lipids and phospholipids. In this reaction, osmium in its +8 valence state converts to a +6 valence state, which is colorless. If two unsaturated bonds are close together there may be cross-linking by OsO_4. Although the complex is colorless at this point, the typical black staining of membranes expected from fixation with osmium requires the production of osmium dioxide ($OsO_2 \cdot 2H_2O$). Osmium dioxide is black, electron dense, and insoluble in aqueous solution; it precipitates as the above unstable compounds break down and becomes deposited on cellular membranes. The breakdown of osmium +6 valence complexes to osmium dioxide (+4 valence state) is facilitated by a reaction with solutions of ethanol.

In addition to its use as a secondary fixative for electron microscope examinations, OsO_4 can also be used to stain lipids in frozen sections. Osmium tetroxide fixation causes tissue swelling which is reversed during dehydration steps. Swelling can also be minimized by adding calcium or sodium chloride to osmium-containing fixatives (Hayat 1981).

Cross-linking fixatives for electron microscopy

Cell organelles such as cytoplasmic and nuclear membranes, mitochondria, membrane-bound secretory granules, and smooth and rough endoplasmic reticulum need to be preserved carefully for electron microscopy. The lipids in these structures are extracted by many fixatives with dehydrants (e.g. alcohols). Therefore for ultrastructural examination it is important to use a fixative that does not solubilize lipids. The preferred fixatives are a strong cross-linking fixative such as glutaraldehyde, a combination of glutaraldehyde and formaldehyde, or Carson's modified Millonig's, followed by post-fixation in an agent that further stabilizes as well as emphasizes membranes such as OsO_4.

Mercuric chloride

Historically, mercuric chloride was greatly favored for its qualities of enhancing the staining properties of tissues, particularly for trichrome stains. However, it is now rarely used in the clinical laboratory due to the health and safety issues involved with the use of a mercury-containing fixative, and also due to the reduced reliance on 'special stains'. A further major disadvantage of mercuric chloride fixation is the inevitable formation of deposits of intensely black precipitates of mercuric pigment in the tissues. This subsequently gives them inferior value for immuno-histochemical and molecular studies. In recently fixed tissues, these precipitates can be readily removed by a Lugol's iodine step in the staining procedure, followed by bleaching of the section in sodium hypochlorite solution (Hypo). However, this is not effective on mercuric chloride fixed tissues which have been stored for a number of years as paraffin blocks. In these tissues, retrospective analysis by immunohistochemistry and molecular techniques becomes unreliable due to the formation of much larger aggregates of mercuric pigment which cannot be removed subsequently by Lugol's iodine. The chemistry of fixation using mercuric chloride is not well understood. It is, however, known that mercuric chloride reacts with ammonium salts, amines, amides, amino acids, and sulfydryl groups, and hardens tissues. It is especially reactive with cysteine, forming a dimercaptide (Hopwood 2002) and acidifying the solution:

$$\text{sulfydryl} -2\,(\text{R–S–H}) + HgCl_2 \rightleftharpoons$$
$$(\text{R–S})_2\text{–Hg} + 2H^+ + 2Cl^-$$

If only one cysteine is present, a reactive group of R–S–Hg–Cl is likely.

Mercury-based fixatives are toxic and should be handled with care. They should not be allowed to come into contact with metal, and should be dissolved in distilled water to prevent the precipitation of mercury salts. Mercury-containing chemicals are an environmental disposal problem. These fixatives penetrate slowly, so specimens must be thin, and mercury and acid formaldehyde hematein pigments may deposit in tissue after fixation. Mercury fixatives (Hopwood 1973) are no longer used routinely except by some laboratories for fixing hematopoietic tissues (especially B5). A potential replacement for mercuric chloride is zinc sulfate. Special formulations of zinc sulfate in formaldehyde replacing mercuric chloride in B5 may give better nuclear detail than formaldehyde alone and improve tissue penetration (Carson 1990).

Special fixatives

Dichromate and chromic acid fixation

Chromium trioxide dissolves in water to produce an acidic solution of chromic acid, with a pH of 0.85.

Chromic acid is a powerful oxidizing agent which produces aldehyde from the 1, 2-diglycol residues of polysaccharides. These aldehydes can react in histochemical stains (PAS and argentaffin/argyrophil) and should increase the background of immunohistochemical staining (Grizzle 1996a).

Actual chromic salts (i.e. chromium ions in +3 valence state) may destroy animal tissues (Kiernan 1999) but chromium ions in their +6 state coagulate proteins and nucleic acids. The fixation and hardening reactions are not understood completely but probably involve the oxidation of proteins, which varies in strength depending upon the pH of the fixative, plus interaction of the reduced chromate ions directly in cross-linking proteins (Pearse & Stoward 1980). Chromium ions specifically interact with the carboxyl and hydroxyl side chains of proteins. Chromic acid also interacts with disulfide bridges and attacks lipophilic residues such as tyrosine and methionine (Horobin 1982). Fixatives containing chromate at a pH of 3.5–5.0 make proteins insoluble without coagulation. Chromate is reported to make unsaturated but not saturated lipids insoluble upon prolonged (>48 hours) fixation and hence mitochondria are well preserved by dichromate fixatives.

Dichromate-containing fixatives have primarily been used to prepare neuroendocrine tissues for staining, especially normal adrenal medulla and related tumors (e.g. phaeochromocytomas). However, reliance on the chromaffin reaction used to identify chromaffin granules following dichromate fixation has greatly diminished, being replaced by immunohistochemistry to a range of neuroendocrine markers, to include neuron-specific enolase, chromagranin A, and synaptophysin (Grizzle 1996a, 1996b).

Fixatives for DNA, RNA, and protein analysis

Lykidis et al. (2007) conducted a comprehensive analysis of 25 fixative compounds, many reputed to provide improved preservation of DNA and RNA and proteins in tissues for immunocytochemical analysis, whilst at the same time ensuring optimal morphological preservation. The compounds included the commercially available HOPE (HEPES-glutamic acid buffer mediated Organic Solvent Protection Effect) fixative and the reversible cross-linker dithio-bis[succinimidyl propionate] (DSP) for immunocytochemistry and expression profiling, in addition to zinc-based fixatives. They concluded that a novel zinc formation (Z7) containing zinc trifluoroacetate, zinc chloride and calcium acetate was significantly better than the standard zinc-based fixative (Z2) and NBF for DNA, RNA and antigen perseveration. DNA and RNA fragments up to 2.4kb and 361bp in length, respectively, were detected by PCR, reverse transcriptase PCR and real-time PCR in the Z7 fixed tissues, in addition to allowing for protein analysis using 2D electrophoresis. Nucleic acids and protein were found to be stable over a period of 6–14 months. Moreover, the fixative is less toxic than formaldehyde formulations. Whilst this fixative appears to show great promise, it should be borne in mind that fixation in NBF will also allow the extraction of similarly sized fragments of DNA and RNA for analysis by PCR-based technologies, within this time frame.

Metallic ions as a fixative supplement

Several metallic ions have been used as aids in fixation, including Hg^{2+}, Pb^{2+}, Co^{2+}, Cu^{2+}, Cd^{2+}, $[UO_2]^{2+}$, $[PtCl_6]^{2+}$, and Zn^{2+}. Mercury, lead, and zinc are used most commonly in current fixatives, e.g. zinc-containing formaldehyde is suggested to be a better fixative for immunohistochemistry than formaldehyde alone. This does however depend upon the pH of the formaldehyde, as well as the zinc formaldehyde (Arnold et al. 1996; Eltoum et al. 2001a).

Compound fixatives

Pathologists use formaldehyde-based fixatives to ensure reproducible histomorphometric patterns. Other agents may be added to formaldehyde to produce specific effects that are not possible with formaldehyde alone. The dehydrant ethanol, for example, can be added to formaldehyde to produce alcoholic formalin. This combination preserves molecules such as glycogen and results in less shrinkage and hardening than pure dehydrants.

Compound fixatives are useful for specific tissues, e.g. alcoholic formalin for fixation of some fatty tissues, such as breast, in which preservation of the lipid is not important. In addition, fixation of gross specimens in alcoholic formalin may aid in identifying lymph nodes embedded in fat. Some combined fixatives including alcoholic formalin are good at preserving antigen immunorecognition, but non-specific staining or background staining in immunohistochemical procedures can be increased. Unreacted aldehyde groups in glutaraldehyde-formaldehyde fixation for example may increase background staining, and alcoholic formalin may cause non-specific staining of myelinated nerves (Grizzle et al. 1995, 1997, 1998a, 1998b; Arnold et al. 1996; Grizzle 1996b).

Factors affecting the quality of fixation

Buffers and pH

The effect of pH on fixation with formaldehyde may be profound depending upon the applications to which the tissues will be exposed. In a strongly acidic environment, the primary amine target groups ($-NH_2$) attract hydrogen ions ($-NH^+_3$) and become unreactive to the hydrated formaldehyde (methylene hydrate or methylene glycol), and carboxyl groups ($-COO^-$) lose their charges ($-COOH$). This may affect the structure of proteins. Similarly the hydroxyl groups of alcohols ($-OH$) including serine and threonine may become less reactive in a strongly acidic environment. The extent of formation of reactive hydroxymethyl groups and cross-linking is reduced in unbuffered 4% formaldehyde (Means & Feeney 1995), which is slightly acidic (French & Edsall 1945), because the major methylene cross-links are between lysine and the free amino group on side chains. The decrease in the effectiveness of formaldehyde fixation and hence cross-linking in such a slightly acid environment has led some

authors to suggest that unbuffered formalin is a better fixative than NBF with respect to immuno-recognition of many antigens (Arnold et al. 1996; Eltoum et al. 2001b). This no doubt aided the detection of antigens before the early 1990s, prior to the advent of heat-induced epitope retrieval methods in immunocytochemistry. However, minimal delay in effectively fixing very labile antigens, such as the estrogen receptor, is vital in the immunohistochemical testing for a range of clinically important prognostic and predictive biomarkers. Whilst formaldehyde fixation remains the recommended method for optimal preservation of morphological features, proteins and nucleic acids in a clinical environment, the most reliable way of achieving optimal formalin fixation is through its buffering at pH 7.2–7.4 (i.e. neutral buffered formalin).

At the acidic pH of unbuffered formaldehyde, hemoglobin metabolic products are chemically modified to form a brown-black, insoluble, crystalline, birefringent pigment. The pigment forms at a pH of less than 5.7, and the extent of its formation increases in the pH range of 3.0 to 5.0. Formalin pigment is recognized easily and should not affect diagnoses except in patients with large amounts of hemoglobin breakdown products secondary to hematopoietic diseases. The pigment is removed easily with an alcoholic solution of picric acid. To avoid the formation of formalin pigment, neutral buffered formalin is used as the preferred formaldehyde-based fixative.

Acetic acids and other acids work mainly through lowering pH and disrupting the tertiary structure of proteins. Buffers are used to maintain optimum pH. The choice of specific buffer depends on the type of fixative and analyte. Commonly used buffers are phosphate, cacodylate, bicarbonate, Tris, and acetate. It is necessary to use low salt-buffered formalin in the new complex tissue processors in order to keep the machine 'clean', and reduce problems in its operation.

Duration of fixation and size of specimens

The factors that govern diffusion of a fixative into tissue were investigated by Medawar (1941). He found that the depth (d) reached by a fixative is directly proportional to the square root of duration of fixation (t) and expressed this relation as:

$$d = k\sqrt{t}$$

The constant (k) is the coefficient of diffusability, which is specific to each fixative. Examples are 0.79 for 10% formaldehyde, 1.0 for 100% ethanol, and 1.33 for 3% potassium dichromate (Hopwood 1969). Thus, for most fixatives, the time of fixation is approximately equal to the square of the distance which the fixative must penetrate. Most fixatives, such as NBF, will penetrate tissue to the depth of approximately 1 mm in one hour; hence for a 10 mm sphere, the fixative will not penetrate to the center until $(5)^2$ or 25 hours of fixation. It is important to note that the components of a compound fixative will penetrate the tissue at different rates, so that these aspects of the fixative will be best manifest in thin specimens.

Gross specimens should not rest on the bottom of a container of fixative: they should be separated from the bottom by wadded fixative-soaked paper or cloth, so allowing penetration of fixative or processing fluids from all directions. In addition, unfixed gross specimens which are to be cut and stored in fixative prior to processing should not be thicker than 0.5cm. When surgical specimens are to be processed to paraffin blocks, the time of penetration by fixative is more critical. Specific issues related to the processing of tissues have been reviewed by Grizzle et al. (2001) and Jones et al. (2001).

Fixation proceeds slowly and the period between the formation of reactive hydroxymethyl groups and the formation of a significant number of cross-links is unknown. Ninety percent of reactive groups can be removed by 4 weeks of washing (Helander 1994), confirming that cross-linking is not a rapid process and may require weeks for completion of potential bonds.

Proteins inactivate fixatives, especially those in blood or bloody fluids. Bloody gross specimens should therefore be washed with saline prior to being put into fixative. The fixative volume should be at least 10 times the volume of the tissue specimen for optimal, rapid fixation. Currently in some laboratories, thin specimens may be fixed in NBF for only 5–6 hours including the short time of fixation in tissue processors. The extent of formation of cross-links during such rapid NBF 'fixation' is uncertain. Consequently, the formation of hydroxymethyl groups may predominate, as opposed to more resilient cross-linking. It has been suggested that rapid fixation is acceptable as long as histochemical staining remains adequate; and that immunohistochemistry and other molecular techniques are probably enhanced by shorter times of fixation using an aldehyde (e.g. formaldehyde)-based fixation. However, recent studies investigating the time taken to adequately fix clinical cases of breast cancer tissue for subsequent immunohistochemical detection of estrogen receptors illustrate that this practice can be detrimental to the optimal preservation of important antigens and should be avoided. Goldstein et al. (2003) found that 6–8 hours was the minimum time required to adequately fix breast tissue for immunohistochemical testing of estrogen receptors, regardless of the size and type of specimen. Consequently, the current guidelines for estrogen receptor and progesterone receptor testing produced by the American Society of Clinical Oncology (ASCO) and College of American Pathologists (CAP) recommend this minimal fixation time in neutral buffered formalin for all clinical breast cancer specimens (Hammond et al. 2010).

Temperature of fixation

The diffusion of molecules increases with rising temperature due to their more rapid movement and vibration; i.e. the rate of penetration of a tissue by formaldehyde is faster at higher temperatures. Microwaves therefore have been used to speed formaldehyde fixation by both increasing the temperature and molecular movements. Increased vapor levels, however, are a safety problem (Grizzle & Fredenburgh 2001, 2005). Most chemical reactions occur more rapidly at higher temperatures and therefore formaldehyde reacts more rapidly with proteins (Hopwood 1985). Closed tissue processors have their processing retort directly above the paraffin holding stations which are held at 60–65°C, making the retort slightly warmer than room temperature.

Concentration of fixative

Effectiveness and solubility primarily determine the appropriate concentration of fixatives. Concentrations of formalin above 10% tend to cause increased hardening and shrinkage (Fox et al. 1985). In addition, higher concentrations result in formalin being present in its polymeric form, which can be deposited as white precipitate, as opposed to its monomeric form $HO(H_2CO)H$, which at 4% provides for greatest solubility (Baker 1958). Ethanol concentrations below 70% do not remove free water from tissues efficiently.

Osmolality of fixatives and ionic composition

The osmolality of the buffer and fixative is important; hypertonic and hypotonic solutions lead to shrinkage and swelling, respectively. The best morphological results are obtained with solutions that are slightly hypertonic (400–450 mOsm), though the osmolality for 10% NBF is about 1500 mOsm. Similarly, various ions (Na^+, K^+, Ca^{2+}, Mg^{2+}) can affect cell shape and structure regardless of the osmotic effect. The ionic composition of fluids should be as isotonic as possible to the tissues.

Additives

The addition of electrolytes and non-electrolytes to fixatives improves the morphology of the fixed tissue. These additives include calcium chloride, potassium thiocyanate, ammonium sulfate, and potassium dihydrogen phosphate. The electrolytes may react either directly with proteins causing denaturation, or independently with the fixatives and cellular constituents (Hayat 1981). The choice of electrolytes to be added to fixatives used on a tissue processor may vary. Fixatives buffered with electrolytes such as phosphates may cause problems with some processors due to precipitation of the salts. The

addition of non-electrolyte substances such as sucrose, dextran, and detergent has also been reported to improve fixation (Hayat 1981).

Selecting or avoiding specific fixatives

The choice of a fixative is a compromise, balancing their beneficial and detrimental effects. Kiernan (1999) originally produced a table of the actions of fixatives; this was later modified and published by Eltoum et al. (2001b), and Table 4.1 is a further modification of the latter.

However, specific fixatives are unsuitable for most uses and should be avoided. The main problem with fixatives used in histological staining is the loss by solution/extraction of molecules that are targets of specific histochemical methods. Typically, some molecules are soluble in aqueous fixatives (e.g. glycogen), while others are soluble in organic-based fixatives (e.g. lipids). Some fixatives may chemically modify targets of histochemical staining and thus affect the quality of special stains (e.g. glutaraldehyde for silver stains); this includes modification of staining secondary to changes in pH induced by fixation. A good discussion of the effects of fixation on histochemistry is by Sheehan and Hrapchak (1980).

The table of Sheehan and Hrapchak (1980) modified by (Eltoum et al. 2001b) has been changed so that harmful methods of fixation could be identified rapidly. Table 4.2 of this chapter is a further modification of the table.

Fixation for selected individual tissues

Eyes

The globe must be firmly fixed in order to cut good sections for embedding. Eyes may be fixed in NBF, usually for about 48 hours; to speed fixation one or two small windows can be cut into the globe (avoid the retina and iris) after 24 hours. After gross description, the anterior (iris) and posterior (e.g. optic nerve) are removed with a new, sharp razor blade and the components of the globe are fixed for an

Table 4.2 Incompatible stains and fixatives

Target of special stain	Type of special stain	Fixative best avoided	Preferred fixative
Amebas	Best's carmine	Alcohol or alcoholic formalin	Aqueous fixative
Cholesterol and cholesterol esters	Schultz's method	10% NBF (frozen section)	Bouin's; Zenker's
	Digitonin	10% NBF (frozen section)	Bouin's; Zenker's
Chromaffin granules	Ferric ferricyanide reduction test	Orth's; Möller's	
	Gomori-Burtner methenamine silver Periodic acid-Schiff (PAS)	Orth's; Möller's	
	Mallory's aniline blue collagen stain	10% NBF; Bouin's; Heidenhain's mercuric chloride	Dichromate and alcohol bases
Connective tissue	Wilder's reticulum	10% NBF; Zenker's; Helly's	No picric acid fixatives
	Masson's trichrome	Bouin's	NBF tissues must be post-fixed with (Bouin's)
	Mallory's analine blue collagen stain	Zenker's	All except preferred
Copper	Mallory's stain	Alcohol-based fixatives	Formalin
Degenerating myelin	Marchi's method	Orth's for 48 hours; 10% NBF	All except preferred
DNA/RNA	Feulgen	Ethanol	Bouin's, strong acids
Elastic fibers	Gomori's aldehyde fuchsin	10% NBF	No chromates
Fats/lipids	Nile blue sulfate	Formal calcium	All except preferred
	Osmic acid (frozen section)	10% NBF	All except preferred
	Oil red O (frozen section)	10% NBF	Zenker's; Helly's
	Sudan black B (frozen section)	10% NBF	Zenker's; Helly's
Fibrin	Mallory's phosphotungstic acid hematoxylin	Zenker's	Bouin's
	Weigert's stain for fibrin	Absolute ethanol; Carnoy's alcoholic formalin	Bouin's
Glycogen	Bauer-Feulgen	Carnoy's or Gendre's	Aqueous fixative
	PAS	Acid alcoholic formalin	Aqueous fixative
	Best's carmine	Absolute alcohol; Carnoy's	Aqueous fixative
Glycoproteins	Müller-Mowry colloidal iron	Alcoholic formalin Carnoy's	Chromates
Hemoglobin	Lepehne's (frozen section)	Short time in 10% NBF	Zenker's
	Dunn-Thompson	10% NBF	Bouin's, Zenker's, Helly's

Table 4.2 (continued)

Target of special stain	Type of special stain	Fixative best avoided	Preferred fixative
Hepatitis B surface antigen	Orcein Aldehyde fuchsin		No chromates No chromates
Iron	Mallory's stain	Alcohol-based fixatives	Formalin
Juxtaglomerular cells of kidney	Bowie's stain	Helly's	All except preferred
Melanin pigments	DOPA oxidase	Fresh frozen or formalin	All except preferred
Mitochondria		Carson-Millonig's	Dehydrants, ethanol methanol, acetone
Mucoproteins	PAS		Glutaraldehyde
Neuroendocrine granules	Rapid argyrophil Fontana-Masson	10% NBF	Ethanol, methanol, acetone
Pancreas α, β, & δ cells	Trichrome-PAS	10% NBF or Helly's	Zenker's, Bouin's Alcohol based
Paneth cell granules	Phloxine tartrazine	10% NBF	Acid
Peripheral nerve elements	Bielschowski's for neurofibrils and axis cylinders	3–6 weeks in 10% NBF	All except preferred
	Bodian's for myelinated and non-myelinated nerve fibers	9 parts ethanol, 1 part formalin	All except preferred
	Nonidez's for neurofibrils and axis cylinders	100 ml 50% ethanol plus 25 g chloral hydrate	All except preferred
	Rio-Hortega for neutrofibrils	10% NBF	All except preferred
	Immunohistochemistry biotin-streptavidin	Formal zinc	Alcoholic formalin
Phospholipids	Smith-Dietrich (frozen section)	Formal calcium	All except preferred
	Baker's acid hematin (frozen section)	10% NBF	All except preferred
Pituitary β cells	Congo red for β cells	10% NBF	
	Gomori's aldehyde fuchsin for β cells	Bouin's	NBF requires mordant
Silver stains	Fontana-Masson-Grimelius		Glutaraldehyde
Spirochetes	Giemsa		Bouin's; Zenker's Bouin's
	Gram's technique		Zenker's Bouin's
	Levaditi		Zenker's
	Warthin-Starry	10% NBF	All except preferred
Uric acid crystals	Gomori's methenamine silver for urate	Absolute ethanol	All except preferred
	Gomori's chrome alum hematoxylin-phloxine	Bouin's	Avoid chromates

additional 48 hours, or more, in buffered formaldehyde, before being processed. Embedding may be in celloidin or paraffin. Perfusion fixation of the eye is recommended for studies of the canal of Schlemm and/or the aqueous outflow pathways.

Brain

The problem of fixing a whole brain is to render it firm enough to investigate the neuroanatomy and to produce sections to show histopathology and to respond to immunochemistry if required. Conventionally this fixation takes at least 2 weeks. Adickes et al. (1997) proposed a perfusion technique which allows all of the above to be accomplished and the report issued in 5–6 days. This method depends on the perfusion of the brain via the middle cerebral arteries. Fixatives may also be enhanced by the use of microwave technology (Anonymous 2001; Kok & Boon 2003; Leong 2005). Alcoholic formalin should not be used for fixation if immunohistochemistry is to be performed using biotin-avidin (streptavidin) methods (Grizzle et al., unpublished data).

Breast

Clinical samples should be fixed in 10% NBF for between a minimum of 6–8 hours and a maximum of 72 hours, and should be sliced at 5mm intervals after appropriate gross inspection and margins designation. Time from tissue acquisition to fixation should be as short as possible in order to prevent lysis of clinically important biomarkers, such as estrogen receptors, progesterone receptors and the human epidermal growth factor receptor-2 (HER2). They should be placed in a sufficient volume of NBF to allow adequate tissue penetration. If the tumor specimen has come from a remote geographical location, it should be bisected through the tumor on removal and sent to the laboratory immersed in a sufficient volume of NBF (Hammond et al., 2010).

Lungs

Lung biopsies are typically fixed in NBF. The lungs from autopsies may be inflated by and fixed in NBF via the trachea or major bronchi, and in our experience these lungs can be cut within 2 hours. Gross sections are fixed overnight and sections to be processed and cut the next day.

Lymphoid tissue

Special care should be taken with all lymphoid tissue, as many organisms (e.g. *Mycobacterium tuberculosis* and viruses) may sequester themselves in the lymphoid reticular system. The lymphoid tissue is usually sliced and a representative sample of fresh tissue taken for special studies (e.g. flow cytometry or molecular analysis). The rest of the lymph node is fixed in NBF, though some laboratories fix part of the tissue in B5 or zinc.

Testis

Biopsies of the testes are fixed routinely in NBF.

Muscle biopsies

Biopsies of muscle are received fresh. A portion is separated for enzyme histochemistry. The tissue for routine histological assessment is fixed in NBF and embedded so the fibers of the specimens are viewed in cross-section and longitudinally. After processing this is stained with H&E, a trichrome stain, and Congo red if amyloid is suspected.

Renal biopsies

Renal core biopsies should be subdivided into three and each piece should contain adequate numbers of glomeruli. Each portion is then preserved, depending upon the method to be used for analysis:

- NBF for routine histology
- Buffered glutaraldehyde (pH 7.3) for ultrastructural analysis
- Snap frozen in isopentane and liquid nitrogen for immunofluorescence examination.

Useful formulae for fixatives

Gray (1954) lists over 600 formulations for various fixatives. The following is a list of the fixatives and formulae most commonly used by biomedical scientists and histotechnologists. Many of these formulae are based on those presented in standard textbooks of histochemistry (Sheehan & Hrapchak 1980; Carson 1990; Kiernan 1999). They vary slightly from text to text, but these variations are unlikely to cause problems.

For routine histology, 10% neutral buffered formalin (NBF) is frequently used for initial fixation and for the first station on tissue processors. NBF is composed of a 10% solution of phosphate buffered formaldehyde. Formaldehyde is commercially supplied as a 37–40% solution and in the following formulae is referred to as 37% formaldehyde.

Neutral buffered 10% formalin

Tap water	900 ml
Formalin (37% formaldehyde solution)	100 ml
Sodium phosphate, monobasic, monohydrate	4 g
Sodium phosphate, dibasic, anhydrous	6.5 g

The pH should be 7.2–7.4

There are other formulations of NBF and related fixatives. NBF purchased from commercial companies may vary widely in its aldehyde content, and commercial companies may add material such as methanol (Fox et al. 1985) or other agents to stabilize NBF preparations.

Carson's modified Millonig's phosphate buffered formalin

Formaldehyde (37–40%)	10 ml
Tap water	90 ml
Sodium phosphate, monobasic	1.86 g
Sodium hydroxide	0.42 g

Deionized water can be used if tap water is hard and/or contains solids. The pH should be 7.2–7.4. This formula is reported to be better for ultrastructural preservation than NBF.

Sometimes the term 'formal' is used to refer to 10% formalin or 37% formaldehyde.

Formal (10% formalin), calcium acetate

Tap water	900 ml
Formaldehyde (37%)	100 ml
Calcium acetate	20 g

This is a good fixative for preservation of lipids.

Formal (10% formalin), saline

Tap water	900 ml
Formaldehyde (37%)	100 ml
Sodium chloride	9 g

Formal (10% formalin), zinc, unbuffered

Tap water	900 ml
Formaldehyde (37%)	100 ml
Sodium chloride	4.5 g
Zinc chloride or (zinc sulfate)	1.6 g (or 3.6 g)

Zinc formalin is reported to be an excellent fixative for immunohistochemistry.

Formalin, buffered saline

Tap water	900 ml
Formaldehyde (37%)	100 ml
Sodium chloride	9 g
Sodium phosphate, dibasic	12 g

Formalin, buffered zinc

10% neutral buffered formalin	1000 ml
Zinc chloride	1.6 g

Mercuric fixatives

A problem with fixation in mercury solutions is that several types of pigment may combine with the mercury. These pigments are removed from sections by using iodine treatment followed by sodium thiosulfate.

Zenker's solution

Distilled water	250 ml
Mercuric chloride	12.5 g
Potassium dichromate	6.3 g
Sodium sulfate	2.5 g

Just before use add 5 ml of glacial acetic acid to 95 ml of above solution. This is a good fixative for bloody (congested) specimens and trichrome stains.

Helly's solution

Distilled water	250 ml
Mercuric chloride	12.5 g

Potassium dichromate   6.3 g
Sodium sulfate   2.5 g

Just before use add 5 ml of 37% formaldehyde to 95 ml of above solution. It is excellent for bone marrow extramedullary hematopoiesis and intercalated discs.

Schaudinn's solution

Distilled water	50 ml
Mercuric chloride	3.5 g
Absolute ethanol	25 ml

Ohlmacher's solution

Absolute ethanol	32 ml
Chloroform	6 ml
Glacial acetic acid	2 ml
Mercuric chloride	8 g

This fixative penetrates rapidly.

Carnoy-Lebrun solution

Absolute ethanol	15 ml
Chloroform	15 ml
Glacial acetic acid	15 ml
Mercuric chloride	8 g

This fixative penetrates rapidly.

B5 fixative

Stock solution:

Mercuric chloride	12 g
Sodium acetate	2.5 g
Distilled water	200 ml

Add 2 ml of formaldehyde (37%) to 20 ml of stock solution just before use.

Frequently used for bone marrow, lymph nodes, spleen, and other hematopoietic tissues.

Dichromate fixatives

There is a variation among the names attributed to the formulae of dichromate fixatives but not in the formulae themselves. Time of fixation (24 hours) is critical for dichromate fixatives. Tissue should be washed after fixation and transferred to 70% ethanol. Failure to wash the tissue after fixation may cause pigments to be precipitated. Extensive shrinkage occurs when tissues are processed to paraffin blocks.

Miller's or Möller's solution

Potassium dichromate	2.5 g
Sodium sulfate	1 g
Distilled water	100 ml

Möller's or Regaud's solution

Potassium dichromate	3 g
Distilled water	80 ml

At time of use add 20 ml of formaldehyde (37%).

Orth's solution

Potassium dichromate	2.5 g
Sodium sulfate	1 g
Distilled water	100 ml

At time of use add 10 ml of formaldehyde (37%).

Lead fixatives

See special fixatives.

Picric acid fixatives

Many picric acid fixatives require a saturated aqueous solution of picric acid. Aqueous picric acid 2.1% will produce a saturated solution and 5% picric acid a saturated solution in absolute ethanol.

Bouin's solution

Saturated aqueous solution of picric acid	1500 ml
Formaldehyde (37%)	500 ml
Glacial acetic acid	100 ml

Bouin's solution is an excellent general fixative for connective tissue stains. The yellow color can be removed with 70% ethanol, lithium carbonate, or another acid dye, separately or during the staining sequence. Bouin's solution destroys membranes; therefore intact nuclei cannot be recovered from Bouin's fixed tissue and there may be extensive shrinkage of larger specimens.

Fixation for fatty tissue

Bouin's solution	75 ml
95% ethanol	25 ml

May require up to 48 hours for good sections of lipomas or well-differentiated liposarcomas.

Note

This chapter is an introduction to fixation. More detailed and advanced issues related to fixation are included in several other texts/references (Sheehan & Hrapchak 1980; Eltoum et al. 2001a, 2001b; Grizzle et al. 2001). As discussed, various formulae may vary within a few percentages, but most of these formulae produce equivalent results.

References

Adickes, E.D., Folkerth, R.D., Sims, K.L., 1997. Use of pro-fusion fixation for improved neuropathologic fixation. Archives of Pathology and Laboratory Medicine 121, 1199–1206.

Anonymous, 2001. Preserve for microwave fixation, vol. 2001. Energy Beam Sciences. Online. Available: http://www.ebsciences.com/microwave/preserve.htm.

Arnold, M.M., Srivastava, S., Fredenburgh, J., et al., 1996. Effects of fixation and tissue processing on immunohistochemical demonstration of specific antigens. Biotechnic and Histochemistry 71, 224–230.

Baker, J.R., 1958. Principles of biological microtechnique: a study of fixation and dyeing. Methuen & Co Ltd, London.

Bayliss High, O.B., Lake, B., 1996. Lipids. In: Bancroft, J.D., Stevens, A. (Eds.), Theory and practice of histological techniques. Churchill-Livingstone, Edinburgh, pp. 213–242.

Bhakuni, V., 1998. Alcohol-induced molten globule intermediates of proteins: are they real folding intermediates or off pathway products? Archives of Biochemistry and Biophysics 357, 274–284.

Carson, F.L., 1990. Histotechnology: a self-instructional text. American Society of Clinical Pathologists, Chicago, IL.

Dapson, R.W., 1993. Fixation for the 1990s: a review of needs and accomplishments. Biotechnic and Histochemistry 68, 75–82.

Eltoum, I.-E., Fredenburgh, J., Grizzle, W.E., 2001a. Advanced concepts in fixation: effects of fixation on immunohistochemistry and histochemistry, reversibility of fixation and recovery of proteins, nucleic acids, and other molecules from fixed and processed tissues, special methods of fixation. Journal of Histotechnology 24, 201–210.

Eltoum, I., Fredenburgh, J., Myers, R.B., Grizzle, W., 2001b. Introduction to the theory and practice of fixation of tissues. Journal of Histotechnology 24, 173–190.

Fox, C.H., Johnson, F.B., Whiting, J., Roller, P.P., 1985. Formaldehyde fixation. Journal of Histochemistry and Cytochemistry 33, 845–853.

Fraenkel-Conrat, H., Mecham, D.K., 1949. The reaction of formaldehyde with proteins. VII. Demonstration of intermolecular cross-linking by means of osmotic pressure measurements. Journal of Biological Chemistry 177, 477–486.

Fraenkel-Conrat, H., Olcott, H.S., 1948a. The reaction of formaldehyde with proteins. V. Cross-linking between amino and primary amide or guanidyl groups. Journal of the American Chemical Society 70, 2673–2684.

Fraenkel-Conrat, H., Olcott, H.S., 1948b. Reactions of formaldehyde with proteins. VI. Cross-linking of amino groups with phenol, imidazole, or indole groups. Journal of Biological Chemistry 174, 827–843.

Fraenkel-Conrat, H., Cooper, M., Olcott, H.S., 1945. The reaction of formaldehyde with proteins. Journal of the American Chemical Society 67, 950–954.

Fraenkel-Conrat, H., Brandon, B.A., Olcott, H.S., 1947. The reaction of formaldehyde with proteins. IV. Participation of indole groups. Gramacidin. Journal of Biological Chemistry 168, 99–118.

Potassium dichromate	6.3 g
Sodium sulfate	2.5 g

Just before use add 5 ml of 37% formaldehyde to 95 ml of above solution. It is excellent for bone marrow extramedullary hematopoiesis and intercalated discs.

Schaudinn's solution

Distilled water	50 ml
Mercuric chloride	3.5 g
Absolute ethanol	25 ml

Ohlmacher's solution

Absolute ethanol	32 ml
Chloroform	6 ml
Glacial acetic acid	2 ml
Mercuric chloride	8 g

This fixative penetrates rapidly.

Carnoy-Lebrun solution

Absolute ethanol	15 ml
Chloroform	15 ml
Glacial acetic acid	15 ml
Mercuric chloride	8 g

This fixative penetrates rapidly.

B5 fixative

Stock solution:

Mercuric chloride	12 g
Sodium acetate	2.5 g
Distilled water	200 ml

Add 2 ml of formaldehyde (37%) to 20 ml of stock solution just before use.

Frequently used for bone marrow, lymph nodes, spleen, and other hematopoietic tissues.

Dichromate fixatives

There is a variation among the names attributed to the formulae of dichromate fixatives but not in the formulae themselves. Time of fixation (24 hours) is critical for dichromate fixatives. Tissue should be washed after fixation and transferred to 70% ethanol. Failure to wash the tissue after fixation may cause pigments to be precipitated. Extensive shrinkage occurs when tissues are processed to paraffin blocks.

Miller's or Möller's solution

Potassium dichromate	2.5 g
Sodium sulfate	1 g
Distilled water	100 ml

Möller's or Regaud's solution

Potassium dichromate	3 g
Distilled water	80 ml

At time of use add 20 ml of formaldehyde (37%).

Orth's solution

Potassium dichromate	2.5 g
Sodium sulfate	1 g
Distilled water	100 ml

At time of use add 10 ml of formaldehyde (37%).

Lead fixatives

See special fixatives.

Picric acid fixatives

Many picric acid fixatives require a saturated aqueous solution of picric acid. Aqueous picric acid 2.1% will produce a saturated solution and 5% picric acid a saturated solution in absolute ethanol.

Bouin's solution

Saturated aqueous solution of picric acid	1500 ml
Formaldehyde (37%)	500 ml
Glacial acetic acid	100 ml

Bouin's solution is an excellent general fixative for connective tissue stains. The yellow color can be removed with 70% ethanol, lithium carbonate, or another acid dye, separately or during the staining sequence. Bouin's solution destroys membranes; therefore intact nuclei cannot be recovered from Bouin's fixed tissue and there may be extensive shrinkage of larger specimens.

Hollande's solution

Distilled water	1000 ml
Formaldehyde (37%)	100 ml
Acetic acid	15 ml
Picric acid	40 g
Copper acetate	25 g

A useful fixative for gastrointestinal biopsies and endocrine tissue; specimens are washed before exposure to NBF.

Dehydrant fixatives

Dehydrant fixatives act to remove free and bound water, causing a change to the tertiary structure of proteins so that they precipitate, leaving the nucleic acids relatively unchanged. Ultrastructure is destroyed by any of these four dehydrants due to the extraction of lipids, and each may cause excessive shrinking of tissue components after more than 3–4 hours of fixation. Each of these fixatives can be modified by adding other chemicals to produce specific effects.

1. Ethanol, absolute
2. Ethanol, 95%
3. Ethanol, 70–95%
4. Methanol, 100%
5. Acetone, 100%

Methanol is useful for touch preparations and smears, especially blood smears. Many alcohol mixtures may undergo slow reactions among ingredients upon long-term storage; in general most alcohol-based fixatives should be prepared no more than 1–2 days before use. Acetone fixation should be short (1 hour) at 4°C only on small specimens. Acetone produces extensive shrinkage and hardening, and results in microscopic distortion. It is used for immunohistochemistry, enzyme studies, and in the detection of rabies. Cold acetone is especially useful to 'open' the membranes of intact cells (e.g. grown on coverslips or microscope slides) to facilitate entrance of large molecules (e.g. antibodies for immunohistochemical studies). 'Trade secret' ingredients stabilize commercial formulations.

Clarke's solution

Absolute ethanol	60 ml
Glacial acetic acid	20 ml

This solution produces good general histological results for H&E stains. It has the advantage of preserving nucleic acids while lipids are extracted. A short fixation is recommended and tissues are transferred to 95% ethanol following fixation.

Carnoy's fixative

Acetic acid	10 ml
Absolute ethanol	60 ml
Chloroform	30 ml

Carnoy's fixative is useful for RNA stains, e.g. methyl green pyronine, and for glycogen preservation. It shrinks and hardens tissues and hemolyzes red blood cells. It may destroy the staining of acid-fast bacilli. It is useful in cytology to clear heavily blood-stained specimens.

Methacarn

Acetic acid	10 ml
100% methanol	60 ml
Chloroform	30 ml

Causes less hardening and less shrinkage than Carnoy's, but with the same pattern of staining.

Dehydrant cross-linking fixatives

Compound fixatives with both dehydrant and cross-linking actions include alcohol-formalin mixtures. Alcohol-formalin fixation or post-fixation can be advantageous in large specimens with extensive fat. Lymph nodes can be detected much more easily in specimens with alcohol-formalin fixation due to the extraction of lipids and to texture differences compared with tissues fixed in NBF. The preparation of alcohol-formaldehyde solutions is complex, especially buffered forms of this compound fixative. It is probably best to purchase commercial preparations of buffered alcohol-formaldehyde. For use in post-fixation (e.g. after 10% NBF), Carson (1990) recommends the following formula:

Absolute ethanol	650 ml
Distilled water	250 ml
Formaldehyde (37%)	100 ml

Carson recommends this formula because she noted that the concentration of ethanol should be less than 70% to prevent the precipitation of phosphates in 10% NBF saturated tissues. For initial fixation the following formulae can be used:

Alcoholic formalin

Ethanol (95%)	895 ml
Formaldehyde (37%)	105 ml

Alcohol-formalin-acetic acid fixative

Ethanol (95%)	85 ml
Formaldehyde (37%)	10 ml
Glacial acetic acid	5 ml

Methanol may be substituted for ethanol with care; similarly, various mixtures of ethanol, acetic acid, and formalin may be used.

Alcoholic Bouin's (Gendre's solution)

This fixative is similar to Bouin's except it is less aqueous and there is better retention in tissues of some carbohydrates (e.g. glycogen). Fixation should be between 4 hours and overnight followed by washing in 70% ethanol, followed by 95% ethanol (several changes). This is the one alcoholic fixative that improves upon aging (Lillie & Fullmer 1976).

Gendre's solution

95% ethanol saturated with picric acid (5 g per 100 ml)	800 ml
Formaldehyde (37%)	150 ml
Glacial acetic acid	50 ml

To increase the effectiveness of alcoholic Bouin's, if there is no time for aging, the following formula has been recommended (Gregory 1980):

Equivalent to aged alcoholic Bouin's

Picric acid	0.5 g
Formaldehyde (37%)	15 ml
95% ethanol	25 ml

Glacial acetic acid	5 ml
Ethyl acetate	25 ml
Tap water	30 ml

Another alcoholic form of Bouin's solution is as follows:

Stock Bouin's solution	75 ml
95% ethanol	25 ml

This solution is excellent for lymph nodes (24 hours) and for fatty tissue (48 hours).

A closely related fixative is:

Rossman's solution

Tap water	10 ml
Formaldehyde (37%)	10 ml
Absolute ethanol	80 ml
Lead nitrate	8 g

Fix for 24 hours at room temperature. This is a good fixative for connective tissue mucins and umbilical cord.

For metabolic bone disease

Phosphate buffer

Tap water	1000 ml
$NaH_2PO_4 \cdot H_2O$	1.104 g
$NaHPO_4$ (anhydrous)	4.675 g

Fixative

Phosphate buffer	900 ml
Formaldehyde (37%)	100 ml

Adjust pH to 7.35.

Fixation and decalcification

Bouin's decalcifying solution

Saturated aqueous solution of picric acid (10.5 g per 500 ml)	500 ml
Formaldehyde (37%)	167 ml
Formic acid	33 ml

Fixation for fatty tissue

Bouin's solution	75 ml
95% ethanol	25 ml

May require up to 48 hours for good sections of lipomas or well-differentiated liposarcomas.

Note

This chapter is an introduction to fixation. More detailed and advanced issues related to fixation are included in several other texts/references (Sheehan & Hrapchak 1980; Eltoum et al. 2001a, 2001b; Grizzle et al. 2001). As discussed, various formulae may vary within a few percentages, but most of these formulae produce equivalent results.

References

Adickes, E.D., Folkerth, R.D., Sims, K.L., 1997. Use of pro-fusion fixation for improved neuropathologic fixation. Archives of Pathology and Laboratory Medicine 121, 1199–1206.

Anonymous, 2001. Preserve for microwave fixation, vol. 2001. Energy Beam Sciences. Online. Available: http://www.ebsciences.com/microwave/preserve.htm.

Arnold, M.M., Srivastava, S., Fredenburgh, J., et al., 1996. Effects of fixation and tissue processing on immunohistochemical demonstration of specific antigens. Biotechnic and Histochemistry 71, 224–230.

Baker, J.R., 1958. Principles of biological microtechnique: a study of fixation and dyeing. Methuen & Co Ltd, London.

Bayliss High, O.B., Lake, B., 1996. Lipids. In: Bancroft, J.D., Stevens, A. (Eds.), Theory and practice of histological techniques. Churchill-Livingstone, Edinburgh, pp. 213–242.

Bhakuni, V., 1998. Alcohol-induced molten globule intermediates of proteins: are they real folding intermediates or off pathway products? Archives of Biochemistry and Biophysics 357, 274–284.

Carson, F.L., 1990. Histotechnology: a self-instructional text. American Society of Clinical Pathologists, Chicago, IL.

Dapson, R.W., 1993. Fixation for the 1990s: a review of needs and accomplishments. Biotechnic and Histochemistry 68, 75–82.

Eltoum, I.-E., Fredenburgh, J., Grizzle, W.E., 2001a. Advanced concepts in fixation: effects of fixation on immunohistochemistry and histochemistry, reversibility of fixation and recovery of proteins, nucleic acids, and other molecules from fixed and processed tissues, special methods of fixation. Journal of Histotechnology 24, 201–210.

Eltoum, I., Fredenburgh, J., Myers, R.B., Grizzle, W., 2001b. Introduction to the theory and practice of fixation of tissues. Journal of Histotechnology 24, 173–190.

Fox, C.H., Johnson, F.B., Whiting, J., Roller, P.P., 1985. Formaldehyde fixation. Journal of Histochemistry and Cytochemistry 33, 845–853.

Fraenkel-Conrat, H., Mecham, D.K., 1949. The reaction of formaldehyde with proteins. VII. Demonstration of intermolecular cross-linking by means of osmotic pressure measurements. Journal of Biological Chemistry 177, 477–486.

Fraenkel-Conrat, H., Olcott, H.S., 1948a. The reaction of formaldehyde with proteins. V. Cross-linking between amino and primary amide or guanidyl groups. Journal of the American Chemical Society 70, 2673–2684.

Fraenkel-Conrat, H., Olcott, H.S., 1948b. Reactions of formaldehyde with proteins. VI. Cross-linking of amino groups with phenol, imidazole, or indole groups. Journal of Biological Chemistry 174, 827–843.

Fraenkel-Conrat, H., Cooper, M., Olcott, H.S., 1945. The reaction of formaldehyde with proteins. Journal of the American Chemical Society 67, 950–954.

Fraenkel-Conrat, H., Brandon, B.A., Olcott, H.S., 1947. The reaction of formaldehyde with proteins. IV. Participation of indole groups. Gramacidin. Journal of Biological Chemistry 168, 99–118.

French, D., Edsall, J.T., 1945. The reactions of formaldehyde with amino acids and proteins. Advances in Protein Chemistry 2, 277–333.

Goldstein, N.S., Ferkowicz, M., Odish, E., et al., 2003. Minimum formalin fixation time for consistent estrogen receptor immunohistochemical staining of invasive breast cancer. American Journal of Clinical Pathology 120, 86–92.

Gray, P., 1954. The microanatomist's formulary and guide. The Blakiston Co., McGraw-Hill, New York, NY.

Gregory, R.E., 1980. Alcoholic Bouin fixation of insect nervous systems for Bodian silver staining. I. Composition of 'aged' fixative. Stain Technology 55, 143–149.

Grizzle, W.E., 1996a. Theory and practice of silver staining in histopathology. Journal of Histotechnology 19, 183–195.

Grizzle, W.E., 1996b. Silver staining methods to identify cells of the dispersed neuroendocrine system. Journal of Histotechnology 19, 225–234.

Grizzle, W.E., Fredenburgh, J., 2001. Avoiding biohazards in medical, veterinary and research laboratories. Biotechnic and Histochemistry 76, 183–206.

Grizzle, W.E., Fredenburgh, J., 2005. Safety in biomedical and other laboratories. In: Patrinos, G., Ansorg, W., (Eds.), Molecular diagnostics, Ch. 33, pp. 421–428.

Grizzle, W.E., Myers, R.B., Oelschlager, D.K., 1995. Prognostic biomarkers in breast cancer: factors affecting immunohistochemical evaluation. Breast 1, 243–250.

Grizzle, W.E., Myers, R.B., Manne, U., 1997. The use of biomarker expression to characterize neoplastic processes. Biotechnic and Histochemistry 72, 96–104.

Grizzle, W.E., Myers, R.B., Manne, U., et al., 1998a. Factors affecting immunohistochemical evaluation of biomarker expression in neoplasia. In: Hanausek, M., Walaszek, Z. (Eds.), John Walker's methods in molecular medicine–tumor marker protocols, vol. 14. Humana Press, Totowa, NJ, pp. 161–179.

Grizzle, W.E., Myers, R.B., Manne, U., Srivastava, S., 1998b. Immunohistochemical evaluation of biomarkers in prostatic and colorectal neoplasia. In: Hanausek, M., Walaszek, Z. (Eds.), John Walker's methods in molecular medicine–tumor marker protocols, vol. 14. Humana Press, Totowa, NJ, pp. 143–160.

Grizzle, W.E., Stockard, C., Billings, P., 2001. The effects of tissue processing variables other than fixation on histochemical staining and immunohistochemical detection of antigens. Journal of Histotechnology 24, 213–219.

Gustavson, K.H., 1956. The chemistry of tanning processes. Academic Press, New York, NY.

Habeeb, A.F., 1966. Determination of free amino groups in proteins by trinitrobenzenesulfonic acid. Analytical Biochemistry 14, 328–336.

Hammond, E.H., Hayes, D.F., Dowsett, M., et al., 2010. American Society of Clinical Oncology/College of American Pathologists guideline recommendations for immunohistochemical testing of estrogen/progesterone receptors in breast cancer. J Clin Oncol 28, 2784–2795.

Hayat, M.A., 1981. Principles and techniques of electron microscopy. Biological applications, second ed. University Park Press, Baltimore, MD, Vol. 1.

Helander, K.G., 1994. Kinetic studies of formaldehyde binding in tissue. Biotechnic and Histochemistry 69, 177–179.

Herskovits, T.T., Gadegbeku, B., Jaillet, H., 1970. On the structural stability and solvent denaturation of proteins. I. Denaturation by the alcohols and glycols. Journal of Biological Chemistry 245, 2588–2598.

Hopwood, D., 1969. Fixatives and fixation: a review. Histochemical Journal 1, 323–360.

Hopwood, D., 1973. Fixation with mercury salts. Acta Histochemica (Suppl) 13, 107–118.

Hopwood, D., 1985. Cell and tissue fixation, 1972–1982. Histochemical Journal 17, 389–442.

Hopwood, D., 2002. Fixation and fixatives. In: Bancroft, J.D., Gamble, M. (Eds.), Theory and practice of histological techniques. Churchill Livingstone, London, pp. 63–84.

Hopwood, D., Milne, G., Penston, J., 1990. A comparison of microwaves and heat alone in the preparation of tissue for electron microscopy. Journal of Histochemistry 22, 358–364.

Horobin, R.W., 1982. Histochemistry: an explanatory outline of histochemistry and biophysical staining. Gustav Fischer, Stuttgart.

Jewell, S.D., Srinivasan, M., McCart, L.M., et al., 2002. Analysis of the molecular quality of human tissues: an experience from the Cooperative Human Tissue Network. American Journal of Clinical Pathology 118, 733–741.

Jones, W.T., Stockard, C.R., Grizzle, W.E., 2001. Effects of time and temperature during attachment of sections to microscope slides on immunohistochemical detection of antigens. Biotechnic and Histochemistry 76, 55–58.

Kiernan, J.A., 1999. Histological and histochemical methods: theory and practice, third ed. Butterworth-Heinemann, Oxford, UK.

Kok, L.P., Boon, M.E., 2003. Microwaves for the art of microscopy. Coulomb Press, Leyden.

Leong, A.S.-Y., 2005. Microwave technology for light microscopy and ultrastructural studies. Milestone, Bangkok.

Lhotka, J.F., Ferreira, A.V., 1949. A comparison of deformalinizing technics. Stain Technology 25, 27–32.

Lillie, R.D., Fullmer, H.M., 1976. Histopathologic technic and practical histochemistry, fourth ed. McGraw-Hill, New York.

Lykidis, D., Van Noorden, S., Armstrong, A., et al., 2007. Novel zinc-based fixative for high quality DNA, RNA and protein analysis. Nucleic Acids Research 35, e85, doi: 10.1093/nar/gkm433.

McGhee, J.D., von Hippel, P.H., 1975a. Formaldehyde as a probe of DNA structure. I. Reaction with exocyclic amino groups of DNA bases. Biochemistry 14, 1281–1296.

McGhee, J.D., von Hippel, P.H., 1975b. Formaldehyde as a probe of DNA structure. II.

Reaction with endocyclic imino groups of DNA bases. Biochemistry 14, 1297–1303.

McGhee, J.D., von Hippel, P.H., 1977a. Formaldehyde as a probe of DNA structure. 3. Equilibrium denaturation of DNA and synthetic polynucleotides. Biochemistry 16, 3267–3276.

McGhee, J.D., von Hippel, P.H., 1977b. Formaldehyde as a probe of DNA structure. 4. Mechanism of the initial reaction of formaldehyde with DNA. Biochemistry 16, 3276–3293.

Means, G.E., Feeney, R.E., 1995. Reductive alkylation of proteins. Analytical Biochemistry 224, 1–16.

Medawar, P.B., 1941. The rate of penetration of fixatives. Journal of the Royal Microscopical Society 61, 46–57.

O'Leary, T.J., Mason, J.T., 2004. A molecular mechanism of formalin fixation and antigen retrieval. American Journal of Clinical Pathology 122, 154; author reply 154–155.

Papanikolau, Y., Kokkinidis, M., 1997. Solubility, crystallization and chromatographic properties of macromolecules strongly depend on substances that reduce the ionic strength of the solution. Protein Engineering 10, 847–850.

Pearse, A.G., 1980. Histochemistry, theoretical and applied, Vol. I. Churchill Livingstone, Edinburgh.

Pearse, A.G.E., Stoward, P.J., 1980. Histochemistry, theoretical and applied. Vol. 1. Preparative and optical technology. Vol. 2. Analytical technique. Vol. 3. Enzyme histochemistry. Churchill-Livingstone, Edinburgh.

Rait, V.K., O'Leary, T.J., Mason, J.T., 2004. Modeling formalin fixation and antigen retrieval with bovine pancreatic ribonuclease A: I – structural and functional alterations. Laboratory Investigations 84, 292–299.

Rait, V.K., Zhang, Q., Fabris, D., et al., 2005. Conversions of formaldehyde-modified 2-deoxyadenosine 5′-monophosphate in conditions modeling formalin-fixed tissue dehydration. Journal of Histochemistry and Cytochemistry 54, 301–310.

Sheehan, D.C., Hrapchak, B.B., 1980. Theory and practice of histotechnology, second ed. C.V. Mosby, St. Louis, MO.

Singer, S.J., 1962. The properties of proteins in nonaqueous solvents. Advances in Protein Chemistry 17, 1–68.

Shi, S.R., Key, M.E., Kalra, K.L., 1991. Antigen retrieval in formalin fixed, paraffin tissues: an enhancement method for immunohistochemical staining based on microwave oven heating of tissue sections. J Histochem Cytochem 39, 741–748.

Steg, A., Wang, W., Blanquicett, C., et al., 2006. Multiple gene expression analyses in paraffin–embedded tissues by TaqMan low-density array: application to hedgehog and wnt pathway analysis in ovarian endometrioid adenocarcinoma. Journal of Molecular Diagnostics 8, 76–83.

Taylor, C.R., Burns, J., 1974. The demonstration of plasma cells and other immunoglobulin-containing cells of formalin-fixed and paraffin-embedded tissues using peroxidase-labelled antibody. J Clin Pathol 27, 14–20.

Tome, Y., Hirohashi, S., Noguchi, M., Shimosato, Y., 1990. Preservation of cluster 1 small cell lung cancer antigen in zinc-formalin fixative and its application to immunohistological diagnosis. Histopathology 16, 469–474.

The gross room/surgical cut-up 5

S. Kim Suvarna • Christopher Layton

Introduction

The dissection and preparation of any specimen for histological/microscopic analysis involves more than simply the tissue processing and section cutting. Whilst the dissection and laboratory area are often perceived as the key elements of the department, it must be clearly understood that there are many other steps that follow specimen receipt. Some are specific to tissue selection and handling, and others are clearly support role in type. It is also implicit that a good laboratory will be adequately staffed by appropriately trained scientific/medical and support staff (secretarial, medical laboratory assistants, administration, etc.), as they interface at multiple levels with pathological sample handling. Indeed, a poorly staffed department will perform weakly – at best.

Safety first and last

The histopathology department is rich in hazards (e.g. biological, chemical, radiation). These are also risks reflecting the range of materials used to store, process and analyze tissues. These may be toxic, flammable, allergic, carcinogenic, electrical, etc. Furthermore, the presence of sharp cutting implements, complex machinery and the movement of the specimens around the laboratory needs staff to be fully trained and aware of all these potential hazards. Every laboratory should have accessible and clear standard operating procedures (SOPs, see Chapter 1), of which many will reflect national/international guidelines (websites 1–3). Ongoing safety education is required and caution should be employed at every step of specimen handling for safe laboratory practice (websites 2 and 4).

Specimen reception

A separate room is required for specimen reception, acting as the interface between hospital staff (or other visitors) and the pathological laboratory. Appropriate benching and good lighting must be available, along with good ventilation, safety equipment, disinfectants, absorption granules and protective clothing. In the event of specimen spillage (i.e., body fluids, fixative leakage or other mishap), the immediate response by staff will limit any potential local health risk, and also prevent risk to other laboratory personnel.

The key point of this room is to receive samples safely and securely. The specimen should be confirmed in terms of the identity and to be assigned a unique laboratory specimen identifier – usually a complex number. Correlation of the specimen against the clinical request form is mandatory, along with checking of appropriate clinical details mentioned against the specimen. Corroborative data in the form of the hospital number/registration index, national patient identifier number, the full name, date of birth and address are also valid ways of verifying the identity of any specimen. Multiple sources of cross reference are advocated, and if there is any doubt with regard to the probity of specimen then it should not be passed onwards until the clinician concerned has confirmed the appropriate details and probity of the sample.

In many situations the two-person rule is best followed, with two independent laboratory practitioners verifying the various details of the specimen – at all the different stages of examination. Confirmation of a minimum of three unique identifiers (as detailed above) is advisable. Once validated and identified, the case can be passed to the dissection room for examination, specimen description and block sampling.

The usual method of specimen identification is simply the year (expressed usually in two digits) with a sequential numbering system starting with one (1) and proceeding up to the final specimen of each year. There may be a check digit, usually in the form of a letter applied, but this simple system allows surgical pathology samples to be processed with ease and to be correlated against paraffin blocks, photographs and other tests (see below). Thus, case 2345 L/12 is the two thousand, three hundred and forty-fifth sample of the year 2012. The letter suffix (L) is a computer check datum to verify that the numerical data is valid.

Particular attention must be paid to cases with unusual names, or contrastingly, very common names. Names which have a variety of different spellings and any specimens that have incomplete information should be very carefully considered before being accepted.

In some cases multiple specimens from a single patient may be received on the same day for analysis. Some laboratories prefer to annotate each sample with a separate number. However, a single laboratory number may suffice, but with sub-parts of the specimen being separately designated (e.g., sample A, sample B, etc.). Within this framework, if multiple blocks were taken from a sub-part of the specimen then these can be designated with individual numbers/letters in a similar ascending fashion. Thus, a gastrectomy sample with lymph node groups and the spleen could have one case number, multiple sub-part specimens and multiple blocks that can be correlated against the surgeon's operative dissection. For example, using the number described above, the spleen in this case could be being designated 2345 L/12.C.2 (C. indicating the sub-part of the third sample = spleen; and the block number = 2).

Barcodes can be used where appropriate facilities exist, but in general terms many laboratories still have paper request forms that will accompany the specimen as it passes through the laboratory and towards final report emission.

Surgical cut-up/specimen dissection/grossing

The ideal layout of this room is a matter of debate, varying between different laboratories and pathologists' needs. There are multiple different design solutions existing around the general principles of a histology laboratory (Rosai 2004, Cook 2006, websites 2, 4), but it is imperative that the dissection area must have good lighting, good ventilation, non-absorbent wipe-clean surfaces, appropriate protective clothing for the laboratory personnel, gloves and other equipment (photography, tissue macerators, disposal bins). The dissection room should be a comfortable environment permitting undisturbed work by the pathologist and support technical staff. Given that the range of specimens received in most laboratories is wide, the technical staff will have to be familiar with the various requirements of different specimens that guide their subsequent handling and pathological preparation.

It is a matter of preference whether the operators within this environment sit or stand, and ideally both options should be available. Modern dissection areas often have integrated dissection desks, enclosed fluid/fixative feeds and laminar downdraft ventilation (website 5) in order to protect both the dissector and support staff from formalin vapor. All tools and materials should be ergonomically accessible. The room should have good natural and/or electric lighting (Fig. 5.1).

Thinking before dissection

Prior to fixation it may be relevant to reserve some tissue from the specimens for microbiology assessment (being placed into appropriate culture media) and/or electron microscopy (requiring

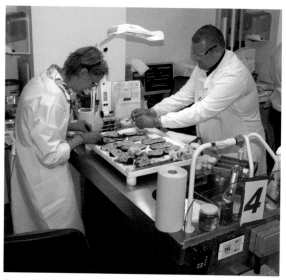

Figure 5.1 A pathology dissection station with a downdraft ventilated bench and clear dissection zone. Note the well-lit and ergonomic layout for the grossing pathologist and the technician support. (Grateful thanks are expressed to Dr Caroline Verbeke and Mr Jonathan Sheriff for their assistance and consent for the illustration.)

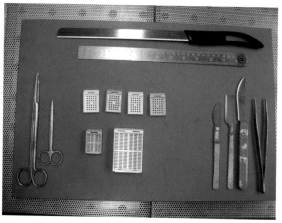

Figure 5.2 Cut-up/grossing tools. A range of small and large bladed tools are advocated along with forceps, ruler and a fluid-resistant dissecting surface. An appropriate measure and access to photography are needed. Varying sizes of cassette (centrally) are available, in a range of colors and sizes, to permit handling of varying amounts of sample and also to indicate handling issues that follow tissue processing.

glutaraldehyde fixation). Fresh tissue can be taken for DNA extraction, cytogenetics and molecular pathology techniques. Other specialized tests (e.g., mass spectroscopy) may also require tissue retention before standard formalin fixation. Some samples need fixation and then decalcification in EDTA (*see section later in the book*).

Some specimens are only examined by means of macroscopic assessment, possibly with photography and other physical techniques. Examples include various mechanical/prosthetic implants, metal bodies, bullets, gallstones and medical devices. These must be dealt with according to the needs of the request/case. It should be noted that some specimens may require retention for a prolonged period of time – as in cases of forensic/criminal investigation.

This dissection/blocking/grossing/cut-up facility must have an appropriate storage area immediately to hand. This allows clearance of examined samples promptly, without the dissecting area becoming cluttered.

The individual choice of dissecting tools will reflect the type of specimen being considered

(Fig. 5.2). However, a range of cutting blades is advised, enabling the dissector to deal with small specimens through to complex and large resections. Very large knives are particularly useful for obtaining full transverse sections of organs (lungs, liver, etc.). The smaller blades are useful for precise trimming of tissues. However, before any knife is put to the specimen, it is emphasized that the tissue specimen should be well fixed. Forceps and absorbent cloths should be available. The blocks taken (vi) should not completely fill the cassette (Fig. 5.3) as this would impede processing fluid access to the tissue. Thus, tissue cassettes are generally made of plastic and conform to a variety of size standards across the developed world nowadays. Most standard blocks allow a sample of about $20 \times 20 \times 3$ mm thick tissue to be contained and processed. There is variation in cassette size that does allow larger blocks to be selected (Fig. 5.2). This is particularly useful for histological examination of large surgical resections where the global geography of the specimen is needed for analysis. Examples could include rectal cancer resection, radical prostatectomy and autopsy lung tissue for industrial disease. However,

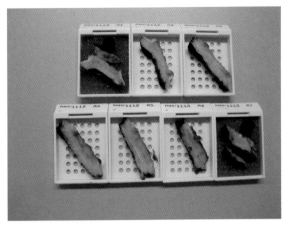

Figure 5.3 Tissue blocks are placed into the cassette. Note they should not fill the cassette, and must permit room for processing fluid circulation. The orientation of the blocks is enhanced by a sponge securing the specimens in sequential position and a colored agar marker allows designation of the order of slices taken. The samples have been marked with different colored inks to permit designation of the sidedness of the samples and the resection margins.

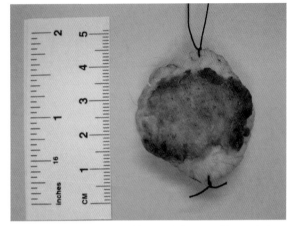

Figure 5.4 A medium-sized skin sample is seen with a central lesion. This could be described as 'A skin ellipse x by y by z mm depth is seen with an orientation suture, designated 12 o'clock. The sample shows a central yellow-brown nodule z mm that is k mm clear of the closest margin'. It is sectioned into parallel slices and then placed into a cassette (see Fig. 5.3).

some general rules can be developed to specimen handling/sampling.

The specimens should be analyzed with only one pot open at any one time. The request and specimen identity should be checked. The sample should be described in terms of the shape, size and defining characteristics of the specimen. This means that small biopsies, for example endoscopic mucosal samples, may simply be afforded a simple descriptor in the form of the number of pieces and the size (SI units, usually mm) of the largest piece of tissue. An example could be 'three pieces of brown tissue, the largest 3 mm diameter'.

Medium and large specimens (Fig. 5.4) need more detailed and careful description of the various anatomical components, together with identification of macroscopic landmarks, orientation markers/sutures and the lesion/s as relevant. The background tissues, beyond the lesion under consideration, also require description. The sampling of any large case/resection should follow local/national guidelines in order to provide the relevant information for subsequent clinical management of the patient (website 6).

Any macroscopic description is usually dictated for subsequent secretarial transcription, or on occasion can be simply written down for typing later. Canned/proforma reports may be of value to standardize the approach to samples. The departmental computer system can be set to track specimen movement through the laboratory, from receipt to final pathologist report authorization. Photographing the macroscopic specimen is particularly important in cases of complex surgical excision (e.g. Wertheim's hysterectomy, pneumonectomy, AP resection, etc.), and may be of use in later analysis/case discussion (Fig. 5.5). The availability of cheap and reliable digital photography has been a major bonus to the laboratory, permitting verification of the image being captured. Nevertheless, specialist photography may still be required for cases that might end up as visual teaching presentation, journal/book illustration publication, or in a medico-legal setting. Consideration of the potential to recognize a patient's sample should be made, with some guidance existing on the subject (website 7).

If one knows beforehand of additional tests that are automatically required on some specimens (such as liver core biopsies requiring multiple ancillary

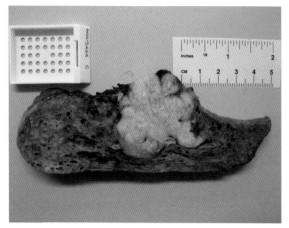

Figure 5.5 A lung lobectomy sample, sliced to show the hilar and mediastinal plane of resection, highlighting tumor adjacent to the margin. Block sampling at this interface and background tissue sampling against standard protocols will allow full analysis. Note the numbered cassette along with the ruler for full case identification and analysis.

histochemical stains) then different color cassettes/ markers can be used in order to designate additional actions that should follow as an automatic laboratory consequence (Fig. 5.2). The different colored cassettes may also indicate the types of section and sections required, as well as the speed/urgency of any specimen.

Following dissection, the residual tissues must be stored in a ventilated secure archive format, and waste materials must be disposed of according to local health and safety regulations (websites 4, 5, 8).

Specimen dissection plans

Small samples

Small biopsy samples rarely need dissection, and can be simply processed, embedded and then sectioned as they present themselves. In some cases orientation of the specimen can be facilitated by means of a dissecting microscope or magnifying lens – such as when considering morphological abnormalities of small bowel biopsies. However, the majority of small biopsies can be adequately examined at multiple levels allowing the pathologist to

mentally reconstruct the three-dimensional quality of the tissue during microscopic examination.

These small samples may benefit from being placed in a nylon bag, between metal disks with fine mesh, within paper, etc., in order to prevent them falling through the cassette perforations and being lost. In some cases, eosin is used as a marker for small samples, in order to highlight them on the background of paper, embedding bench or equivalent. It is recommended that a count of the small tissue biopsy fragments is taken at the description/ grossing stage in order to verify that all the tissue has survived processing prior to section cutting.

Core biopsies

These are treated in a somewhat similar manner, although their embedding requires being laid out in longitudinal fashion so that the plane of section cuts along the majority of the tissue. Larger cores (with diameters of 4–5 mm or greater) may occasionally benefit by division into two halves along the long axis. Alternatively it may be easier to simply provide multiple levels with retention of tissue in between the levels, for adequate analysis. Multiple cores often require each core being placed into individual cassettes.

Skin biopsies

These include simple punch biopsies (handled akin to cores) and shave biopsies that should be mounted on edge in order to provide an adequate view of the epidermis, dermis and subcuticular substrates. A marker item placed into the cassette (e.g., plastic bead or colored paper) will identify such samples to embedding personnel. Alternatively, some laboratories use cheese paste to help maintain specimen orientation (Tripathi et al. 2008). The protein in the paste helps hold the tissue orientation during processing (Fig. 5.6).

Skin samples also include the more complex intermediate and large specimens for removal of defined lesions, right up to radical skin cancer resections including deep soft/bony tissues.

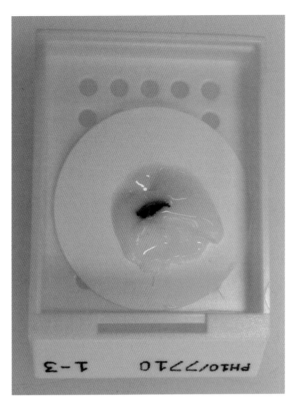

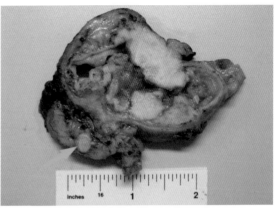

Figure 5.7 A large bowel specimen is seen with anatomical complexity requiring a good description and multiple blocks to be taken for full analysis. This sample shows the resection, opened to visualize the cancer. The specimen has been photographed to facilitate understanding of the local resection margins and the serosal surface (inked). The entire tumor and local bowel can be blocked into a large cassette, if desired. A lymph node (arrowed) is clearly involved by tumor in the fatty serosal tissues, but the fatty mesentery can be removed for fat-clearance nodal identification and analysis.

Figure 5.6 Cheese paste is seen holding the thin fragment of inked skin on edge and in position securely. The cheese protein matrix will survive tissue processing!

The intermediate and larger samples of skin are often presented as an ovoid/ellipse/piece of skin/subcutis, mostly with a central lesion (see Fig. 5.4). These must be described in terms of the width and breadth of the specimen together with a depth. The lesion characteristics (nodule, ulcer, papule, color/margin, etc.) should be discussed. Specimens of these skin resections are often best managed in sequential/serial transverse section, with Indian ink/other dyes being applied to different surfaces in order to confirm the orientation/boundaries of the specimen (Fig 5.3). Markers can be placed into cassettes in order to confirm pieces of tissue with orientation markers, although it is generally found that specimens start with small apical transverse sections through to the broadest point across the waist of the specimen and then taper off towards the other end.

Very large resections of skin with soft tissues may require photography and then targeted block sampling. This should also allow for the appropriate assessment of any tumor/lesion with deep and lateral margin correlation along with multiple blocks of the pathology in order to allow for disease variations that may be present. These samples, and indeed their smaller counterparts, should be blocked to permit reporting against national/international standards.

Bowel specimens

These generally are medium and large tissue resections along the length of the gastrointestinal tract (e.g. partial colectomy/gastrectomy). They are best sampled with multiple (usually n ≥ 3) blocks of any lesion in relation to the adjacent mucosa, wall and serosal aspect tissues (Fig. 5.7), although large geographic blocks can be employed. The margins often need inking and the background tissues including resection margins are often included as part of the relevant dissection protocol (Allen 2006, Allen & Cameron 2004, website 6). Particular attention is paid to the lymph nodes, and these can be either manually dissected in groups, or can be identified from fat-clearance protocols (Prabhudesai et al. 2005) as described below. It is vital that the nodes are assessed in terms of their proximity to the lesion along with their different 'level' stages. Many cases require consideration of the high tie (i.e. the most proximal node in the resection) lymph node (or equivalent).

Fat clearance

Finding lymph nodes within a large amount of fatty mesenteric/soft tissue can be problematic, and the ability to remove the adipose substrate from any specimen will lead to an enhanced rate of node detection and thereby sampling. One aspect of the histological tissue handling in the cut-up room allows such node identification (Prabhudesai et al. 2005). The fatty tissue is usually sliced into 10 mm fragments and placed into large cassettes, thereby increasing the access of solvents to the specimen. Fat removal occurs as part of the processing of tissues, but the blocks of fatty parenchyma are normally removed from the processing chamber before the tissues are impregnated finally with wax. At this stage the lymph nodes can now be readily identified by transillumination of the tissue sample from below (Fig. 5.8). The sampled nodes can then be placed back in the tissue processor in a smaller cassette, with normal embedding, sectioning and staining to follow.

Lung tissues

These generally are performed as localized biopsies or lobectomy/pneumonectomy specimens. The background pleura and lung must be evaluated along with any lesions as required in standard pro-forma sampling protocols (Allen 2006, Allen & Cameron 2004, website 6). In general terms, multiple blocks for any tumor (usually n ≥ 3) along with sampling of pleural/mediastinal/bronchial margins

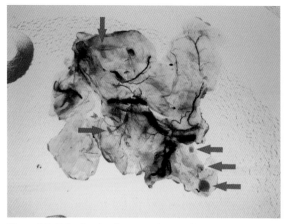

Figure 5.8 Following fat clearance, the transilluminated sample is searched for nodes (arrowed). These are then extracted and placed into smaller cassettes for routine histology assessment after the final stage of processing and embedding.

are needed. Nodes are often presented in groups separately, although careful dissection of the hilar tissues should allow further node harvest from these tissues (Fig. 5.5).

Gynecological samples

Common samples, such as cone biopsies from the cervix, need appropriate inking of margins and orientation, often in a serial block fashion across the specimen with specimen photography. This allows the three-dimensional assessment of dysplasia or invasive neoplasia in relation to the various surgical margins. Uterine samples are usually sampled in terms of background cervix, endometrium and myometrial tissues together with some representative sampling of common benign lesions (fibroids/leiomyomas/etc.). Sampling will be guided by local practice together with national guidelines (Allen 2006, Allen & Cameron 2004, website 6). Dysplastic and malignant lesions often require multiple blocks, resection margins together with careful examination of related lymph nodes (usually presented, and therefore blocked, separately). Specific tissues such as tubes and ovaries should follow similar standard guidelines in terms of the sampling pattern, number of blocks and related tissue samples. It is emphasized that pluripotential differentiation of tumors within the female genital tract requires multiple blocks of a tumor to be taken for full analysis.

Breast resections

These are also common resections, usually with the need for inked margins, in relation to the orientation of the specimen. Multiple blocks of the tumor are usually required. Background tissues at multiple points should be also assessed and the lymph nodes (if present) are often examined in tiered/grouped fashion in order to assess tumor spread up towards the highest-level nodal size. Fat clearance may be required to capture all the nodes in the axillary tail.

Soft tissue resections

These should be examined with multiples blocks of tissue, background parenchyma and the margins. Some experts advocate 1 block for every 10 mm diameter of tumor, up to 10 blocks – although more may be required on occasion. Careful slicing and examination of the specimens macroscopically will allow sampling and consideration of all peripheral boundaries. Furthermore, given the pervasive nature of soft tissue tumors, this widespread sampling is usually required. Tumor sampling before fixation for molecular/genetic analysis may be required.

Other samples

The chapter is not sufficient to discuss all resections and specimen subtypes, and the groups above are illustrative only. The reader is referred to relevant governing bodies/organizations that have produced protocols for the analysis of other specimens (Allen 2006, Allen & Cameron 2004, website 6).

References

Allen, D.C., 2006. Histopathology reporting. Guidelines for surgical cancer, second ed. Springer, London.

Allen, D.C., Cameron, R.I. (Eds.), 2004. Histopathology specimens: clinical, pathological and laboratory aspects. Springer , London.

Cook, D.J., 2006. Some aspects of the organisation of a histology laboratory. In: Cellular pathology, second ed. Scion, Bloxham, Oxfordshire, pp. 357–367.

Prabhudesai, A.G., Dalton, R., Kumar, D., Finlayson, A.G., 2005. Mechanised one-day fat clearance method to increase the lymph node yield in rectal cancer specimens. British Journal of Biomedical Science 62, 120–123.

Rosai, J., 2004. Introduction and gross techniques in surgical pathology. Rosai and Ackerman's surgical pathology, ninth ed. Mosby, Edinburgh, pp. 1–24, 25–36.

Tripathi, M., Sethuraman, C., Lindley, R., Ali, R.B., 2008. Comparison of use of cream cheese and agar gel for orientation of skin biopsies. XXIX Symposium of the ISDP, Graz, Austria, October 2–4, 2008. American Journal of Dermatopathology 30, 514–533.

Websites

1. Clinical Pathology Accreditation (UK) Ltd. http://www.cpa-uk.co.uk/.

2. Institute of Biomedical Science. Good professional practice for biomedical scientists. http://www.ibms.org/go/professional:good-professional-practice.

3. National Pathology Accreditation Advisory Council. Requirements for Pathology Laboratories (2007, second ed.). http://www.health.gov.au/internet/main/publishing.nsf/Content/D34B4BC09A2A254FCA25728400126ED2/$File/dhapathlabs.pdf.

4. Health and Safety Executive. http://www.hse.gov.uk/index.htm.

5. Ventilation in the histopathology laboratory. http://www.afosgroup.com/news/Ventilation%20in%20the%20Histopathology%20Laboratory.pdf.

6. Datasets and tissue pathways. Royal College of Pathologists. http://www.rcpath.org/index.asp?PageID=254.

7. Making and using visual and audio recordings of patients – guidance for doctors. http://www.gmc-uk.org/guidance/ethical_guidance/making_audiovisual.asp.

8. The Human Tissue Act 2004 (Ethical Approval, Exceptions from Licensing and Supply of Information about Transplants) (Amendment) Regulations 2008. http://www.legislation.gov.uk/uksi/2008/3067/pdfs/uksi_20083067_en.pdf.

Tissue processing 6

Lena T. Spencer • John D. Bancroft

INCORPORATING

Microarray

Wanda Grace Jones

Introduction

After the removal of a tissue sample from the patient, a series of physical and chemical processes must take place to ensure that the final microscopic slides produced are of a diagnostic quality. Tissues are exposed to a series of reagents that fix, dehydrate, clear, and infiltrate the tissue. The tissue is finally embedded in a medium that provides support for microtomy. The quality of the structural preservation of tissue components is determined by the choice of exposure times to the reagents during processing. Every step in tissue processing is important; from selection of the sample, determining the appropriate protocols and reagents to use, to staining and final diagnosis. Producing quality slides for diagnosis requires skills that are developed through continued practice and experience. As new technology and instrumentation develops, the role of the histology laboratory in patient care will continue to evolve, providing standardization of processes, increased productivity, and better utilization of the resources available. This chapter will provide an overview of the steps in the process and the reagents needed to prepare tissue for microscopic evaluation.

Labeling of tissues

A unique accession number or code should be assigned to every tissue sample as discussed in Chapter 5. This unique number should accompany the specimens throughout the entire laboratory process and may be electronically or manually generated. New technology has made bar code quick response (QR) and character recognition systems readily available in most laboratories. Automated pre-labeling systems that permanently etch or emboss tissue cassettes and slides, as well as chemically resistant pens, pencils, slides and labels, are routinely used in pathology laboratories. Regardless of whether an automated or manual labeling system is used, adequate policies and procedures must be in place to ensure positive identification of the tissue blocks and slides during processing, diagnosis, and filing.

Principles of tissue processing

Tissue processing is designed to remove all extractable water from the tissue, replacing it with a support medium that provides sufficient rigidity to enable sectioning of the tissue without parenchymal damage or distortion.

Factors influencing the rate of processing

When tissue is immersed in fluid, an interchange occurs between the fluid within the tissue and the surrounding fluid. The rate of fluid exchange is dependent upon the exposed surface of the tissue that is in contact with the processing reagents. Several factors influence the rate at which the interchange occurs: namely, agitation, heat, viscosity and vacuum.

Agitation

Agitation increases the flow of fresh solutions around the tissue. Automated processors incorporate vertical or rotary oscillation, or pressurized removal and replacement of fluids at timed intervals as the mechanism for agitation. Efficient agitation may reduce the overall processing time by up to 30%.

Heat

Heat increases the rate of penetration and fluid exchange. Heat must be used sparingly to reduce the possibility of shrinkage, hardening or embrittlement of the tissue sample. Temperatures limited to 45°C can be used, but higher temperatures may be deleterious to subsequent immunohistochemistry.

Viscosity

Viscosity is the property of resistance to the flow of a fluid. The smaller size of the molecules in the solution, the faster the rate of fluid penetration (low viscosity). Conversely, if the molecule size is larger, the rate of exchange is slower (high viscosity). Most of the solutions used in processing, dehydration and clearing, have similar viscosities, with the exception of cedar wood oil. Embedding mediums have varying viscosities. Paraffin has a lower viscosity in the fluid (melted) state, enhancing the rapidity of the impregnation.

Vacuum

Using pressure to increase the rate of infiltration decreases the time necessary to complete each step in the processing of tissue samples. Vacuum will remove reagents from the tissue, but only if they are more volatile than the reagent being replaced. Vacuum used on the automated processor should not exceed 50.79 kPa to prevent damage and deterioration to the tissue. Vacuum can also aid in the removal of trapped air in porous tissue. Impregnation time for dense, fatty tissue can be greatly reduced with the addition of vacuum during processing.

Stages of tissue processing

- Fixation – stabilizes and hardens tissue with minimal distortion of cells.
- Dehydration – removal of water and fixative from the tissue.
- Clearing – removal of dehydrating solutions, making the tissue components receptive to the infiltrating medium.
- Infiltrating – permeating the tissue with a support medium.
- Embedding – orienting the tissue sample in a support medium and allowing it to solidify.

Fixation

Preserving cells and tissue components with minimal distortion is the most important aim of processing tissue samples. Fixation stabilizes proteins, rendering the cell and its components resistant to further autolysis by inactivating lysosomal enzymes. It also changes the tissues' receptiveness to further processing. Fixation must finish before subsequent steps in the processing schedule are initiated.

If fixation is not complete prior to processing, stations should be designated on the processor for this purpose. If the tissue is inadequately fixed, the subsequent dehydration solutions may complete the process, possibly altering the staining characteristics of the tissue. The size and type of specimen in the tissue cassette determines the time needed for complete fixation and processing. The tissue should be dissected to 2–4 mm in thickness. Care must be taken not to overfill the cassette, as this would impede the flow of reagents around the tissue. If possible, larger and smaller pieces of tissue should be separated and processed using different schedules. The most commonly used reagent for the fixation of histological specimens is 10% neutral buffered formalin (NBF) – see Chapter 4.

Post-fixation treatment

Special fixation techniques may require additional steps before processing is initiated. Picric acid fixatives (Bouin's) form water-soluble picrates making it necessary to place the tissue cassettes directly into 70% alcohol for processing. Alcoholic fixatives, such as Carnoy's fluid, should be placed directly into 100% alcohol. To help in the visualization of small fragments of tissue during embedding, a few drops of 1% eosin can be added to the specimen container 30 minutes prior to processing. The pink color of the tissue remains during processing, but washes out during subsequent staining.

Dehydration

The first stage of processing is the removal of 'free' unbound water and aqueous fixatives from the tissue components. Many dehydrating reagents are hydrophilic ('water loving'), possessing strong polar groups that interact with the water molecules in the tissue by hydrogen bonding. Other reagents affect dehydration by repeated dilution of the aqueous tissue fluids. Dehydration should be accomplished slowly. If the concentration gradient is excessive, diffusion currents across the cell membranes may increase the possibility of cell distortion. For this reason, specimens are processed through a graded series of reagents of increasing concentration. Excessive dehydration may cause the tissue to become hard, brittle and shrunken. Incomplete dehydration will impair the penetration of the clearing reagents into the tissue, leaving the specimen soft and non-receptive to infiltration. There are numerous dehydrating agent; ethanol, ethanol acetone, methanol, isopropyl, glycol and denatured alcohols.

Dehydrating fluids

Ethanol (C_2H_5OH)

Ethanol is a clear, colorless, flammable liquid. It is hydrophilic, miscible with water and other organic solvents, fast-acting and reliable. Aside from its human health-risk potential, ethanol is taxable, controlled by many governments, and therefore requires careful record keeping. Graded concentrations of ethanol are used for dehydration; the tissue is immersed in 70% ethanol in water, followed by 95% and 100% solutions. Ethanol ensures total dehydration, making it the reagent of choice for the processing of electron microscopy specimens. For delicate tissue it is recommended that the processing starts in 30% ethanol.

Industrial methylated spirit (denatured alcohol)

This fluid has the same physical property as ethanol. Denatured alcohol consists of ethanol, with the addition of methanol (about 1%), isopropyl alcohol or a combination of alcohols. For purposes of tissue processing it is used in the same manner as ethanol.

Methanol (CH_3OH)

Methanol is a clear, colorless and flammable fluid that is miscible with water, ethanol and most organic solvents. It is highly toxic but can be substituted for ethanol in processing protocols.

Propan-2-ol, isopropyl alcohol ($CH_3CHOHCH_3$)

Isopropyl alcohol is miscible with water, ethanol and most organic solvents. It is used in microwave processing schedules. Isopropyl alcohol does not cause over-hardening or shrinkage of the tissue.

Butyl alcohol (butanol) (C_4H_9OH)

Used primarily for plant and animal histology. Butyl alcohol is a slow dehydrant causing less shrinkage and hardening of the tissue.

Acetone (CH_3COCH_3)

Acetone is a clear, colorless, flammable fluid that is miscible with water, ethanol and most organic solvents. It is rapid in action, but has poor penetration and causes brittleness in tissues if its use is prolonged. Acetone removes lipids from tissue during processing.

Additives to dehydrating agents

When added to dehydrating agents, phenol acts as a softening agent for hard tissues such as tendon, nail, and dense fibrous tissue and keratin masses. Phenol (4%) should be added to each of the 95% ethanol stations. Alternatively, hard tissue can be immersed in a glycerol/alcohol mixture.

Universal solvents

Universal solvents are no longer used for routine processing due to their hazardous properties, and they should be handled with extreme care. Universal solvents both dehydrate and clear tissues during tissue processing. Dioxane, tertiary butanol and tetrahydrofuran are considered to be universal solvents. They are not recommended for processing delicate tissues due to their hardening properties.

Clearing

Clearing reagents act as an intermediary between the dehydration and infiltration solutions. They should be miscible with both solutions. Most clearants are hydrocarbons with refractive indices similar to protein. When the dehydrating agent has been entirely replaced by most of these solvents the tissue has a translucent appearance: hence the term 'clearing agent'.

The criteria for choosing a suitable clearing agent are:

• rapid penetration of tissues
• rapid removal of dehydrating agent
• ease of removal by melted paraffin wax
• minimal tissue damage
• low flammability
• low toxicity
• low cost

Most clearing agents are flammable liquids, which warrant caution in their use. The boiling point of the clearing agent gives an indication of its speed of replacement by melted paraffin wax. Fluids with a low boiling point are generally more readily replaced. Viscosity influences the speed of penetration of the clearing agent. Prolonged exposure to most clearing agents causes the tissue to become brittle. The time in the clearing agent should be closely monitored to ensure that dense tissue blocks are sufficiently cleared and smaller more fragile tissue blocks are not damaged. Cost should be considered, especially as it relates to disposal of the reagent. Since most clearing agents are aromatic hydrocarbons or short-chain aliphatic hydrocarbons, environmental issues must be addressed. Most institutions have a policy for the storage, disposal and safety requirements for all flammables used in the laboratory.

Clearing agents suitable for routine use

Xylene

Xylene is a flammable, colorless liquid with a characteristic petroleum or aromatic odor, which is miscible with most organic solvents and paraffin wax. It is suitable for clearing blocks that are less than 5 mm in thickness and rapidly replaces alcohol from the tissue. Overexposure to xylene during processing can cause hardening of tissues. It is most commonly used in routine histology laboratories and is also recyclable.

Toluene

This has similar properties to xylene, although it is less damaging with prolonged immersion of tissue. It is more flammable and volatile than xylene.

Chloroform

Chloroform is slower in action than xylene but causes less brittleness. Thicker tissue blocks can be processed, greater than 1 mm in thickness. Tissues placed in chloroform do not become translucent. It is non-flammable but highly toxic, and produces highly toxic phosgene gas when heated. It is most commonly used when processing specimens of the central nervous system.

Xylene substitutes

Xylene substitutes are aliphatic hydrocarbons that exist in long- and short-chained forms. They differ in the number of carbon atoms within the carbon chain. Short-chained aliphatics have the same evaporation properties as xylene, and have no affinity for water. Long-chained aliphatics do not evaporate rapidly and may cause contamination of the paraffin wax on tissue processors.

Citrus fruit oils – limonene reagents

Limonene reagents are extracts from orange and lemon rinds; they are non-toxic and miscible with water. Disposal is dependent upon the water treatment centers and local/national standards. The main disadvantages are that they can cause sensitization and have a strong pungent odor that may cause headaches. Also, small mineral deposits such as copper or calcium may dissolve and leach from tissues. They are extremely oily and cannot be recycled.

Infiltrating and embedding reagents

Paraffin wax

Paraffin wax continues to be the most popular infiltration and embedding medium in histopathology laboratories. Paraffin wax is a mixture of long-chained hydrocarbons produced in the cracking of mineral oil. Its properties are varied depending on the melting point used, ranging from 47 to 64°C. Paraffin wax permeates the tissue in liquid form and solidifies rapidly when cooled. The tissue is impregnated with the medium, forming a matrix and preventing distortion of the tissue structure during microtomy. It has a wide range of melting points, which is important for use in the different climatic regions of the world. To promote desirable ribboning during microtomy, paraffin wax of suitable hardness at room temperature should be chosen. Heating the paraffin wax to a high temperature alters the properties of the wax. Higher melting point paraffin wax provides better support for harder tissues,

e.g. bone, can allow production of thinner sections, but may cause difficulty with ribboning. Lower melting point paraffin wax is softer and provides less support for harder tissues. It is more difficult to obtain thinner sections but ribboning is easier. Paraffin wax is inexpensive, provides quality sections and is easily adaptable to a variety of uses. Paraffin wax is compatible with most routine and special stains, as well as immunohistochemistry protocols.

Paraffin wax additives

Paraffin waxes that contain plasticizers or other resin additives are commercially available, providing a selection that is appropriate for most laboratories. These additives create paraffin waxes with selectable hardness compatible with the tissue to be embedded. The amount of additive will impact the rate of infiltration. Substances added to paraffin wax in the past include beeswax, rubber, ceresin, plastic polymers and diethylene glycol distearate. Many of these additives had a higher melting point than paraffin wax, consequently making the tissue more brittle.

Alternative embedding media

There are occasions when paraffin wax is an unsuitable medium for the type of tissue being processed including:

- Processing reagents remove or destroy tissue components that are the object of investigation, e.g. lipids
- Sections are required to be thinner, e.g. lymph nodes
- The use of heat may adversely affect tissues or enzymes
- The infiltrating medium is not sufficiently hard to support the tissue

Resin

Resin is used exclusively as the embedding medium for electron microscopy (see Chapter 22), ultra-thin sectioning for high resolution and also for undecalcified bone (see Chapter 16).

Agar

Agar gel alone does not provide sufficient support for sectioning tissues. Its main use is as a cohesive agent for small friable pieces of tissue after fixation, a process known as double embedding. Fragments of tissue are embedded in melted agar, allowed to solidify and trimmed for routine processing. A superior, more refined, method is to filter the fixative containing small, friable tissue fragments through a Millipore filter using suction. Molten agar is then carefully poured into the filter apparatus, the agar is left to solidify and the resultant agar pellet is removed and routinely processed and embedded in paraffin wax.

Gelatin

Gelatin is primarily used in the production of sections of whole organs using the Gough-Wentworth technique and in frozen sectioning. It is rarely used.

Celloidin

The use of celloidin or LVN (low viscosity nitrocellulose) is discouraged because of the special requirements needed to house the processing reagents and the limited use these types of sections have in neuropathology. It is rarely used.

Paraffin wax embedding

Embedding involves the enclosing of properly processed, correctly oriented specimens in a support medium that provides external support during microtomy. The embedding media must fill the matrix within the tissue, supporting cellular components. The medium should provide elasticity, resisting section distortion while facilitating sectioning.

Most laboratories use modular embedding centers, consisting of a paraffin dispenser, a cold plate, and a heated storage area for molds and tissue cassettes. Paraffin wax is dispensed automatically from a nozzle into a suitably sized mold. The tissue is oriented in the mold; a cassette is attached, producing a flat block face with parallel sides. The mold is placed on a small cooling area to allow the paraffin wax to solidify. The quick cooling of the wax ensures a small crystalline structure, producing fewer artifacts when sectioning the tissue.

Orientation of tissues

Specimen orientation during embedding is important for the demonstration of proper morphology. Incorrect orientation may result in diagnostic tissue elements being damaged during microscopy or not being evident for pathology review. Products are available that help ensure proper orientation: marking systems, tattoo dyes, biopsy bags, sponges, and papers. Orientation of the tissue should offer the least resistance of the tissue against the knife during sectioning. A margin of embedding medium around the tissue assures support of the tissue.

Tissues requiring special orientation include:

- Tubular structures: cross section of the wall and lumen should be visible; arteries, veins, fallopian tube and vas deferens samples.
- Skin biopsies; shave punch or excisions, cross section of the epidermis, dermis and subcutaneous layers must be visible.
- Intestine, gallbladder, and other epithelial biopsies: cut in a plane at right angles to the surface, and oriented so the epithelial surface is cut last, minimizing compression and distortion of the epithelial layer.
- Muscle biopsies: sections containing both transverse and longitudinal planes.
- Multiple pieces of a tissue are oriented side by side with the epithelial surface facing in the same direction.

Automated tissue processing

The basic principle for tissue processing requires the exchange of fluids using a series of solutions for a predetermined length of time in a controlled environment. For decades, the instrumentation used in tissue processing remained relatively unchanged. Recent advances now include specialty microwave ovens, the emergence of constant throughput processors, and processors with multi-sectioned retorts.

Tissue processors

The carousel-type processor (tissue transfer) and the self-contained fluid exchange systems were the first automated tissue processors used in the histology laboratory. The carousel-type processor transports tissue blocks contained in baskets through a series of reagents housed in stationary containers. The length of time the specimens were submerged in each reagent container was electronically controlled. Earlier models accomplished this step by notching the face of a clock disk. Vertical oscillation or the mechanically raising and lowering of the tissue into the reagent containers provided the agitation needed for the processing of the tissue.

The enclosed, self-contained vacuum tissue processor later became the mainstay of most laboratories. A microprocessor was used to program this instrument. Tissues were loaded into a retort chamber where they remained throughout the process. Reagents and melted paraffin wax were moved sequentially into and out of the retort chamber using vacuum and pressure. Each step could be customized by controlling time, temperature, or pressure/vacuum (P/V). The advantages of this system are that vacuum and heat can be used at any stage, customized schedules for tissue processing are possible, and there is fluid spillage containment and elimination of fumes. These processors usually employ alarm systems and diagnostic programs for troubleshooting any instrumentation malfunction. Newer instrumentation have divided retorts that allows for different programs to run simultaneously, allowing for better utilization of the equipment and providing the opportunity to divide tissue by size. Many processors have solution management systems, allowing reagents to be monitored for purity and to be used for a greater period of time without adversely harming the tissue.

Microwave processors

Microwave ovens specially designed for tissue processing are now common. The microwave oven shortens the processing time from hours to minutes.

Microwave exposure stimulates the diffusion of the solutions into the tissue by increasing the internal heat of the specimen, thus accelerating the reaction. Tissues are manually transferred from container to container of reagent. Most laboratory microwave ovens contain precise temperature controls, timers, and fume extraction systems. The processing time depends on the thickness and density of the specimen. Reagents used for microwave processing include ethanol, isopropanol and proprietary mixtures of alcohol, and paraffin. Graded concentration of solutions is not required. Clearing agents are not necessary because the temperature of the final paraffin step facilitates evaporation of the alcohols from the tissue. Xylene and formalin are not used in this process, which eliminates toxic fumes and carcinogens. Properly controlled processing provides uncompromised morphology and antigenicity of the specimens. Increased efficiency through improved turnaround times, environmentally friendly reagents, and greater profitability due to reduction in number and volume of reagents are advantages of this system. Disadvantages of the system include the fact that the process is labor intensive because the solutions are manually manipulated, temperatures must be maintained between 70 and 85°C, and the size of tissue sample is critical (2 mm). Also the cost of laboratory-grade microwaves may be prohibitive, and proper use of the microwave oven requires careful calibration and monitoring.

Alternative rapid processors

Advances in technology have led to the development of a 'continuous input rapid tissue processor'. The enclosed processor uses microwave technology, vacuum infiltration and proprietary reagents which are described as being 'molecular-friendly'. A robotic arm moves the tissue cassettes through four stations which contain acetone, isopropanol, polyethylene glycol, mineral oil and paraffin. Microwaves and agitation are used to accelerate the diffusion of solvents in tissue. A patented microwave technology is utilized, which operates at a continuous low power instead of pulsing high levels of microwave energy.

The retort chamber is cylindrical; microwaves circle around the cavity, taking advantage of the physical principle of the 'whispering chamber' effect that eliminates hot and cold spots. The advantage of this system is the acceptance of tissues into the system every 15 minutes, improving turnaround time. The reagents used are environmentally safe, eliminating toxic vapors in the laboratory. The morphology and quality of the specimens is consistent with that of traditional tissue processing. The disadvantages include the cost of the processor, and the grossing of the tissue sample that requires standardization of specimen dissection.

Advantages of newer technology in processing

- custom programs specific to tissues being processed, addition of vacuum, agitation or heat at any stage
- rapid schedules
- fluid and fume containment
- environmentally friendly reagents
- time delay for start of processing schedules
- reagent management

Processor maintenance

Every institution should have a policy outlining the rotation and changing of solutions on the tissue processor. The numbers, sizes, types of tissue processed and the reagents used will play a role in the determination of this policy. Solutions should be carefully monitored to ensure quality. Every manufacturer has a handbook outlining an appropriate maintenance schedule.

Important maintenance tips

- Any spillage or overflow should be cleaned immediately
- Accumulation of wax on any surface should be removed

- The temperature of the paraffin wax bath should be set to 3°C above the melting point of the paraffin wax and monitored daily
- Timings should be checked when placing tissue cassettes in the processor, especially when delayed schedules are selected
- Warm water flushes should be incorporated, keeping the lines free of salts, protein and debris

Automated processing schedules

Although overnight schedules for tissue processing remain popular in many laboratories, schedules have changed to reflect the emphasis on reducing turnaround time for specimen reporting. Rapid processing for small biopsies or stat specimens can easily be accommodated.

Overnight processing

For many laboratories, this is considered to be the routine processing schedule. Tissues continue fixation by being immersed in 10% formalin, buffered or unbuffered. The process may include alcoholic formalin, varying concentrations of alcohol, xylene, or a xylene substitute, followed by infiltration in paraffin wax. Schedules are customized for the tissues being processed. Factors influencing the processing schedule include end time required, reagents used, the inclusion of heat and vacuum and the size and number of tissue cassettes processed. The schedule in Table 6.1 can be modified, adjusting times for the various stations, keeping in mind the end time needed for process completion.

Processing breast specimens

Standardization of the fixation and processing of breast tissue has become a focus of laboratory regulatory agencies. Pre-analytic, analytic and post-analytic variables are addressed in the findings. The purpose of the guidelines is to improve the accuracy of hormone receptor testing and the utility of these prognostic and predictive markers for assessing breast carcinomas.

Table 6.1	Overnight processing schedule			
Station	Reagents	Time	P/V	Temp
1	10% Formalin	1 h	On	38°C
2	10% Formalin	1 h	On	38°C
3	50% Alcohol/formalin	1 h	On	38°C
4	70% Alcohol	1 h	On	38°C
5	95% Alcohol	1 h	On	38°C
6	95% Alcohol	40 min	On	38°C
7	100% Alcohol	1 h	On	38°C
8	100% Alcohol	40 min	On	38°C
9	Xylene	1 h	On	38°C
10	Xylene	30 min	On	38°C
11	Paraffin	30 min	On	60°C
12	Paraffin	30 min	On	60°C
13	Paraffin	30 min	On	60°C
14	Paraffin	30 min	On	60°C

Due to the pressures of compliance with the new standards and guidelines, histology laboratories are revisiting their processing schedules, and adapting or adjusting new protocols for breast tissue. Currently, breast tissue should be received in the histology laboratory within one hour of removal from the patient, sectioned at 5 mm intervals and placed in 10% neutral buffered formalin and fixed for no less than six hours and not more than 72 hours before processing. Table 6.2 provides a processing schedule that is adjustable to address the parameters of these guidelines.

Schedule for processing eyes

Eyes require special processing (Table 6.3) dictated by the delicate nature of some parts of the structures and toughness of others. Ideally, a separate processor should be dedicated for tissues that require special handling because of the reagents used. The eye must be thoroughly fixed, prior to dissection, and subsequent processing. Phenol is added to the lower-percentage alcohols to soften the sclera and lens. Reagents are selected that provide the best dehydration and clearing of the tissue; chloroform has been used as the clearing agent because it is less harsh than xylene and causes minimal shrinkage, keeping the retina attached. Large tissue cassettes and molds are specifically made for use in processing eyes.

Rapid processing schedules for small biopsies

Recently excised endoscopic biopsies and needle biopsies can be adequately processed in 2–5 hours using heat (37 to 45°C) and vacuum. Tissues requiring dissection should be trimmed to 2 mm in thickness. Most small specimens will fix prior to processing. If fixation is not complete, processing should begin in a station containing 10% NBF. Table 6.4 shows an example of a shortened process for an enclosed processor. With the enclosed processor, drain time is approximately 3–5 minutes at each station. The program can be amended, changing times at various stations. Drain times should be taken into consideration when determining the end time. After each run the instrument must be cleaned to purge the lines of any residual paraffin. The clean cycle will flush the lines using xylene, 100% alcohol, and water.

Table 6.2 Processing schedule for breast tissue

Station	Reagents	Time	P/V	Temp
1	10% Formalin	3 h	On	38°C
2	10% Formalin	3 h	On	38°C
3	50% Alcohol/formalin	2 h	On	38°C
4	70% Alcohol	30 min	On	38°C
5	95% Alcohol	45 min	On	38°C
6	95% Alcohol	45 min	On	38°C
7	100% Alcohol	45 min	On	38°C
8	100% Alcohol	45 min	On	38°C
9	Xylene	40 min	On	38°C
10	Xylene	40 min	On	38°C
11	Paraffin	30 min	On	60°C
12	Paraffin	20 min	On	60°C
13	Paraffin	20 min	On	60°C
14	Paraffin	40 min	On	60°C

Table 6.3 Eye processing schedule

Station	Reagents	Time
1	10% Formalin	0 h
2	4% Phenol/70% alcohol	1 h
3	4% Phenol/70% alcohol	1 h
4	95% Alcohol	1 h
5	95% Alcohol	1 h
6	100% Alcohol	1.5 h
7	100% Alcohol	1.5 h
8	100% Alcohol/chloroform	2 h
9	Chloroform	2 h
10	Chloroform	2 h
11	Paraffin	2 h
12	Paraffin	3 h

Table 6.4 Short processing schedule for biopsies

Station	Reagents	Time	P/V	Temp
1	10% Formalin	10 min	On	38°C
2	10% Formalin	10 min	On	38°C
3	70% Alcohol	10 min	On	38°C
4	95% Alcohol	10 min	On	38°C
5	95% Alcohol	10 min	On	38°C
6	100% Alcohol	10 min	On	38°C
7	100% Alcohol	10 min	On	38°C
8	Xylene	10 min	On	38°C
9	Xylene	10 min	On	38°C
10	Paraffin	10 min	On	60°C
11	Paraffin	10 min	On	60°C

Manual tissue processing

Manual tissue processing has stopped in most laboratories. There are circumstances requiring the tissue sample to be manually processed, including:

- Power failure or equipment malfunction.
- Large tissue samples requiring more time than can be allocated on an automated processor.
- Small biopsies, such as transplant specimens needing a rapid diagnosis, although the above 2–5 hour schedule often suffices.

Restoration of tissue dried in processing

Despite precautions taken during processing, technical or mechanical malfunctions and human error may occur, resulting in tissue drying out prior to paraffin wax impregnation. The tissue will never be regarded as normal, but the following treatment may help provide slides of adequate diagnostic quality.

Tissue restoration

70% ethanol	70 ml
Glycerol	30 ml
Dithionite	1 g

Tissues remain in the solution for several hours or overnight. Processing begins with the dehydrating solutions and continues to completion. Tissue may be difficult to section; coated or plus slides should be used.

Safety

Chapter 2 deals with the safe handling of common histological reagents and chemicals. Every histology laboratory should have a chemical hygiene plan that incorporates specific work practices to protect workers from potentially hazardous chemicals. Material safety sheets should be available for chemicals used in the laboratory. Basic information contained in the sheets includes maximum exposure limits, target organs, storage, disposal and how to handle spillages. Material safety data sheets (MSDS) should be saved and placed in an easily accessible place for quick reference.

Recycling reagents

Distillation equipment is used in many laboratories to recycle alcohol and xylene. Equipment used for recycling solvents uses fractional distillation. Heat is used to separate different waste products in the solvents by their boiling points, the component with the highest boiling point being purified. Advantages include reduced cost, a rapid/efficient process which eliminates the need to have chemicals removed by a waste disposal company, and avoidance of sending environmentally unsafe chemicals to landfills for disposal. The recycled reagents must be tested for quality.

Quality control

Temperature of all paraffin wax dispensers, flotation water baths and automated processors are carefully monitored, maintained and documented. The histology laboratory should have a policy and procedure manual that addresses quality issues and corrective actions taken.

Summary

Technological advances have been made in the instrumentation of tissue processors, in part due to increased workload, the demand for faster turnaround time for diagnostic samples and the reduction in workforce. The addition of microprocessors, microwaves, and environmentally friendly chemicals are only a few of the improvements that continue to advance tissue processing.

Tissue microarray

Lena T. Spencer, John D. Bancroft

Tissue microarray (TMA) was developed as a method to evaluate numerous samples of tissue in a short period. Battifora (1986) first introduced this concept and then Kononen et al. (1998) used this mechanism for examining several histological sections at the same time by arraying them in a single

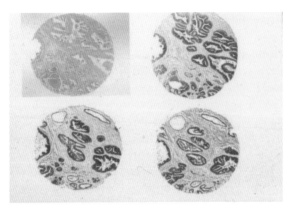

Figure 6.1 Tissue microarray slide.

paraffin block. Today, TMA uses multiple tissues samples that can be arranged in a single paraffin block using precision tools to prepare the recipient block (Fig. 6.1).

Purpose

Histological techniques are taking an important role in the development of molecular biology and TMA has become a powerful diagnostic tool, conserving tissue samples and saving time for both research (including cancer) and clinical work. TMA has applications in clinical pathology and serves as quality control for new antibodies. The production of antibodies is an expensive and lengthy process, and TMA is a unique tool which can aid the streamlining of the cumbersome validation and quality control of archival tissue as well as daily immunohistochemistry (IHC) controls.

Advantages of the technique

TMA enables researchers and pathologists to study and evaluate many diseases at an early stage. A hollow needle is used to take 100 or more tissue core samples from specific areas of pre-existing blocked tissue and then, placed in a single array block. Sections are then taken from this block, the exact

number depending on the size of the cores and the experience of the technologist, ultimately producing a single slide containing hundreds of tissue cores for the pathologist to review. This technique can be used for a wide range of staining procedures, including IHC, *in situ* hybridization (ISH), fluorescent *in situ* hybridization (FISH), special stain control samples, and quality control sections for H&E stains. Only a small amount of reagent is used to analyze each slide, making TMA cost-effective, particularly with IHC and *in situ* hybridization techniques. TMAs have been widely used in IHC for several years for quality control and assurance. They may demonstrate the antibody thresholds on a single slide which optimizes where the high and low signal intensities are seen.

Types of tissue microarrays

Prevalence TMAs are assembled from tumor samples of one or several types without attached clinical and pathological information. They are used to determine the prevalence of a given alteration in a specific area of interest in a tumor.

Progression TMAs contain samples of different stages of one tumor type and are used to discover associations between tumor genotype and phenotype. For example, a breast cancer progression TMA could contain samples of normal breast from patients with and without a history of breast cancer, different non-neoplastic breast diseases, ductal and lobular carcinoma *in situ*, invasive cancer of all stages, grades and histological subtypes as well as metastases and recurrences after initially successful treatment.

Prognosis TMAs contain samples from tumors available with clinical follow-up data and represent a fast and reliable method for the evaluation of clinical importance of new detected disease-related genes. Validation studies using prognosis TMAs can establish the associations between molecular findings and clinical outcomes.

Experimental TMAs are constructed from cell lines or samples from TMA archives for testing new antibodies and looking for gene targets.

Designing the grid

The design of the grid varies, depending on the purpose of the array, and needs considerable thought before tissue transfer occurs. The pathologist and technologist determine the guidelines according to the purpose and utilization of each specific laboratory. An array uses a series of 50 or more samples, set into one or several blocks. It is important to plan and record in advance how many samples will be arrayed, and to create a map or grid sheet which will be easy to follow and refer to later (Fig. 6.2). A large number of samples (high density) can be arrayed in a 37 × 24 × 5 mm block and a smaller number of samples (low density) in a 24 × 24 × 5 mm block.

Normal tissue controls and control cell lines are often placed in columns between the tumors and other normal tissue can be sited asymmetrically at one end of the block. Placing a notch at the end of the cassette block helps to confirm later that the orientation of the block is correct. Archived blocks can be used as a source of control tissue without destructive sampling. Making the tissue array is a multistep project. Selecting the slides, collecting the blocks, and designing the grid consume the time rather than the array process itself. Standardizing the construction of the grid makes it easier to follow, but it can still take several weeks to a month before the array process begins. The organization of the blocks and slides is critical throughout the TMA process.

Fixation and processing of tissues and controls

Fixation and processing of the sampled tissues is assumed to be standard, and these realities are discussed fully in Chapter 4 and earlier in this chapter. Some antigens are not well demonstrated using 10% NBF as a fixative and pre-treatment methods such as proteolytic enzyme digestion or retrieval can be performed, as necessary.

Preparation of the donor block

The file slides and blocks are reviewed to determine which blocks will be arrayed. The area of interest to be sampled is usually marked by circling with a pilot pen or permanent fine point marker, although some pathologists prefer to mark the blocks rather than the slides. Once the slides are reviewed and marked, the block is usually matched to the corresponding glass slide (Figs 6.3 and 6.4). It is important that the block is marked in the same area of interest as the marked slide. Donor blocks must be at least 1 mm thick to be suitable for array construction; if a marked area is less than 1 mm thick, two cores from this site are stacked on top of each other.

When marking the slides and blocks, the following colors can be used as indicators (Fig. 6.5):

- Red – Cancer
- Green – Normal
- Black – Pre-invasive

It is important to keep the blocks and slides together. A filing system where a sectioned H&E case study slide is filed behind the archived control block is ideal.

Needle sizes

The size of the punch is critical in planning the TMA. There are four different sizes of punches; 0.6, 1.0, 1.5 and 2.0 mm. The 1.0 or 1.5 mm needles are recommended for general use, but the 0.6 mm needles can be used if you are placing 200 or more samples into the blocks. The use of 2.0 mm needles is not recommended, as damage can occur to the donor blocks. The spacing between the cores must be planned carefully; spaces of 0.1 mm are ideal.

Database for tissue microarray analysis

(Shanknovich et al., 2003)

The first step in the construction of a TMA is the selection of cases from a database and creation of a

TISSUE MICROARRAY GRID/MAP FORM

Cassette (place notch at this end of cassette)

	1	2	3	4	5	6	7	8	9	10
A										
B										
C										
D										
E										
F										
G										
H										
I										
J										
K										
L										

Investigator's name: _____

Date received: _____

Fixation type: _____

Tissue type: Human/Rodent/Cell lines

Tech initials: _____

Date completed: _____

In our laboratory, we have found that color coding the grid sheet and TMA slide can make it easier for the pathologist and investigator to review the slide

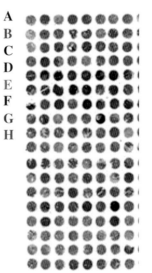

Figure 6.2 Tissue microarray grid/map form.

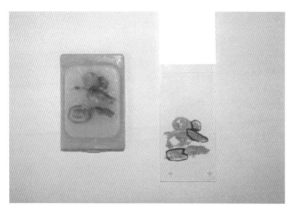

Figure 6.3 Shows an H&E slide and the paraffin block area are matched.

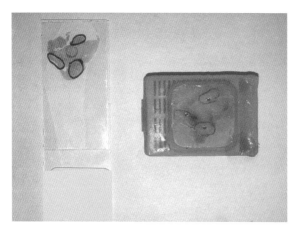

Figure 6.4 The slide is reviewed and the area(s) of interest for the TMAs are circled.

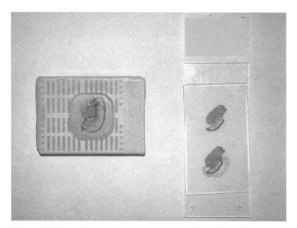

Figure 6.5 Specific areas of interest can be identified with different colored markings; cancer areas are marked red, normal tissue green, and invasive areas black.

template or spreadsheet which identifies the position for each case and controls in the TMA block. During the viewing and photographing of a tested slide, the cores are referred to by their position, and each case in the database can be identified by the unique positions of each core on the template.

Later, after the sections are stained, one image per core is taken and saved as a compressed file, then logged as its own position identifier. Image acquisition often takes less than one minute, including field selection, manual focusing, and identification. It is sensible to save a set of images for each stain in an identified folder. Several images from different stains can be viewed on the screen, scored, and the data entered manually onto the spreadsheet adjacent to the image cell. This method allows examination, consideration and scoring of multiple cores and multiple stains of the same case with ease, allowing flexibility which is impossible at the microscope – where it requires changing slides, stains, light sources and identifying the correct area of tissue. Co-investigators can check scoring, and images can be printed and shared over an electronic network for large trials and also as an educational tool.

Arrayers

There are several different arrayers on the market today (see Figs 6.6–6.9).

Automated arrayer

The automated arrayer is easy to use and includes a specimen tracking software system. The instrument marks, edits, and saves punch coordinates using an on-screen display and software tools. The automated arrayer is ideal for a laboratory with a high volume of TMAs, as 120–180 cores can be 'punched' per hour.

Manual arrayer

A manual arrayer relies on the designed map or grid sheet and direct visual identification and manual

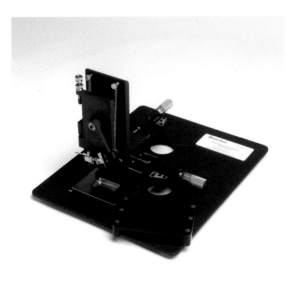

Figure 6.6 Manual tissue arrayer MTAI, manufactured by Beecher Instruments, Inc.

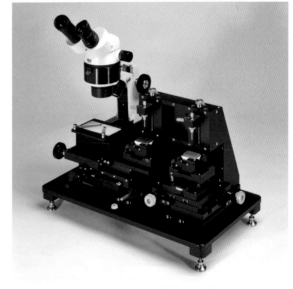

Figure 6.8 Manual tissue arrayer MTAIII with microscope, manufactured by Beecher Instruments, Inc.

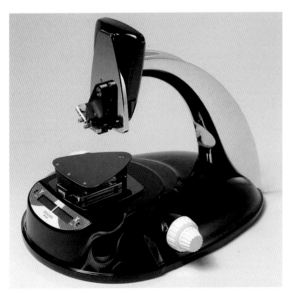

Figure 6.7 Manual tissue arrayer MTAII, manufactured by Beecher Instruments, Inc.

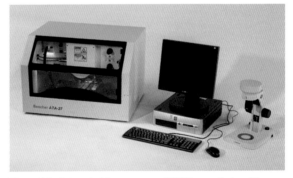

Figure 6.9 Automated tissue arrayer ATA27, manufactured by Beecher Instruments, Inc.

special stain controls, or QC controls for H&E staining, an inexpensive pen extractor is suitable.

Portable quick ray

This device is portable, easy to handle and economical. Its applications are the same as above but the needles are replaced by tips 1, 2, 3 or 5 mm in diameter. The recipient block is pre-prepared and sectionable with cores fitting easily into the holes. The block is then placed into an embedding mold with its cut

selection of the punching by the technologist, after the pathologist has marked the areas of interest on the slide. The number of cores punched per hour depends on the experience of the worker, but averages 30–70 cores. To prepare microarray blocks for surface face down and molten paraffin added to fill the mold before being allowed to solidify. The TMA is then ready to section.

Preparation of the recipient and donor array block

A blank paraffin block is prepared and used as the recipient for the tissue samples. It is best to use soft paraffin and make sure there are no holes in the block caused by air bubbles. The number of specimens per array depends on the size of the punches and the desired array density. The 1.0 mm needle is favored as it gives a desirable core and leaves little distortion in the donor block (Table 6.5).

To ensure the alignment of the punches, first move the recipient punch into position and make a mark in the paraffin. The same task is performed for the donor punch. Moving the needles uses the X or Y micrometer adjustment controls. The position of the punches over the block can be made by gently pushing down on them until a mark is made in the paraffin. One continues to make adjustments with the micrometer knobs until the desired position is attained.

The empty recipient block is placed in the holder and the attachment screws are tightened to keep this block from slipping. The recipient block is placed with its notched edge to the left of the block holder. Making a hole in the first position begins the array process. The smaller needle is used to create the hole. First the depth stop is adjusted and its nut is

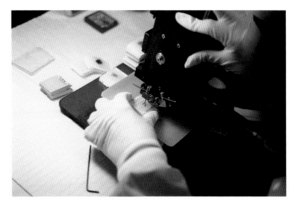

Figure 6.10 In the preparation stage of making the TMA at the arrayer the bridge is placed over the recipient block.

tightened to stop the needle at the correct depth. The needle is pushed downwards by hand, and the depth stop limits this motion. The handle in the needle is used to rotate the needle. The downward pushing pressure is then relieved and springs will pull the needle upwards. The stylet is used to empty the needle but this must not be removed from the needles during the array process. The donor block bridge is placed over the recipient block and the turret is moved to switch the larger needle into a vertical sampling position (Fig. 6.10). The donor block is moved under the sampling needle and the larger needle is used to retrieve the sample. The needle is pushed downwards to retrieve the sample. The depth stop does not block the needle motion in the donor block and care must be taken to prevent the needle from entering too deep. It is best to have three punches from the same site, making the tissue sample well represented for the evaluation of prognostic markers. Use of a four block indexer allows four replicate blocks to be made at the same time. The donor core can be cut if it is too tall to fit in the recipient punch by ejecting the core with the stylus and placing it on a clean flat surface. A clean razor blade is used to cut the core to the desired length and it is then placed into the recipient block using a pair of forceps (Fig. 6.11).

The ability to study archival tissue specimens is important and cores can be stored in labeled Eppendorf tubes for use in future arrays.

Table 6.5 Typical core spacing and number of cores using various needle sizes

Needle size	Spacing between samples	Array format	Number of cores
0.6 mm	0.2 mm	20 × 20 cores	400
1.0 mm	0.3 mm	16 × 13 cores	208
1.5 mm	0.4 mm	11 × 9 cores	99

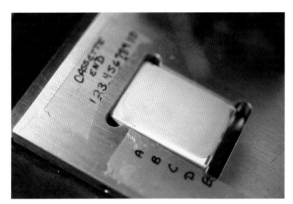

Figure 6.11 The donor tissue has been placed in the appropriate location in the recipient block.

Smoothing and sectioning

The array block must be smooth and level before sectioning. The easiest way to do this is to heat a clean microscopic slide to around 70–80°C and touch it to the array block surface. The surface of the block will begin to melt. Move the slide in a circular motion and place the slide and block in the refrigerator or freezer.

Microtomy

The water bath is set at 37°C. Gently face off the array block on a dedicated microtome and cut a hundred or more sections at 4–5 μm. One should place the sections on positively charged slides in the same orientation. It is advised to stain one slide for H&E and place the remaining unstained slides in a box for storage at −20°C.

Sections can be cut a day or two before they are stained, but to avoid contamination they are stored in slide boxes. Sectioned TMA blocks should be dipped in paraffin to seal the surface to avoid loss of antigens. Note that excessive soaking or freezing can cause the tissue to swell and keep the array block from ribboning well.

The tissue block can be cored several times with minimal distortion and on further sectioning of the whole block it is still possible in the majority of cases to make a diagnosis.

Troubleshooting and tips

- Core does not come out of the punch easily – suggesting that the punch tip is bent or distorted. It is advised to change the punch.
- Tissue core was pushed too deep. Advise removal of the sample with the small punch and place a new sample in the same position.
- Insufficient spacing of cores. This can cause minor cracks or stress on the core when sectioning.
- Thinning of TMA cores in block. This can be a result of repeated sectioning of the same block, where cores are uneven in the block, and one should not use this block.
- Loss of tissue on water bath. This may be due to folds, wrinkles, and mishandling of ribbon.
- Re-facing block – if additional sections are required after the block has been filed it is important for continuity to reposition the block as close as possible to its original position on the microtome; hence the importance of using a dedicated microtome.
- Re-facing angle. Incautious consideration shortens the life of the tissue microarray block, which is called thinning. It is important to make sure the cassette is completely flat on top of the mold.

Maintenance of the arrayer

During the array process, it is advised to clean any residual paraffin from the punches, sampling block and block holders, wiping all with a 5 × 5 cm gauze sponge. Parts should not be soaked in xylene, but one should oil X-Y or Z rails once every few months.

The punches need to be periodically replaced as they are made of a thin tube. They can easily bend or the tip of the punch may become dulled after several hundred punches. The replacement punch is correctly positioned when the groove in the punch hub is firmly placed against the metal rod in the v-block, making sure it does not wobble. Alignment of the replacement punches should be checked prior to beginning an array.

Additional reading for tissue processing

Bancroft, J.D., Cook, H.C., 1994. Manual of Histological Techniques and their Diagnostic Application. Churchill Livingstone, Edinburgh.

Boon, M.E., Kok, L.P., 1989. Microwave Cookbook of Pathology. Coulomb Press, Leiden.

Carson, F.L., 1997. Histotechnology: A Self-Instructional Text, second ed. ASCP Press, Chicago.

Carson, F.L., Hladic, C., 2010. Histotechnology: A Self-Instructional Text, third ed. ASCP Press, Chicago.

Culling, C.F.A., Allison, R.T., Barr, W.T., 1985. Cellular Pathology Technique, third ed. Butterworths, London.

Kok, L.P., Boon, M.E., 1992. Microwave Cookbook of Microscopists, third ed. Coulomb Press, Leiden.

Luna, L.G., 1992. Histopathologic Methods and Color Atlas of Special Stains and Tissue Artifacts. Johnson Printers, Downers Grove.

Morales, A.R., Nassiri, M., Kanhoush, R., et al., 2004. Experience with an automated microwave-assisted tissue processing method. Validation of histologic quality and impart on the timeliness of diagnostic surgical pathology. A/CP; 121-528-56.

Sheehan, D.C., Hrapchak, B., 1980. Theory and Practice of Histotechnology, second ed. C.V. Mosby Co., St Louis.

Slap, S.E., 1993. Microwave processing techniques for microscopy. Online. Available: http://www.ebsciences.com/papers/mw_tech.htm.

Vernon, S.E., Continuous Throughput Rapid Tissue Processing Revolutionizes Histopathology WorkFlow, 2005. LABMEDICINE 36 (May (5)), 300–302.

References for microarray

Battifora, H., 1986. The mulitumor (sausage) tissue block: Novel method for immunohistochemical antibody testing. Laboratory Investigation 55, 244.

DeMarzo, A.M., Fedor, H., 2003. Tissue microarrays: principles and practice. NSH Workshop, Louisville, KY.

Jones, M.L., 2009. Real time rapid tissue processing. NSH workshop, Birmingham, AL.

Jones, M.L., 2011. Microarray and your lab, Sakura Webinar, February.

Kononen, J., Bubendorf, L., Kallioniemi, A., et al., 1998. Tissue microarrays high throughput molecular profiling of tumor specimens. Nat Med 4, 844–847.

Shaknovich, R., Celestine, A., Lin, Y., Cattoretti, G., 2003. Novel relational database for tissue microarray analysis. Laboratory Medicine, 127 (4): 492–494.

Additional reading for microarray

Brady, J., The Science Advisory Board, Tissue microarrays: Bringing histology up to speed. http://www.scienceboard.net/community/perspectives.63.html.

Enghardt, M.H., Aghassi, N.B., Bond, C.J., Elston, D.M., 1995. A simplified multitissue control block. The Journal of Histotechnology 18, 51–55.

Flores, G., 2005. Tissue microarrays go coreless. The Scientist 19, 38.

Jensen, T.A., Hammand, M.E.H., 2001. The tissue microarray – a technical guide for histologists. The Journal of Histotechnology 24, 283–287.

Mihatsch, M.J., Sauter, G., Kallioniemi, O.P., 1998. Tissue microarrays high throughput molecular profiling of tumor specimens. Nat Med 4, 844–847.

Shaknovich, R., Celestine, A., Lin, Y., Cattoretti, G., 2003. Novel relational database for tissue microarray analysis. Lab Med 127 (Apr (4)), 492–494.

Microtomy: 7
Paraffin and frozen

Lena T. Spencer • John D. Bancroft

Introduction

The basic principles of microtomy are applicable to both paraffin and frozen sections. This chapter will discuss the techniques necessary to provide quality microscopic slides for clinical and research histology.

Microtomy

Microtomy is the means by which tissue is sectioned and attached to a surface for further microscopic examination. Most microtomy is performed on paraffin wax embedded tissue blocks. The basic instrument used in microtomy is the microtome; an advancing mechanism moves the object (paraffin block) for a predetermined distance until it is in contact with the cutting tool (knife or blade). The specimen moves vertically past the cutting surface and a tissue section is produced. Good technique is achieved through ongoing practice.

Types of microtome

There are several types of microtome, each designed for a specific purpose, although many have multi-functional roles.

Rotary microtome

The rotary microtome is often referred to as the "Minot" after its inventor. The basic mechanism requires the rotation of a fine advance hand-wheel by 360° degrees, moving the specimen vertically past the cutting surface and returning it to the starting position. The rotary microtome may be manual (completely manipulated by the operator), semi-automated (one motor to advance either the fine or course hand-wheel), or fully automated (two motors that drive both the fine and the course advance hand-wheel). The mechanism for block advancement may be retracting or non-retracting. Its advantages include the ability to cut thin 2–3 μm sections and its easy adaption to all type of tissue (hard, fragile or fatty) sectioning. Technological advances in the automation of microtomy have improved section quality, increased productivity, and improved occupational safety for the technologist. Eliminating manual hand-wheel operation of the microtome reduces the incidence of repetitive motion disorders, a common occupational health problem in the histology laboratory.

Base sledge microtome

With the sledge microtome, the specimen is held stationary and the knife slides across the top of the specimen during sectioning. Used primarily for large blocks, hard tissues, or whole mounts, it is especially useful in neuropathology and ophthalmic pathology. Three micron sections are difficult to produce. Further information regarding section of undecalcifed bone is available in Chapter 16.

Rotary rocking microtome

Commonly used in cryostats, the retracting action moves the tissue block away from the knife on the upstroke, producing a flat face to the tissue block.

Sliding microtome

The knife or blade is stationary and the specimen slides under it during sectioning. This microtome was developed for use with celloidin-embedded tissue blocks.

Ultra microtome

Used exclusively for electron microscopy (Chapter 22).

Microtome knives

There are many shapes, sizes and materials for microtome knives. Knives were developed to fit specific types of microtome, and to cope with different degrees of hardness of tissues and embedding media. Most steel knives have been replaced with disposal blades, although exceptions include the tool-edge knives for resin, and steel knives for some cryostats.

Disposable blades

The introduction of disposable stainless steel blades has revolutionized microtomy in the laboratory. Disposable blades are used for routine microtomy and cryotomy, providing a sharp cutting edge that can produce almost flawless 2–4 µm sections. Disposable blade holders are incorporated into the microtome or an adaptor may be purchased. The blades may be purchased in dispensers, with or without a special polytetrafluoroethylene (PTFE) coating, allowing ribbons to be sectioned with ease, reducing resistance during microtomy:

- The clearance angle should be adjusted in small increments to eliminate problems that occur with the ribboning of the tissue.
- Over-tightening the disposable blade in the clamping device may cause cutting artifacts, such as thick and thin sections.
- The clamping device must be clean and free of defects. During sectioning the hand-wheel must be turned slowly.
- Extremely hard tissues may pose a problem for disposable blades.

Reliability of a constant sharp edge, ease of use, low or high profiles adaptable to a variety of tissue and paraffin types, and low cost relative to steel knife sharpening make these blades a mainstay in most laboratories.

Glass and diamond knives

Glass and diamond knives are used in electron microscopy and with plastic resin embedded blocks.

Paraffin section cutting

Equipment required

Tools needed for microtomy:

- Flotation (water) bath
- Slide drying oven or hot plate
- Fine pointed or curved forceps
- Sable or camel haired brush
- Scalpel
- Slide rack
- Clean slides
- Teasing needle
- Ice tray
- Chemical-resistant pencil or pen

Flotation (water) bath

A thermostatically controlled water bath is used for floating out tissue ribbons after sectioning. The temperature of the water in the bath should be 10°C below the melting point of the paraffin to be sectioned. Care should be taken to prevent water bubbles from being trapped under the section. This can be accomplished by using distilled water in the bath. Alcohol or a small drop of detergent may be added to the water to reduce the surface tension, allowing the section to flatten out with greater ease.

Drying oven or hot plate

Drying ovens incorporate fans that keep the warm air circulating around the slides. The temperature setting should be approximately that of the melting point of the paraffin. If the oven is too hot there may be distortion to the cells, causing dark pyknotic nuclei or nuclear bubbling; cells that are completely devoid of nuclear detail. Drying times vary depending on the type of tissue, the number of slides to be dried and size of the drying device. Many automated stainers have drying ovens as part of the instrument, so the time and temperature is easily regulated. Special care should be taken when drying delicate tissues or tissues from the central nervous system; a lower temperature is required to prevent splitting and cracking of the section; 37°C for 24 hours is recommended.

Brush and forceps

Forceps, brushes or teasing needles are helpful in the removal of folds, creases and bubbles that may form during the floating out of the section on the water bath. They are also helpful for manipulating the section as it passes across the edge of the blade.

Slides

For normal routine work, 76 × 25 mm slides are universally used. Although slides are available in a variety of thicknesses, those specified as 1.0–1.2 mm in thickness are preferred because they do not break as easily. Most slide racks are made to accommodate this slide size. Larger slides are available for use with specialty tissues such as eyes or brains. Unique identification numbers or codes, patient name or other information should be etched, embossed or written on each slide. Automated instruments that imprint the patient's information on the glass slide are readily available. Chemical-resistant pens and pencils are routinely used to label the slide.

Slides that are positively charged or pre-treated with an adhesive resist detachment of the tissue from the slide during staining. Colored, frost-ended slides may be used to identify special handling (decal, special stains, immunohistochemistry, etc.).

Section adhesives

Provided clean slides are used and sections are adequately dried, the problem of sections detaching

from the slide during staining should not occur. There are occasions when sections may detach from the slide:

- Exposure to strong alkali solutions during staining
- Cryostat sections for immunofluorescence, immunohistochemistry or intra-operative consultation
- Central nervous system (CNS) tissues
- Sections that are submitted to extreme temperatures
- Tissues containing blood and mucous
- Decalcified tissues

Adhesives may alleviate the problem of tissue loss. Protein adhesives such as albumen, gelatin and starch may be prone to bacterial growth or heavy staining; close monitoring will prevent these problems. Adhesives that may be used:

Poly-L-lysine (PLL)

Poly-L-lysine is bought as a 0.1% solution, which is further diluted for use, 1 in 10 with distilled water. Slides are coated with the diluted solution and allowed to dry. The effectiveness of the coating to adhere the tissue to the slide will diminish within a few days.

3-aminopropyltriethoxysilane (APES)

Slides are dipped in a 2% solution of APES in acetone, drained, dipped in acetone, and drained again; the process is complete when the slides are dipped in distilled water. Slides are placed upright in a rack to dry. These slides are useful for cytology, especially specimens that may be bloody or contain proteinaceous material.

Charged or plus slides

Laboratories often use slides that have been manufactured with a permanent positive charge. Placing a positive charge on the slides is accomplished by coating the slide with a basic polymer in which a chemical reaction occurs, leaving the amino groups linked by covalent bonds to the silicon atoms of the glass. These slides have proven to be superior in their resistance to cell and tissue loss during staining or pre-treatments such as enzyme and antigen retrieval.

Practical microtomy

The expertise that must be gained to become a competent microtomist cannot be achieved from textbooks. Practical experience under the guidance of a skilled tutor is the best way to gain the confidence and coordination necessary to manipulate the microtome and the sections produced. Techniques will be described, providing information and helpful hints for use during microscopy.

Setup of the microtome

Maintenance of the microtome is important to the production of quality slides for diagnosis. The manufacturer's recommendation regarding the proper care of the instrument should be closely followed. A departmental policy should be implemented outlining daily, weekly, quarterly and yearly preventive maintenance procedures.

The water bath and the microtome should be ergonomically positioned to reduce stress and tension on the employee's neck and shoulders. The water bath may be filled with distilled or tap water, and adjusted to the proper temperature of the paraffin. Care should be taken to reduce air bubbles that may distort the tissue section.

The blade should be sharp and defect free. The blade or knife holder should be adjusted to optimize the clearance angle, the distance between the lower facet angle and the surface of the block face. The recommended angle varies from 2–4° for paraffin to 5–7° for frozen sections. The correct angle reduces friction as the blade passes through the block, preventing compression of the section. Determining the exact angle is largely a matter of trial and error. Clamps and screws must be firmly tightened. If a disposable blade is to be used, care should be taken to ensure enough pressure is being exerted on the blade to provide support, but it should not be over-tightened, since this causes thick and thin sectioning.

Sectioning

Trimming the tissue blocks

The paraffin block may be faced or "rough cut" by setting the micrometer at 15–30 μm or by advancing the block using the coarse feed mechanism. Aggressive trimming will cause "moth holes" artifacts. Care must be taken to ensure that the block clamped in the chuck has been retracted so there is no contact with the blade on the initial down-stroke. It is possible to damage the tissue by gouging or scoring when trimming the block.

Cutting sections

Blocks should be arranged in numerical order on an ice tray, cooling both the tissue and the paraffin, giving them a consistent temperature. A small amount of water is absorbed into the tissue, causing slight swelling, and making sectioning easier. Oversoaking may cause expansion and distortion of the tissue section. Proper processing greatly reduces or eliminates the need to pre-soak blocks. Routine surgical material should be cut at 3–4 μm. The micrometer setting does not guarantee that each section will be that exact thickness. Thickness depends on many factors, including temperature, knife angle and cutting speed. Experience will determine the speed of the stroke, but in general, one should use a smooth, slow stroke. If there is difficulty cutting a smooth flat section, warming the block face with warm water, or gently exhaling breath onto the block surface during sectioning, may help. This has the effect of expanding the block, giving a slightly thicker section. Ideally, successive sections will stick edge-to-edge due to local pressure with each stroke, forming a ribbon. If the entire block is to be sectioned and retained, the ribbons are stored in a receptacle for future use. Ribbons of sections are the most convenient way of handling sections. When a ribbon of several sections has been cut, the first section is held by forceps, or teasing needle, and the last section eased from the knife edge with a small brush.

Floating out sections

The floating out of the ribbon must be smooth, with the trailing end of the ribbon making contact with the water first. The slight drag produced when the rest of the ribbon is laid on the water is sufficient to remove most, if not all, of the folds that occur. Sections are floated on the water bath, shiny side down. Folds in the section may be removed by simply teasing with the forceps. Approximately 30 seconds should be long enough for a ribbon to flatten, since prolonged time on the water causes excessive expansion, distorting the tissue. Individual sections or ribbons may be floated onto the slide. Circular structures such as eyes may be difficult to flatten. Various techniques are useful in these situations, such as placing the section on a slide which has been pre-flooded with 50% alcohol. The slide is gently immersed in the water bath and the section of eye will float on the surface. The presence of the alcohol will set up diffusion currents that help to flatten the tissue section. The water bath should be cleaned after each block is cut, removing debris and tissue fragments by dragging tissue paper across the surface. Cleanliness cannot be overemphasized; debris ("pick-up") material from different blocks is a serious problem.

Drying sections

The small amount of water held under the section will allow further flattening to occur when heat is applied to dry the section. The temperature should be at the melting point of the paraffin. Automated stainers have drying ovens as part of the instrumentation. Slides may be attached to the stainer with individual slide holders or in racks that are designed for the instrument. It is important to eliminate overheating during the slide drying stage, as cellular details may be compromised. Hot plates may cause localized overheating of the slide. When delicate tissues are to be dried, less distortion will occur if

the temperature is reduced and the time prolonged. Overnight drying at 37°C is recommended for many tissues.

Cutting hard tissues

Since the introduction of disposable blades, cutting hard tissues is less problematic. The reason for cutting difficulties is more likely poor fixation or over-processing. Prolonged soaking of the block, or exposing the block surface to running tap water for 30 minutes, may often overcome many of the problems associated with cutting hard tissues. A slight reduction in the knife angle may also yield results. If these remedies fail, softening agents may be used on the surface of the block.

Surface decalcification

When small foci of calcium are present in the tissue section, cutting a quality section may be difficult. The block may be removed from the chuck after rough cutting the tissue and placed face down in a dish that contains a small amount of decalcification solution.

The time for exposure to the decal will vary depending on the tissue; closely monitor the progress of the decal. The block is rinsed well, blotted dry, chilled and returned to the microtome. An immediate section should be taken since the decalcification achieved will be limited. Diagnostic materials may be compromised if over-decalcification occurs. It must be noted that the staining properties of the tissue may be affected after this treatment and allowances must be made to achieve optimum results.

Problems and solutions

Table 7.1 addresses the most common problems encountered during microtomy and possible solutions.

Frozen and related sections

This section provides a discussion of the methods used to produce sections without the use of

Table 7.1 Problems and solutions for paraffin sectioning

Causes	Solutions
Ribbon/consecutive sections curved	
1. Block edges not parallel	1. Trim block until parallel
2. Dull blade edge	2. Replace blade or move to a different area
3. Excessive paraffin	3. Trim away excess paraffin
4. Tissue varying in consistency	4. Re-orient block
Thick and thin sections	
1. Paraffin too soft for tissue or conditions	1. Cool block with ice or re-embed in higher MP wax
2. Insufficient clearance angle	2. Increase clearance angle
3. Faulty microtome mechanisms	3. Maintain microtome – lubricate and calibrate. Check for obvious faults with microtome, parts may be worn
4. Blade or block loose in holders	4. Tighten block and blade
Chatter – thick and thin zones parallel to blade edge	
1. Blade or block loose in their holders	1. Tighten blade and block holders
2. Excessively steep clearance angle or knife tilt	2. Reduce angle
3. Tissue or paraffin too hard for sectioning	3. Use softening fluid
4. Calcified areas in tissue	4. Rehydrate and surface decalcify
5. Over-dehydration of the tissue	5. Re-embed in fresh paraffin
6. Dull blade	6. Replace or use new area of blade; also clean blade edge to remove excess paraffin
Splitting of sections at right angles to knife edge	
1. Nicks in blade	1. Use different part of blade or replace
2. Hard particles in tissue	2. If calcium deposit – surface decal
3. Hard particles in paraffin	3. If mineral or other particle, remove with fine sharp pointed scalpel
Sections will not form ribbons	
1. Paraffin too hard for sectioning conditions	1. Re-embed in lower melting point paraffin
2. Debris on knife edge	2. Clean with xylene moist cloth
3. Clearance angle incorrect	3. Adjust to optimal angle
Sections attach to block on return stroke	
1. Insufficient clearance angle	1. Increase clearance angle
2. Debris on blade edge	2. Clean with xylene moist cloth
3. Debris on block edge	3. Trim edges of block
4. Static electricity on ribbon	4. Humidify the air around the microtome; place static guard or dryer sheets near microtome
Incomplete section	
1. Incomplete impregnation of the tissue with paraffin	1. Re-process tissue block
2. Tissue incorrectly embedded	2. Re-embed tissue; make sure orientation is correct and tissue is flat in mold
3. Sections superficially cut	3. Re-face block, cut deeper into the tissue

Table 7.1 *(continued)*	
Causes	**Solutions**
Excessive compression	
1. Dull blade	1. Replace blade
2. Paraffin too soft for the tissue	2. Cool block face and re-cut
Sections expand or disintegrate on water bath	
1. Poor impregnation of tissue	1. Re-process tissue
2. Water temperature too high in flotation bath	2. Turn down the temperature of the flotation bath.
Sections roll into a coil instead of remaining flat on knife edge	
1. Blade dull	1. Use a new blade
2. Rake angle too small	2. Reduce blade tilt if clearance angle is excessive
3. Section too thick	3. Reduce section thickness

dehydrating and clearing solutions, and in the case of frozen sections, without embedding media. Frozen sections have important clinical and research applications. Clinically the use of frozen sections for intra-operative consultation, Mohs procedures for surgical margins and sentinel node evaluation has great significance in patient care and maintenance.

Uses of frozen sections

The production of frozen sections has many applications in routine histology laboratories:

- rapid production of sections for intra-operative diagnosis
- diagnostic and research enzyme histochemistry for labile enzymes
- immunofluorescent methodology (Chapter 18)
- immunohistochemistry techniques when heat and fixation may inactivate or destroy the antigens (Chapters 18 and 20)
- diagnostic and research non-enzyme histochemistry, e.g. lipids and some carbohydrates (Appendix II and Chapter 12, respectively)
- silver demonstration methods, particularly in neuropathology (Chapter 17)

Theoretical considerations

The principle of cutting frozen sections is simple: when the tissue is frozen, the interstitial water in the tissue turns to ice, and in this state the tissue is firm, with the ice acting as the embedding medium. The consistency of the frozen block may be altered by varying the temperature of the tissue. Reducing the temperature will produce a harder block; raising the temperature makes the tissue softer. The majority of non-fatty unfixed tissues section well at −25°C. The sectioning of fixed tissue requires a block temperature of approximately −10°C or warmer. There is more water in fixed tissue; consequently, the tissue will have a harder consistency, requiring a higher temperature to obtain the ideal consistency for sectioning.

The cryostat

To produce thin, high-quality, frozen sections, the tissue must be properly frozen and embedded correctly, the conditions of the cryostat must be optimal, the block temperature must be correct for the tissue being cut and the blade must be clean and properly secured. The best-quality frozen sections are produced from fresh unfixed tissue which has been rapidly frozen.

The cryostat is a refrigerated cabinet in which a specialty microtome is housed. All the controls for the microtome are operated outside the cabinet. The first cryostats were introduced in 1954. Improvements in design have facilitated sectioning and safety:

- electronic temperature control
- electronically controlled advance and retraction of the block
- specimen orientation facility
- digital visualization of chuck and cabinet temperature
- mechanical cutting speed control and section thickness
- automatic defrost mechanism
- automated decontamination and sterilization

Freezing of fresh unfixed tissue

Tissue for freezing should be fresh. The specimen should be frozen as rapidly as is possible without creating freeze artifacts. Techniques for suitable freezing include:

- liquefied nitrogen (−190°C)
- isopentane (2-methylbutane) cooled by liquid nitrogen (−150°C)
- dry ice (−70°C)
- carbon dioxide gas (−70°C)
- aerosol sprays (−50°C)

When freezing tissue for frozen sections, freeze artifact may occur. The water in the tissue freezes and forms ice crystals, and the crystal size and the quantity of crystals is proportional to the speed at which the tissue is frozen. The tissue is cut and placed on a room temperature slide; at this point the tissue is thawed. The thawing of the ice crystals produces freeze artifact that appears as holes or a discontinuation of the tissue architecture when viewed microscopically.

The best frozen sections are obtained when the tissue is frozen very quickly. The method of choice is isopentane and liquid nitrogen. The problem with using liquid nitrogen alone is the formation of

nitrogen vapor bubbles around the tissue, acting as an insulator and so inhibiting rapid, even cooling of the tissue. This can produce freeze artifact in the tissue, which may make diagnostic interpretation difficult, especially in muscle biopsies. The problem can be overcome by snap freezing the tissue in an agent with a high thermal conductivity which has been cooled to approximately −160°C by immersion of the liquid nitrogen in isopentane. A beaker of isopentane is suspended in a flask of liquid nitrogen. When the temperature of the isopentane reaches −160°C the tissue is submerged in the isopentane (affixed to a cork disk, aluminum foil or a cryostat chuck). Insufficient time in the freezing medium can lead to freeze artifact, while prolonged freezing may crack the block, compromising the sample and causing sectioning problems. The tissue may be rolled in talc prior to snap freezing to reduce freezing artifact.

Solid carbon dioxide (dry ice) may be used for freezing tissue blocks. Two pieces of dry ice are held in gloved hands against the cryostat block holder containing the tissue, which has been oriented in a cryoembedding medium, such as OCT. As the tissue freezes, a white line will be seen passing through the tissue. The dry ice should then be removed, to avoid over-freezing the tissue. This method is not economical, since the dry ice will return to the gaseous state upon storage. The need for regular deliveries and the wastage of large amounts of dry ice are disadvantages of this method.

Carbon dioxide gas from a CO_2 cylinder has been successful in the past. Tissue blocks are frozen by adapting a conventional freezing microtome with a gas supply or by using a special adaptor for the CO_2 tank that holds the tissue chuck.

Aerosol sprays have gained popularity as a means of freezing small tissue blocks. These sprays are available from a number of vendors, and have the advantage of being readily available and easily stored. A major problem is the environmental issues of aerosol emissions, and the safety problem of inhaling the aerosol while cutting the tissue.

Tissue can be successfully frozen directly in the cryostat, using the freeze bar and the heat extractor. The tissue is frozen simultaneously from the block face and the block holder. Freeze artifact may be reduced if all objects are kept cold and ready for use. This method is very quick and is often used for intra-operative frozen sections.

Fixed tissue and the cryostat

For most diagnostic purposes in a routine laboratory, cryostat sections of unfixed tissue are suitable, although certain methods require post-fixation in cold formal calcium. However, the effect of freezing unfixed tissue is the diffusion of labile substances. This is enhanced when the section is cut in the cryostat, producing heat which causes slight thawing of the cut section. This may not cause a problem for diagnosis, but it can affect the accurate localization of some abundant enzymes, such as acid and alkaline phosphatases. To accurately localize these hydrolytic enzymes and other antigens, it is useful to fix the tissue prior to sectioning in the cryostat. Tissue prepared in this manner must be fixed under controlled conditions. The tissue must be absolutely fresh and placed in formal calcium at 4°C for 18 hours. The technique is outlined below.

Gum sucrose

Gum acacia	2 g
Sucrose	60 g
Distilled water	200 ml

Store at 4°C

Method

1. Fix fresh tissue block in formal calcium, at 4°C for 18 hours.
2. Rinse in running water, or for a short time in distilled water if the tissue fragment is small or fragile, e.g. jejunal biopsy.
3. Blot dry.
4. Place tissue in the gum sucrose solution at 4°C for 18 hours, or less with small fragments.
5. Blot dry
6. Freeze tissue onto the block holder.

Following fixation, the block is frozen slowly to avoid damage caused by the rapid expansion of ice within the tissue. Freezing the block by standing it in the cryostat cabinet gives acceptable results for the majority of fixed tissue. The length of time required for this procedure limits its value as a diagnostic tool.

Cryostat sectioning

Cabinet temperature

The temperature of the microtome and the cryostat chamber should be monitored. Many cryostats have digital displays of the block temperature and the cabinet temperature. The temperature should be suitable for the tissue type and the type of preparation to be cut. Most unfixed material will section well between −15 and −23°C. Tissues containing large amounts of water will section best at the warmer temperature, and harder tissues and those that contain fat require a colder temperature. Table 7.2 gives an indication of the optimal cutting temperatures for a variety of tissue types. If sections are shattered, with chatter lines, this is an indication that the block is too cold. Most fixed tissues will section best within the range of −7 to −12°C, depending on the hardness of the tissue. Small blocks of undecalcified cancellous bone can be sectioned, but care must be taken to remove any cortical bone fragments, prior to freezing.

Microtome

If cutting problems are encountered, the microtome should be defrosted and oiled according to manufacturer's recommendation. A policy should be in place that outlines a routine maintenance schedule for each cryostat, including a section on decontamination of the instrument.

Cryoembedding medium

There are many different cryoembedding media commercially available. The properties of each should be carefully considered before use, including the temperature, freezing mode and type of tissue that is being frozen.

Blade or knife

Stainless steel knives may be necessary in research and animal pathology laboratories. The type of tissue and the procedures to be performed may dictate the use of a steel knife. If a knife is used,

Table 7.2 Optimal tissue freezing temperatures

Tissue	−7 to −10°C	−10 to −13°C	−13 to −16°C	−16 to −20°C	−20 to −25°C	−25 to −30°C
Adrenal			X			
Bladder		X				
Bone marrow					X	
Brain	X					
Breast					X	
Breast with fat						X
Cervix				X		
Fat					X	X
Heart				X		
Intestinal				X		
Kidney			X			
Liver	X	X				
Lung				X		
Lymphoid			X			
Muscle			X			
Ovary				X		
Pancreas				X		
Prostate				X		
Rectal			X			
Skin			X			
Spleen	X					
Testicular		X	X			
Thyroid		X				
Uterine scrapings	X					
Uterus			X			

sharpening techniques should be discussed in the procedure manual. A sharp edge is paramount in obtaining a quality frozen section. The microtome blade angle and block face angle should be closely monitored. Disposable blades have become routine in most clinical laboratories; they produce a perfect edge and are instantly available. In addition to the advantage of sharpness, the blades are rapidly cooled because of their size. Tissues which are extremely hard or dense may be troublesome to a disposal blade.

Anti-roll plate

This piece of equipment, which is attached to the front of the microtome blade adaptor, is intended to stop the natural tendency of frozen sections to curl upwards on sectioning. The device is usually made of Plexiglas or a hard plastic material. The anti-roll plate is aligned parallel to the blade edge and fractionally above it. The plate can be raised or lowered against the knife, to increase the angle between the knife and the blade. It is the micro-adjusting of the anti-roll plate that determines the success of sectioning the tissue block. Anti-roll adjustments include:

- correct height of blade edge
- correct angle of blade
- edge of plate should not be nicked or damaged
- cabinet temperature

If the anti-roll plate is not working correctly, a sable hair brush can be used to manipulate the section.

Sectioning technique

Frozen sectioning often requires practice to master the technique. Speed, tissue type, and temperature of the block and the cabinet play important roles in frozen sectioning. The cut section will rest on the surface of the blade holder after cutting; a room temperature slide is held above the section, where electrostatic attraction causes the tissue to adhere to the slide. If tissues are being cut that will require harsh or lengthy staining procedures, positively charged or coated slides should be used. If coated slides are required, there are several methods, gelatin-formaldehyde or poly-L-lysine (0.01% aqueous solution). Difficult sections may also be cut and placed on the slide by use of a tape transfer system. This system is valuable for tissue sections that will not adhere to the slide.

Gelatin-formaldehyde mixture

1% gelatin	5 ml
2% formaldehyde	5 ml

Coat slides with the above mixture. Allow to dry at 37°C over 1 hour or overnight before picking up sections. Another suitable adhesive is poly-L-lysine.

Poly-L-lysine coating

0.01% poly-L-lysine (PLL) aqueous

1. Wash slides in detergent for 30 minutes.
2. Wash slides in running tap water for 30 minutes.
3. Rinse slides in distilled water twice, 1 minute each.
4. Wash slides in 95% alcohol twice, 5 minutes each.
5. Air dry slides for 10 minutes.
6. Smear 20 ml of PLL over each slide.
7. Air dry and store dust free.

This is often used as a section adhesive in immunohistochemistry.

Rapid biopsy for intra-operative diagnosis

Frozen sections provide a valuable tool in the rapid diagnosis of tissues during surgery. The pathologist selects a piece of tissue; the tissue is frozen using one of the several techniques that have previously been discussed. The slide is immediately submerged in cold acetone or 95% alcohol. The sections are stained immediately by a rapid hematoxylin and eosin (H&E), methylene blue or polychrome stain. With properly cut and stained slides a rapid diagnosis can be made for the operating suite.

Ultracryotomy

Ultracryotomy is used primarily in research laboratories. It involves rapid freezing of fixed or unfixed tissue by using isopentane and liquid nitrogen and cutting sections at 50 to 150 nm. Much success has been gained by pre-fixing the tissue in glutaraldehyde prior to sectioning.

Equipment

There are two basic types of equipment for frozen ultra-thin sectioning. The first uses a standard or slightly modified ultra-microtome in a deep freeze, and the second utilizes a microtome specially designed for ultra-thin sectioning at low temperatures. The temperature control on these ultracryotomes is between −20 and −212°C. The sections are cut with a glass knife and picked up on grids. A cutting temperature of approximately −180°C is suitable for most tissues. These sections are useful in the localization of enzyme activity at the ultrastructural level.

Freeze drying and freeze substitution

Freeze drying is the technique of rapid-freezing (quenching) of fresh tissue at −160°C, and the subsequent removal of water molecules (in the form of ice) by sublimation in a vacuum at a higher temperature (−40°C). The blocks are then raised to room temperature and fixed by vapor or embedded in a suitable medium. This technique is usually restricted to research laboratories. The technique minimizes:

- loss of soluble substances
- displacement of cell constituents
- chemical alteration of reactive groups
- denaturation of proteins
- destruction or inactivation of enzymes

There are four stages to freeze drying:

Quenching

Quenching instantly stops chemical reactions and diffusion in the tissue. It converts the tissue into a solid state in which unbound water in the tissue is changed into small ice crystals, which are subsequently removed in the drying phase.

Drying

This stage in the technique is the most time-consuming because the tissues contain 70–80% water by weight that has to be removed without damage to the tissue. Drying is divided into three distinct steps:

- Introduction of heat to the tissue to cause sublimation of ice
- Transfer of water vapor from the ice crystals through the dry portion of the tissue
- Removal of water vapor from the surface of the specimen

Drying of tissue takes place when heat is supplied to the frozen tissue in a vacuum of 133 mPa or greater. The heat vaporizes the water molecules that pass through the tissue to the surface. For drying to continue there must be efficient removal of the water molecules from the surface of the specimen. The water molecules leaving the tissue are removed by a vapor trap: either a "cold finger" trap filled with liquid nitrogen or a chemical trap containing a dehydrant chemical such as phosphorus pentoxide.

Fixation and embedding

When the tissue is completely dry, it is allowed to come to room temperature. At atmospheric pressure it will not absorb moisture unless drying is incomplete, when the tissue will rapidly reabsorb the water. The dried piece of tissue is extremely friable, and any undue pressure on it will cause the tissue to disintegrate into a fine powder. The delicate tissue is ready for embedding and sectioning or for fixing in a suitable vapor.

Vapor fixation

A number of fixatives can be used in their vapor form, including formaldehyde, glutaraldehyde, and osmium tetroxide. The most important is formaldehyde. This gives excellent preservation of the tissue components, and the tissue can be used for all histochemical techniques, with the exception of enzymes. Following fixation, the tissue is embedded in paraffin.

Applications and uses of freeze-dried material

Initially, the technique of freeze drying was used as a method of demonstrating fine structural details. Other applications include:

- immunohistochemistry methods
- demonstration of hydrolytic enzymes
- fluorescent antibody studies and formaldehyde-induced fluorescence
- autoradiography
- microspectrofluorimetry of autofluorescent substances
- mucosubstances
- scanning electron microscopy
- formaldehyde-induced fluorescence
- proteins

Fluorescent antibody studies

These studies are usually carried out on cryostat sections. Many polypeptides and polypeptide hormones are better demonstrated on freeze-dried sections.

Autoradiography

This technique provides excellent results with freeze-dried sections, and accurate localization of soluble substances can be achieved. Water-soluble isotopes can be used if the sections are dry-mounted onto the slides.

Microspectrofluorimetry of autofluorescent substances

This technique requires sections that are unaltered by processing methods. Frozen sections give adequate results, but are affected by thawing of the water in the section. The effect of the embedding medium on freeze-dried sections appears to cause less damage.

Formaldehyde-induced fluorescence (FIF)

Formaldehyde-induced fluorescence (FIF) is used in the demonstration of biogenic amines. This technique is known as the Falck method (1962), and it involves the use of blocks of tissue that are freeze-dried and subjected to formal vapor at a temperature between 60°C and 80°C, under controlled humidities. FIF is used to demonstrate 5-hydroxytryptamine, epinephrine (adrenaline), norepinephrine (noradrenaline) and other catecholamines. When these amines react with formalin they are converted to fluorescent compounds (Chapter 19).

Mucosubstances

Formal vapor fixation after freeze-drying produces good staining of mucosubstances. The reactivity of mucins appears unaltered, while the localization is improved compared to frozen or paraffin sections. The uses of freeze-dried sections are recommended for the accurate demonstration and localization of glycogen.

Proteins

Many proteins can be satisfactorily demonstrated on suitably fixed freeze-dried sections. Formal vapor fixation may remove some protein sections.

Scanning electron microscopy (SEM)

Standard processing procedures do not work well for electron microscopy. Processing causes alterations: water present in the tissue will evaporate when placed in vacuum conditions, which leads to distortion of the tissue. Frozen tissues under vacuum will slowly freeze dry, and the sublimation of the ice from the tissue surface will distort the picture.

Frozen section substitution

The technique of frozen section substitution involves the rapid freezing of the tissue to −160°C in isopentane supercooled by liquid nitrogen. Cryostat sections are cut at 8–10 μm and placed in a cold container maintained at cryostat temperature. The sections are transferred to water-free acetone and cooled to −70°C for 12 hours. The sections are floated onto slides and allowed to dry. The histochemical method is applied. For most diagnostic purposes, cryostat sections preserve most tissue components. This method is convenient and labor-saving, and is easy to implement in the laboratory. Freeze drying and freeze substitution is too labor-intensive, time-consuming and capricious for clinical diagnostic use. These techniques are more commonly used in research.

Additional reading

Bancroft, J.D., 1975. Histochemical Technique, second ed. Butterworths, London.

Bancroft, J.D., Cook, H.C., 1994. Manual of Histological Techniques and their Diagnostic Application. Churchill Livingstone, Edinburgh.

Bancroft, J.D., Hand, N.M., 1987. Enzyme Histochemistry. Royal Microscopical Society Handbook 14. Oxford Science, Oxford.

Brown, R.W., 2009. Histologic Preparations: Common Problems and Their Solutions. CAP Press, Chicago, pp. 16–34.

Carson, F.L., 1997. Histotechnology, A Self-Instructional Text, second ed. ASCP Press, Chicago, pp. 35–42.

Carson, F.L., Hladic, V., 2010. Histotechnology, A Self-Instructional Text, third ed. ASCP Press, Chicago, pp. 25–42.

Falck, B., 1962. Observations on the possibilities of the cellular localization of monoamines by a fluorescence method. Acta Physiologica Scandinavica 56 (Suppl), 197.

Fedor, N., Sidman, R.L., 1958. Histological fixation by a modified freeze substitution method. Journal of Histochemistry and Cytochemistry 6, 401.

Luna, L.G., 1992. Histopathologic Methods and Color Atlas of Special Stains and Tissue Artifacts. Johnson Printers, Downers Grove, pp. 758–766.

Mailhiot, M.A., 2005. Microtomy, It's All about Technique! National Society for Histotechnology.

Merryman, H.T., 1960. Principles of freeze drying. Annals of the New York Academy of Sciences 85, 630.

Pearse, A.G.E., 1963. Rapid freeze drying of biological tissues with a thermoelectric unit. Journal of Scientific Instruments 40, 176.

Pearse, A.G.E., 1980. Histochemistry, Theoretical and Applied, fourth ed, Vol. 1. Churchill Livingstone, Edinburgh.

Pearse, A.G.E., Bancroft, J.D., 1966. Journal of the Royal Microscopical Society 85, 385.

Sheehan, D.C., Hrapchak, B., 1980. Theory and Practice of Histotechnology, second ed. C.V. Mosby Co., St Louis, pp. 79–82.

Simpson, W.L., 1941. Experimental analysis of Altman's technique of freeze drying. Anatomical Record 80, 329.

Plastic embedding for light microscopy

8

Neil M. Hand

Introduction

Paraffin wax is a suitable embedding medium for most tissues, combining adequacy of tissue support with ease of sectioning on a standard microtome. Section thicknesses of about 5 µm are satisfactory for most diagnostic purposes, although with skill and experience thinner sections may be produced. However, there are three main areas where paraffin wax is an unsuitable embedding medium for light microscopy studies. Firstly, it may not offer sufficient support for some tissues. Secondly, it does not permit very thin sections to be cut (these two factors are inter-related). Thirdly, labile substances such as enzymes are destroyed. In these circumstances, the use of plastic instead of paraffin wax may provide superior histological preparations. This chapter will focus mainly on the use of plastic techniques for light microscopy, as details of those for electron microscopy demand specific and different protocols, which are described in Chapter 22. The main applications of the use of plastic embedding are outlined below.

Ultrastructural studies

In the early development of electron microscopy, extremely hard ester waxes were used with limited success. They were unsuitable for ultrastructural studies as they did not offer sufficient support for ultra-thin sections (approximately 30–80 nm), and because they were unable to withstand the high-energy electron beam that passes through the section within the electron microscope (see Chapter 22). The introduction of plastic/resin embedding media during the 1950s provided improved results and stimulated the development of electron microscopy. Nunn (1970) and Glauert (1987) discuss the properties of embedding media suitable for ultrastructural studies.

Hard tissues and implants

In extremely hard tissues such as undecalcified bone, especially where the sample is large and/or when dense cortical bone is present, the difference in hardness between the tissue and the medium in which it is embedded may be so great that sectioning is exceptionally difficult, resulting in only poor-quality fragmented sections being obtained. Therefore the use of a harder embedding medium such as a plastic can enable superior sections to be cut, compared to the use of paraffin wax. This may be achieved either in the form of a section using a motorized microtome, or as a slice which is then ground down to the required thickness. The latter (known as a ground section) requires specialized equipment and procedures that are different from those used for conventional microtomy. Ground sections are useful if inorganic material such as a stent (vascular implant) is present, or the tissue is tooth, as these are virtually impossible to section by traditional means. These applications are discussed more fully in Chapter 16.

High-resolution light microscopy

It has long been appreciated that where an accurate diagnosis and prognosis may depend on the detection of some subtle histological or cytological change, sections thinner than the usual 5 μm greatly facilitate accurate examination. The two best-known examples are for renal biopsy and interpretation of hematopoietic tissue, where the reduction of paraffin section thickness to about 2 μm has led to easier and more accurate diagnosis through the detection of minor histological abnormalities which are obscured in thicker sections. Experience has proved that even thinner sections, combined with high-quality optics, will provide a more accurate assessment by light microscopy of minor histological abnormalities in the renal biopsy. Unfortunately, even with the greatest skill and experience, it has (until recently with the waxes available) been extremely difficult to produce good-quality sections thinner than about 3 μm. As a result the possibilities for high-resolution light microscopy have been limited, and though slightly thinner sections can be produced nowadays with superior waxes and microtomes, the artifacts produced in wax sections limits potential morphological improvements. These artifacts are often less obvious if a plastic is employed as the embedding medium.

Pathologists experienced in the use of electron microscopy have long been aware of the increased amount of cytological detail detectable in 0.5–1 μm plastic-embedded tissue sections produced prior to ultra-thin sectioning for ultrastructural studies. It was the realization of the diagnostic value of high-resolution light microscopy in identifying certain nuclear and cytoplasmic characteristics, which are usually obscured in thicker sections, that led to an interest in plastic embedding for specific uses in diagnostic histopathology. In practice, tissue sections other than those from a renal biopsy are frequently cut at 2–3 μm (referred to as semi-thin sections), to combine satisfactory resolution with sufficient staining intensity and contrast. As applications and histological procedures have developed, there have been a variety of techniques and uses applied to plastic sections for high-resolution light microscopy, some of which will be discussed in this chapter.

Plastic embedding media

Plastics are classified according to their chemical composition into epoxy, polyester, or acrylic. The change in the physical state of an embedding medium from liquid to solid is called polymerization and is brought about by joining molecules together to produce a complex macromolecule made up of repeating units. The macromolecule, termed polymer (derived from the Greek word *poly* meaning 'many' and *mer* meaning 'part'), is synthesized from simple molecules called monomers ('single part'). Several ingredients are required to produce a plastic suitable as an embedding medium for biological material and subsequent histological examination. Some of these ingredients can present potential health and safety problems, and it is important that all chemicals used in the formulation of plastics are handled in accordance with local and legal safety requirements. The chemical reactions between the various ingredients in plastic embedding kits, including the process of polymerization, are complex and more akin to data found in the polymer industry. However, as it is useful to understand the fundamental role of particular components, an outline is discussed below.

Epoxy plastics

Various epoxy plastics have found their widest application as embedding media for ultrastructural studies, because the polymerized plastic is sufficiently hard to permit sections as thin as 30–40 nm to be cut, and it is stable in an electron beam. Embedding schedules for the different epoxy resins used in electron microscopy are given in Chapter 22, and only a brief outline of their properties and uses is given here. Epoxy plastics derive their name from the active group through which they polymerize (Fig. 8.1).

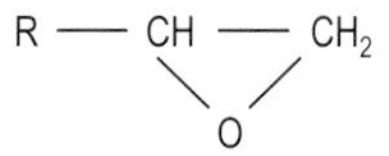

$$R \text{---} CH \text{---} CH_2$$
$$\diagdown \diagup$$
$$O$$

Figure 8.1 The active epoxide group in all epoxy plastics.

Epoxide or oxirane groups can be attached to an almost infinite number of chemical structures in single or multifunctional conformations. Three types of epoxy plastic are used in microscopy: those based on either bisphenol A (Araldite), glycerol (Epon), or cyclohexene dioxide (Spurr). The names in parentheses are those in common usage by microscopists and do not convey any structural information.

Epoxy embedding plastics are a carefully balanced mixture of epoxy plastic, catalyst, and accelerator, each component having a direct influence on the physical and mechanical properties of the cured plastic. The catalyst system used is of the anhydride/amine type and causes curing of the resin through the formation of ester cross-links. The anhydride catalyst can be either a long-chain aliphatic anhydride, e.g. dodecenyl succinic anhydride (DDSA), or an aromatic fused ring anhydride, e.g. methyl nadic anhydride (MNA). The long-chain anhydrides act as internal plasticizers which make blocks more flexible and generally tough, whereas MNA is a rigid molecule that results in stiffening and hardening of cured blocks. Both catalysts increase the hydrophobicity of the plastic, but this property can be reduced by oxidizing the alkyl chains and aromatic rings with peroxides.

The amines used as accelerators are either mono- or poly-functional. As amines form adducts with epoxide groups, the use of poly-functional amines, e.g. dimethylamino methyl phenol (DMP 30), can result in the formation of three-dimensional structures, which are slow to diffuse and hence slow to infiltrate tissue. Thus the mono-functional amines, ethanolamine and benzyl dimethyl amine (BDMA), are more conducive to faster infiltration times. The only other common additive in epoxy plastic mixtures is dibutyl phthalate (DBP), which is present as an external plasticizer to soften the blocks, especially in 'Araldite' formulations.

The rate at which each epoxy plastic infiltrates the tissue depends on the density of the tissue and the size of the diffusing molecules. Infiltration by Araldite is slow, partly because of the formation of amine adducts, but also because the epoxy plastic itself is a large molecule. The glycerol-based epoxy plastics (Epon) have a lower viscosity but are often sold as mixtures of isomers, and care should be exercised in choosing the most suitable fraction of isomers. Cyclohexene dioxide-based plastics (Spurr) can be obtained pure and infiltrate the fastest, having a low viscosity (7 centipoise at 25°C). Infiltration at higher temperatures is faster, although agglomerates can form and these negate any increase in the diffusion coefficient.

The physical properties of epoxy plastics are considerably affected by their rate of polymerization. In industry, the same formulations as used in microscopy are cured at temperatures in excess of 150°C for up to several days, whereas tissue blocks at 60°C are considerably undercured. Rapid curing for 1 hour at 120°C produces large numbers of cross-links, but hard brittle blocks; 18 hours at 60°C results in tougher blocks that are more suitable for sectioning and subsequent microscopy. Care is needed to provide a section with the right level of cross-linking to allow staining later. Sodium methoxide can be used to reduce the cross-link density of the cured plastic by trans-esterifying the ester cross-links. This allows the plastic to expand more in solvents and improves access to the tissue for stains and antibodies.

Stability in an electron beam arises from two main factors. Both aromatic and unsaturated groups can stabilize the radicals formed by electron impact, either within the aromatic ring or along an unsaturated aliphatic chain, thus preventing chain fission and depolymerization. Further stability is induced by cross-links that minimize the effects of any depolymerization that occurs by preventing creep.

Epoxy plastics have some disadvantages: they are hydrophobic and subsequent oxidation by peroxide to correct this may produce tissue damage. Both epoxide groups and anhydrides can react under mild conditions with proteins, which may reduce the antigenicity of embedded tissue, and may in addition cause sensitization of workers who absorb them by skin contact or inhalation. The components of many epoxy plastics are toxic, and one, vinylcyclohexane dioxide (VCD), is known to be carcinogenic. Hence gloves should always be worn when handling these plastics, and adequate facilities must be provided for the removal of the chemical vapors and the disposal of toxic waste (Causton 1981).

Cutting and staining epoxy sections for light microscopy

Ultra-thin section cutting and staining for electron microscopy are discussed in detail in Chapter 22. It is not possible to obtain satisfactory sections of thickness 0.5–1 µm on a standard microtome using a steel knife, so semi-thin sections are produced using a glass or diamond knife, and cut on a motorized microtome. Using specialized strips of glass and equipment, two types of glass knives can be prepared: either the more common triangular shape Latta-Hartmann knife or the Ralph knife, which has a longer cutting edge.

To an observer experienced in its interpretation, there is little doubt that for high-resolution light microscopy, toluidine blue is the most useful and informative stain applied to tissue sections embedded in an epoxy plastic. If the stain is heated and used at high alkaline pH, it easily penetrates the plastic and stains various tissue components a blue color of differing shades and intensities, with no appreciable staining of the embedding medium. The staining intensity of tissue components by toluidine blue largely reflects its electron density, and the ultrastructural appearances on subsequent electron microscopy can be partly predicted by the appearances at light microscopy level. For those who prefer polychromatic stains, various formulations, e.g. Paragon, can be used which resemble H&E staining. Many staining techniques can be applied after the surface resin has been 'etched' using alcoholic sodium hydroxide (Janes 1979), but the results are not always reliable. Another type of pre-treatment consists of oxidizing osmium-fixed tissue without etching (Bourne & St John 1978) so that aqueous solutions can be stained more consistently.

A few reports have described the application of immunohistochemistry to epoxy sections for light microscopy studies following treatment with sodium ethoxide/methoxide (Giddings et al. 1982; McCluggage et al. 1995; Krenacs et al. 2005), but this practice is seldom used. In general, for the majority of occasions when high-resolution light microscopy is required, it is preferable to use acrylic plastic sections because of their potential easier handling and quality of staining achieved, although some techniques such as immunohistochemistry (as discussed later) have presented tough challenges.

Polyester plastics

These plastics were originally introduced for electron microscopy in the mid-1950s, but were soon superseded by the superior epoxides for ultrastructural purposes. Nowadays they are rarely used for microscopy, although Mawhinney and Ellis (1983) have reported on the use of embedding undecalcified bone for light microscopy studies.

Acrylic plastics

The acrylic plastics used for microscopy are esters of acrylic acid ($CH_2 \cdot \cdot CH \cdot COOH$) or more commonly methacrylic acid ($CH \cdot \cdot C(CH_3) \cdot COOH$), and are often referred to as acrylates and methacrylates, respectively. They are used extensively for light microscopy, but some have been formulated so that electron microscopy can be performed, either in addition or exclusively. Numerous mixes can be devised to produce plastics that provide a wide range of properties, and consequently there is a diverse range of potential uses. Butyl, methyl, and glycol methacrylate (the latter is chemically the monomer 2-hydroxyethyl methacrylate or HEMA) were all introduced for electron microscopy, but are now rarely used (unless as a component of a mix) because the plastic disrupts in the electron beam. However, greater success has been achieved in the production and staining of semi-thin sections for high-resolution light microscopy.

Conventional acrylics are cured by complex free-radical chain reactions. The intermediate chemicals formed have an incomplete number of electrons. The monomer is exposed to a source of radicals, usually produced from the breakdown of a catalyst such as benzoyl peroxide. This decomposes to produce phenyl (benzoyl-peroxy) radicals that transfer to the double bond of the acrylic monomer, and which then itself breaks to become a radical in turn. This now acts as an active site, attracting and joining another monomer by repeating the process of opening the carbon-carbon double bond and forming a covalent link. In this way a polymer is formed by joining monomeric units together to produce a long aliphatic chain. Finally, to complete the polymer, a phenyl radical instead of another monomer molecule attaches to the active site to block and terminate further reactions. Both oxygen and acetone prevent attachment of radicals and therefore should be avoided during the curing process.

Radicals can be produced spontaneously by light or heat, and consequently acrylic plastics and their monomers should be stored in dark bottles in a cool place. Acrylics contain a few parts per million of hydroquinone to prevent premature polymerization, and for most applications this can remain when preparing the embedding mixes. Benzoyl peroxide is the most common source of radicals, since it breaks down at 50–60°C, but the addition of a tertiary aromatic amine, e.g. *N,N*-dimethylaniline or dimethyl *p*-toluidine, can cause the peroxide to break down into radicals at 0°C, so that the plastic can be cured at low or room temperature. Dry benzoyl peroxide is explosive and is therefore supplied damped with water, or as a paste mixed with dibutyl phthalate, or as plasticized particles. In some mixes, the water is required to be removed and care must be taken to dry aliquots away from direct sunlight or heat. Azobisisobutyronitrile and Perkadox 16 are other catalysts that have been used, but by far the most popular is benzoyl peroxide. Light-sensitive photocatalysts such as benzil and benzoin (various types) are used for polymerization of acrylics at subzero temperature using short wavelength light.

In addition to the monomer and catalyst, several other ingredients are often necessary in acrylic plastics. An amine will stimulate polymerization to proceed at a faster rate, and consequently these chemicals are termed either activators or more commonly accelerators. Other activators include sulfinic acid and some barbiturates. To improve the sectioning qualities of acrylic blocks, softeners or plasticizers are often added to the mix. Examples are 2-butoxyethanol, 2-isopropoxyethanol, polyethylene glycol 200/400 and dibutyl phthalate. Some acrylic mixes require a small amount of a cross-linker to stabilize the matrix of the plastic against physical damage caused by either the electron beam (Lowicryl plastics) or staining solutions (Technovit 8100). An example of a cross-linking agent is the difunctional ethylene glycol dimethacrylate, which provides flexible hydrophilic cross-links. Unlike epoxides, the viscosity of acrylics is low and hence short infiltration times are possible, although the size and nature of tissue, together with the processing and embedding temperature, will affect the times required.

Poly (2-hydroxyethyl methacrylate) 'glycol methacrylate' (GMA) has proved to be a popular embedding medium for light microscopy since it is extremely hydrophilic, allowing many tinctorial staining methods to be applied, yet tough enough when dehydrated to section well on most microtomes. Various mixes have been reported, with a result that some may be either prepared from the ingredients or purchased as a commercial kit, but many are based on the recipe published by Ruddell (1967). Although the mixes all contain the monomer HEMA, the proportion and variety of this and other ingredients may be different, leading to dissimilar characteristics between various kits. The monomer can be contaminated with methacrylic acid, which may result in some background staining, but this can be reduced by purchasing low-acid HEMA or a high-quality proprietary kit such as JB4, JB4 Plus (Polysciences Inc., USA), Technovit 7100, or Technovit 8100 (Kulzer, Germany). Butyl methacrylate is now rarely used for any histological purpose unless as an ingredient in an acrylic mix, e.g. Unicryl (British BioCell International, UK), since it has proved unreliable and produces considerable tissue artifact during polymerization.

There are also available aromatic polyhydroxy dimethacrylate resins (Histocryl, LR White & LR Gold from London Resin Company, UK). Histocryl is intended for light microscopy purposes but LR White and LR Gold can be used both for light and electron microscopy since they combine hydrophilicity with electron beam stability. LR White may be polymerized by the addition of dimethyl *p*-toluidine, whereas LR Gold is cured by the addition of benzil and exposure to a quartz halogen lamp specifically for sub-zero temperature embedding. Other acrylic plastics cured at low temperature include Lowicryl HM20, HM23 (hydrophobic) and K4M, K4M Plus, K11M (hydrophilic), and Unicryl (formerly called Bioacryl). The Lowicryls may be cured by the addition of a benzoin photocatalyst exposed to ultraviolet light. Though in some cases these plastics can be employed for light microscopy studies, they are really intended and are more suitable for electron microscopy. Lowicryl K4M Plus is a light curable epoxy-acrylate product combining rapid polymerization of an acrylic with the high strength of an epoxy. Various plastic embedding kits have been marketed under different names (especially the Technovit range), which has caused confusion (Hand 1995a), and there is a constant introduction of new proprietary kits, each with claims suggesting their suitability for specific studies, which often makes it difficult for the scientist to know which to choose. Currently many of these kits are available from TABB, UK and/or Polysciences, USA.

For many years methyl methacrylate (MMA) has been widely used because of its hardness as the ideal embedding medium for undecalcified bone, other hard tissues, and tissues with stents or implants, and again there are proprietary kits such as Technovit 9100, (Kulzer) OsteoBed (Polysciences) and Acrylosin (Dorn & Hart Microedge Inc.) for these purposes. However, by using the MMA monomer in specially devised mixes and in specific ways, it has been shown that tinctorial and immunohistochemical staining on semi-thin sections for high-resolution light microscopy is possible.

Applications of acrylic sections

The development of acrylic plastic embedding media has usually been stimulated by a requirement for a specific application. Most applications are for light microscopy, but as understanding of the formulation of acrylics has increased, so too have various plastics been introduced which may also be useful for some electron microscopy studies. Some of these plastics, such as the Lowicryls, have been developed mainly for electron microscopy alone (Carlemalm et al. 1982; Acetarin et al. 1986), whereas LR White and Unicryl (Scala et al. 1992) can be used for either purpose. However, for various technical reasons, not all dual-purpose plastics are practical for routine high-resolution light microscopy studies.

Hydrophilic plastics such as GMA and LR White allow tissue to be stained without removal of the embedding medium, and have therefore become popular for routine use. Many 'simple' staining techniques may be applied, but some may require modification or present special difficulties to those used on paraffin sections. All acrylic hydrophilic media are insoluble, and consequently all staining occurs with the plastic *in situ*. This can cause problems in two ways, either because the medium itself becomes stained, which may affect the final appearance, or because the matrix acts as a physical barrier to particular molecules. The most obvious example where the latter occurs is the difficulty that large molecules have in penetrating the plastic matrix during immunohistochemical staining. The alternative use of hydrophobic MMA without the addition of cross-linking agents as an embedding medium permits the plastic to be dissolved, and for certain techniques this is an extremely useful property. However, hydrophobic plastics such as Lowicryl HM20 and HM23 that contain cross-linking agents are insoluble.

Acrylic plastics may be polymerized in different ways by using a chemical accelerator, heat, or light. The optimum method depends on several factors, including the study required and the practicality of the method chosen. Polymerization can also be induced at low temperature, and with some Lowicryl plastics, processing and embedding can be accomplished at temperatures down to −70°C. K4M is the most popular, and is said at −35°C to enhance ultrastructural preservation and immunohistochemical staining.

Tinctorial staining

Acrylics have become popular for high-resolution light microscopy mainly because of the ease with which sections can be stained. Excellent staining may be achieved on tissue embedded in any of the various GMA mixes/kits and other acrylics such as LR White, even though the plastic cannot be removed. Numerous (but not all) routine histological staining methods may be applied, including H&E, PAS, van Gieson, alcian blue, Perls', elastic methods, Giemsa, and silver techniques for reticulin. Modifications from the standard methods for paraffin sections may be necessary and, because London Resins (Histocryl, LR White, and LR Gold) are all softened by alcohol with the possibility of section loss from the slide, alcoholic staining solutions such as those used in elastic methods should be avoided. Consequently, even hematoxylin staining on London Resins should be progressive to avoid differentiation with acid alcohol, whereas regressive staining on GMA is (with care) possible. The plastic embedding medium (especially GMA) may also become stained, but in some techniques this can be reduced by various washing procedures.

An alternative approach is to use MMA where the plastic can easily be removed prior to staining, using similar procedures and solutions but with slightly extended times to those used routinely for dewaxing paraffin sections. It is beyond the scope of this chapter to describe in detail numerous staining methods on different acrylics, but generally best results are achieved using either a method previously published or one that is recommended by other histologists. It should be noted that tinctorial staining of tissue embedded in MMA is possible (where no cross-linker has been added) without removing the plastic, and this is often useful for sections of undecalcified bone MMA prepared as described in Chapter 16. However, this type of procedure is unsuitable for semi-thin sections described in this chapter for high-resolution light microscopy.

Enzyme histochemistry

The ability to process, embed, and polymerize some acrylic plastics at low temperature enables several enzymes to be preserved and demonstrated in tissue sections. Many enzymes are destroyed by routine fixation and processing, but under controlled

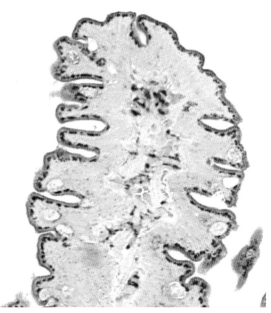

Figure 8.2 Section of jejunum fixed in formal calcium and embedded in glycol methacrylate (JB4) showing hydrolytic acid phosphatase activity in the macrophages (lamina propria) and lysozymes in the villi using hexazonium pararosanilin. Original magnification × 325. (Reproduced with permission from Hand, N.M., 1999. Plastic embedding for light microscopy. A guide for the histotechnologist. *Tech Sample*. Histotechnology No. HT-6. 29-35. © American Society of Clinical Pathologists.)

conditions several (mainly hydrolytic) enzymes may be localized, including those illustrated in Figures 8.2 and 8.3. Fixation, processing, and polymerization are all usually carried out at 4°C, and sections are dried on to a coverglass or slide at room temperature overnight (rather than at 60°C) prior to performing enzyme histochemical staining.

A variety of aldehyde fixatives have been advocated, but in this author's experience 10% formal calcium as recommended by Dawson (1972) has proved successful. Enhanced staining can be further achieved if the tissue is subsequently washed at 4°C in 3% buffered sucrose solution. Hand (1988) has also shown that enzyme activity may also be affected during processing, infiltration, embedding, and polymerization, and therefore to achieve best results the effects of these stages on a particular enzyme should first be ascertained. Polymerization is normally carried out at 4°C using a chemical

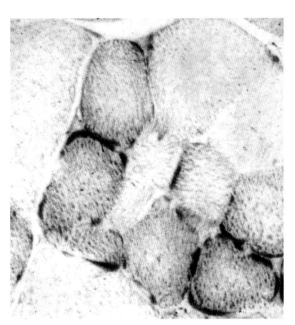

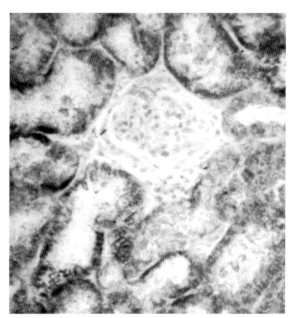

Figure 8.3 Section of transversely cut muscle fixed in formal calcium and embedded in glycol methacrylate (JB4), showing oxidative NADH diaphorase staining in mitochondria using methyl-thiazolyldiphenyl tetrazolium (MTT).

Figure 8.4 Section of unfixed kidney embedded in LR Gold which has been photo-polymerized, showing succinate dehydrogenase activity in mitochondria using tetra-nitro blue tetrazolium (TNBT).

accelerator, but for methods utilizing sub-zero temperatures either an excess of catalyst or a photocatalyst has been employed.

The use of GMA for enzyme histochemical studies is preferred, as this acrylic is probably the easiest to handle and produces the best results. Various enzyme histochemical investigations have been described using several different techniques on plastic-embedded tissue including the identification of cell types (Beckstead 1983), cephaloridine nephrotoxicity in rats (Bennett 1982), and assessment of malabsorption on jejunum (Hand 1987).

A further development described by Thompson and Germain (1983) employed processing fresh (unfixed) tissue stabilized with polyvinyl pyrollidine (MW 44,000) at −25°C and embedded in LR Gold. Polymerization was induced by irradiating the plastic containing the photocatalyst benzil with blue light from a quartz halogen lamp. This specialized procedure offers the potential to demonstrate enzymes, including those that are sensitive to fixation, but in reality the only additional enzyme demonstrated to those that survive mild fixation

has been the oxidative enzyme succinate dehydrogenase (Fig. 8.4). Other enzymes that have been demonstrated in fixed tissue include acid phosphatase, adenosine triphosphatase (membrane), alkaline phosphatase, chloroacetate esterase, dipeptidyl (amino) peptidase IV, lactase, lactate dehydrogenase, leucine aminopeptidase, α-galactosidase, glucose-6-phosphate, phosphate dehydrogenase, α-glucuronidase, γ-glutamyl transpeptidase, NADH, α-naphthyl acetate, non-specific esterase, 5α-nucleotidase, peroxidase, and sucrase. Following successful staining, care must be taken to ensure that enzyme diffusion and loss do not occur during the washing and mounting procedures.

Immunohistochemistry

During the past 30 years, numerous reports have been published describing the application of immunohistochemistry to acrylic-embedded tissue sections, with even a GMA kit developed specifically for this use (ImmunoBed from Polysciences Inc., USA). However, immunohistochemical staining still remains a controversial topic because the results have been mainly idiosyncratic and disappointing, leading many laboratories to abandon this type of investigation for diagnostic purposes. Further confusion has been compounded by the wide variety of plastics and techniques advocated, but a major cause of unreliable immunostaining is that many of the acrylics are insoluble in their polymerized form. Although it would be too simplistic an explanation to imply that all the problems are due to the insolubility of the polymer involved, there is no doubt that the presence of the embedding medium can present formidable difficulties (Gerrits 1988).

Many papers based on the classic publications of Beckstead (1985) and Casey et al. (1988) have tried to create mild conditions by fixing, processing, and then polymerizing the plastic at low temperature in an attempt to protect sensitive antigens, and produce a 'looser' matrix that would be more conducive to allowing large immunological reagents to penetrate through to antigen sites. Unfortunately, this is not always easy to control, and further cross-linking can continue after 'polymerization' to produce super-polymerization that will inhibit access of reagents to the antigens. In addition, it has long been recognized that tissue antigens may be chemically altered by the reagents in the plastic embedding medium (Takamiya et al. 1980). A more recent novel application of immunostaining using specialized procedures with GMA has been described by Howat et al. (2005) for tissue microarrays.

A variety of complex and sophisticated staining protocols using 3,3'-diaminobenzidine tetrahydrochloride (DAB) as the chromogen have also been suggested. One particular procedure recommended by Newman et al. (1983) for LR White used an enhancement technique, where DAB was intensified using a gold-sulfide-silver method to detect immunohistochemical reactivity. Using small molecular weight antibodies and chromogens such as aminoethylcarbazole (AEC) are suggested to improve immunostaining with ImmunoBed (Polysciences).

Though immunohistochemistry is possible on all acrylic plastics, the non-routine procedures required, coupled with frequently poor results, do not encourage this type of histological examination for light microscopy. Against this background, an alternative concept employing a plastic based on MMA was developed (Hand et al. 1989; Hand & Morrell 1990). Tissue can be fixed in formalin under routine conditions and then processed and embedded at room temperature. The plastic is polymerized using a chemical accelerator, e.g. *N,N*-dimethylaniline, although other amines have been successfully used. The embedding procedure is similar to that used for GMA blocks using an open moulding tray system inside a glass desiccator. The main difference from other acrylics is that the polymerized plastic is soluble, and therefore can be removed prior to staining, which is particularly advantageous for immunohistochemical staining. Routine tinctorial staining is obviously possible, although the procedure is probably not suitable for the localization of many enzymes. To date, over 100 antibodies have been successfully demonstrated with excellent results, including those illustrated in Figures 8.5–8.7. Further details are discussed later in this chapter relating to immunohistochemical staining on MMA sections.

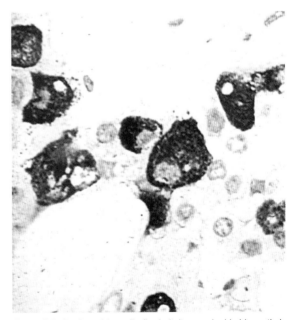

Figure 8.5 Section of formalin-fixed pituitary embedded in methyl methacrylate showing localization of adrenocorticotropin hormone (ACTH) with immunoperoxidase staining. Chromogen 3,3 α-diaminobenzidine tetrahydrochloride (DAB).

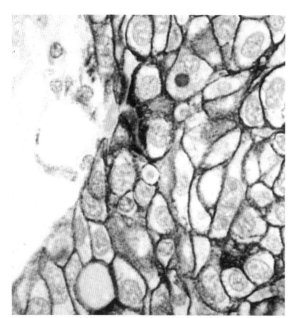

Figure 8.6 Section of formalin-fixed ovarian tumor embedded in methyl methacrylate showing immunoperoxidase staining of cytokeratin 7 following pretreatment using microwave antigen retrieval. Chromogen DAB. (Reproduced, with permission, from Hand, N.M., Blythe, D., Jackson, P., 1996. Antigen unmasking using microwave heating on formalin fixed tissue embedded in methyl methacrylate. Journal of Cellular Pathology 1, 31–37. © Greenwich Medical Media Ltd, London.)

In situ hybridization

Only a few methods have been described for *in situ* hybridization on various plastic sections using either isotopic or non-isotopic techniques. Studies by Church et al. (1997, 1998) and Doverty (2005, 2007), both using non-isotopic methods on MMA sections, have demonstrated *Sox* gene mRNA in chick tissue, and kappa (κ) and lambda (λ) mRNA in bone marrow trephines, respectively.

Acrylic plastic processing schedules

Processing and embedding schedule for glycol methacrylate using ingredients *(Ruddell 1967)*

Solution a

2-hydroxyethyl (glycol) methacrylate	80 ml
2-butoxyethanol	16 ml
Dried benzoyl peroxide	0.27 g

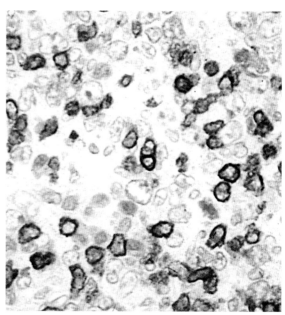

Figure 8.7 Section of formalin-fixed lymph node embedded in methyl methacrylate showing immunoperoxidase staining of T lymphocytes with anti-CD3 following pretreatment with trypsin digestion and subsequent heat-induced antigen retrieval using a pressure cooker. Chromogen DAB. (Reproduced, with permission, from Hand, N.M., 1999. Plastic embedding for light microscopy. A guide for the histotechnologist. *Tech Sample*. Histotechnology No. HT-6. 29–35. © American Society of Clinical Pathologists.)

Solution b

Polyethylene glycol 400	15 parts
N,N-dimethylaniline	1 part

Fixation

Fix tissues in formalin, e.g. formal saline, neutral buffered formalin, or buffered paraformaldehyde.

Processing and embedding

1. If necessary, rinse tissue in an appropriate buffer for 15 minutes.
2. Dehydrate through 70%, 90%, and 100% ethanol. For an average block of 10 × 5 × 2 mm, use two 15 minutes changes in each solution.
3. Infiltrate in two changes of solution a, each for 1 hour.
4. Embed in the following mixture:

Solution a	42 parts
Solution b	1 part

5. Polymerize at room temperature, standing the mould in cold water to dissipate heat generated by

the exothermic reaction. Polymerization should be complete in 2–4 hours.

Notes

a. Specimens should only be processed under a fume hood with extraction.

b. Processing is best achieved if the specimens are agitated continuously on a roller mixer.

c. Small aliquots of benzoyl peroxide should be dried carefully away from direct heat and sunlight as it is potentially explosive. It must be completely dissolved in the infiltrating solution and this may take up to 30 minutes.

d. Several block moulding systems are commercially available, but the open polypropylene moulding tray system enables the tissue to be attached directly onto a block stub (Polysciences Inc., USA). To achieve good polymerization, the mould should be placed inside a glass desiccator and oxygen excluded by filling the chamber with oxygen-free nitrogen. The chamber is then sealed.

e. The acrylic plastic mixes are best prepared in the quantity required, preferably using a large capped glass vial. It is advisable to measure the quantities by volume.

f. Any waste solutions containing plastic components must be handled and discarded in accordance with local and legal requirements.

benzoyl peroxide plasticized (C) in 100 ml of solution A or the equivalent, until the solid is completely dissolved). Most tissues require at least 3 hours' infiltration depending on the nature and size of the tissue. Hard dense tissues such as bone are best infiltrated overnight at 4°C.

4. Embed in fresh embedding medium (add 1 ml of solution B to 25 ml of freshly catalyzed solution A or the equivalent) at room temperature in a mould. The time needed for full polymerization varies with the temperature, atmospheric oxygen, etc., but at room temperature (22°C) it may take 1–2 hours. For enzyme histochemical investigations, better results will be obtained using pre-chilled solutions throughout, with processing and embedding at 4°C. In these circumstances, polymerization may take 6–12 hours.

Notes

See Notes a, b, c, d, e, and f from previous GMA schedule. Tissues may be taken directly into several changes of freshly catalyzed solution A from buffer, omitting the alcohols, but it may be necessary to extend the time of this partial dehydration with at least three changes. This procedure may produce better results with some enzyme methods, and lipids are also better retained.

Standard processing and embedding schedule for JB4 embedding medium

JB4 embedding medium is supplied as a kit, comprising two stock solutions (A and B) and separate plasticized benzoyl peroxide (C). Solution A is the infiltrating/embedding medium and solution B is the accelerator.

Fixation

Any, preferably formalin or paraformaldehyde.

Processing and embedding

1. If necessary, rinse tissue in an appropriate buffer for 15 minutes.

2. Dehydrate through 70%, 90%, and 100% ethanol as described for the previous GMA schedule.

3. Infiltrate tissue in two changes of freshly prepared catalyzed solution A (prepared by mixing 1.25 g of

Modified processing and embedding schedule for JB4 embedding medium

This particular schedule is especially useful for hematological bone marrow trephines to provide a firmer support medium.

Fixation

Fix tissues in formalin, e.g. formal saline, neutral buffered formalin, or buffered paraformaldehyde.

Processing and embedding

1. If necessary, rinse tissue in an appropriate buffer for 15 minutes.

2. Dehydrate through 70%, 90%, and 100% ethanol using two changes in each solution of 30 minutes.

3. Infiltrate tissue in two changes of freshly prepared catalyzed solution A (prepared by mixing 120 mg of benzoyl peroxide plasticized in 9 ml of solution A and 1 ml of methyl methacrylate monomer until

the solid is completely dissolved) for 1 hour, followed by infiltration overnight at room temperature.

4. Embed in pre-chilled embedding medium (10 ml of catalyzed solution A and 450 μl of JB4 solution B) at room temperature in a mould. The time needed for full polymerization varies with the temperature, atmospheric oxygen, etc., but at room temperature (22°C) may be 1–2 hours.

Notes

See Notes a, b, c, d, e, and f from previous GMA schedule.

Processing and embedding schedule for methyl methacrylate

This schedule can be used for routine tinctorial and immunohistochemical staining, although other schedules and mixtures have been published. Care should be taken when handling MMA as it has a pungent odor and is flammable.

Infiltration solution

Methyl methacrylate monomer (unwashed)	15 ml
Dibutyl phthalate	5 ml
Dried benzoyl peroxide	1 g

Fixation

Fix tissues in formalin, e.g. 10% formalin, 10% formal saline, or 10% formal calcium, 24–48 hours.

Processing and embedding

1. Dehydrate through 50%, 70%, and 90% ethanol. For an average block of 10 × 5 × 2 mm, use 1-hour changes in each solution.
2. Complete dehydration through two changes of 100% ethanol, each for 1 hour.
3. Infiltrate in two changes of infiltration solution, each for 1 hour.
4. Infiltrate in a further change of infiltration solution overnight.
5. Embed in 10 ml aliquots of infiltration solution to which 125 μl of *N,N*-dimethylaniline is added. Polymerization will occur in 3–4 hours. D. Blythe (personal communication) recommends 250 μl of *N,N*-dimethylaniline for bone marrow trephines, where polymerization is achieved in 1.5–2 hours.

Notes

a. Aliquots of benzoyl peroxide should be dried carefully away from direct heat and sunlight as it is potentially explosive. It is important that no water is present before dissolving the catalyst (2 minutes) in the infiltrating solution.

b. Also see Notes a, b, d, e, and f from previous GMA schedule.

Standard processing and embedding schedule for LR White

LR White is usually supplied as a pre-mixed solution that includes catalyst in three grades (hard, medium, and soft) to match as closely as possible the hardness of the tissue being processed. (To avoid spontaneous polymerization in hot climates, it is possible to purchase the monomer and catalyst separately.) A dropper bottle containing accelerator is also supplied.

Fixation

Fix tissues in formalin or paraformaldehyde.

Processing and embedding

1. If necessary, rinse tissue in an appropriate buffer for 15 minutes.
2. Dehydrate through 70%, 90%, and 100% ethanol, using two changes of each solution for 15 minutes for a block of 12 × 10 × 3 mm.
3. Infiltrate with LR White, three changes of 60 minutes each or leave overnight, depending on nature and size of tissue block. Hard tissues such as bone and teeth benefit from vacuum infiltration during the last change of resin.
4. Polymerize using 'heat' or 'cold' (accelerator) curing. To 'heat' cure, place the moulds in an incubator between 55°C and 60°C for 20–24 hours. For 'cold' curing add 1 drop of accelerator per 10 ml of resin; polymerization should occur in 15–20 minutes.

Notes

a. When 'heat' curing it is important to limit the contact of oxygen with the resin while polymerization occurs. The most convenient way of achieving this is to use gelatin capsules for small pieces of tissue, or the commercial block stub and moulding tray systems for larger pieces.

Alternatively a nitrogenous environment can be utilized.

b. Processing is best achieved if the specimens are agitated continuously on a roller mixer.

c. Small aliquots of benzoyl peroxide should be dried carefully, away from direct heat and sunlight as it is potentially explosive. It must be completely dissolved in the infiltrating solution and this may take up to 30 minutes.

d. Polymerization time and temperature are fundamental to the physical character of the final block. Increased temperature or time will produce highly cross-linked blocks that are brittle and may be difficult to stain.

Cutting acrylic plastic sections

Semi-thin sections of GMA, MMA, and LR White of thickness 2–3 µm may be cut with a steel knife on a standard microtome, but better-quality semi-thin sections will be obtained using a glass knife on a motorized microtome. Either the triangular Latta-Hartmann or longer-edged Ralph knife is suitable, but the choice depends mainly on the mould/block size. For most routine purposes, 2–3 µm sections are satisfactory and these can be picked up using a fine pair of forceps. GMA sections will flatten immediately on contact with water at room temperature, and if a water bath is used the sections may be picked up on slides similar to paraffin sections. Using the MMA mix described, the water bath will require to be heated at 65–70°C for these sections to flatten. LR White sections are floated out on 70% alcohol or 30–40% acetone on a hot-plate at 60°C. It is advisable that all acrylic sections are picked up on grease-free slides that have been coated with an adhesive such as 2% APES, and allowed to drain before drying on a hot-plate at 60°C for at least 30 minutes. Many histotechnologists have commented that MMA sections, especially when used for unde-calcified bone marrow trephines, become detached from the slide. Whilst this is true with many MMA formulations, if the recipe described in the series of articles by Hand and in the processing schedule on page 133 is used, then this is less likely. The use of Superfrost Plus slides (without adhesive) for bone samples has proved satisfactory (D. Blythe, personal communication).

Staining acrylic plastic sections

As previously described, GMA and LR White sections are stained with the plastic matrix present. LR White is softened by alcohol, so after completion of staining it is recommended that sections are blotted and dried on a hot-plate at 60°C for a few minutes before being dipped in xylene and mounted. MMA sections require the plastic embedding medium to be removed prior to staining, and this may be easily achieved by immersing the slides in xylene for 10–20 minutes at 37°C. Numerous H&E protocols can be used, but the following has proved satisfactory for GMA and LR White. For MMA sections, 30 minutes in hematoxylin and 5 minutes in 1% buffered eosin staining is preferred, but sections should be washed rapidly in water and ethanol as eosin is quickly removed.

Hematoxylin and eosin method

1. Stain in Harris's or Gill's alum hematoxylin for 10–20 minutes.
2. Wash in tap water.
3. If necessary, differentiate in 1% acid alcohol for 2–3 seconds.
4. Blue in tap water.
5. Wash in water for 15 minutes.
6. Stain in filtered 1% aqueous eosin in 1% calcium chloride for 3 minutes.
7. Wash in tap water for 30 seconds.
8. Blot dry.
9. Rinse in ethanol for 20 seconds.
10. Rinse in xylene.
11. Mount in DPX.

Note

Omit steps 3 and 9 for LR White.

Immunohistochemical staining on MMA sections

Sections can be stained with a protocol and procedure that follows closely that which is used for paraffin sections, using a routine immunoperoxidase technique such as the sensitive avidin-biotin type technique and polymer-based immunohistochemical procedures. DAB can be used as the chromogen and intensification is not required for visualization. Incubations are carried out at room temperature and essentially the reagents and times of the various stages are as usual, although optimal staining of some antigens may require changes in pre-treatment and/or dilution of the antibody. In addition to the application of a wide range of polyclonal and monoclonal antibodies, rabbit monoclonal antibodies have also recently been successful (L. Doverty, personal communication). To avoid poor or erroneous results, it is important during staining that sections are not allowed to dry out, which occurs faster than for paraffin sections.

As with paraffin sections, one of the most problematic aspects of immunostaining is the use of pre-treatment. Enzyme digestion with trypsin has been used for some antigens, but the introduction of heat-mediated procedures, using either a microwave oven (Hand et al. 1996) or a pressure cooker (Hand & Church 1998) with sodium citrate solution has helped significantly to improve and standardize staining. However, some details of the precise procedure may differ from those for paraffin sections, and for some antigens a combination of pre-treatments may be required to achieve best results. Heat-mediated pre-treatment also retrieves antigenicity better in archive material (Hand et al. 1996). For greater detail, the reader is advised to refer to a number of articles (Hand 1995b; Blythe et al. 1997; Hand & Church 1997), although a development of the studies by Blythe et al. has now led to pretreatment using pressure cooking and polymer-based detection reagents (D. Blythe, personal communications).

In recent years an amplification procedure based on tyramide has been introduced to immunohistochemistry, resulting in a highly sensitive intensification technique. Although the procedure was originally intended for paraffin sections and is useful when certain antibodies produce only a weak signal using a conventional technique, it has also been successfully applied to MMA-embedded tissue (Jackson et al. 1996).

The protocols and techniques previously outlined can produce excellent immunohistochemical staining and have been used routinely, especially on undecalcified hematological bone marrow trephines (Blythe et al. 1997) and hair follicles (Randall & Foster 2007).

Processing and embedding schedule for Lowicryl K4M
(Al-Nawab & Davies 1989)

The following schedule has been used on a renal needle biopsy where 2 μm and 90 nm sections were then cut for light microscopy and electron microscopy studies, respectively.

Fixation

4% paraformaldehyde for 2 hours at room temperature.

Dehydration

1. 50% methanol at −20°C for 30 minutes.
2. 80% methanol at −20°C for 60 minutes.
3. 90% methanol at −20°C for 60 minutes.

Infiltration

4. 1 part methanol and 1 part Lowicryl K4M at −20°C for 30 minutes.
5. 1 part methanol and 2 parts Lowicryl K4M at −20°C for 60 minutes.
6. 100% Lowicryl K4M at −20°C for 60 minutes.
7. 100% Lowicryl K4M at −20°C overnight.

Polymerization

Embed the tissue in fresh Lowicryl K4M in gelatin capsules and photo-polymerize at 35°C overnight using indirect (diffuse) ultraviolet irradiation from a Philips TLAD 15 W/05 fluorescent lamp (wavelength peak at 360 nm). The capsules are suspended in ethanol baths with their lower poles immersed in alcohol to dissipate any heat build-up during the polymerization process, and then removed and irradiated at room temperature for a further 1–2 days to improve sectioning properties.

Future of acrylic plastic embedding

As histological diagnosis becomes ever more demanding with increasing use of sophisticated techniques, so too has the technology of plastic embedding procedures been advanced. New embedding media are constantly being developed, and there is recognition that the flexibility of acrylics can sometimes provide the most suitable embedding medium for a particular investigation. Many applications are for high-resolution light microscopy, but some may be used for electron microscopy. Studies such as those reported by Bowdler et al. (1989) and Al-Nawab and Davies (1989) have combined both light microscopy and electron microscopy on the same biopsy using LR White and Lowicryl K4M, respectively, hence demonstrating direct comparisons between immunohistochemical techniques at light microscopy with those at the electron microscopy level. The recent introduction of Lowicryl K4M Plus combines both acrylic and epoxy properties but remains as yet not fully evaluated.

Special acrylic plastics have been formulated for low-temperature processing and embedding of tissue, especially for electron microscopy, as temperatures above 50°C are known to promote denaturation of proteins, causing loss of enzyme activity and reduction in antigenicity. Three low-temperature embedding procedures have been used with Lowicryl plastics: freeze substitution, freeze drying, and progressive lowering temperature (PLT). Processing machines are now available that can shorten as well as standardize processing times, and reduce occasions when tissue is required to be handled.

This chapter has focused mainly on the use of semi-thin acrylic sections for high-resolution light microscopy where a wide range of techniques have been applied. How future plastic embedding media and their techniques impact on routine histological practice is questionable, but for some specialized procedures the use of plastic embedding media continues to remain necessary and/or beneficial.

References

Acetarin, J.-D., Carlemalm, E., Villiger, W., 1986. Developments of new Lowicryl resins for embedding biological specimens at even lower temperatures. Journal of Microscopy 143, 81–88.

Al-Nawab, M.D., Davies, D.R., 1989. Light and electron microscopic demonstration of extracellular immunoglobulin deposition in renal tissue. Journal of Clinical Pathology 42, 1104–1108.

Beckstead, J.H., 1983. The evaluation of lymph nodes, using plastic sections and enzyme histochemistry. American Journal of Clinical Pathology 80, 131–139.

Beckstead, J.H., 1985. Optimal antigen localization in human tissues using aldehyde-fixed plastic-embedded sections. Journal of Histochemistry and Cytochemistry 33, 954–958.

Bennett, R., 1982. The use of histochemical techniques on 1 micron methacrylate sections of kidney in the study of cephaloridine nephrotoxicity. In: Bach, P.H., Bonner, F.W., Bridges, J.W., Locks, E.A. (Eds.), Nephrotoxicity: assessment and pathogenesis. John Wiley, Chichester.

Blythe, D., Hand, N.M., Jackson, P., et al., 1997. The use of methyl methacrylate resin for embedding bone marrow trephine biopsies. Journal of Clinical Pathology 50, 45–49.

Bourne, C.A.J., St John, D.J.B., 1978. Application of histochemical and histological stains to epoxy sections: pre-treatment with potassium permanganate and oxalic acid. Medical Laboratory Sciences 35, 397–398.

Bowdler, A.L., Griffiths, D.F.R., Newman, G.R., 1989. The morphological and immunocytochemical analysis of renal biopsies by light and electron microscopy using a single processing method. Histochemical Journal 21, 393–402.

Carlemalm, E., Garavito, R.M., Villiger, W., 1982. Resin development for electron microscopy and an analysis of embedding at low temperature. Journal of Microscopy 126, 123–143.

Casey, T.T., Cousar, J.B., Collins, R.D., 1988. A simplified plastic embedding and immunologic technique for immunophenotypic analysis of human haematopoietic and lymphoid tissues. American Journal of Pathology 131, 183–189.

Causton, B.E., 1981. Resins: toxicity, hazards and safe handling. Proceedings of the Royal Microscopical Society 16 (4), 265–271.

Church, R.J., Hand, N.M., Rex, M., Scotting, P.J., 1997. Non-isotopic in situ hybridization to detect chick *Sox* gene mRNA in plastic-embedded tissue. Histochemical Journal 29, 625–629.

Church, R.J., Hand, N.M., Rex, M., Scotting, P.J., 1998. Double labelling using non-isotopic in situ hybridisation and immunohistochemistry on plastic embedded tissue. Journal of Cellular Pathology 3, 11–16.

Dawson, I.M.P., 1972. Fixation: What should the pathologist do? Histochemical Journal 4, 381–385.

Doverty, L., 2005. Cyclin D1 expression in multiple myeloma: positive or negative prognostic factor? Abstract no. 91 of papers presented to the Institute of Biomedical Science Congress 2005.

Doverty, L., 2007. Immunocytochemistry and in-situ hybridisation on bone marrow trephine biopsy (electronic letter). Available: http://jcp.bmj.com/content/59/9/903/reply#jclinpath_el_401

Gerrits, P.O., 1988. Immunohistochemistry on glycol methacrylate tissue: possibilities and limitations. Journal of Histotechnology 11, 243–246.

Giddings, J., Griffin, R.C., MacIver, A.G., 1982. Demonstration of immunoproteins in araldite-embedded tissues. Journal of Clinical Pathology 35, 111–114.

Glauert, A.M., 1987. Fixation, dehydration and embedding of biological specimens. Elsevier North-Holland, Amsterdam.

Hand, N.M., 1987. Enzyme histochemistry on jejunal tissue embedded in resin. Journal of Pathology 40, 346–347.

Hand, N.M., 1988. Enzyme histochemical demonstration of lactase and sucrase activity in resin sections: the influence of fixation and processing. Medical Laboratory Sciences 45, 125–130.

Hand, N.M., 1995a. The naming and types of acrylic resins. UK NEQAS Newsletter 6, 15 (letter).

Hand, N.M., 1995b. Diagnostic immunocytochemistry on resin-embedded tissue. UK NEQAS Newsletter 6, 13–16.

Hand, N.M., 1999. Plastic embedding for light microscopy. A guide for this histotechnologist. *Tech Sample*. Histotechnology No HT-6. 29–35. American Society of Clinical Pathologists.

Hand, N.M., Church, R.J., 1997. Immunocytochemical demonstration of hormones in pancreatic and pituitary tissue embedded in methyl methacrylate. Journal of Histotechnology 20, 35–38.

Hand, N.M., Church, R.J., 1998. Superheating using pressure cooking: its use and application in unmasking antigens embedded in methyl methacrylate. Journal of Histotechnology 21, 231–236.

Hand, N.M., Morrell, K.J., 1990. Immunocytochemistry on plastic sections for light microscopy. Proceedings of the Royal Microscopical Society 25 (2), 111.

Hand, N.M., Morrell, K.J., MacLennan, K.A., 1989. Immunohistochemistry on resin embedded tissue for light microscopy: a novel post-embedding procedure. Proceedings of the Royal Microscopical Society 24 (1), A54–A55.

Hand, N.M., Blythe, D., Jackson, P., 1996. Antigen unmasking using microwave heating on formalin fixed tissue embedded in methyl methacrylate. Journal of Cellular Pathology 1, 31–37.

Howat, W.J., Warford, A., Mitchell, J.N., et al., 2005. Resin tissue microarrays: a universal format for immunohistochemistry. Journal of Histochemistry and Cytochemistry 53, 1189–1197.

Jackson, P., Blythe, D., Quirke, P., 1996. Amplification of immunocytochemical reactions by the catalytic deposition of biotin on tissue sections. Journal of Pathology 179 (Suppl), 23A.

Janes, R.B., 1979. A review of three resin processing techniques applicable to light microscopy. Medical Laboratory Sciences 36, 249–267.

Krenacs, T., Bagdi, E., Stelkovics, E., et al., 2005. How we process trephine biopsy specimens: epoxy resin embedded bone marrow biopsies. Journal of Clinical Pathology 58, 897–903.

Mawhinney, W.H.B., Ellis, H.A., 1983. A technique for plastic embedding of mineralised bone. Journal of Clinical Pathology 36, 1197–1199.

McCluggage, W.G., Roddy, S., Whiteside, C., et al., 1995. Immunohistochemical staining of plastic embedded bone marrow trephine biopsy specimens after microwave heating. Journal of Clinical Pathology 48, 840–844.

Newman, G.R., Jasani, B., Williams, E.D., 1983 The visualisation of trace amounts of diaminobenzidine (DAB) polymer by a novel gold-sulphide-silver method. Journal of Microscopy 132 (2), RP1–RP2.

Nunn, R.E., 1970. Electron microscopy: preparation of biological specimens. Butterworths, London.

Randall, K.J., Foster, J.R., 2007. The demonstration of immunohistochemical biomarkers in methyl methacrylate-embedded plucked human hair follicles. Toxicologic Pathology 35, 952–957.

Ruddell, C.L., 1967. Embedding media for 1–2 micron sectioning. 2-hydoxyethyl methacrylate combined with 2-butoxethanol. Stain Technology 42, 253–255.

Scala, C., Cenacchi, G., Ferrari, C., et al., 1992. A new acrylic resin formulation: a useful tool for histological, ultrastructural, and immunocytochemical investigations. Journal of Histochemistry and Cytochemistry 40, 1799–1804.

Takamiya, H., Batsford, S., Vogt, A., 1980. An approach to post-embedding staining of protein (immunoglobulin) antigen embedded in plastic. Journal of Histochemistry and Cytochemistry 28, 1041–1049.

Thompson, G., Germain, J.P., 1983. Histochemistry and immunocytochemistry of fixation labile moieties in resin embedded tissue. Journal of Pathology 142 (2), A6.

How histological stains work 9

Richard W. Horobin

Introduction

All histological staining methods, from acid dyeing to silver impregnation, are based on the same physicochemical principles, as will be described in this chapter. Examples are provided from several of the application areas discussed in this book. Methods using dyestuffs are emphasized, so some background information concerning dyes is provided at the end of the chapter. A generic troubleshooting guide is also appended.

The key questions to bear in mind when seeking to understand histological stains are as follows:

a. Why do *any* tissue components stain?

b. Why do stained components *remain* stained?

c. Why are *all* components not stained?

The answers are often complex, reflecting the multiphase nature of the staining process, in which solid cells and tissues interact with solutions of staining reagents. Thus enzyme histochemistry is not 'merely' biochemistry, nor is the periodic acid-Schiff (PAS) procedure merely organic chemistry, nor immunostaining merely immunochemistry. In addition to biochemistry, chemistry and immunochemistry, such staining methods are also influenced by selective uptake of reagents into tissues, and selective losses of products and/or reagents from the tissues. Such uptakes and losses depend on both affinity and rate factors. Nomenclature note: *staining* always involves the visual labeling of some biological entity by attaching, or depositing in its vicinity, a marker of characteristic color or form. The *stain* is the marker, or the reagent used to generate the marker.

A general theory of staining

Why are stains taken into the tissues?

Stain uptake is often due to dye-tissue or reagent-tissue affinities. In the histological staining literature, to say a tissue component has a high affinity for a dye may merely mean that, under the conditions of use, the component becomes intensely stained. Affinity is however also used to describe those attractive forces thought to bind dye to tissue.

Physical chemists use the term affinity in the former sense, and their usage is adopted here. So in this chapter affinity describes the tendency of a stain to transfer from solution onto a section. The affinity's magnitude depends on every factor favoring or hindering this movement. Stain-tissue, stain-solvent, and stain-stain interactions must all be considered, as indeed must solvent-solvent interactions. This approach initially assumes staining continues until equilibrium is reached, but in practice this is often not achieved. Moreover uptake of dyes and reagents is often multistep, in both space and time. A reagent may initially enter tissues due to, say, coulombic attractions. Once inside it may form covalent bonds with some tissue grouping. Intensity of staining may also be limited by the solubility of a stain in solvent and tissue environments.

Various contributions to stain-tissue affinity are outlined in Table 9.1, and are discussed below. Practical staining processes commonly involve several such factors.

Table 9.1 Factors contributing to dye-tissue affinities

Interactions	Practical examples where the factor is important
Reagent-tissue interactions	
Coulombic attractions	Acid and basic dyes, and other ionic reagents, including inorganic salts
Van der Waals' forces	Most important with large molecules such as the elastic fiber stains, and final reaction products such as bisformazans in enzyme histochemistry
Hydrogen bonding	Staining of glycogen by carminic acid, and collagen by Sirius red
Covalent bonding	Methods such as the Feulgen nuclear, PAS, & mercury orange for thiols
Solvent-solvent interactions	
The hydrophobic effect	Staining systems using aqueous solutions of dyes or other organic reagents; enzyme substrates for example
Reagent-reagent interactions	Metachromatic staining with basic dyes, inorganic pigments in Gomori-type enzyme histochemistry, silver impregnation

Reagent-tissue interactions

Coulombic attractions, which have also been termed salt links or electrostatic bonds, are widely discussed reagent-tissue interactions. These arise from electrostatic attractions of unlike ions, e.g. the colored cations of basic dyes and tissue structures rich in anions such as phosphated DNA, or sulfated mucosubstances (Lyon 1991; Prentø 2009). In practice, the amount of dye ion binding to a tissue substrate depends not only on the charge signs of dye and tissue but also on their magnitude, on the amount of non-dye electrolyte present in the dyebath, and on the ability of the tissue substrate to swell or shrink (Scott 1973; Bennion & Horobin 1974; Goldstein & Horobin 1974b; Horobin & Goldstein 1974).

Such phenomena are important for all ionic reagents, not just dyestuffs, an example being the periodate anions used as the oxidant in the periodic acid-Schiff procedure (Scott & Harbinson 1968). Even initially uncharged tissue substrates acquire ionic character after binding ionic reagents, e.g., glycogen staining by the PAS procedure and with Best's carmine.

Van der Waals' forces include such intermolecular attractions as dipole-dipole, dipole-induced dipole and dispersion forces. These occur between all reagents and tissue substrates, but since molecules with extensively delocalized electronic systems tend to have larger dipoles and are more polarizable, van

der Waals' forces are usually most critical when tissues or stains contain such moieties.

Consequently proteins rich in tyrosine and tryptophan residues, and nucleic acids with their heterocyclic bases, favor van der Waals' attractions, as do the large aromatic systems of stains such as bisazo dyes and bistetrazolium salts, halogenated dyes (such as rose Bengal and phloxine), and enzyme substrates based on naphthyl and indoxyl with extended conjugation (Horobin & Bennion 1973). For instance, van der Waals' attractions contribute substantially to stain-tissue affinity when staining elastic fibers – rich in aromatic desmosine and isodesmosine residues – with polyaromatic acid and basic dyes such as Congo red and orcein.

Hydrogen bonding is a dye-tissue attraction arising when a hydrogen atom lies between two electronegative atoms (e.g. oxygen or nitrogen), though it is covalently bonded only to one. Water is hydrogen bonded extensively to itself, forming the clusters important for the hydrophobic effect discussed below, and also to other molecules with hydrogen bonding groups, such as many dyes and tissue components. As there are many more molecules of water present than dye, hydrogen bonding is not usually important for stain-tissue affinity when aqueous solvents are used. An exception arises when hydrogen bonding is particularly favored by the substrate, as is the case with connective tissue fibers (Prentø

2007). In wholly or partially non-aqueous solutions, hydrogen bonding can also be significant, as with Best's carmine stain for glycogen (Horobin & Murgatroyd 1970).

Covalent bonding between tissue and stain also occurs, which bonds may be regarded merely as another source of stain-tissue affinity. Practical reactive methods, e.g. the Feulgen nuclear and the periodic acid-Schiff procedures, are described elsewhere in this volume. The polar covalent bonds between metal ions and 'mordant' dyes are a special case. Dye-tissue binding due to such bonds has been termed *mordanting,* but is of uncertain status. The characteristic staining properties of mordant dyes may have other, or at least additional, causes. For instance, unlike most cationic dyes used as biological stains, cationic metal-complex dyes are usually markedly hydrophilic (Bettinger & Zimmermann 1991) and consequently resist extraction into alcoholic dehydration fluids (Marshall & Horobin 1973).

Solvent-solvent interactions

A major contribution to stain-tissue affinity when using organic reagents or dyes in aqueous solution is the *hydrophobic effect*. This is the tendency of hydrophobic groupings (such as leucine and valine side chains of proteins; or biphenyl and naphthyl groupings of enzyme substrates and dyes) to come together, even though initially dispersed in an aqueous environment. The process occurs because water is a highly structured liquid. Many water molecules are held together by hydrogen bonding (see above) in transient clusters, whose formation is favored by the presence of hydrophobic groups. Processes breaking clusters into individual water molecules occur spontaneously, because these events increase the entropy of the system. Consequently, removing cluster-stabilizing hydrophobic groups from contact with water, by placing them in contact with each other, is thermodynamically favored. For background on the hydrophobic effect see textbooks of biochemistry or chemical thermodynamics (Tanford 2004). The effect becomes more important as the substrate and reagent become more hydrophobic, as with staining of fats

by Sudan dyes. When these hydrophobic dyes are applied from substantially aqueous solutions, the hydrophobic effect will be a major contribution to affinity. It should be noted that the hydrophobic effect is sometimes termed hydrophobic bonding, even though no special bonds are involved (only water-water hydrogen bonds and, sometimes, stain-tissue van der Waals' attractions).

Some staining procedures involving Sudan dyes use solvents in which water is absent, or is only a minor constituent. Here the second law of thermodynamics – the tendency of a system to change spontaneously to maximize its disorder (i.e., for *entropy* to increase as described in texts of chemical thermodynamics) – may again be invoked. Dye dispersed through fat *and* solvent constitutes a more disordered system than dye restricted to a single phase. Consequently, dye becomes dispersed and staining occurs. Of course, such increases in entropy involving substrate and dye occur in all types of staining system.

Stain-stain interactions

Dye-dye interactions can also contribute to affinity. Dye molecules tend to attract each other, forming aggregates. Even in dilute solutions, and especially in aqueous solutions where the hydrophobic effect is important, dimers or larger aggregates of dye ions are often present. van der Waals' attractions (see above) between dye molecules will be important in both aqueous and non-aqueous solutions. Dye aggregation increases with concentration, e.g. when high dye concentrations build up on tissue sections. With basic (cationic) dyes this occurs on substrates of high negative charge density, e.g. sulfated polysaccharides in mast cell granules, a classic site for *metachromatic staining* by dyes such as toluidine blue. This phenomenon occurs because dye aggregates have spectral properties different from the monomeric dye. That dye-dye interactions contribute to affinity in tissue sections was demonstrated quantitatively by Goldstein (1962).

Other examples of stain-stain interactions contributing to affinity include metallic nano- and micro-crystals generated by gold or silver impregnation, metal sulfide precipitates formed in Gomori-type enzyme histochemistry, and the purple azure-eosin charge transfer complex produced during Romanowsky-Giemsa staining of cell nuclei (Horobin 2011).

Some unusual possibilities

Some stains are not taken up by their tissue targets. In *negative staining* the shapes of structures are disclosed by outlining or filling them with a stain. Examples include visualizing individual microorganisms using nigrosine, and demonstrating canaliculi of bone matrix using picro-thionine.

Sometimes stains are taken into live creatures, in ways that reflect the biochemical composition and physiological activities of the living cell or organism. Traditionally termed *vital staining* or supravital staining, this is now usually described as the *use of fluorescent probes*. Over the past 20 years this methodology has undergone a renaissance; for a recent overview see Celis (2006).

Solubility, a related property

A little-discussed, but nevertheless important, property of stains is their solubility. For instance, when staining fat with Sudan dyes, an upper limit of staining intensity is set by the solubility of the dyes in the target substance, and is also influenced by the solubility in the staining bath solvent. Solubility is also involved in dye retention after staining: see below. The solubility of a staining reagent has complex causes. Put simply, the stronger the reagent-reagent interactions, the lower the solubility. For a general discussion of solubility see physicochemical texts such that of Letcher (2007).

Why is stain retained in tissue after its removal from the staining bath?

This occurs because the stains either have a very high affinity for tissue elements and/or low affinity for processing fluids and mounting media, or at least dissolve in these latter materials very slowly.

To illustrate these points, consider some common stains.

Pigments such as the Prussian blue generated in the Perls' method for iron, and the lead sulfide produced in Gomori-style enzyme histochemistry, are virtually insoluble in standard solvents. This is also true for microcrystals of silver and gold produced by metal impregnation. Some organic pigments are less satisfactory. Thus, azo dyes, formazans and substituted indigos produced as final reaction products in enzyme histochemistry have low solubility in water, but may dissolve in hydrophobic media such as alcohols, xylene, and polystyrene. In such cases hydrophilic mounting media are used, and staining of lipid-rich tissue elements should be regarded as possibly artifactual.

Solubilities of formazans and azodyes are sometimes reduced by *in situ* conversion to metal complexes. Other routine metal complex stains are the aluminum, chromium and iron complexes of hematein, and the chromium complex of gallocyanine. These metal complex dyes are not readily removed from tissues by routine processing fluids or mounting media (see above).

This contrasts with routine basic (cationic) dyes such as crystal violet or methylene blue, which freely and rapidly dissolve in the lower alcohols. Routine acid (anionic) dyes, such as eosin Y or orange G, are often less soluble in alcohols, as indeed are hydrophilic basic dyes with large aromatic systems, such as alcian blue. Non-ionic dyes such as Sudan fat stains are soluble in common dehydrating agents and clearing solvents, and in resin mountants. Note: structures of exemplar hydrophilic and lipophilic basic dyes are shown in Figure 9.1.

Sections stained with routine basic dyes must therefore be dehydrated rapidly through the alcohols, or by the use of non-alcoholic solvents, or by air-drying, whereas dehydration is less critical with acid dyes. Sections stained with either acid or basic dyes are usually mounted in non-aqueous media to prevent extraction of dye. Alternatively, dyes may be immobilized, for example, by formation of metal coordination compounds, phosphotungstates or

Alcian blue 8G

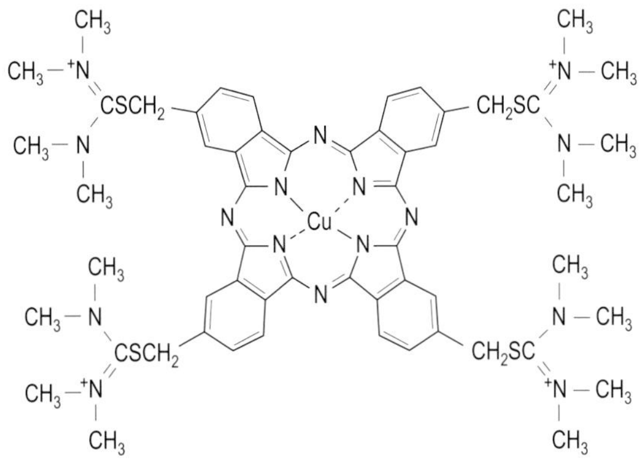

Crystal violet

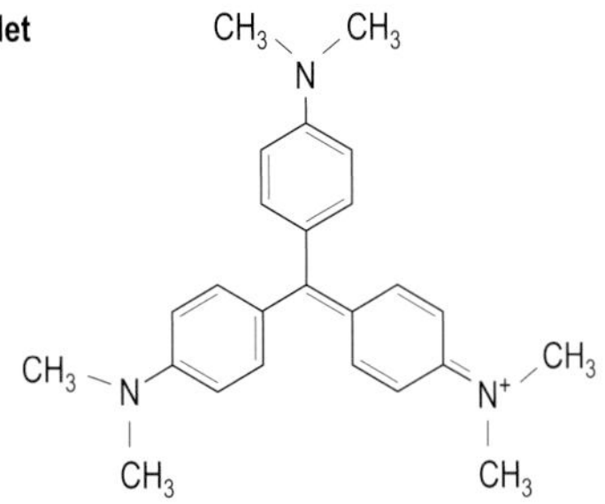

Dye	Ionic weight	Log P
Alcian blue 8G	1380	−9.7
Crystal violet	372	+1.9

Figure 9.1 Structural formulae of two widely used basic dyes, plus numerical descriptions of certain of their physicochemical properties.

iodine complexes. Non-ionic dyes must be mounted in aqueous media.

Why are the stains not taken up into every part of the tissue?

This question of selectivity is fundamental to histochemistry, and even routine oversight methods such as hematoxylin and eosin (H&E), Papanicolaou and Romanowsky-Giemsa stains distinguish nuclei from cytoplasm. So we must discover what factors control such selectivities.

Numbers and affinities of binding sites

Both these factors influence staining. However, in the absence of quantitative investigation, they are not readily distinguishable – so will here be discussed as a single effect. Stain-tissue affinities and numbers of binding sites present in tissues can vary independently.

Sudan dyes can be used as an example. These have a high affinity for fat but low affinity for the surrounding hydrated proteins. Alternatively one may consider staining systems in which covalent bonds are formed. Reagents give colored products only with a limited range of tissue chemical groupings. Thus, the acid hydrolysis-Schiff reagent sequence of the Feulgen nucleal technique gives red derivatives only with DNA.

An understanding of staining systems often requires consideration of patterns of affinities. With the traditional acid dye-basic dye pairs (H&E, Papanicolaou, and Romanowsky) the negatively charged acid dyes have high affinities for tissue structures carrying cationic charges (proteins, under acidic conditions). However they have low affinities for structures carrying negative charges (those rich in sulfated glycosaminoglycans, or in phosphated nucleic acids), with the opposite being the case for basic dyes. This produces two-tone staining patterns in which cytoplasm contrasts with nuclear material.

Practical staining conditions maximize selective affinities. Basic dyes are applied from neutral or acidic solutions, since under alkaline conditions proteins carry an overall negative charge and so may also bind basic dyes. Affinities are also influenced by varying the concentration of inorganic salt present. The various aluminum-hematoxylin, for instance, differ substantially in this regard. The critical electrolyte concentration methodology (Scott 1973) and several other empirical procedures are based on control of electrolyte content. However, staining that distinguishes two structures is still possible even when stain-tissue affinities and the number of stain-binding sites are the same. This is because rate of reagent uptake, or rate of subsequent reaction, or rate of loss of reagent or product, may not be the same in the two structures.

Rates of reagent uptake

Progressive dyeing methods may be rate controlled, for instance mucin staining using alcian blue or colloidal iron. Selectivity requires short periods of dyeing during which only fast-staining mucins acquire color (Goldstein 1962, Goldstein & Horobin 1974a). If staining is prolonged, additional basophilic materials such as nuclei and RNA-rich cytoplasms can also stain. Dyes used in this way are often large in size, and hence diffuse slowly, maximizing the control possible via differential rate effects.

Rate of reaction

Selective staining by reactive reagents, yielding colored derivatives, may depend on differential *rates of reaction*. For instance, periodic acid can oxidize a variety of substrates present in tissues. However, in histochemical applications of the periodic acid-Schiff procedure short oxidation time limits subsequent coloration to fast-reacting 1,2-diol groupings of polysaccharides. Enzyme histochemistry provides further examples of reaction rate controlling selectivity. When incubating at low pH, hydrolysis of an organic phosphate is rapid in tissues containing acid phosphatases whereas in structures containing alkaline phosphatases, with higher pH optima, hydrolysis rates are slow.

Rate of reagent loss

Differentiation or *regressive staining* involves selective losses of stain from tissues. Many dyeing methods exploit this phenomenon, for example staining of muscle striations with iron-hematoxylin, and of myelin sheaths with luxol fast blue. In such procedures an initial non-selective staining is followed by extraction in a solvent. Dye is first lost from permeable structures such as collagen fibers. Relatively impermeable structures such as the A and Z bands of muscle, and myelin sheaths, retain stain longest.

Rate control of reagent loss is critical in a very different methodology, namely silver staining of nerve fibers. During an impregnation step, silver ions bind non-selectively to many tissue groupings. Subsequently, the tissue is treated with a developer capable of reducing silver cations to silver metal. The rate of reaction with this reducing agent is critical. If the rate is too fast, because of high concentration or high reactivity of the reagent, silver grains are deposited non-selectively throughout the tissue. If reduction is too slow, no staining occurs because most silver ions diffuse away into the solvent before they are reduced. Selective staining occurs when silver ions diffuse from the background quickly, being retained in less permeable entities (e.g., nerve fibers, nucleoli, red blood cells) where they are then reduced (Peters 1955a, 1955b).

Such rate-controlled methods are fraught by a wide range of technical artifacts. Indeed, any factor affecting rate of reagent loss (e.g., variation in section thickness, temperature, stirring of the reagent solution, presence of cavities in the tissue) can alter the staining result.

Metachromasia and related phenomena

Even when neither affinity nor rate controls the staining pattern, selective coloration can still be obtained. For instance basic dyes such as methylene blue and toluidine blue are absorbed by a variety of basophilic substrates in the tissues. Chromatin stains orthochromatically blue, but cartilage matrix, mast cell granules, and mucins stain metachromatically reddish purple (reviewed by Pearse 1968) due to formation of dye aggregates in these polyanion-rich sites.

What are the effects on staining of prior tissue modification?

Modifications include fixation, whose effects on staining are adventitious, as well as blocking and extraction techniques intended to alter staining patterns. Modifications due to resin embedding are discussed separately below.

Effects of fixation

Fixation is carried out to prevent losses of tissue constituents into processing and staining solutions, and to reduce postmortem morphological changes of the tissue. Fixation converts soluble tissue components into insoluble derivatives, resistant to autolysis or attack by bacteria and fungi. For a general account of fixation see Chapter 4; here only influences on staining are discussed.

A given substance is often retained to different extents by different fixative agents, and nothing can be stained that is not retained. For instance, many lipids are well preserved after fixation in osmium tetroxide or dichromates, poorly preserved after formalin, and actively extracted during alcoholic or acetone fixation. Staining lipids after alcoholic fixation is therefore ineffective.

However, whilst retention of a substance is necessary, mere retention may be insufficient for subsequent histochemical demonstration. For instance, although glutaraldehyde often retains more protein than do other fixative agents, its use in immunostaining and enzyme histochemistry (and most antigens and all enzymes are proteins) is limited. The same chemical reactions that insolubilize proteins also modify haptenic and enzymic activity. Alcohol and acetone, on the other hand, although poor at retaining proteins in the tissues, are also poor at destroying the activity of whatever antigen or enzyme is retained. Thus both retention and reactivity of substances affect staining, and both may be fixative dependent.

Fixation has more subtle influences on staining patterns, of which, acid and basic dyeing provide instructive examples. As shown by Singer (1952), such staining is generally enhanced by the protein denaturation produced by fixatives. Moreover the acidophilia-basophilia balance of a tissue is also influenced. Thus formalin and osmium tetroxide usually reduce tissue acidophilia, while acidic dichromate solutions usually increase tissue acidophilia (Baker 1958).

Effects of histochemical blocking and extraction

Such processes underlie certain control procedures. Tissue components are modified in ways which should eliminate staining. Consequently any subsequent staining indicates lack of staining specificity.

However reality may be more complex than expectation, in various ways.

Thus, blockade may be incomplete, as occurs with van Slyke's nitrous acid reagent used to convert the tissue amino groups causing acidophilia to non-ionizing hydroxyl groups. However, the efficacy of this reagent is tissue and fixative dependent, and can confuse an uncritical bench worker. Analogous effects occur with histochemical extraction procedures. Thus, removal of RNA from ribosomes by RNase is also fixative dependent, and does not occur readily after formalin fixation.

Unexpected tissue modifications due to blockade and extractive procedures also occur, removing substances additional to those intended. When using trichloroacetic or perchloric acids to extract nucleic acids, losses of polysaccharides and some proteins can also occur. Analogous problems arise during enzymic extractions when trace enzyme impurities are present. Polysaccharides may also be lost by chemical solvolysis during 'methylation' of tissue acids by methanolic-HCl, and DNA and RNA are extracted by the acetic anhydride-pyridine used to blockade nuclear histones. Indeed material can be extracted by staining solutions, especially if acidic or alkaline or when tissues are poorly fixed.

In addition to these narrow chemical effects, all such procedures modify the physical properties of a tissue section, such as its permeability. After exposure to swelling agents or proteases, tissues may stain more rapidly: for example, nuclei may be stained by alcian blue and cytoplasms by the 'collagen' dye of a trichrome stain.

What are the effects of specimen geometry on staining?

Here 'specimen' means the biological material actually in contact with the staining solution such as a dewaxed section, a cervical smear, or a lymph node dab. When looking at a screen or down a microscope it is easy to forget that a specimen has thickness, not just breadth and width. Many people find it hard to believe that differences in thickness of a few μm or less influence staining patterns. However, dispersed cells prepared by smearing often stain differently to cells of the same type cut from a tissue block, and thin sections stain differently from thick. Indeed, sections with irregular surface profiles will stain differently to the same biological material cut in sections with smooth surfaces.

Simple geometrical influences

All things being equal, thin specimens stain faster than thick; specimens with irregular surfaces stain faster than smooth; and dispersed specimens stain faster than uniform slabs. In a given staining procedure, therefore, dispersed specimens such as smears or dabs require shorter staining times than sections of similar cells cut from a solid tissue. Moreover, cryosections (which usually have irregular surfaces) will typically stain faster than smoother paraffin sections. It should be noted that resin sections typically have smoother profiles (see below).

In systems with rate-controlled staining mechanisms, such effects can interfere with selectivity. Some trichrome stains require shorter staining times with cryosections than with paraffin sections, otherwise cryosections become overstained by the higher ionic weight dye.

More complex effects of specimen geometry

More complex geometries may originate in the biological structures, or may arise during specimen preparation. The latter, artifactual, geometries are considered first.

A well-known modification of section geometry induced by microtomy is chatter. This results in sections containing alternating thick and thin strips. Possible consequences for staining include the occurrence of alternate strips of strong and weak staining or, with some trichromes, alternate strips of varying color.

Complex geometries also arise in smear preparations. For instance, smears from epithelia often contain multicellular clumps of cells as well as monocellular dispersions. Cells at the centers of such clumps are less accessible to stains than are peripheral cells. Consequently, in rate-controlled methods such as the Papanicolaou and Romanowsky

stains, centrally situated cells can be overstained by the smallest dye present, as illustrated by Boon and Drijver (Plates 6.4 and 24.4; 1986).

A section's profile is also influenced by fixation. Coagulant fixatives such as Carnoy's fluid tend to shatter cells and tissues, giving rise to more dispersed specimens, whilst fixatives such as formalin give more integral forms. For a direct illustration of this, see Horobin (Fig. 14, 1982). Consequently, if a rate-controlled trichrome stain gives rise to the correct color balance when applied to formalin-fixed tissue, it will tend to show overstaining by the collagen fiber stain (usually the larger dye) if applied without modification to material fixed in Carnoy's fluid.

The size of biological structures relative to section thickness can also be significant. Consider secretion granules with diameters much larger or much smaller than the section thickness. All large granules will be sliced through, with their contents exposed on a surface of the section, whereas some small granules will be intact, enclosed within the section. This will strongly influence accessibility for larger stains: for example, immunostaining in which stains are macromolecular. The 'two types of secretion granule' reported in a number of immunostaining studies may therefore represent intact versus sliced granules. Such effects can be even more pronounced in resin sections: see below.

Geometrical complexity also arises from swelling of cell and tissue components in staining solvents. Materials rich in glycosaminoglycans (e.g. mucus and cartilage matrix) swell markedly in aqueous solutions; and collagen fibers swell grossly at extremes of pH. Swelling can increase rates of staining of these structures, compared to unswollen material. This probably contributes to the high selectivity of aqueous alcian blue for mucins, nuclear staining usually being absent after short staining times; and to the high selectivity of strongly acidic picro-trichrome stains for collagen fibers. Since alcohol does not induce such swelling, these effects may partially account for changes in staining when a dye is used in alcoholic rather than aqueous solution. Luxol fast blue, for instance, stains myelin selectively from aqueous solution, but from alcoholic solutions gives selective staining of collagen fibers. Such effects are often more marked in resin sections, as noted later.

What are the effects of resin embedding on staining?

Typically, resin embedding involves infiltration of biological material with a reactive monomer, most commonly an acrylate or epoxide. Subsequent polymerization yields a block of resin enclosing the specimen. Sections cut from such blocks are termed resin, or plastic, sections. The presence of resin, in addition to the biological material, during the staining process gives rise to changes in staining pattern. If resin is removed prior to staining, as is usually done with methylmethacrylate sections, staining patterns closely resemble those of paraffin sections, so are not discussed here. Specimens may also be embedded in a preformed polymer, usually nitrocellulose (i.e. celloidin). These sections are routinely stained with the polymer present, and behave much like resin sections.

Resins as stain excluders

As resin sections contain both biological material and resin, penetration of staining reagents is usually slower than into paraffin or cryosections. If resin cross-linking is increased, rates of stain penetration fall still further.

Resin embedding often has more complicated effects than a mere reduction in staining rate. Resin usually infiltrates biological specimens unevenly, with dense or hydrophilic structures being poorly infiltrated. This is because even 'water-miscible' or 'low-viscosity' resin systems use monomers which are slightly lipophilic and quite viscous. Consequences of uneven resin infiltration are complex. For instance, in glycol methacrylate-embedded specimens, structures such as dense secretion granules are often poorly infiltrated, so they may be resin free and stain readily. If the surrounding cytoplasm is better infiltrated with resin, granules may consequently stand out more clearly and crisply than in paraffin sections.

Resins as stain binders

Resins can themselves bind stains. For instance, glycol methacrylate monomer is sometimes contaminated with methacrylic acid, resulting in formation of carboxylated glycol methacrylate resins. Such anionic resin can give strong background basophilia, which does not occur when the pure monomer is used. However, background staining due to binding of lipophilic dyes, such as aldehyde fuchsin or Janus green, to glycol methacrylate is unavoidable because the resin itself is somewhat lipophilic, despite the resin monomer being water miscible (Horobin et al. 1992). In addition to background artifacts, stain-resin binding can give negative staining artifacts since the amount of reagent reaching the biological staining target may be reduced by binding to resin. An example is the weak enzyme histochemical staining seen with certain lipophilic enzyme substrates.

Glycol methacrylate, the major constituent of many light microscopic resin embedding kits, exhibits another dye-binding artifact, namely the 'irreversible' binding of certain dyes. This arises with dyes of moderate size, e.g. aluminum hematoxylin or eosin. These can enter the resin and modify the polymer structure, making it less permeable. This antiplasticizing effect traps the dye, although, it can sometimes be removed by differentiating in solvents with plasticizing action, such as ethanol.

How stain chemistry influences staining patterns

With small reagents, which diffuse rapidly through resins, staining methods developed for paraffin or cryostat sections can be used without modification. When working with routine glycol methacrylate embedding media, 'small' means <550 daltons (Da), and includes such common substances as methylene blue, naphthyl phosphate, and Schiff reagent. Conversely, large reagents may be totally excluded from the resin, restricting staining to resin-free structures. When using glycol methacrylate resins 'large' reagents are those with sizes >1000 Da, and include alcian blue, Sirius red, and labeled antibodies.

The possibility of stains binding to lipophilic embedding media, resulting in both positive and negative staining artifacts, was noted above. Such problems occur only with lipophilic reagents (Horobin et al. 1992). When glycol methacrylate resin is being used, 'lipophilic' implies reagents whose log P > 1 (see below for an explanation of this parameter). Examples include eosin, which has to be differentiated with alcohol, and Gomori's aldehyde fuchsin, which cannot be satisfactorily differentiated.

By considering both size and hydrophilicity-lipophilicity, guidelines may be specified for staining specimens in water-miscible resins such as glycol methacrylate:

- Small hydrophilic stains, e.g. methylene blue and Schiff reagent, behave much as they do in paraffin or cryosections, though staining a little more slowly.

- Stains of moderate size and/or lipophilicity, e.g. eosin Y and aluminum hematoxylin, often stain more slowly in resin. They also color the resin, and removing this background requires differentiation with plasticizing solvents such as ethanol.

- Lipophilic stains, e.g. Gomori's aldehyde fuchsin, give strong coloration of the resin, which may prove difficult to remove without generalized de-staining of the tissues.

- Staining of tissues by large hydrophilic stains (e.g. alcian blue, Sirius red, or a labeled antibody) is limited to structures poorly infiltrated with resin.

How resin chemistry influences staining patterns

Occurrence of high temperatures within tissue blocks during embedding is considered to cause loss of antigenicity and enzymic activity. Consequently low-temperature embedding is used to increase the sensitivity of immunohistochemical and enzyme histochemical methods with resin-embedded tissues. It is also probable that organic solvents and reagents used for dehydration, infiltration, and polymerization cause increased protein denaturation. Hence, partial dehydration and short infiltration times

have been adopted to enhance staining sensitivity. However, these variations may also lower the amount of resin in a section, and so reduce stain exclusion.

The properties of the resin itself also influence staining processes, with ionic character, cross-linking, and lipophilicity already being mentioned. Carry-over of plasticizers and polymerization catalysts into the resin block is another factor. Variations in amount and type of plasticizer influence the permeability of resin to stains. The presence of a basic polymerization catalyst results in binding of anionic staining reagents (e.g. acid dyes) to the resin at low pH, when the base is protonated and so cationic.

Some dyestuff properties

Some general influences of dye chemistry on staining

When those physicochemical features of dyes that influence dye-tissue affinity and staining rates are described using numerical parameters, systematic correlations can be demonstrated between dye chemistry and staining outcomes. The physicochemical parameters include electric charge; overall size (as represented by ionic or molecular weight); and hydrophilic/lipophilic character (modeled by the log P value, i.e. the logarithm of the octanol-water partition coefficient). To appreciate the advantages of numerical parameters, inspect Figure 9.1, where chemical information concerning two widely used basic dyes is presented in two modes, graphical and numerical.

When considering relative sizes of dyes, information provided graphically by structural formulae is satisfactory. One can see that alcian blue is a much larger dye than crystal violet. The fact that the staining pattern of alcian blue is highly dependent on staining time (Goldstein & Horobin 1974a) is thus not surprising. The relative hydrophilic/lipophilic character of the two dyes cannot however be readily assessed by visual inspection of formulae, whilst the log P values of the two dyes are clearly very different. Negative values imply hydrophilicity, and positive values imply lipophilicity. In keeping with this concept, sections stained with alcian blue are dehydrated through the alcohols with no removal of dye, but crystal violet is easily lost into the alcohols.

Several dye properties are usually necessary for predicting the performance of a stain. As detailed discussion is inappropriate, merely note that quantitative structure-staining correlations based on such structure parameters can illuminate diverse issues in histotechnology, from fixation effects in the staining of phospholipids (Horobin 1989), through staining mechanisms of trichromes (Horobin & Flemming 1988) to assessing effects of resin embedding on histochemical staining procedures (Horobin et al. 1992). For overviews see Horobin (2004, 2010a). In fact such correlations have also proved applicable to vital staining by fluorescent probes; for summaries of which see Horobin (2001, 2010b).

Effects of dye impurities on staining

Almost all dyes used as stains are impure, which has provoked many experimental investigations and polemical editorials. But what is meant by an 'impure' dye?

A batch of dye is considered impure if it does not contain the compound named on the label, or if it contains substantial amounts of other colored substances additional to the named dye. Alternatively, an impure batch may contain very little dye, with most of the contents being inorganic salt. Dyes that are pure when purchased may decompose on storage, or after being made up into a staining solution, or even during staining itself. Impurities influence staining in two ways. First they may alter staining intensity. Typically staining is reduced, but very occasionally impurities result in a more intense color. Second, impurities may change staining patterns, the nature and mechanisms of such effects depending on the type of impurity, the particular staining procedure, and the tissue substrate.

Unfortunately there is no simple way to identify, and so avoid, such impure products. A practical tip

is to purchase dye lots certified by the *Biological Stain Commission*. These have been tested in the *Commission's* laboratory, and met purity and staining efficacy criteria. Surprisingly, *Commission* certified dyes are on average no more expensive than non-certified dyes. (For an example of the benefits of certified dyes, see Henwood 2003.) Another practical tip is to check if staining problems are due to impure stains by retaining samples of effective dye lots. Faced with an unexpected staining pattern, a specimen can then be stained with the effective dye. If this gives satisfactory coloration, there may be problems due to dye impurity.

What can you do about impure dye batches? Few have the resources, or the inclination, to engage in analysis or purification. The most useful advice is to buy another batch of dye, preferably *Biological Stain Commission* certified. If analysis or purification does prove necessary, there is an extensive literature, which may be accessed for individual dyes via the monographs of the 10th edition of *Conn's Biological Stains* (Horobin & Kiernan 2002), or more generally via an earlier review article by the present author (Horobin 1969).

Dye nomenclature

Names of individual dyes, and terms used to describe dye properties, are sometimes inconsistent and are often confusing. As dyes are complex molecules, nearly all have trivial names that do not explicitly describe their structures. Most biological stains were first manufactured as textile dyes, when each manufacturer gave the dye their own trade name. A biologist may therefore say 'Use Congo blue', to which his colleagues reply 'But we haven't got any of *that*'. And yet they have, but on their shelves it is labeled trypan blue. Even worse is the surfeit of suffixes. Sometimes these are merely flourishes of a copywriter's pen, so pyronines G and Y are synonyms. Sometimes suffixes indicate dye content, and a standard product may be labeled 'A 100' whilst a grade containing a higher content of dye is termed 'A 150' or merely 'A extra'. Sometimes, however, suffixes indicate substantial chemical

Table 9.2 Some descriptive terms used in classifying dyestuffs used as biological stains	
Categories of terms	**Examples of terms (and of dyes)**
Describing the origins of a dye	Natural (hematoxylin and carmine), synthetic or aniline (almost any other)
Describing physicochemical properties of a dye	Fluorescent (acridine orange), leuco (leuco methylene blue), metachromatic (toluidine blue), neutral (azure-eosinate)
Giving some kind of description of the dye's structure	Azo (orange G), metal complex (aluminum or iron complexes of hematein), xanthene (pyronine Y)
Describing the dye's usage in biological staining	Fat (oil red O), fluorescent probe (YOYO-1), mucin (alcian blue)
Describing the dye's usage in textile dyeing	Acid (eosin), basic (safranine), direct (Congo red)
Describing the supposed mode of action of the dye	Mordant (gallocyanine chrome alum), reactive (mercury orange)

differences: e.g. rhodamines B and 6G, respectively, describe zwitterionic and cationic dyes.

To reduce confusion, industrial dye users established the *Color Index* (Society of Dyers and Colourists 1999). Dyes are given unique code numbers – the *Color Index*, or C.I., number – and code names. Thus eosins G, WG, and Y are identified as a single dye, C.I. 45380, Acid Red 87, whilst eosin B is a chemically different dye, C.I. 45400, Acid Red 91.

Dyes synthesized for biological staining are named equally idiosyncratically. A traditional example is Gomori's aldehyde fuchsin, and a recent one YOYO-1. Since these products are not of industrial significance, most do not have a *Color Index* entry. In such cases the puzzled should peruse *Conn's Biological Stains* (see Lillie 1977 and Horobin & Kiernan 2002 for the 9th and 10th editions, respectively).

Various terms used to classify dyestuffs are given in Table 9.2, and comments on points sometimes confused in the histochemical literature follow here. *Acid* and *basic* dyes are not acids and bases but salts, whose colored species are anionic and cationic, respectively. *Neutral* dyes are not non-ionic, but salts in which both the anion and cation are dyes. *Vital stains*, used to stain living cells, are nowadays often called *fluorescent probes* or *biosensors*. Note finally that all dyes can be given multiple descriptors. Thus alcian blue 8G is a *synthetic basic* dye, structurally a

metal complex, though not a *mordant dye*, of copper with *phthalocyanine*, substituted by *thioguanidinium groups*, and is routinely used as a *mucin stain*.

Problem avoidance and troubleshooting

Avoiding problems and recognizing and correcting errors are perennial laboratory concerns. Typical strategies are sketched below, and detailed information for several dozen routine and special histopathology stains has been assembled in monograph form (Horobin & Bancroft 1998).

Strategies for avoiding problems – to minimize the need for troubleshooting

Issues concerning staining procedures

- Stains used must be compatible with the fixative and embedding medium. *Case example*: water-miscible resin sections do not allow selective staining of elastic fibers with aldehyde fuchsin.

- Use a routine, preferably a standardized, staining protocol. *Tip*: see the listing of such protocols at the back of Horobin and Bancroft (1998).

- Use controls to detect problems proactively, not merely to investigate mistakes retrospectively. *Tip*: keep samples of effective batches of stain to use when you suspect inadequate stain purity.
- Consider whether you have necessary skills and knowledge or, if not, is a mentor available? *Tip:* many silver stains are tricky; expect problems with their use.

Issues concerning staining reagents

- Obtain reliable stains and reagents. *Tip*: use *Biological Stain Commission* certified dyes, as they are on average less impure whilst being no more expensive.
- Ensure stains remain reliable. *Tips*: store Schiff reagent in a gas-tight container; store dye solutions in lightproof containers.

Cues for recognizing errors – before mistakes can be rectified, they must be noticed

- Stain or staining solution is not as expected in terms of color, solubility, or stability. *Case example*: some alcian blue samples dissolve, but then precipitate from solution within an hour or less.
- The expected structures stain, but only weakly. *Case example*: unexpectedly weak staining of calcium by alizarin red S results from extraction of tissue calcium ions into aqueous fixatives.
- Color of staining is unexpected. *Case example*: excessively red staining seen with Gomori's trichrome may arise from insufficiently acidic staining solutions.
- Unexpected structures stain. *Case example*: granular material stained by the Feulgen nucleal procedure may be carbonate deposits.
- Nature of the staining is unusual. *Case example*: if differential staining of Gram positive and negative organisms is poor, the preparation may be too thick.

- And there are always *other* problems! *Case examples*: loss of sections from slides in the Grocott hexamine silver method for fungi, due to overheating; and black deposits on slides and sections in the Von Kossa procedure, due to contaminated glassware.

Once an error has been noticed, and a plausible cause identified, a solution can be sought. This is sometimes simple. Perhaps the trickiest situations arise when staining specimens prepared in another laboratory. Again a variety of practical problem-solving suggestions, for a range of routine and special histopathology stains, is given in Horobin and Bancroft (1998).

References

Baker, J.R., 1958. Principles of biological microtechnique. Methuen, London.

Bennion, P.J., Horobin, R.W., 1974. Some effects of salts on staining: the use of the Donnan equilibrium to describe staining of tissue sections with acid and basic dyes. Histochemistry 39, 71–82.

Bettinger, C.H., Zimmermann, H.W., 1991. New investigations on hematoxylin, hematein, and hematein-aluminium complexes. 2. Hematein-aluminium complexes and hemalum staining. Histochemistry 96, 215–228.

Boon, M.E., Drijver, J.A., 1986. Routine cytological staining techniques: theoretical background and practise. Macmillan, London.

Celis, J.F. (Ed.), 2006. Cell biology: a laboratory handbook, vol 1, third ed. Elsevier, Amsterdam.

Chayen, J., Bitensky, L., 1991. Practical histochemistry, second ed. Wiley, Chichester.

Goldstein, D.J., 1962. Correlation of size of dye particle and density of substrate, with special reference to mucin staining. Stain Technology 37, 79–93.

Goldstein, D.J., Horobin, R.W., 1974a. Rate factors in staining with alcian blue. Histochemical Journal 6, 157–174.

Goldstein, D.J., Horobin, R.W., 1974b. Surface staining of cartilage by alcian blue, with reference to the role of microscopic aggregates in histological staining. Histochemical Journal 6, 175–184.

Henwood, A., 2003. Current applications of orcein in histochemistry. A brief review with some new observations concerning influence of dye batch variation and aging of dye solutions on staining. Biotechnic and Histochemistry 78, 303–308.

Horobin, R.W., 1969. The impurities of biological dyes: their detection, removal, occurrence and histological significance – a review. Histochemical Journal 1, 231–265.

Horobin, R.W., 1982. Histochemistry: an explanatory outline of histochemistry and biophysical staining. Butterworths, Fischer: Stuttgart, and London.

Horobin, R.W., 1988. Understanding histochemistry: selection, evaluation and design of biological stains. Horwood, Chichester.

Horobin, R.W., 1989. A numerical approach to understanding fixative action: being a reanalysis of the fixation of lipids by the dye-glutaraldehyde system. Journal of Microscopy 154, 93–96.

Horobin, R.W., 2001. Uptake, distribution, and accumulation of dyes and fluorescent probes within living cells. A structure-activity modelling approach. Advances in Colour Science and Technology 4, 101–107.

Horobin, R.W., 2004. Staining by numbers: a tool for understanding and assisting use of routine and special histo-pathology stains. Journal of Histotechnology 27, 23–28.

Horobin, R.W., 2010a. 'Special stains' influence of dye chemistry on staining. Connection 14, 121–126.

Horobin, R.W., 2010b. Can QSAR models describing small-molecule xenobiotics give useful tips for predicting uptake and localization of nanoparticles in living cells? And if not, why not? Chapter 11. In: Weissig V., D'Souza G.G.M. (Eds.), Organelle specific pharmaceutical nanotechnology. Wiley, Hoboken NJ, pp. 193–206.

Horobin, R.W., 2011. How Romanowsky stains work and why they remain valuable – including a proposed universal Romanowsky staining mechanism and a rational trouble shooting scheme. Biotech Histochem 86, 36–51.

Horobin, R.W., Bancroft, J.D., 1998. Troubleshooting histology stains. Churchill Livingstone, New York.

Horobin, R.W., Bennion, P.J., 1973. The interrelation of the size and substantivity of dyes: the role of van der Waals' attractions and hydrophobic bonding in biological staining. Histochemie 33, 191–204.

Horobin, R.W., Flemming, L., 1988. One-bath trichrome staining: investigation of a general mechanism based on a structure-staining correlation analysis. Histochemical Journal 20, 29–34.

Horobin, R.W., Goldstein, D.J., 1974. The influence of salt on the staining of sections with basic dyes; an investigation into the general applicability of the critical electrolyte concentration theory. Histochemical Journal 6, 599–609.

Horobin, R.W., Kiernan, J.A., 2002. Conn's biological stains. A handbook of dyes and fluorochromes for use in biology and medicine, tenth ed. BIOS Scientific Publishers, Oxford.

Horobin, R.W., Murgatroyd, L.B., 1970. The staining of glycogen with Best's carmine and similar hydrogen bonding dyes. A mechanistic study. Histochemical Journal 3, 1–9.

Horobin, R.W., Gerrits, P.O., Wright, D.J., 1992. Staining sections of water-miscible resins. 2. Effects of staining-reagent lipophilicity on the staining of glycolmethacrylate-embedded tissues. Journal of Microscopy 166, 199–205.

Kiernan, J.A., 2007. Histological and histochemical methods: theory and practice, fourth ed. Scion, Bloxham.

Letcher, T. (Ed.), 2007. Developments and applications in solubility. Royal Society of Chemistry, London.

Lillie, R.D., 1965. Histopathologic technic and practical histochemistry, third ed. McGraw-Hill, New York.

Lillie, R.D., 1977. H.J. Conn's biological stains, ninth ed. Williams & Wilkins, Baltimore.

Lyon, H., 1991. Theory and strategy of histochemistry: a guide to the selection and understanding of techniques. Springer-Verlag, Berlin.

Mann, G., 1902. Physiological histology. Methods and theory. Clarendon, Oxford.

Marshall, P.N., Horobin, R.W., 1973. The mechanism of action of 'mordant' dyes – a study using preformed metal complexes. Histochemie 35, 361–371.

Pearse, A.G.E., 1968. Histochemistry, theoretical and applied, vol. 1, third ed. Churchill Livingstone, Edinburgh.

Peters, A., 1955a. Experiments on the mechanism of silver staining. 1. Impregnation. Quarterly Journal of Microscopical Science 96, 84–102.

Peters, A., 1955b. Experiments on the mechanism of silver staining. 2. Development. Quarterly Journal of Microscopical Science 96, 103–115.

Prentø, P., 2007. The structural role of glycine and proline in connective tissue fiber staining with hydrogen bonding dyes. Biotechnic and Histochemistry 82, 170–173.

Prentø, P., 2009. Staining of macromolecules. Biotechnic and Histochemistry 84, 139–158.

Scott, J.E., 1973. Affinity, competition and specific interactions in the biochemistry and histochemistry of polyelectrolytes. Biochemical Society Transactions 1, 787–806.

Scott, J.E., Harbinson, J., 1968. Periodic oxidation of acid polysaccharides. Inhibition by the electrostatic field of the substrate. Histochemie 14, 215–220.

Sheehan, D.C., Hrapchak, B.B., 1987. Theory and practice of histotechnology, second ed. Battelle Press, Columbus, OH.

Singer, M., 1952. Factors which control the staining of tissue sections with acid and basic dyes. International Review of Cytology 1, 211–255.

Society of Dyers and Colourists, 1999. Colour Index International, third ed. Issue 3 on CD ROM. The Society of Dyers and Colourists, Bradford, UK.

Tanford, C., 2004. Ben Franklin stilled the waves: an informal history of pouring oil on water with reflections on the ups and downs of scientific life in general. Oxford University Press, Oxford.

Zollinger, H., 2003. Colour chemistry, third ed. Wiley-VCH, and VHCA: Zurich, Weinheim.

Further reading

Few accounts of histology staining consider the physicochemical unity underlying the technical diversity of the various staining technologies. There are many published protocols but a paucity of critical reviews and summations. Thus encyclopedic texts like the present one and earlier examples such as those of Lillie (1965), Pearse (1968), and Sheehan and Hrapchak (1987) summarize a remarkable amount of information and provide extensive bibliographies. Some staining manuals also set out to integrate theoretical background with procedural information, e.g. Chayen and Bitensky (1991) and Kiernan (2007). A few authors have attempted to provide modern physicochemical accounts of staining methods as a whole; for instance Horobin (1982, 1988), Horobin and Bancroft (1998), Lyon (1991), and Prentø (2009). Some classic works can also be recommended: read Baker (1958) for his early integrative account and his elegant English; read Lillie (1965) for his hard-won personal experience and historical long view; and then read Mann (1902) to be astonished at why it took us so long to follow up his experimental investigations. Finally, those wishing to learn more about dyestuffs have several modern texts available. The book written by Zollinger (2003) does, unusually, include a section explicitly considering biological stains and staining.

The hematoxylins and eosin

10

John D. Bancroft • Christopher Layton

Introduction

The hematoxylin and eosin stain (H&E) is the most widely used histological stain. Its popularity is based on its comparative simplicity and ability to demonstrate clearly an enormous number of different tissue structures. Hematoxylin can be prepared in numerous ways and has a widespread applicability to tissues from different sites. Essentially, the hematoxylin component stains the cell nuclei blue-black, showing good intranuclear detail, while the eosin stains cell cytoplasm and most connective tissue fibers in varying shades and intensities of pink, orange, and red. While automated staining instruments and commercially prepared hematoxylin and eosin solutions are more commonly used in today's laboratories for routine staining, students of histological techniques should have a basic knowledge of the dyes and preparation techniques in order to troubleshoot and/or modify procedures for specialized use. It should be noted that hematoxylin has additional uses beyond just the hematoxylin and eosin combination.

Eosin

Eosin is the most suitable stain to combine with an alum hematoxylin to demonstrate the general histological architecture of a tissue. Its particular value is its ability, with proper differentiation, to distinguish between the cytoplasm of different types of cell, and between the different types of connective tissue fibers and matrices, by staining them differing shades of red and pink.

The eosins are xanthene dyes and the following types are easily obtainable commercially: eosin Y (eosin yellowish, eosin water-soluble) C.I. No. 45380 (C.I. Acid Red 87); ethyl eosin (eosin S, eosin alcohol-soluble) C.I. No. 45386 (C.I. Solvent Red 45); eosin B (eosin bluish, erythrosin B) C.I. No. 45400 (C.I. Acid Red 91).

Of these, eosin Y is much the most widely used, and despite its synonym it is also satisfactorily soluble in alcohol; it is sometimes sold as 'water and alcohol soluble'. As a cytoplasmic stain, it is usually used as a 0.5 or 1.0% solution in distilled water, with a crystal of thymol added to inhibit the growth of fungi. The addition of a little acetic acid (0.5 ml to 1000 ml stain) is said to sharpen the staining. Differentiation of the eosin staining occurs in the subsequent tap water wash, and a little further differentiation occurs during the dehydration through the alcohols. The intensity of eosin staining, and the degree of differentiation required, is largely a matter of individual taste. Suitable photomicrographs of H&E-stained tissues are easier to obtain when the eosin staining is intense and the differentiation slight (at least double the routine staining time is advisable). Ethyl eosin and eosin B are now rarely used, although occasional old methods specify their use: for example, the Harris stain for Negri bodies. Alternative red dyes have been suggested as substitutes for eosin, such as phloxine, Biebrich scarlet, etc.; however, although these substitutes often give a more intense red color to the tissues, they are rarely as amenable to subtle differentiation as eosin and are generally less valuable.

Under certain circumstances eosin staining is intense and difficulty may be experienced in obtaining adequate differentiation; this may occur after mercuric fixation. Over-differentiation of the eosin may be continued until only the red blood cells and granules of eosinophil polymorph are stained red. This is, occasionally, used to facilitate the location and identification of eosinophils. Combining eosin Y and phloxine B (10 ml 1% phloxine B, 100 ml 1% eosin Y, 780 ml 95% alcohol, 4 ml glacial acetic acid) produces a cytoplasmic stain, which more dramatically demonstrates various tissue components. Muscle is clearly differentiated from collagen, and red cells stain bright red. According to Luna (1992), eosin dye content should be 88% and not contain sodium sulfate (sometimes used as filler). When using this dye in solution, a fine granular precipitate forms, and the staining of the cytoplasm will be poor.

Hematoxylin

Hematoxylin is extracted from the heartwood ('logwood') of the tree *Hematoxylon campechianum* that originated in the Mexican State of Campeche, but which is now mainly cultivated in the West Indies. The hematoxylin is extracted from logwood with hot water, and then precipitated out from the aqueous solution using urea (see prior editions). Hematoxylin itself is not a stain. The major oxidization product is hematein, a natural dye that is responsible for the color properties. Hematein can be produced from hematoxylin in two ways.

Natural oxidation ('ripening') by exposure to light and air

This is a slow process, sometimes taking as long as 3–4 months, but the resultant solution seems to retain its staining ability for a long time. Ehrlich's and Delafield's hematoxylin solutions are examples of naturally ripened hematoxylins.

Chemical oxidation

Examples are sodium iodate (e.g. Mayer's hematoxylin) or mercuric oxide (e.g. Harris's hematoxylin). The use of chemical oxidizing agents converts the hematoxylin to hematein almost instantaneously, so these hematoxylin solutions are ready for use immediately after preparation. In general, they have a shorter useful life than the naturally oxidized hematoxylins, probably because the continuing oxidation process in air and light eventually destroys much of the hematein, converting it to a colorless compound. Hematein is anionic, having a poor affinity for tissue, and is inadequate as a nuclear stain without the presence of a mordant. The mordant/metal cation confers a net positive charge to the dye-mordant complex and enables it to bind to anionic tissue sites, such as nuclear chromatin. The type of mordant used influences strongly the type of tissue components stained and their final color. The most useful mordants for hematoxylin are salts of aluminum, iron, and tungsten, although hematoxylin solutions using lead as a mordant are occasionally used (for example in the demonstration of argyrophil cells). Most mordants are incorporated into the hematoxylin staining solutions, although certain hematoxylin stains required the tissue section to be pre-treated with the mordant before staining; such as Heidenhain's iron hematoxylin. Hematoxylin solutions can be arbitrarily classified according to which mordant is used:

- alum hematoxylins
- iron hematoxylins
- tungsten hematoxylins
- molybdenum hematoxylins
- lead hematoxylins
- hematoxylin without mordant.

Alum hematoxylins

This group comprises most of those that are used routinely in the hematoxylin and eosin stain, and produce good nuclear staining. The mordant is aluminum, usually in the form of 'potash alum' (aluminum potassium sulfate) or 'ammonium alum' (aluminum ammonium sulfate). All stain the nuclei a red color, which is converted to the familiar blue-black when the section is washed in a weak alkali solution. Tap water is usually alkaline enough to produce this color change, but occasionally alkaline solutions such as saturated lithium carbonate, 0.05% ammonia in distilled water, or Scott's tap water substitute (see Appendix III) are necessary. This procedure is known as 'blueing'.

The alum hematoxylins can be used *regressively*, meaning that the section is over-stained and then differentiated in acid alcohol, followed by 'blueing', or *progressively*, i.e. stained for a predetermined time to stain the nuclei adequately but leave the background tissue relatively unstained. The times for hematoxylin staining and for satisfactory differentiation will vary according to the type and age of alum hematoxylin used, the type of tissue, and the personal preference of the pathologist. For routine hematoxylin and eosin staining of tissues, the most commonly used hematoxylins are Ehrlich's, Mayer's, Harris's, Gill's, Cole's, and Delafield's. Carazzi's hematoxylin is occasionally used, particularly for urgent frozen sections.

Ehrlich's hematoxylin (Ehrlich 1886)

This is a naturally ripening alum hematoxylin which takes about 2 months to ripen; the ripening time can be shortened somewhat by placing the unstoppered bottle in a warm sunny place such as a window-ledge, and is shorter in the summer than in winter. Once satisfactorily ripened, this hematoxylin solution will last in bulk for years, and retains its staining ability in a Coplin jar for some months. Ehrlich's hematoxylin, as well as being an excellent nuclear stain, also stains mucins including the mucopolysaccharides of cartilage; it is recommended for the staining of bone and cartilage (Chapter 16).

Preparation of solution

Hematoxylin	2 g
Absolute alcohol	100 ml
Glycerin	100 ml
Distilled water	100 ml
Glacial acetic acid	10 ml
Potassium alum	15 g approx.

The hematoxylin is dissolved in the alcohol, and the other chemicals are added. Glycerin is added to slow the oxidation process and prolong the hematoxylin shelf life. Natural ripening in sunlight takes about 2 months, but in an emergency the stain can be chemically ripened by the addition of sodium iodate,

using 50 mg for every gram of hematoxylin; this will inevitably shorten the bench life of the stain. By definition this chemically oxidized variant is not a true Ehrlich's hematoxylin and will not have the same longevity as naturally oxidized Ehrlich's hematoxylin. One should always filter before use.

Ehrlich's hematoxylin, being a strong hematoxylin solution, stains nuclei intensely and crisply, and stained sections fade much more slowly than those stained with other alum hematoxylins. It is particularly useful for staining sections from tissues that have been exposed to acid. It is suitable for tissues that have been subjected to acid decalcification or, more valuably, tissues that have been stored for a long period in formalin fixatives which have gradually become acidic over the storage period, or in acid fixatives such as Bouin's fixative. Ehrlich's hematoxylin is not ideal for frozen sections.

Delafield's hematoxylin (Delafield 1885)

A naturally ripened alum hematoxylin, Delafield's has similar longevity to Ehrlich's hematoxylin.

Preparation of solution

Hematoxylin	4 g
95% alcohol	125 ml
Saturated aqueous ammonium alum (15 g/100 ml)	400 ml
Glycerin	100 ml

The hematoxylin is dissolved in 25 ml of alcohol, and then added to the alum solution. This mixture is allowed to stand in light and air for 5 days, then filtered, and to it are added the glycerin and a further 100 ml of 95% alcohol. The stain is allowed to stand exposed to light and air for about 3–4 months or until sufficiently dark in color, then is filtered and stored. Filter before use.

Mayer's hematoxylin (Mayer 1903)

This alum hematoxylin is chemically ripened with sodium iodate. It can be used as a regressive stain like any alum hematoxylin. However, it is also useful as a progressive stain, particularly in situations where a nuclear counterstain is needed to emphasize a cytoplasmic component which has been demonstrated, by a special stain, and where the acid-alcohol differentiation might destroy or de-color the stained cytoplasmic component. It is used as a nuclear counterstain in the demonstration of glycogen, in various enzyme histochemical techniques, and in many others. The stain is applied for a short time (usually 5–10 minutes), until the nuclei are stained, and is then 'blued' without any differentiation.

Preparation of solution

Hematoxylin	1 g
Distilled water	1000 ml
Potassium or ammonium alum	50 g
Sodium iodate	0.2 g
Citric acid	1 g
Chloral hydrate SLR	50 g or
Chloral hydrate AR	30 g

The hematoxylin, potassium alum, and sodium iodate are dissolved in the distilled water by warming and stirring, or by allowing to stand at room temperature overnight. The chloral hydrate and citric acid are added, and the mixture is boiled for 5 minutes, then cooled and filtered. If higher-purity chloral hydrate AR grade is used, the amount may be reduced, as shown above. The stain is ready for use immediately. Filter before use.

Harris's hematoxylin (Harris 1900)

This alum hematoxylin was traditionally chemically ripened with mercuric oxide. As mercuric oxide is highly toxic, environmentally unfriendly, and has detrimental and corrosive long-term effects on some automated staining machines, sodium or potassium iodate is frequently used as a substitute for oxidation. Harris is a useful general-purpose hematoxylin and gives particularly clear nuclear staining, and for this reason has been used, as a progressive stain, in diagnostic exfoliative cytology. In routine histological practice, it is generally used regressively, but can be useful when used progressively. When using Harris's hematoxylin as a progressive stain, an acetic acid-alcohol rinse provides a more controllable method in removing excess stain from tissue components and the glass slide. The traditional hydrochloric acid-alcohol acts quickly and indiscriminately, is more difficult to control, and can result in a light nuclear stain. A 5–10% solution of acetic acid, in 70–95% alcohol, detaches dye molecules from the cytoplasm/nucleoplasm while keeping nucleic acid complexes intact (Feldman & Dapson 1985).

Preparation of solution

Hematoxylin	2.5 g
Absolute alcohol	25 ml
Potassium alum	50 g
Distilled water	500 ml
Mercuric oxide	1.25 g or
Sodium iodate	0.5 g
Glacial acetic acid	20 ml

The hematoxylin is dissolved in the absolute alcohol, and is then added to the alum, which has previously been dissolved in the warm distilled water in a 2-liter flask. The mixture is rapidly brought to the boil and the mercuric oxide or sodium iodate is then slowly and carefully added. Plunging the flask into cold water or into a sink containing chipped ice rapidly cools the stain. When the solution is cold, the acetic acid is added, and the stain is ready for immediate use. The glacial acetic acid is optional but its inclusion gives more precise and selective staining of nuclei.

As with most of the chemically ripened alum hematoxylins, the quality of the nuclear staining begins to deteriorate after a few months. This deterioration is marked by the formation of a precipitate in the stored stain. At this stage, the stain should be filtered before use, and the staining time may need to be increased. For the best results, it is wise to prepare a fresh batch of stain every month, although this may be uneconomical unless only small quantities are prepared each time.

Cole's hematoxylin (Cole 1943)

This is an alum hematoxylin, artificially ripened with an alcoholic iodine solution.

Preparation of solution

Hematoxylin	1.5 g
Saturated aqueous potassium alum	700 ml
1% iodine in 95% alcohol	50 ml
Distilled water	250 ml

The hematoxylin is dissolved in warm distilled water and mixed with the iodine solution. The alum solution is added, and the mixture brought to the boil, then cooled quickly and filtered. The solution is ready for immediate use, but may need filtering after storage, for the same reason as described above for Harris's hematoxylin. Filter before use.

Carazzi's hematoxylin *(Carazzi 1911)*

Carazzi's is an alum hematoxylin which is chemically ripened using potassium iodate.

Preparation of solution

Hematoxylin	5 g
Glycerol	100 ml
Potassium alum	25 g
Distilled water	400 ml
Potassium iodate	0.1 g

The hematoxylin is dissolved in the glycerol, and the alum is dissolved in most of the water overnight. The alum solution is added slowly to the hematoxylin solution, mixing well after each addition. The potassium iodate is dissolved in the rest of the water with gentle warming and is then added to the hematoxylin-alum-glycerol mixture. The final staining solution is mixed well and is then ready for immediate use; it remains usable for about 6 months. Care must be taken in preparing the hematoxylin to avoid over-oxidation; it is safer if heat is not used to dissolve the reagents. Filter before use.

Like Mayer's hematoxylin, Carazzi's hematoxylin may be used as a progressive nuclear counterstain using a short staining time, followed by blueing in tap water. It is particularly suitable, since it is a pale and precise nuclear stain and does not stain any of the cytoplasmic components.

Gill's hematoxylin *(Gill et al. 1974 modified)*

Preparation of solution

Hematoxylin	2 g
Sodium iodate	0.2 g
Aluminum sulfate	17.6 g
Distilled water	750 ml
Ethylene glycol (ethandiol)	250 ml
Glacial acetic acid	20 ml

The distilled water and ethylene glycol are mixed, and then the hematoxylin is added and dissolved. The ethylene glycol is an excellent solvent for hematoxylin and it prevents the formation of surface precipitates (Carson 1997). Sodium iodate is added for oxidation, and the aluminum sulfate mordant is then added and dissolved. Finally, the glacial acetic acid is added and stirred for 1 hour. The solution is filtered before use. Carson reported that, although the stain can be used immediately, it provides a better intensity if allowed to ripen for 1 week in a 37°C incubator. It should be noted that the popularity of Gill's solution has made it one of the more commercially successful formulas.

Double or triple hematoxylin concentrations may be used as preferred. These are usually referred to as Gill's I (normal), Gill's II (double), and Gill's III (triple), with the Gill III being the most concentrated. Gill's hematoxylin is more frequently used for routine H&E staining than Mayer's hematoxylin, and is more stable than Harris's hematoxylin, as auto-oxidation is inhibited to the extent that no measurable changes occur over many months. Disadvantages associated with Gill's hematoxylin include staining of gelatin adhesive and even the glass itself. Some mucus may also stain darkly, as compared to Harris's, where mucus generally remains unstained, and the glass usually fails to attract the stain. Feldman and Dapson (1987) theorized that the aluminum sulfate mordant is responsible. Certain charged sites in the tissue, in the adhesive, and on the glass are masked by the Harris mordant, leaving them unavailable for staining. Gill's mordant system fails to do that, and the sites attract the dye-mordant complex.

Staining times with alum hematoxylins

It is not possible to give other than a rough guide to suitable staining times with alum hematoxylins because the time will vary according to the following factors:

1. Type of hematoxylin used, e.g. Ehrlich's 20–45 minutes, Mayer's 10–20 minutes.
2. Age of stain. As the stain ages, the staining time will need to be increased.
3. Intensity of use of stain. A heavily used hematoxylin will lose its staining powers more rapidly and longer staining times will be necessary.
4. Whether the stain is used progressively or regressively, e.g. Mayer's hematoxylin used

Table 10.1 Staining times with alum hematoxylins	
Cole's	20–45 min
Delafield's	15–20 min
Ehrlich's (progressive)	20–45 min
Mayer's (progressive)	10–20 min
Mayer's (regressive)	5–10 min
Harris's (progressive in cytology)	4–30 s
Harris's (regressive)	5–15 min
Carazzi's (progressive)	1–2 min
Carazzi's (regressive)	45 s
Carazzi's (frozen sections, see text)	1 min
Gill's I (regressive)	5–15 min

progressively 5–10 minutes, used regressively 10–20 minutes.

5. Pre-treatment of tissues or sections, e.g. length of time in fixative or acid decalcifying solution, or whether paraffin or frozen sections.
6. Post-treatment of sections, e.g. subsequent acid stains such as van Gieson.
7. Personal preference.

The times given in Table 10.1 are only a general indication of a suitable range for each type of stain; the optimal time must be determined by trial and error. Except where stated, these figures refer to normally fixed paraffin sections. As a rule, the times need to be considerably shortened for frozen sections, and increased for decalcified tissues and those that have been stored for a long time in non-buffered formalin.

Disadvantages of alum hematoxylins

The major disadvantage of alum hematoxylin nuclear stains is their sensitivity to any subsequently applied acidic staining solutions. The most common examples are in the van Gieson and other trichrome stains. The application of the picric acid-acid fuchsin mixture in van Gieson's stain removes most of the hematoxylin so that the nuclei are barely discernible. In this case satisfactory nuclear staining can be achieved by using an iron-mordanted

hematoxylin such as Weigert's hematoxylin (see below), which is resistant to the effect of picric acid. A suitable, and now more popular, alternative is the combination of a celestine blue staining solution with an alum hematoxylin. Celestine blue is resistant to the effects of acid, and the ferric salt in the prepared celestine blue solution strengthens the bond between the nucleus and the alum hematoxylin to provide a strong nuclear stain which is reasonably resistant to acid.

Celestine blue-alum hematoxylin procedure

Celestine blue solution

Celestine blue B	2.5 g
Ferric ammonium sulfate	25 g
Glycerin	70 ml
Distilled water	500 ml

The ferric ammonium sulfate is dissolved in the cold distilled water with stirring, the celestine blue is added to this solution, and the mixture is boiled for a few minutes. After cooling, the stain is filtered and glycerin is added. The final stain should be usable for over 5 months. Filter before use.

Method

1. Dewax sections, rehydrate through descending grades of alcohol and take to water.
2. Stain in celestine blue solution for 5 minutes.
3. Rinse in distilled water.
4. Stain in an alum hematoxylin (e.g. Mayer's or Cole's) for 5 minutes.
5. Wash in water until blue.
6. Proceed with required staining technique.

Routine staining procedures using alum hematoxylins

Hematoxylin and eosin stain for paraffin sections

Method

1. Dewax sections, rehydrate through descending grades of alcohol to water.
2. Remove fixation pigments if necessary.
3. Stain in an alum hematoxylin of choice for a suitable time.
4. Wash well in running tap water until sections 'blue' for 5 minutes or less.

5. Differentiate in 1% acid alcohol (1% HCl in 70% alcohol) for 5–10 seconds
6. Wash well in tap water until sections are again 'blue' (10–15 minutes), *or*
7. Blue by dipping in an alkaline solution (e.g. ammonia water), followed by a 5-minute tap water wash.
8. Stain in 1% eosin Y for 10 minutes.
9. Wash in running tap water for 1–5 minutes.
10. Dehydrate through alcohols, clear, and mount.

Results

Nuclei	blue/black
Cytoplasm	varying shades of pink
Muscle fibers	deep pink/red
Red blood cells	orange/red
Fibrin	deep pink

Notes

Note that structures and substances other than nuclei may be hematoxyphilic to varying degrees. Examples include fungal hyphae, which are faintly hematoxyphilic, and calcium deposits, which are often deep blue-black.

Rapid hematoxylin and eosin stain for urgent frozen sections

1. Freeze suitable tissue block onto a chuck.
2. Cut cryostat sections at 3–6 μm thickness.
3. Fix section in 10% neutral buffered formalin at room temperature for 20 seconds.
4. Rinse in tap water.
5. Stain in double strength Carazzi's hematoxylin for 1 minute.
6. Wash well in tap water for 10–20 seconds.
7. Stain in 1% aqueous eosin for 10 seconds.
8. Rinse in tap water.
9. Dehydrate, clear, and mount.

Papanicolaou stain for cytological preparations

The universal stain for cytological preparations is the Papanicolaou stain. Harris's hematoxylin is the optimal nuclear stain and the combination of OG 6 and EA 50 gives the subtle range of green, blue, and pink hues to the cell cytoplasm.

Most laboratories use commercial stains and each will consider their modification of the original technique to be the optimum. The result, however, should retain the transparent quality of the cytoplasmic stain, and the nuclear chromatin should be easily distinguished.

Papanicolaou formula

Harris's hematoxylin

Orange G 6

10% aqueous Orange G	50 ml
Alcohol	950 ml
Phosphotungstic acid	0–15 g

EA 50

0.04 M light green SF	10 ml
0.3 M eosin Y	20 ml
Phosphotungstic acid	2 g
Alcohol	750 ml
Methanol	250 ml
Glacial acetic acid	20 ml

Filter all stains before use.

Papanicolaou staining method

1. Remove polyethylene glycol fixative in 50% alcohol, 2 minutes.
2. Hydrate in 95% alcohol, 2 minutes, and 70% alcohol, 2 minutes.
3. Rinse in water, 1 minute.
4. Stain in Harris's hematoxylin, 5 minutes.
5. Rinse in water, 2 minutes.
6. Differentiate in 0.5% aqueous hydrochloric acid, 10 seconds approx.
7. Rinse in water, 2 minutes.
8. 'Blue' in Scott's tap water substitute, 2 minutes.
9. Rinse in water, 2 minutes.
10. Dehydrate, 70% alcohol for 2 minutes.
11. Dehydrate, 95% alcohol, 2 minutes.
12. Dehydrate, 95% alcohol, 2 minutes.
13. Stain in OG 6, 2 minutes.
14. Rinse in 95% alcohol, 2 minutes.
15. Rinse in 95% alcohol, 2 minutes.
16. Stain in EA 50, 3 minutes.
17. Rinse in 95% alcohol, 1 minute.

The staining times can be adjusted to suit personal preference for a darker or paler stain. Alternatives to Scott's tap water substitute include 0.1% ammoniated water or a weak aqueous solution of lithium carbonate.

Results

The nuclei should appear	blue/black
Cytoplasm (non-keratinizing squamous cells)	blue/green
Keratinizing cells	pink/orange

Note

Change stains frequently.

Iron hematoxylins

In these hematoxylin solutions, iron salts are used both as the oxidizing agent and as mordant. The most commonly used iron salts are ferric chloride and ferric ammonium sulfate, and the most common iron hematoxylins are:

- Weigert's hematoxylin
- Heidenhain's hematoxylin
- Loyez hematoxylin for myelin
- Verhöeff's hematoxylin for elastin fibers.

Over-oxidation of the hematoxylin is a problem with these stains, so it is usual to prepare separate mordant/oxidant and hematoxylin solutions and mix them immediately before use (e.g. in Weigert's hematoxylin) or to use them consecutively (e.g. Heidenhain's and Loyez hematoxylins). Because of the strong oxidizing ability of the solution containing iron salts, it is often used as a subsequent differentiating fluid after hematoxylin staining, as well as for a mordanting fluid before it.

The iron hematoxylins are capable of demonstrating a much wider range of tissue structures than the alum hematoxylins, but the techniques are more time-consuming and usually incorporate a differentiation stage which needs microscopic control for accuracy. The use of iron hematoxylin-based methods for the specific identification of phospholipids is briefly discussed in Appendix II.

Weigert's hematoxylin (Weigert 1904)

This is an iron hematoxylin in which ferric chloride is used as the mordant/oxidant. The iron and the hematoxylin solutions are prepared separately and are mixed immediately before use. They are prepared as follows.

Weigert's iron hematoxylin

Preparation of solutions

a. Hematoxylin solution

Hematoxylin	1 g
Absolute alcohol	100 ml

This is allowed to ripen naturally for 4 weeks before use.

b. Iron solution

30% aqueous ferric chloride (anhydrous)	4 ml
Hydrochloric acid (concentrated)	1 ml
Distilled water	95 ml

This solution is filtered and added to an equal volume of the hematoxylin solution immediately before the stain is used. The mixture should be a violet-black color and must be discarded if it is brown. The main use of Weigert's hematoxylin is as a nuclear stain in techniques where acidic staining solutions are to be applied to the sections subsequently (e.g. van Gieson stain). A staining time of 15–30 minutes is usual. In this role, Weigert's hematoxylin has been largely replaced by the more convenient celestine blue-alum hematoxylin procedure. It remains a useful stain, with eosin, for CNS tissues. For the purist who prefers a black nuclear counterstain with a van Gieson technique, the ferrous hematein technique of Slidders (1969) is satisfactory.

Heidenhain's hematoxylin

(Heidenhain 1896)

This iron hematoxylin uses ferric ammonium sulfate as oxidant/mordant, and the same solution is used as the differentiating fluid. The iron solution is used first and the section is then treated with the hematoxylin solution until it is overstained, and is then differentiated with iron solution under microscopic control.

Heidenhain's hematoxylin can be used to demonstrate many structures according to the degree of differentiation. After staining, all components are black or dark gray-black. The hematoxylin staining is removed progressively from different tissue structures at different rates using the iron alum solution. Mitochondria, muscle striations, nuclear chromatin, and myelin can all be demonstrated; the black color disappears first from mitochondria, then from muscle striations, then from nuclear chromatin. Differentiation that is more prolonged will remove the stain from almost all structures, although red blood cells and keratin retain the stain the longest. More easily controllable differentiation can be achieved if the differentiating iron alum solution is diluted with an equal volume of distilled water or an alcoholic picric acid solution.

Heidenhain's iron hematoxylin

Preparation of solutions

a. Hematoxylin solution

Hematoxylin	0.5 g
Absolute alcohol	10 ml
Distilled water	90 ml

The hematoxylin is dissolved in the alcohol, and the water is then added. The solution is allowed to ripen naturally for 4 weeks before use.

b. Iron solution (5% iron alum)

Ferric ammonium sulfate	5 g
Distilled water	100 ml

It is important that only the clear violet crystals of ferric ammonium sulfate be used.

Method

1. Dewax sections, rehydrate through descending grades of alcohol to water.
2. Mordant in iron solution (5% iron alum) for 1 hour (see Note a).
3. Rinse in distilled water.
4. Stain in Heidenhain's hematoxylin solution for 1 hour (see Note a).
5. Wash in running tap water.
6. Differentiate in the iron solution (5% iron alum), or the iron solution diluted with an equal volume of distilled water. Alternate a rinse in differentiator with a rinse in tap water. The degree of differentiation is controlled microscopically until the desired structure is clearly demonstrated (see Note b).
7. Wash in running tap water for 10 minutes.
8. Dehydrate, clear, and mount.

Results

Mitochondria, muscle striations, myelin, chromatin, etc., gray-black.

Notes

a. The time needed in the mordant and stain will vary according to the fixative used; for most purposes, 1 hour in each solution is satisfactory, but tissues fixed in dichromate solutions need longer. The following times are a rough guide. Tissues fixed in formalin solutions, formal sublimate, Susa, Bouin's, and Carnoy's, 1 hour. Tissues fixed in Helly's or Zenker's, 3 hours. Tissues fixed in osmium tetroxide and Fleming's fluid, up to 24 hours.

b. Differentiation is difficult to judge, the authors recommend dipping the slide in and out of the 5% iron alum until the background of the slide is clear, then check microscopically. If the differentiation proceeds beyond the desired end, the section can be restained in the hematoxylin solution for the same length of time and differentiation attempted again.

c. Cytoplasmic counterstains are rarely necessary, although they may be used to accentuate nuclear chromatin, particularly in the demonstration of chromosomes or mitoses. Aqueous eosin or Orange G is satisfactory.

d. Sections stained with Heidenhain's iron hematoxylin are resistant to fading only if the section is washed well after the differentiation stage to remove all traces of iron alum.

Loyez hematoxylin

(Loyez 1910)

This iron hematoxylin uses ferric ammonium sulfate as the mordant. The mordant and hematoxylin solutions are used consecutively, and differentiation is by Weigert's differentiator (borax and potassium ferricyanide). It is used to demonstrate myelin and can be applied to paraffin, frozen, or nitrocellulose sections. Two methods are similar to that of Loyez. The Heidenhain myelin stain (not to be confused with Heidenhain's iron hematoxylin) is essentially the Loyez technique but judicious selection of staining time removes the need for separate differentiation. The second variant is the short Weil technique in which the mordant and dye are mixed before use, rather than used consecutively. Both these techniques are shorter than the Loyez.

Verhöeff's hematoxylin

(Verhöeff 1908)

This iron hematoxylin is used to demonstrate elastic fibers. Ferric chloride is included in the hematoxylin staining solution, together with Lugol's iodine, and 2% aqueous ferric chloride is used as the differentiator. Coarse elastic fibers stain black.

Other elastin methods may stain finer fibers, but for the high contrast required for photomicrography the intense black staining produced by Verhöeff's is ideal. Verhöeff's is also used to stain elastin fibers as part of the Movat's pentachrome.

Tungsten hematoxylins

There is only one widely used tungsten hematoxylin, although there are many variants on the original Mallory phosphotungstic acid hematoxylin (PTAH) technique. Mallory (1897, 1900) combined hematoxylin with 1% aqueous phosphotungstic acid, the latter acting as the mordant. It is possible to prepare a staining solution using hematein instead of hematoxylin; the oxidation process is unnecessary and the staining solution can be used immediately, but its activity is comparatively short-lived. The hematoxylin can be oxidized chemically by using a potassium permanganate solution; again, the solution is usable within 24 hours. The most satisfactory method of preparation, albeit time-consuming, is to allow natural ripening of the tungsten hematoxylin solution in light and air. The PTAH solution produced may take some months to ripen, but will remain usable for many years. Its use is applicable to both CNS material and general tissue structure, and to tissues fixed in any of the standard fixatives. Staining times will vary according to the method

of preparation, the fixative used, and the tissue structure to be demonstrated. Staining is more precise after the section has been treated with an acid dichromate solution, and after a Mallory bleach procedure (which also aids differential staining).

PTAH staining technique solution using hematein
(Shum & Hon 1969)

Solution A

Hematein	0.8 g
Distilled water	1 ml

Grind the 0.8 g hematein to a paste with 1 ml distilled water. (The paste should be chocolate brown. Lighter colors are usually indicative of an unsuitable batch of hematein and should be discarded.)

Solution B

Phosphotungstic acid	0.9 g
Distilled water	9 ml

Mix solution A and solution B, bring to the boil, then cool and filter.

Method

1. Dewax, rehydrate through descending grades of alcohol to water.
2. Treat with acid permanganate (see below) for 5 minutes.
3. Rinse in tap water.
4. Bleach with 5% aqueous oxalic acid.
5. Wash well in tap water.
6. Stain in PTAH solution for 12–24 hours at room temperature.
7. Wash in distilled water.
8. Dehydrate rapidly, clear, and mount.

The solution may be used at 56°C for several hours, but staining for the longer time at room temperature gives results that are more precise and is preferable.

PTAH solution, chemically oxidized with potassium permanganate

Solution

Hematoxylin	0.5 g
Phosphotungstic acid	10 g
Distilled water	500 ml
0.25% aqueous potassium permanganate	25 ml

The hematoxylin is dissolved in 100 ml of the distilled water, and the phosphotungstic acid in the remaining 400 ml; the two solutions are mixed and the potassium permanganate solution is added. The stain can be used next day, but peak staining activity is not reached until after 7 days. Continuing oxidation of the hematoxylin means that this stain has a comparatively short life.

PTAH solution, naturally oxidized

Preparation of solutions

a. Acid dichromate solution

10% HCl in absolute alcohol	12 ml
3% aqueous potassium dichromate	36 ml

b. Acid permanganate solution

0.5% aqueous potassium permanganate	50 ml
3% sulfuric acid	2.5 ml

c. Staining solution

Hematoxylin	0.5 g
Phosphotungstic acid	5 g
Distilled water	500 ml

The solids are dissolved in separate portions of the distilled water, and then mixed as in the recipes above. The stain is allowed to ripen naturally in a loosely stoppered bottle in a warm, light place for several months.

Method

1. Dewax, rehydrate through descending grades of alcohol to water.
2. Place in acid dichromate solution for 30 minutes.
3. Wash in tap water.
4. Treat with acid permanganate solution for 1 minute.
5. Wash in tap water.
6. Bleach in 1% oxalic acid.
7. Rinse in tap water.
8. Stain in Mallory's PTAH stain overnight.
9. Dehydrate through ascending grades of alcohol, clear, and mount.

Results

Muscle striations, neuroglia, fibers, fibrin and amoebae	dark blue
Nuclei, cilia, red blood cells	blue
Myelin	lighter blue
Collagen, osteoid, cartilage, elastic fibers	deep brownish-red
Cytoplasm	pale pinkish-brown

Notes

The acid dichromate treatment (post chroming) can be omitted if fixation has been by a chromate-containing fixative.

Dehydration should be rapid since water and alcohol may remove some of the stain. If the sections are too blue, some degree of differentiation can be achieved during dehydration. Dehydration may be commenced in 95% alcohol, and CNS sections may need thorough washing in 95% alcohol for several minutes to remove excess red stain. The times in dichromate, permanganate, and stain may need to be modified depending on the nature of the tissue and the feature to be demonstrated

Molybdenum hematoxylins

Hematoxylin solutions that use molybdic acid as the mordant are rare, and the only technique that gained any acceptance was the Thomas (1941) technique which was mentioned by McManus and Mowry (1964). They recommend the method for the demonstration of collagen and coarse reticulin; although more valuable and widely accepted techniques for these connective tissue fibers exist, the Thomas method also stains argentaffin cell granules and may have a potential use for this purpose.

Phosphomolybdic acid hematoxylin stain (Thomas 1941)

Preparation of solutions

a. Hematoxylin solution

Hematoxylin	2.5 g
Dioxane	49 ml
Hydrogen peroxide	1 ml

b. Phosphomolybdic acid solution

Phosphomolybdic acid	16.5 g
Distilled water	44 ml
Diethylene glycol	11 ml

The phosphomolybdic acid solution is filtered and 50 ml of the filtrate is added to the hematoxylin solution. The resultant solution, which should be dark violet in color, is allowed to stand for 24 hours before use.

Method

1. Dewax, rehydrate through descending grades of alcohol to water.
2. Stain with phosphomolybdic acid hematoxylin for 2 minutes.
3. Wash with distilled water.
4. Drop picro-acetic alcohol (see Note a) onto section, then wash away immediately with distilled water.
5. Rinse in tap water, dehydrate through 95% and absolute alcohol, clear, and mount.

Results

Collagen and coarse reticulin	violet to black
Argentaffin cells	black
Nuclei	pale blue
Paneth cells	orange

Notes

a. Picro-acetic alcohol (picric acid 0.5 g, glacial acetic acid 0.5 ml, 70% alcohol 100 ml) acts as a differentiator; this can be omitted.
b. Tissues fixed in dichromate do not give good results.

Lead hematoxylins

Hematoxylin solutions that incorporate lead salts have recently been used in the demonstration of the granules in the endocrine cells of the alimentary tract and other regions. The most practical diagnostic application is in the identification of endocrine cells in some tumors, but it is also used in research procedures such as in the localization of gastrin-secreting cells in stomach (Beltrami et al. 1975). It has largely been superseded by immunohistochemistry.

Hematoxylin without a mordant

Freshly prepared hematoxylin solutions, used without a mordant, have been used to demonstrate various minerals in tissue sections. Mallory (1938) described a method for lead, and later published a similar method capable of demonstrating iron and copper (Mallory & Parker 1939); these methods have now been superseded by techniques that are more specific. The basis of the Mallory methods is the ability of unripened hematoxylin to form blue-black lakes with these metals. The methods are given by Lillie and Fulmer (1976).

One final hematoxylin method is worthy of note. The Weigert-Pal technique discussed in previous editions of this book, for the demonstration of myelin, is a hematoxylin method in which the tissue block is mordanted in a chromate solution before embedding and sectioning. Further mordanting of the section in a copper acetate solution is often performed before the hematoxylin is applied. It is likely that the major mordant is a chromium compound. The uses of hematoxylin stains are briefly summarized in Table 10.2.

Quality control in routine H&E staining

Accurate diagnosis depends on a pathologist or cytologist examining stained microscope slides – usually H&E paraffin sections, the H&E staining having been carried out in bulk by an automated staining machine. The need for consistency of staining is vital to avoid difficult histological interpretation. In general, automated staining machines allow accurate and consistent staining, differentiation, and dehydration by adjusting the times of each step. However, variability in the stains may necessitate adjustment of the staining times. In staining machines, the problems are usually associated with the hematoxylin staining rather than eosin. Variation in batch number of the hematoxylin, a change of supplier, and pH differences are the most common variables. A different person following the same preparation instructions can also result in a stain such as hematoxylin having slightly different staining properties each time it is made up. The age of the stain, and the degree of usage, will also affect the staining properties. New batches of stain must be checked for efficacy against current or earlier batches, and staining times must be adjusted to give uniformity. It is also important to realize that other factors, such as fixation, variations in processing schedules, section thickness,

Table 10.2 The uses of hematoxylin stains

Hematoxylin	Applications	Oxidant	Mordant
Ehrlich	Nuclear stain used with eosin. Stains some mucins	Natural	Alum
Delafield	Nuclear stain used with eosin	Natural	Alum
Mayer	Nuclear stain used with eosin. Nuclear counterstain	Sodium iodide	Alum
Harris	Nuclear stain used with eosin	Mercuric oxide	Alum
Cole	Nuclear stain used with eosin	Iodine	Alum
Carazzi	Nuclear stain used with eosin (used with frozen sections)	Potassium iodate	Alum
Gill	Nuclear stain used with eosin	Sodium iodate	Alum
Weigert	Nuclear stain used with acid dyes	Natural	Iron
Heidenhain	Intranuclear detail, muscle striations	Natural	Iron
Verhöeff	Elastic fibers	Natural	Iron
Loyez	Myelin	Natural	Iron
Mallory PTAH	Fibrin, muscle striations, glial fibers	Natural	Tungsten
Thomas	Collagen, endocrine cell granules	Hydrogen peroxide	Molybdenum
Solcia	Endocrine cell granules	No oxidant	Lead
Mallory	Iron, copper, lead	No oxidant	No mordant
Weigert-Pal	Myelin (in block preparation)	No oxidant	Chromium-copper

and excessive hot-plate temperatures, may all lead to variation in staining.

Difficult sections

The problem of using hematoxylin as a nuclear counterstain when other acidic dyes are to be used (for example van Gieson) has already been mentioned. A similar problem occurs when attempting to stain paraffin sections when the tissue has been fixed for a long time in a formalin fixative that has gradually become more acid. Tissues and/or paraffin wax blocks sent from countries with hot climates

compound the problem. This may occur, particularly in tropical countries, because tissues may be fixed in poor-quality, unbuffered, non-neutral formalin fixative that deteriorates in the heat, and progressively becomes more acidic. The major problem is getting adequate nuclear staining with hematoxylin without also staining the cytoplasm; this phenomenon gives a uniformly muddy purple to the finished section after eosin has been applied.

There are two main ways in which diagnostically acceptable H&E sections can be obtained in these circumstances. One is the use of the celestine blue-alum hematoxylin sequence, and the other is the use of an iron hematoxylin such as Weigert's.

References

Beltrami, C.A., Fabris, G., Marzola, A., et al., 1975. Staining of gastrin cells with lead hematoxylin. Histochemical Journal 7, 95.

Carazzi, D., 1911. Eine neue Hämatoxylinlösung. Zeitschrift für wissenschaftliche Mikroskopie und für mikrosko-pische Technik 28, 273.

Carson, F.L., 1997. Histotechnology: a self-instructional text. American Society for Clinical Pathology, Chicago, 6, 93.

Cole, E.C., 1943. Studies in hematoxylin stains. Stain Technology 18, 125.

Delafield, J., cited by Prudden, J.M., 1885. Zeitschrift für wissenschaftliche. Mikroskopie und für mikroskopische Technik 2, 228.

Ehrlich, P., 1886. Fragekasten. Zeitschrift für wissenschaft-liche. Mikroskopie und für mikroskopische Technik 3, 150.

Feldman, A., Dapson, R., 1985. Newsletter, Winter. ANATECH.

Feldman, A., Dapson, R., 1987. Newsletter, Winter. ANATECH.

Gill, G.W., Frost, J.K., Miller, K.A., 1974. A new formula for half-oxidised hematoxylin solution that neither overstains or requires differentiation. Acta Cytologica 18, 300.

Harris, H.F., 1900. On the rapid conversion of hematoxylin into haematein in staining reactions. Journal of Applied Microscopic Laboratory Methods 3, 777.

Heidenhain, M., 1896. Noch einmal über die Darstellung der Centralkörper durch Eisenhämatoxylin nebst einigen allgemeinen Bemerkungen über die Hämatoxylinfarben. Zeitschrift für wissenschaftliche. Mikroskopie und für mikroskopische Technik 13, 186.

Lillie, R.D., Fulmer, H.M., 1976. Histopathologic technic and practical histochemistry, fourth ed. McGraw-Hill, New York.

Loyez, M., 1910. Coloration des fibers nerveuses par la méthode à l'hématoxyline au fer après inclusion à la celloidine. Compte Rendu des Séances de la Société de Biologie 69, 511.

Luna, L., 1992. Histopathologic methods and color atlas of special stains and tissue artefacts. Johnson Printers, Downers Grove, IL, 67, 73, 77, 78.

McManus, J.F.A., Mowry, R.W., 1964. Staining methods, histologic and histochemical. Harper & Row, London, p. 268.

Mallory, F.B., 1897. On certain improvements in histological technique. Journal of Experimental Medicine 2, 529.

Mallory, F.B., 1900. A contribution to staining methods. Journal of Experimental Medicine 5, 15.

Mallory, F.B., 1938. Pathological technique. Saunders, Philadelphia.

Mallory, F.B., Parker, F., 1939. Fixing and staining methods for lead and copper in tissues. American Journal of Pathology 15, 517.

Mayer, P., 1903. Notiz über Hämatein und Hämalaun. Zeitschrift für wissenschaftliche Mikroskopie und für mikroskopische Technik 20, 409.

Shum, M.W., Hon, J.K.Y., 1969. A modified phosphotungstic acid hematoxylin stain for formalin fixed tissue. Journal of Medical Laboratory Technology 26, 38.

Slidders, W., 1969. A stable iron-hematoxylin solution for staining the chromatin of cell nuclei. Journal of Microscopy 90, 61.

Thomas, J.A., 1941. Un nouveau colorant éléctrif des structures collagènes et réticulaires: l'hématoxyline phos-phomolybdique au dioxane. Technique de coloration. Comptes Rendus des Séances de la Société de Biologie et de ses Filiales 135, 935.

Verhöeff, F.H., 1908. Some new staining methods of wide applicability. Including a rapid differential stain for elastic tissue. Journal of the American Medical Association 50, 876.

Weigert, K., 1904. Eine kleine Verbesserung der Hämatoxylin van-Gieson-methode. Zeitschrift für wissenschaftliche Mikroskopie und für mikroskopische Technik 21, 1.

Connective and mesenchymal tissues with their stains

11

John D. Bancroft • Christopher Layton

Introduction

Connective tissue is one of the four tissue types found throughout the body. The term 'connect' comes from the Latin word *'connectere'* meaning 'to bind'. Its main function is to connect together and provide support to other tissues of the body. During embryonic development, the ectoderm and endoderm are divided by a germ layer called the mesoderm, generically known as mesenchyme. This comes from the Greek words *'mesos'* meaning middle and *'enchyma'* meaning infusion. It is from the mesenchyme that the connective tissues develop.

In almost any type of connective tissue there are three elements: the cells, the fibers, and the amorphous ground substance. The identification of the cells may be based upon their appearance in areolar and loose tissues that can be considered the main 'packing' material in the adult. This can also be considered as a prototype of the connective tissue. The connective tissues are divided into the following groups:

- Connective tissue proper – includes loose or areolar, dense, regular and adipose irregular, reticular
- Cartilage – hyaline elastic and fibrocartilage
- Bone – spongy or cancellous and dense or cortical
- Blood
- Blood-forming – hematopoietic.

Connective tissue usually consists of a cellular portion in a surrounding framework of a non-cellular substance. The ratio of cells to intercellular substance varies from one type of connective tissue to another, as does the primary function of the connective tissue. For example, bone has only a few cells in a usually dense, rigid intercellular substance, with its main function being that of providing strength and support. The cell types of connective tissue can include entities such as fibroblasts, mast cells, histiocytes, adipose cells, reticular cells, osteoblasts and osteocytes, chondroblasts and chondrocytes, blood cells, and blood-forming cells. Some connective tissue has little substance and consists primarily of cells whose functions are not those of production of intercellular substance, such as adipose tissue. Since they do not connect or support the other body tissues they are included under connective tissues as they probably derive from the same parent cell. The parent cell of the entire series is the embryonic mesenchyme cell, which is rarely found in adults.

The intercellular substance is usually composed of both amorphous (non-sulfated and sulfated mucopolysaccharides) and formed elements (collagen, reticular fibers and elastic fibers). These are the non-living parts of the connective tissues. The nature of the intercellular substance varies according to its function. It may be extremely hard and dense, in cortical bone, or soft as in umbilical cord. Its microscopic appearances are also variable, some being fibrillar, whereas others are completely homogeneous. Intercellular substances may be readily classified into two main groups by their microscopic appearance:

- formed or fibrous types
- amorphous or gel types

Formed or fibrous intercellular substances

A frequent fault among histologists is to speak of collagen, reticulin, and elastin, when in reality they mean collagenic fibers, reticular fibers, and elastic fibers. The former terms relate to the protein compound that is predominant in the particular fiber and should not be used to describe the connective tissue fiber itself.

Collagenic fibers

These are the most frequently encountered of all the fibrous types of intercellular substance, and are found in large quantities in most sites in the body. They may occur as individual fibers, as in loose areolar tissues, arranged in an open weave system, or as large bundles of fibers clumped together to form structures of great tensile strength, such as tendon. Individual collagenic fibers are never seen to branch, although some bundles of fibers do branch frequently. When viewed by polarized light, they are strongly birefringent, but lack dichroism.

Types of collagen

Four major types of collagen and several minor types have been characterized and described. The production of the different types is under genetic control, each reflecting slight variations in the α-chain composition. They all display the same characteristic amino acid content.

Type I

This collagen forms the thick collagenous fibers that have been demonstrated histologically and form the bulk of the body's collagen. This type accounts for most of the organic matrix of bases, but is also a major structural protein in the lung. It appears under the electron microscope as bundles of tightly packed, thick fibrils (75 nm diameter) with little interfibrillar substance. The fibrils show the characteristic 64 nm axial periodicity (Fig. 11.1). The prominence of the 'cross-banding' in Type I collagen is thought to be due to the lack of interference from interfibrillar ground substance. However, the presence of a partially processed form of Type III precollagen, pN collagen III (i.e. collagen III with an aminoterminal), helps to regulate the diameter of fibrils formed by collagen Type I, by forming co-polymers with the fibrils. pN collagen III inhibits the rate at which collagen Type I is assembled into fibrils and also decreases the amount of collagen Type I that is incorporated into the fibrils.

Type II

This collagen is found in hyaline and elastic cartilage and is produced by chondroblast activity. The fibers are thin and composed of fibrils arranged in a meshwork with copious amounts of proteoglycans. Type II collagen is usually not readily visible by light microscopic methods. The Type II fibers found in articular cartilage are thicker and resemble, ultrastructurally, Type I fibers. The cross-banding of Type II collagen is less evident due to the masking effect of the abundant interfibrillar material. Treatment with hyaluronidase may unmask Type II fibers to render them accessible for immunohistochemical evaluation.

Type III

This collagen is found only in those tissues that also contain Type I collagen (e.g. lung, liver, spleen, kidney, etc.). Fibers classically known as 'reticular fibers' contain Type III collagen. Ultrastructural studies of reticular fibers reveal loosely packed fibrils surrounded by abundant carbohydrate-rich interfibrillar material. The argyrophilia of reticular fibers is due to the proteoglycan content of the fibers and is not dependent upon the proteins of the fibrils themselves. Type III collagen appears to provide a limited amount of support, but also to allow some motility and the easy diffusion and exchange of metabolites. In some references, Type III collagen is often referred to as 'fetal collagen'. This term is, however, misleading as Type III collagen constitutes a significant proportion of the collagen present in adults. Fetal tissues do contain quite large amounts of Type III collagen in comparison to adult tissues

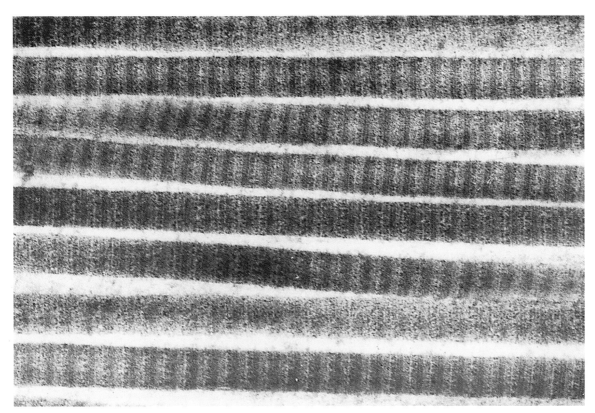

Figure 11.1 Electron micrograph of human collagen showing transverse cross-banding.

from the same site (e.g. 60% of the collagen in fetal skin is Type III, compared to only 20% in adult skin).

Type IV

This collagen has been characterized in structures identified morphologically as basement membranes. It is generally accepted that Type IV collagen does not form fibers or fibrils visible on light microscopic examination. Electron microscopy reveals a random organization of fine fibrils forming a feltwork-like structure in all basement membranes. Type IV collagen is closely associated with significant amounts of carbohydrate complexes, which explains the strong reaction of basement membranes to the periodic acid-Schiff method.

Types V and VI

Type V collagen is produced in small quantities by a wide range of cells, including connective tissue cells, endothelial cells, and some epithelial cells. It remains in close contact with the cell surface and is presumed to be involved in the attachment of cells to adjacent structures and in the maintenance of tissue integrity. Type VI collagen is a disulfide-rich variant which has been identified in boundary zones where interstitial collagenous fibers (Types I and II) are linked to non-collagenous elements.

Staining reactions of collagen

Type I collagen stains strongly with acid dyes, due to the affinity of the cationic groups of the proteins for the anionic reactive groups of the acid dyes. Collagen may be demonstrated more selectively by compound solutions of acid dyes (e.g. van Gieson) or by sequential combinations of acid dyes (e.g. Masson's trichrome, Lendrum's MSB, etc.) The different types of collagen may be differentiated immunohistochemically.

Reticular fibers

These are the fine delicate fibers that are found connected to the coarser and stronger collagenous fibers (Type I fibers). They provide the bulk of the supporting framework of the more cellular organs (e.g. spleen, liver, lymph nodes, etc.), where they are arranged in a three-dimensional network to provide a system of individual cell support (Fig. 11.2). On light microscopic examination, reticular fibers are weakly birefringent, the weak reaction being attributed to their lack of physical size and the masking effect of the interfibrillar substance. They are seen to branch frequently and appear indistinct in H&E-stained preparations. The characteristics of reticulin fibers in human kidney cortex have been studied using immunohistochemical means.

Antibodies directed against Type I and Type III collagens, their corresponding amino peptides and decorin (PG-II) revealed that in this organ the reticulin fibrils consist of hybrids of Type I and Type III collagens. Double immuno-electron microscopy shows that 20–25 nm fibrils consist mainly of Type I collagen, whereas the larger fibrils, 30–35 nm, label simultaneously for Type I and Type III collagens. Most fibrils larger than 40 nm in diameter label for Type III collagen. Reticular fibers may be demonstrated distinctly, in paraffin sections, using one of the many argyrophil-type silver impregnation techniques available or, in frozen section, by the periodic acid-Schiff technique. Both methods of demonstration are dependent upon the reactive groups present in the carbohydrate matrix, and not upon the fibrillar elements of the fiber.

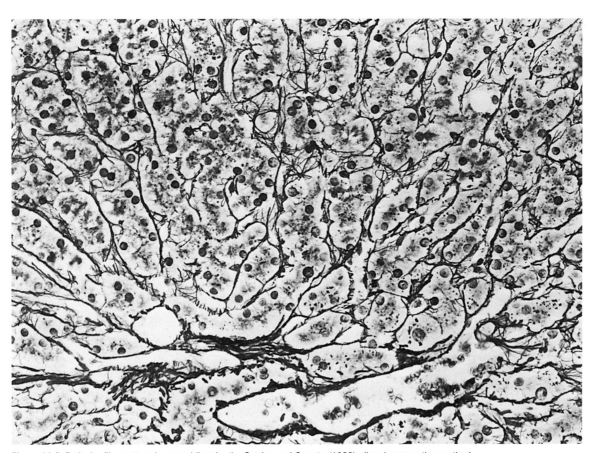

Figure 11.2 Reticular fiber pattern in normal liver by the Gordon and Sweets (1936) silver impregnation method.

Elastic fibers

The elastic system fibers (i.e. oxytalan, elaunin, and elastic fibers) have, respectively, a fibrillar, amorphous, or mixed structure. The elastic fibers may be found throughout the body but are especially associated with the respiratory, circulatory, and integumentary systems. Their appearances under the light microscope may vary considerably according to location, from fine, single fibers, as in the upper dermis, to membrane-like structures ('internal and external elastic laminae') in the large arteries. In the latter situation, the elastic membranes are interrupted by minute holes called fenestrae (Latin *'fenestra'* – window) which permit diffusion of materials through the otherwise impermeable membrane. Recent high-resolution electron microscopic examination has demonstrated that elastic fibers consist of two quite distinct components. There is an amorphous substance which, biochemically, is consistent with the protein elastin, and also a second component, which shows a periodicity of 4–13 nm, that is microfibrillar in nature, and has been termed elastic fiber microfibrillar protein (EFMP). These micro-fibrils, sometimes also called elastin-associated microfibrils (EAMF), are ubiquitous connective tissue structures that are believed to provide tensile strength and flexibility to numerous tissues. They may also act as a scaffold for elastin deposition.

When viewed in transverse section, the central core of the elastic fiber is seen to be composed of the amorphous protein elastin, surrounded by a ring or band of EFMP. The proportions of the two components seem to alter with the age of the fiber (and probably also with the age of the subject). In young fibers, the dominant fraction is the microfibrillar protein. In older fibers, the amorphous protein accounts for over 90% of the fiber content. The basic molecular unit of elastin is a linear polypeptide with a molecular weight of approximately 72 kilodaltons (kDa). This subunit has been referred to as 'soluble elastin' or 'tropoelastin'. One of the characteristic features of elastic fibers is the presence of cross-linking which binds the polypeptide chains into a fiber network. Desmosine and its isomer,

isodesmosine, are the cross-linking compounds involved. The polypeptides are transported out of the fibroblasts or smooth muscle cells and the cross-linking occurs in the extracellular spaces.

Elastic fiber microfibrillar protein has an amino acid content that is quite distinct, biochemically, from that of elastin protein. It is particularly rich in amino acids, which are lacking or present in only small quantities in elastin. The content of cysteine in EFMP is high, reflecting the presence of numerous disulfide linkages that will be of significance when the staining properties of elastic fibers are considered later. Associated with EFMP are a number of carbohydrate complexes, termed 'structural glycoproteins' (Cleary & Gibson 1983); the significance of these in the staining of elastic fibers will also be considered later. For a more detailed account of elastic fiber composition and biochemistry, reference should be made to the work of Cleary and Gibson (1983), Uitto (1979), or Bailey (1978). Elastic fibers are acidophilic, congophilic, and refractile. Following oxidation, they are quite strongly basophilic due to the formation of sulfonic acid groups from the disulfide linkages of the EFMP. Young fibers with a high content of EFMP show a positive periodic acid-Schiff reaction. They may be seen in routine H&E- stained sections, but, for exacting studies, numerous more selective techniques are available. These may be relatively simple, e.g. the Taenzer-Unna orcein method, or more lengthy and complex, e.g. Weigert resorcin-fuchsin methods. With increasing age of the elastic fibers, physical and biochemical changes are seen to occur. These may include splitting and fragmentation, alteration of the ratio of EFMP to elastin, and increases in the levels of glutamic and aspartic acids and calcium. These changes are readily visible in the skin of the subject, which becomes wrinkled and 'loose-fitting'. A more serious problem occurs with the loss of elasticity of the elastic arteries.

Oxytalan fibers

Oxytalan fibers were first described by Fullmer and Lillie (1958) in periodontal membranes. More recently they have been demonstrated in a wide variety of tissues, both normal and abnormal (Alexander & Garner 1977; Cleary & Gibson 1983; Goldfischer et al. 1983). On light microscopic examination, oxytalan fibers may be distinguished from mature elastic fibers by their failure to stain with aldehyde fuchsin solutions, unless they have been previously oxidized by potassium permanganate, performic acid, or peracetic acid. They have also been reported to remain unstained following Verhöeff's hematoxylin, with or without prior oxidation. Following electron microscopic examination by a number of workers, it has been suggested that oxytalan fibers are similar to, if not identical to, EFMP fibers. They appear to be composed of microfibrillar units, 7–20 nm in diameter, with a periodicity of 12–17 nm. Their periodicity is made more conspicuous by pretreatment with ruthenium red. From their morphology, localization, and staining properties, it seems possible that oxytalan fibers may represent an immature form of elastic tissue. It has also been suggested by Goldfischer et al. (1983) that microfibrils and oxytalan fibers may have a role beyond that of elastogenesis and may involve 'anchoring' mechanisms between collagen fibers, stromal cells, lymphatic capillary walls, mature elastic fibers, muscle cells, etc.

Elaunin fibers

Gawlik (1965) first described elaunin fibers; the term 'elaunin' is derived from the Greek 'I stretch'. Unlike oxytalan fibers, elaunin fibers stain with orcein, aldehyde fuchsin, and resorcin–fuchsin without prior oxidation, but do not stain with Verhöeff's hematoxylin.

Classification of fiber types

It is often suggested that the mechanisms of the stains used to classify elaunin and oxytalan fibers are too empirical, that the terms 'elaunin' and 'oxytalan' lack structural or functional significance, and that the three fiber types, oxytalan, elaunin, and elastic, correspond to consecutive stages of normal elastogenesis. It has been shown that there is continuity between the coarse, mature elastic fibers deep in the dermis, through the intermediate elaunin fibers, to the fine oxytalan fibers in the most superficial aspects of the papillary dermis.

Basement membranes

Basement membranes are found throughout the body as a resilient matrix, separating connective tissues from epithelial, endothelial or mesothelial cells, muscle cells, fat cells, and nervous tissues. They support the epithelial cells of mucosal surfaces, glands, and several other structures, for example renal tubules. They also support the endothelial cells lining blood vessels, capillaries, etc. The basement membrane is not homogeneous, but is divided into three zones or layers:

* lamina rara (or lamina lucida)
* lamina densa (basal lamina)
* lamina reticularis.

The lamina rara (lucida) is adjacent to the surface cells and is composed mainly of carbohydrate complexes. This layer is apparently continuous with the glycocalyx of the surface cells and it has been suggested that the lamina rara is produced by the surface cells and not by the underlying connective tissue cells. The lamina densa is composed of a feltwork of microfibrils which have been immunohistochemically identified as predominantly Type IV collagen with a lesser amount of Type V collagen. Type IV collagen is associated with relatively large amounts of structural glycoproteins, mainly laminin and fibronectin, and small amounts of proteoglycans, principally heparan sulfate (Junqueira & Montes 1983; Laurie & Leblond 1983). The lamina reticularis is seen as a layer containing fibrous elements, which are continuous with the underlying connective tissue fibers.

The thickness of the basement membrane varies from site to site; most are in the range 15–50 nm. The glomerular basement membrane (GBM) is particularly thick, up to 350 nm in a healthy adult. The ultrastructural appearance of the GBM also differs from that of other basement membranes, in that the central lamina densa is bordered on both sides by a lamina rara. The sequence of the ultrastructural elements in the GBM is from the capillary lumen outwards: endothelial cell, endothelial-associated lamina rara, lamina densa, epithelial-associated lamina rara, epithelial cell (podocyte). In H&E-stained sections of most tissues, basement membranes are difficult to distinguish; in the glomerulus, they are more conspicuous, particularly in disorders such as membranous nephropathy or diabetes, where they can be markedly thickened. For more critical examination, a number of techniques are available. As a result of their carbohydrate content, the membranes are strongly positive by the periodic acid-Schiff reaction and by any other oxidation-aldehyde demonstration techniques, e.g. methenamine silver, Gridley, Bauer-Feulgen, etc. In sections by the MSB or Azan trichrome methods, the basement membrane stains intensely by the larger molecule, acid dye.

Methenamine silver microwave method

This method delineates the glomerular basement membranes. Methenamine silver demonstrates the carbohydrate component of basement membranes by oxidizing the carbohydrates to aldehydes. Silver ions from the methenamine-silver complex are first bound to carbohydrate components of the basement membrane and then reduced to visible metallic silver by the aldehyde groups. Toning is with gold chloride, and any unreduced silver is removed by sodium thiosulfate. The use of a microwave oven is recommended for the method and the technique should be followed exactly for optimal results. The method below is for five slides. Note: if you do not have five slides, then include blank slides but do not use more than five.

Periodic acid-methenamine silver microwave method for basement membranes (Brinn 1983; Carson 1997)

Fixative
10% neutral buffered formalin is preferred. Mercury-containing fixatives are not recommended.

Sections
Paraffin-processed tissue cut at 2 μm.

Solutions
Stock methenamine silver
3% aqueous methenamine	400 ml
Silver nitrate, 5% aqueous	20 ml

Keep refrigerated at 4°C.

5% borax (sodium borate) solution
Working methenamine silver solution
Stock methenamine silver	25 ml
Distilled water	25 ml
5% borax (sodium borate)	2 ml

1% periodic acid solution
0.2% gold chloride solution
1% gold chloride	1 ml
Distilled water	49 ml

Stock light green solution
Light green SF (yellowish)	1 g
Distilled water	500 ml
Glacial acetic acid	1 ml

Working light green solution
Light green stock solution	10 ml
Distilled water	50 ml

Method
1. Deparaffinize sections and rehydrate to distilled water.
2. Place sections in 1% periodic acid solution for 15 minutes at room temperature.
3. Rinse in distilled water.
4. Place slides (five) in a plastic Coplin jar containing 50 ml of methenamine working solution. Loosely apply the screw cap and place in the microwave oven, and place a loosely capped plastic Coplin jar containing exactly 50 ml (measured) of distilled water in the oven. Microwave on full power for exactly 70 seconds (see Note 2). Remove both jars from the oven, mix the solution with a plastic Pasteur pipette, and let stand. Check the slides frequently until the desired staining intensity is achieved. This will take approximately 15–20 minutes.
5. Rinse slides in the heated distilled water.
6. Tone sections in 0.02% gold chloride for 30 seconds.
7. Rinse slides in distilled water.
8. Treat sections with 2% sodium thiosulfate for 1 minute.
9. Wash in tap water.

10. Counterstain in the working light green solution for, 1½ minutes.
11. Dehydrate with two changes each of 95% and absolute alcohol.
12. Clear with xylene and mount with synthetic resin.

Results

Basement membrane	black
Background	green

If a microwave oven is not used, substitute the following solutions and staining times:

Methenamine silver solution

Stock methenamine silver solution	50 ml
Borax, 5%	5 ml

Preheat the solution and stain slides at 56–60°C for 40–90 minutes.

0.2% gold chloride solution

Gold chloride, 1% solution	10 ml
Distilled water	40 ml

Notes

a. Sharper staining of the basement membrane and less background staining can be obtained with the use of the microwave oven for silver techniques.
b. The temperature is critical and should be just below boiling, or approximately 95°C, immediately after removal from the oven. Each oven should be calibrated for the time required to reach the correct temperature.
c. This is a difficult stain to perform correctly. The glomerular basement membrane should appear as a continuous black line. Stopping the silver impregnation too soon will result in uneven or interrupted staining. The application of too much counterstain will mask the silver stain and decrease contrast.

Connective tissue cells

Connective tissues consist of a non-living framework in which cells function and live. The cellular component is an important aspect of this group of tissues. The parent cell of the entire series of connective tissues is the undifferentiated mesenchymal cell. From this develop many varied cells, each with its different function.

Fibroblasts

The fibroblast is the cell responsible for the production of the collagenic fibers, and also probably the amorphous intercellular substance, which binds the fibers together. Many authors refer to the young active secretory cell as the fibroblast, and reserve the term fibrocyte for the older non-secretory stage of development. The two stages may be distinguished easily by examining the cells. In the active spindle-shaped fibroblast the nucleus contains a prominent nucleolus and is surrounded by abundant, slightly basophilic cytoplasm; the even thinner spindle-shaped fibrocyte has an ovoid flattened nucleus with scanty chromatin and no nucleolus, and the cytoplasm is difficult to distinguish. The fibroblasts are responsible for repair processes in the body and will accumulate at the edges of sites of injury and secrete fibrous intercellular substances that ultimately form scar tissue.

Fat cells

Among the cells that differentiate from the mesenchymal cell, fat cells are exceptional in that their main function is not one of production of intercellular substances or of defense mechanisms, but is one of storage. The first sign of development of a fat cell is the accumulation within its cytoplasm of tiny droplets of lipid material. These gradually increase in size until the cell loses its previous shape and appears as a swollen object with the nucleus forced to one side.

Connective tissues

The physical characteristics of the cells and the intercellular substances vary considerably and they may be divided into groups, according to the ratio of cells to intercellular substance, and the types of cells and intercellular substance:

• areolar tissue
• adipose tissue
• myxoid connective tissue

- dense connective tissue
- cartilage
- bone
- muscle – smooth, voluntary and cardiac
- blood

Areolar tissue

This is probably the most widespread of all the connective tissue types. It connects the epithelial surfaces to the underlying structures; it fills any spaces between organs, and forms the fascia of intermuscular planes. Its construction is such that, although it has considerable strength, it allows movement of adjacent structures relative to each other. The loose pattern of areolar tissue permits free passage of nutrients and waste products. In a stained section, areolar tissue appears as an open-weave network of numerous single or small bundles of collagenic fibers running in all directions, with some elastic fibers and reticular fibers. The most frequent cells are the fibroblasts, which lie adjacent to a fiber or bundle along with small numbers of mast cells and macrophages. There is a liberal supply of arterioles, blood vessels, and lymphatic vessels.

Adipose tissue

Adipose tissue is found among the tissues forming the connective tissues, as it is not directly concerned with support or defense functions. It derives from areolar tissue, and evolves as fat cells to replace almost all other cells and many of the fibers. There is a well-developed network of reticular fibers surrounding the fat cells that are collagenic and the elastic fibers are almost absent. Adipose tissue is well supplied with capillaries and lymphatic capillaries, as it is so closely associated with storage of excess nutriments. Microscopically, it resembles no other body tissue and appears as a collection of cells with flattened eccentric nuclei and, in paraffin wax preparations, clear spaces from where the lipid has been removed during processing.

'Myxoid' connective tissue

One of the less commonly encountered connective tissues, this is not normally found in adult humans. It is found in embryonic specimens and in umbilical cord as 'Wharton's jelly'. It is a cellular tissue with stellate fibroblasts which anastomose and are embedded in a mucinous intercellular matrix containing hyaluronic acid. There are few collagenic fibers apart from those in blood vessels.

Dense connective tissue

Dense connective tissue is often seen as the capsules enclosing organs and, in particular, tubular structures, but is most strikingly characterized in its appearance as tendons and ligaments. These are basically dense masses of collagenic fibers and fibroblasts arranged in an orderly manner, with the cells and fibers being oriented in the same direction (i.e. parallel to the long axis of the tendon). Primarily there is a predominance of fibroblasts, but these secrete increasing amounts of collagen and the bulk of the tendon becomes fibrous. Structures of this composition possess enormous tensile strength and are perfectly suited for connecting the skeletal muscles to the skeleton and so transmitting power. Immature dense connective tissue contains capillaries, but as the fibroblasts mature to become fibrocytes and stop producing intercellular substances, the need for nutriments in quantity is much reduced and the capillary blood supply largely disappears.

Cartilage

The connective tissues discussed previously possess great tensile strength (that is, will resist diverging forces) but, when placed under pressure, they will bend. The structural characteristics of cartilage partially overcomes this problem. It consists of a fairly dense network of collagenic fibers encased in, or bonded with, an amorphous intercellular substance of chondroitin sulfate, which is in the form of a thin gel. Cartilage is distributed throughout the body in sites where the functions it is required to perform are slightly different. Hence, although it has an almost 'standard' form known as hyaline cartilage, it does have two other modified forms, elastocartilage and fibrocartilage. These will be considered later.

Microscopically, hyaline cartilage is composed of a matrix of apparently homogeneous intercellular substance, and is fibrillar in structure, containing large numbers of collagenic fibers. In the matrix are the cellular components of cartilage, the chondrocytes, which reside in spaces in the matrix known as 'lacunae'. There may be one cell or as many as six cells in each lacuna. In a fresh state the chondrocytes will fill the lacunae, whereas in stained sections they will often appear rather shrunken. The cytoplasm contains glycogen and lipid, and the nuclei are spherical with one or more nucleoli. Young immature chondrocytes tend to be rather small and flattened. As they mature they become larger and more rounded. Immediately surrounding the cell lining the lacuna is what appears to be an intercellular substance of a different type from that which comprises the bulk of the matrix.

Hyaline cartilage is the most common cartilage and is found in the larynx, the bronchus, the nose and as the articulatory surface of joints. When thoroughly lubricated with synovial fluid, the surface of articular cartilage will take on the appearance of a high polish and is ideally suited for the bearing surfaces of joints. Although hyaline cartilage is slightly elastic, in some instances this is not adequate. Elastocartilage is found where more elasticity is required. It contains as many collagenic fibers but has the addition of elastic fibers. It is found in the external ear and the epiglottis.

Fibrocartilage is found in sites such as tendon inserts where the tensile strength of hyaline cartilage is insufficient. The collagenic fibers of hyaline cartilage are arranged with no regular pattern; in fibrocartilage they are packed in rows parallel to the direction of the force. Between the collagenic fiber bundles lie fibroblasts and rows of chondrocytes and intercellular substance. Cartilage develops from the mesenchymal cells that differentiate into chondroblasts and lay down intercellular substance. They mature into chondrocytes and the cartilage in this form can live for long periods, as it does in joints.

Mature, hypertrophied chondrocytes will produce alkaline phosphatase, which brings about a reaction whereby insoluble calcium salts are precipitated in the matrix of the cartilage. As the calcification proceeds, the nutriments needed by the chondrocytes are cut off and the cells use up their stored glycogen and die. The calcified cartilage is not a permanent formation as it has no living cellular component, and it soon breaks down and the tissue loses all its supporting structures.

Bone

Cartilage in its several forms is capable of providing support and resisting converging forces. Calcified cartilage is much stronger, but as the process of calcification occurs the chondrocytes are cut off from their nutriments, which come through the permeable intercellular structure, and so they die. A permanent rigid type of connective tissue is required to support the body's weight, to maintain its optimal shape and to shield its delicate structures from external damage; this tissue is bone. The structure of bone is discussed in detail in Chapter 16.

Muscular tissue

The purpose of muscular tissue is to provide the power to enable the body to move and to function. Although muscular tissues are readily divided into three distinct categories, all types are composed of similar constituents and their mode of providing power and movement is also similar. Muscles provide power and movement by contracting their cells, so shortening their overall length, and thus pulling closer together the points to which the muscle is attached. Many cells in the body share this ability to contract and change shape. This phenomenon is due to the presence of three proteins and the interactions between them:

- α-actin
- actin
- myosin

α-Actin forms a base, which allows a strand of actin to become attached. Myosin in turn attaches to this actin strand and is able to move up the strands towards the base by means of a ratchet-like mechanism. Because myosin is double-headed, it interacts simultaneously with two separate actin strands. The movement up the strands from these different base plates pulls the strands together, causing the fiber to contract. A single muscle fiber of skeletal muscle is long and thin and comprises many myofibrils. These subcellular components run parallel to the fiber's long axis. Each myofibril is built up of a large number of identical contractile units called sarcomeres. On full contraction this can shorten by about 30% of its resting length. The three types into which muscular tissues may be classified are:

- involuntary smooth muscle
- voluntary striated muscle
- striated cardiac muscle

Involuntary smooth muscle

Smooth muscle is developed from mesenchymal cells, which elongate themselves to form tapered cells of 20–50 µm in length. The size of the muscle cell, or fiber as it is often called, varies enormously and depends upon the site in which the cells are found. Microscopically, the cells appear eosinophilic with areas of paler staining denoting the presence of glycogen. The cytoplasm contains bundles of myofilaments called myofibrils, which may be up to 1 mm in diameter. These are surrounded by the sarcoplasm, which constitutes the remainder of the cell. The centrally situated nuclei with their fine chromatin pattern are palely stained with hematoxylin and have an elongated appearance; they may contain one or two nucleoli. In cells that contract extensively and regularly, the nuclei may take on a 'concertina' shape which enables them to fit comfortably into the cell when it is in a state of full contraction.

Voluntary striated muscle

Striated or voluntary muscle makes up the bulk of the body's shape and is widely distributed over all parts of the skeleton – hence its alternative name of skeletal muscle. It is the type of muscle over which a person has voluntary control. It is capable of briefly producing tremendous forces when called upon to

do so, and also of maintaining a state of 'semi-contraction' for long periods of time, i.e. holding the body upright while standing. Some functions become almost automatic, although the person still maintains voluntary control, such as respiration, swallowing, blinking, etc. Like smooth muscle, it is composed of elongated eosinophilic cells, but in striated muscle these are much larger and longer, up to 40 mm in length and up to 40 µm in diameter. The cells themselves do not taper towards the ends but are more cylindrical. The nuclei are elongated and stain palely with hematoxylin. There is often more than one nucleus present in each cell and these are situated peripherally and often in contact with the sarcolemma or cell membrane.

The most obvious and striking characteristic of striated muscle is the striations or stripes that cross the cells at right angles to their long axes. On closer examination, and by polarized light, the striations can be seen to be alternating light and dark bands or discs. The darker bands are birefringent and are referred to as A-bands or Q-bands; the paler bands are isotropic and are known as I-bands. On occasions, running through the center of the paler I-bands may be seen a narrow, dark band, known as the Z-line. Studies of relaxed voluntary muscle with the electron microscope have shown the presence of a fourth band, an extremely thin band running through the A-band; this is called the H-line or H-disc (Fig. 11.3). With the aid of the electron microscope it may be seen that these numerous discs or bands are not, in fact, complete structures crossing the muscle cells, but are composed of myofibrils which are striated, and it is the organized arrangement of these striae that gives the appearance of discs. Between these myofibrils is a well-developed system of mitochondria and the sarcoplasmic reticulum. Stored in the sarcoplasm, adjacent to the sarcoplasmic reticulum, is an abundant store of glycogen to provide an immediate source of energy.

Striated cardiac muscle

Cardiac muscle constitutes the bulk of the myocardium. It is not composed of distinctly separate cells which interface with adjacent cells. The cytoplasm contains myofibrils and sarcoplasm and exhibits a

Z-line   H-disc containing
          dark M-line

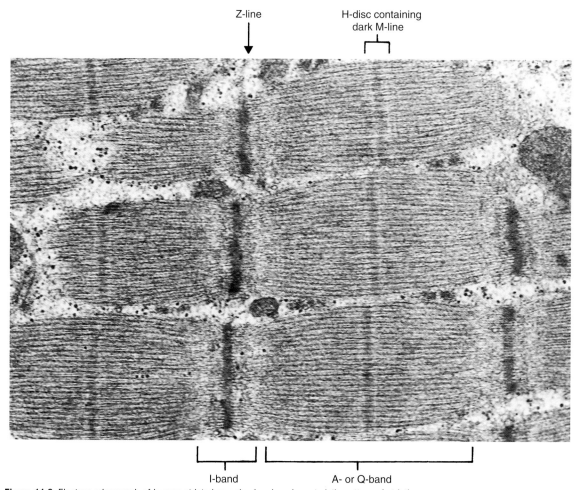

I-band   A- or Q-band

Figure 11.3 Electron micrograph of human striated muscle showing characteristic pattern of striations.

'striated' appearance similar to that of voluntary muscle. The striations are less distinct, as the myofibrils are not arranged to coincide as regularly as in voluntary striated muscle.

One feature unique to cardiac muscle is the presence of intercalated discs. These were originally believed to be another type of striation or stripe. From studies of these bands with the electron microscope it can be seen that these discs represent the end-to-end junction of adjacent cardiac muscle cells. The nuclei are placed centrally in the cells and stain palely with hematoxylin. Situated in the intercellular spaces created between the anastomosing of the cells are the blood vessels, lymphatics, and nerves to maintain and nourish the cardiac muscle.

General structure of muscle

The muscles of the body, whether they are of voluntary, involuntary, or cardiac type, contain considerable amounts of connective tissue. Each complete muscle is surrounded by an envelope of collagenic and elastic fibers known as the 'epimysium'. Arising from the epimysium are numerous bands or sheets of connective tissue which divide the whole muscle into bundles of muscle cells; this is the 'perimysium'. A connective tissue sheath called the 'endomysium' covers each individual muscle cell. This complex system of interconnecting collagenic fibers is continuous with the attachment points of the muscle; the fine sheets of collagenic fibers give way to broader, stronger bands of dense connective tissue which continue to form the tendon.

Fibrin and fibrinoid

Fibrin is an insoluble fibrillar protein formed by polymerization of the smaller soluble fibrillar protein fibrinogen, which is one of the plasma proteins. Fibrin is most commonly seen in tissues where there has been tissue damage; for example in an acute inflammatory reaction, resulting in transudation of fluid and plasma proteins out of damaged vessels. The plasma fibrinogen polymerizes to form insoluble fibrin outside the vessels. Fibrin is an important constituent of the acute inflammatory exudate and may be found wherever there is recent tissue damage.

In paraffin sections fibrin is strongly eosinophilic and stains blue-black with Mallory's phosphotungstic acid hematoxylin (PTAH). Lendrum et al. (1962) devised a trichrome method, the MSB, to demonstrate fibrin and to attempt to distinguish between fibrin of varying ages. 'Fibrinoid' is an eosinophilic material which has identical staining reactions to fibrin, but occurs in tissues in different situations and disorders. It is frequently found within vessel walls where the vessel has undergone acute damage ('necrotising vasculitis'), and sometimes as plugs in capillaries. There is much controversy about the nature of fibrinoid, but many regard it as a mixture of fibrin with other protein components of the plasma. A more detailed discussion of the nature of fibrin, collagen, and basement membranes may be found in the 'Further reading' section.

Connective tissue stains

See Table 11.1.

Trichrome stains

Many techniques available for the differential demonstration of the connective tissues fall into the category of 'trichrome stains'. The term 'trichrome stain' is a general name for a number of techniques for the selective demonstration of muscle, collagen fibers, fibrin, and erythrocytes (Fig. 11.4). By

Table 11.1 Connective tissue stains and their reactions

Tissue	van Gieson	Masson trichrome	MSB	PTAH	PAS	Retic	Meth. silver	Auto fluor.	Refrac.	Biref.	H&E
Muscle	Yellow	Red	Red	Blue	+	Gray	Gray	–	–	–	Deep pink
Collagen	Red	Blue/green	Blue	Orange/red	+	Gray	–	–	–	+	Deep pink
Elastin	Yellow		Blue	Orange/ brown	–	–	–	+	+	–	Pink
Reticulin	Yellow	Blue/green	Blue	Orange/ brown	++	Black	–	–	–	–	–
Basement membranes	Yellow	Blue/green	Blue	Orange	+++	Gray	Black	–	–	–	Pink
Osteoid	Red	Blue/green	Blue	Orange/red	+	Gray	–	–	–	+	Deep pink
Cartilage	Varies	Varies	Varies	Varies	++	Varies	Varies	–	–	–	Purple
Fibrin	Yellow	Red	Red	Blue	+/–	Gray	–	–	–	–	Pink

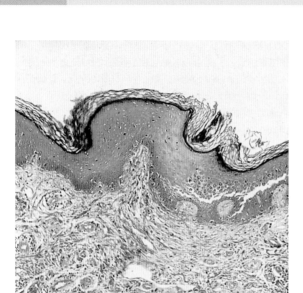

Figure 11.4 Masson trichrome on a section of skin demonstrating collagen in the dermis.

implication three dyes are employed, one of which may be a nuclear stain. The original methods were used to differentiate between collagen and muscle fibers, and some are satisfactory for this application. One of the earlier techniques still in constant use is the van Gieson method.

Factors affecting trichrome staining

Tissue permeability and dye molecular size

Although little work has been published on the permeability of tissues and the 'pore' size of fixed tissues, some deductions may be made from the reactions of various tissue elements with a range of anionic dyes of differing molecular size (Table 11.2). When the protein component of a tissue is exposed to a fixative agent, an interaction between the protein

chains and the fixative occurs. The nature of the reaction and the end result will vary according to the exact composition of the protein and the fixative in use. As a general rule, a three-dimensional, insoluble protein 'network' is formed; and the different proteins will form networks with different physical features. For example, erythrocyte protein will produce a dense network, with only small pores between the protein elements. Muscle cells will form a more open structure with larger pores. Collagen will show the least dense network and is seemingly quite porous.

The structure and density of the protein network may relate directly to the staining reactions of the tissue components. The smaller molecule dyes will penetrate (and stain) any of the three tissue types. Medium-sized dye molecules will penetrate muscle and collagen, but will not react with erythrocytes. The larger dye molecules will penetrate only collagen, leaving muscle and erythrocytes unstained. In practice, the rules seem less rigid and the size of the dye molecule seems to be significant. For example, acid will stain collagen when used in combination with picric acid in van Gieson's stain, but, when used with light green SF in Masson's trichrome, it stains erythrocytes and muscle. Some of the large molecular size dyes, such as sun yellow, pontamine sky blue 6BX, will fail to stain erythrocytes even when the tissues are exposed to the dye solution for long periods due to the incompatibility between the dye molecule size and the permeability of the red cell protein.

The general rule in trichrome staining is that a smaller dye molecule will penetrate and stain a tissue element, but whenever a larger dye molecule can penetrate the same element, the smaller molecule will be replaced by it. Detailed information regarding molecular size of dyes is not readily available. However, the molecular weight may be used as an indication of the relative sizes. It is also possible to calculate the ionic weight of a dye from the molecular weight; this is also of value in estimating relative sizes. Horobin (1980) presents a number of interesting hypotheses relating to tissue structure and its influence on staining mechanisms. For an in-depth review, reference should be made to this work (Chapter 9).

Table 11.2 Dyes in connective tissue stains

Dye	Alternate name	Color index number	Dye formula weight
Picric acid	Trinitrophenol	10305	229
Martius yellow	Acid yellow 24	13015	251
Lissamine fast yellow	Xylene yellow G	18965	551
Sun yellow	Direct yellow 11	4000	837
Orange G	Acid orange 10, Lissamine orange 2G	16230	452
Fast green FCF	Food green 3	42053	809
Fast light green	Cyanol green B, Acid green 50	44090	577
Light green SF	Acid green 5	42095	793
Acid fuchsin	Acid violet 19, Acid magneta	42685	586
Ponceau 2R	Acid red 26	16150	480
Ponceau 3R	Ponceau de xylidine, Acid red 18	16155	494
Azocarmine B	Acid red 103	50085	682
Azofuchsin	Acid red 33	16550	467
Azophloxine	Acid red 1, Amido naphthol red	18050	509
Biebrich scarlet	Acid red 66, Ponceau B	26905	556
Congo red	Direct red 28, Direct red Y	22120	697
Crystal ponceau 6R	Acid red 44	16250	502
Direct garnet	Direct red 10, Congo Corinth	22145	698
Azo eosin	Acid red 4	14710	380
Lissamine red 3GX	Acid red 57, Propalan red 3 GX		527
Sirius	Direct red 80, Chlorantine fast red	35780	1373
Methyl blue	Aniline blue, Acid blue 93, Cotton blue	42780	800
Alkali blue		42750	574
Durazol brilliant blue	Direct blue, Direct blue 109	51310	
Naphthol blue black	Amido black 10B, Acid black 1	20470	617
Pontamine sky blue	6BX Chicago blue 6B, Direct blue 1	24410	993
Isamine blue	Direct blue 41, Pyrrol blue	42700	786
Azocarmine G	Acid red 101	50085	580

Heat

Heat has been shown to increase the rate at which staining occurs and also to influence penetration by the larger dye molecules.

pH

In order to achieve adequate and even staining of connective tissue fibers, dyes utilized in trichrome methods are prepared as low pH solutions (often in the range pH 1.5–3.0).

Nuclear stains for trichrome stains

Due to the acidity of dye solutions used in the differential staining of connective tissue fibers, standard alum hematoxylins are decolorized in the subsequent treatment. Iron hematoxylins are more resistant to acid solutions and are prescribed in most of the techniques.

Effects of fixation

The use of routine, formaldehyde-fixed tissues for trichrome techniques will not produce optimal results. If fixation in formaldehyde has been prolonged the results will be even less satisfactory, due to the saturation of tissue groups with formaldehyde, thus leaving few groups available to react with the trichrome dyes. Treatment of formaldehyde-fixed tissues with picric acid, mercuric chloride solutions, or both, will enhance trichrome intensity and brilliance. Lendrum et al. (1962) recommended 'degreasing' sections for 24–48 hours in trichloroethylene prior to staining. This was claimed to improve further the intensity of the staining reactions. Zenker's solution, formal mercury, Bouin's fixative, or picro-mercuric alcohol are the most satisfactory fixatives for trichrome techniques. The staining reactions following these fixatives will be much brighter and more saturated than formaldehyde fixation. It must be noted that mercury-containing fixatives are now rarely used due to the highly toxic nature of mercury.

---

van Gieson technique (van Gieson 1889)

Sections

Paraffin. For celloidin or low-viscosity nitrocellucose (LVN) sections, see Notes d and e below.

Solution

Saturated aqueous picric acid solution	50 ml
1% aqueous acid fuchsin solution	9.0 ml
Distilled water	50 ml

Method

1. Deparaffinize sections and take to water.
2. Stain nuclei by the celestine blue-hematoxylin sequence.
3. Wash in tap water.
4. Differentiate in acid alcohol.
5. Wash well in tap water.
6. Stain in van Gieson solution for 3 minutes.
7. Blot and dehydrate through ascending grades of alcohol – quickly.

8. Clear in xylene and mount in permanent mounting medium.

Results

Nuclei	blue/black
Collagen	red
Other tissues	yellow

Notes

a. Fixation is not critical, buffered formalin being satisfactory.
b. Washing in water after van Gieson solution should be avoided, the color balance being impaired by this.
c. Nuclear staining should be intense before application of van Gieson solution; the picric acid will act as a differentiator.
d. Celloidin sections are washed in distilled water after van Gieson solution.
e. Celestine blue may stain the celloidin intensely. In such circumstances, Weigert's iron hematoxylin should be used.

Role of phosphotungstic and phosphomolybdic acids (PTA and PMA)

Although phosphomolybdic and phosphotungstic acids do not give identical reactions in trichrome staining techniques, their properties are similar. Experimental work indicates that the principles involved are identical, but it is not suggested that the two substances are interchangeable in any given technique. Throughout the literature on trichrome staining, reference is frequently made to mordanting in phosphotungstic or phosphomolybdic acid. There remains some controversy about the precise roles of these two substances, but it is unlikely that they act as mordants towards the anionic dyes used in these techniques. Everett and Miller (1974) have shown that treatment of formalin-fixed sections with PMA or PTA greatly reduces staining of all tissue components, other than collagen fibers, with aniline blue and other similar anionic dyes. Blocking towards smaller dye molecules such as Biebrich scarlet was shown to be less complete. Binding of PTA to epithelium and connective tissue fibers was demonstrated by the quenching of autofluorescence and by the reduction of the bound PTA to a blue color by means of titanium trichloride solution. These workers postulated that the differential staining by the trichrome methods occurs by binding of aniline blue to basic residues in the connective tissues not already blocked by PTA. Baker (1958) stated that PMA acts as a 'colorless acid dye', of large molecular size and hence slowly diffusing.

Practical uses of PMA and PTA

In trichrome staining, there are three stages at which PMA or PTA may be used: firstly, before treatment with the small-molecule dye; secondly, combined in solution with the small-molecule dye; and thirdly, before treatment with the large-molecule dye. Any combination of these techniques is possible. If a section is first treated with PMA or PTA solution and then with a low concentration of a 'leveling' dye in the same solution, the leveling dye will color nothing but the erythrocytes. In practice, the first treatment with the PMA or PTA is frequently omitted without detriment to the final results. When a section is first treated with a leveling dye or other suitable small-molecule anionic dye and then with PMA or PTA solution, the PMA or PTA competes with the dye and gains access to the collagen easily, expelling the dye in the process. If treatment is stopped at the right moment, only collagen will be free to stain when treated with a 'milling' or other large-molecule dye. If treatment with the large-molecule dye is greatly prolonged, some staining of muscle and cytoplasm may take place. In addition to the rather complex role played by PMA and PTA in connective tissue staining, it must not be forgotten that both are quite capable of acting simply as conventional acidifying agents, a 10% solution of PTA having a pH of less than 1; indeed, PTA is unstable at a pH greater than about 2.

Masson trichrome technique (Masson 1929)

Fixation

Formal sublimate or formal saline.

Sections

All types.

Solution a

Acid fuchsin	0.5 g
Glacial acetic acid	0.5 ml
Distilled water	100 ml

Solution b

Phosphomolybdic acid	1 g
Distilled water	100 ml

Solution c

Methyl blue	2 g
Glacial acetic acid	2.5 ml
Distilled water	100 ml

Method

1. Deparaffinize sections and take to water.
2. Remove mercury pigment by iodine, sodium thiosulfate sequence.
3. Wash in tap water.
4. Stain nuclei by the celestine blue-hematoxylin method.
5. Differentiate with 1% acid alcohol.
6. Wash well in tap water.
7. Stain in acid fuchsin Solution a, 5 minutes.
8. Rinse in distilled water.
9. Treat with phosphomolybdic acid Solution b, 5 minutes.
10. Drain.
11. Stain with methyl blue Solution c, 2–5 minutes.
12. Rinse in distilled water.
13. Treat with 1% acetic acid, 2 minutes.
14. Dehydrate through ascending grades of alcohol.
15. Clear in xylene, mount in permanent mounting medium.

Results

Nuclei	blue/black
Cytoplasm, muscle, and erythrocytes	red
Collagen	blue

Notes

a. The celestin blue-hematoxylin sequence provides a satisfactory alternative to the iron alum hematoxylin used in the original method.
b. Light green may be substituted for methyl blue.

Heidenhain's 'Azan'

Due to prolonged staining times, the 'Azan' technique is not recommended as a general connective tissue method. In the demonstration of 'wire loop lesions', in the diagnosis of lupus nephritis in renal biopsies, the method may be useful.

The demonstration of fibrin

Techniques for the selective demonstration of fibrin are of three types:

- Gram-Weigert
- phosphotungstic acid-hematoxylin
- trichrome methods

Although there would appear to be little similarity between these methods, they all depend for their selectivity upon the use of dyes or dye complexes of suitable molecular size. Trichrome techniques of the Masson type may prove satisfactory for the demonstration of fibrin, although older deposits tend to stain as collagen. Lendrum et al. (1962) showed that modifications to the Masson technique enable older deposits of fibrin to be demonstrated. The main features of the Martius scarlet blue (MSB) technique are the use of a small-molecule yellow dye, together with phosphotungstic acid in alcoholic solution, selectively to stain red cells. Early fibrin deposits may be stained by this dye, although the phosphotungstic acid blocks the staining of muscle, collagen, and most connective tissue fibers. On treatment with the medium-sized molecule red dye, muscle and mature fibrin are stained, gross staining of collagen being prevented by phosphotungstic acid remaining from the first stage. Further treatment with aqueous phosphotungstic acid removes any trace of red from the collagen fibers. Final treatment with a large-molecule blue dye demonstrates collagen and old fibrin deposits.

MSB technique for fibrin *(Lendrum et al. 1962)*

The standard MSB technique employs Martius yellow (acid yellow 24) CI 10315, brilliant crystal scarlet (acid red 44) CI 16250, and soluble blue (methyl blue) (acid blue 93) CI 42780.

Preparation of solutions

Solution a

Martius yellow	0.5 g
Phosphotungstic acid	2 g
95% alcohol	100 ml

Solution b

Brilliant crystal scarlet	1 g
Glacial acetic acid	2 ml
Distilled water	100 ml

Solution c

Phosphotungstic acid	1 g
Distilled water	100 ml

Solution d

Methyl blue	0.5 g
Glacial acetic acid	1 ml
Distilled water	100 ml

Solution e

Glacial acetic acid	1 ml
Distilled water	100 ml

Notes on solutions

Martius yellow is dissolved in alcohol before adding the phosphotungstic acid. A satisfactory substitute for Martius yellow is the larger-molecule dye, lissamine fast yellow, which has the advantage of being less easily removed by the subsequent red dye. A number of medium-sized molecule anionic red dyes may be substituted for the brilliant crystal scarlet, and Ponceau de xylidine and azofuchsin have been found satisfactory. Many large-molecule blue or green dyes may be substituted for the methyl blue, including the following: durazol blue, pontamine sky blue, fast green FCF, and naphthalene black 10B. The replacement of methyl blue by pontamine sky blue reduces the tendency of fibrin coloring by the blue dye, due to the larger molecular size.

Method

1. Deparaffinize sections and take to water.
2. Remove mercury pigment with iodine, sodium thiosulfate treatment.
3. Stain nuclei by the celestine blue-hematoxylin sequence.
4. Differentiate in 1% acid alcohol.
5. Wash well in tap water.
6. Rinse in 95% alcohol.
7. Stain in Martius yellow solution, 2 minutes.
8. Rinse in distilled water.
9. Stain in brilliant crystal scarlet solution, 10 minutes.
10. Rinse in distilled water.
11. Treat with phosphotungstic acid solution until no red remains in the collagen.

12. Rinse in distilled water.
13. Stain in methyl blue solution until collagen is sufficiently stained.
14. Rinse in 1% acetic acid.
15. Dehydrate through ascending grades of alcohol.
16. Clear in xylene and mount in permanent mounting medium.

Results

Nuclei	blue
Erythrocytes	yellow
Muscle	red
Collagen	blue
Fibrin	red (early fibrin may stain yellow and old fibrin, blue)

Notes

a. At step 11 the time required may be up to 10 minutes, although sufficient selectivity may be achieved by using a standard time of 5 minutes.

b. At step 13, examine after 2 minutes and at successive 2-minute intervals; excessive stain cannot readily be removed.

Demonstration of muscle striations

Muscle striations can be demonstrated by hematoxylin and eosin, and trichrome methods. They may also be stained by using Heidenhain's iron hematoxylin and Mallory's phosphotungstic acid hematoxylin. Both these methods will give better definition of muscle striations than the trichromes.

Staining of elastic tissue fibers

Numerous techniques have been evolved for the demonstration of elastic tissue fibers, although few are in current use. Of these, the most popular are Verhöeff's method, the orcein technique, Weigert's resorcin-fuchsin, and the aldehyde fuchsin method. In addition to these methods, use has been made of the dyes chlorazol black E and luxol fast blue, mainly as techniques to determine the mechanism of elastic tissue staining.

General notes on the mechanism of elastic staining

Elastic fibers will stain quite intensely, but not always selectively, by a number of sometimes unrelated techniques, e.g. H&E, hematoxylin-phloxine-saffron, Congo red, periodic acid-Schiff (PAS), Verhöeff's hematoxylin, resorcin-fuchsin, aldehyde fuchsin, Taenzer-Unna orcein, etc. The reaction of elastic fibers with eosin, phloxine, or Congo red may be attributed to coulombic reactions between elastin protein and the acid dyes. The positive PAS reaction, seen particularly in immature, fine fibers, may be accounted for by the presence of carbohydrate-containing glycoproteins, associated with the elastic fiber microfibrillar protein which is a major component of young elastic fibers (and possibly oxytalan and elaunin fibers also).

As stated previously, elastin and the 'pre-elastin' fibers are highly cross-linked by disulfide bridges. Following oxidative treatment, for instance by permanganate in Weigert-type methods and aldehyde fuchsin, or by iodine as in Verhöeff's hematoxylin, these disulfide bridges may be, in part, converted to anionic sulfonic acid derivatives (Horobin & Flemming 1980). These derivatives will be strongly basophilic and capable of relatively selective reactions with the basic dye compounds of the above solutions. These reactions are further enhanced by the high electrolyte concentrations of the staining solutions, which will inhibit dye uptake by chromatin, ribosomal RNA, etc. Goldstein (1962) showed that elastic tissue staining by orcein, resorcin-fuchsin and aldehyde fuchsin was reduced or inhibited by the presence of urea, a strong hydrogen bonding agent, in the stain solution. He further considered that, if hydrogen bonding was responsible for elastic staining, the stain molecule must be the hydrogen donor and the tissue the hydrogen acceptor. For an informative discussion on the mechanisms of elastic fiber staining, the work of Horobin and Flemming (1980) should be consulted.

Verhöeff's method is the classical method for elastic fibers and works well after all routine fixatives. Coarse fibers are intensely stained, but the staining of the fine fibers may be less than satisfactory. The differentiation step is critical to the success of this method, and some expertise is necessary to achieve reproducible results; it is easy to over-differentiate (and lose) the finer fibers. Although some older texts state that the prepared working solution has a usable life of only 2–3 hours, satisfactory results have been obtained using solutions up to 48 hours old.

Verhöeff's method for elastic fibers *(Verhöeff 1908)*

Preparation of stain

Solution a

Hematoxylin	5 g
Absolute alcohol	100 ml

Solution b

Ferric chloride	10 g
Distilled water	100 ml

Solution c, Lugol's iodine solution

Iodine	1 g
Potassium iodide	2 g
Distilled water	100 ml

Verhöeff's solution

Solution a	20 ml
Solution b	8 ml
Solution c	8 ml

Add in the above order, mixing between additions.

Method

1. Deparaffinize sections and take to water.
2. Stain in Verhöeff's solution, 15–30 minutes.
3. Rinse in water.
4. Differentiate in 2% aqueous ferric chloride until elastic tissue fibers appear black on a gray background.
5. Rinse in water.
6. Rinse in 95% alcohol to remove any staining due to iodine alone.
7. Counterstain as desired (van Gieson is conventional, although eosin may be used).
8. Blot to remove excess stain.
9. Dehydrate rapidly through ascending grades of alcohol.
10. Clear in xylene and mount in permanent mounting medium.

Results

Elastic tissue fibers	black

Other tissues according to counterstain.

Notes

a. Pretreatment with 1% potassium permanganate for 5 minutes, followed by oxalic acid, improves sharpness and intensity of staining.

b. Removal of mercury pigment is unnecessary; this being carried out by the iodine in the staining solution.

c. Rinsing in warm tap water improves intense staining of fibers.

Orcein methods

Orcein is a naturally occurring vegetable dye, which has now been synthesized. Variations between batches of dye may produce erratic results with insufficient depth of stain on occasions. The main advantage of this stain is the simplicity of preparation. The choice of fixative appears unimportant.

Weigert's resorcin-fuchsin method

Although the standard Weigert technique employs basic fuchsin, a number of related cationic dyes of the triphenyl-methane group may be substituted. Indeed, the composition of basic fuchsin is variable, at least three dyes being present in many batches of this dye. These variations considerably affect the staining and storage properties of the prepared solution as well as the stain imparted to elastic fibers. Another variable is the impurities in the ferric chloride. Even fresh ferric chloride contains the ferrous salt, which does not produce a satisfactory staining solution. Ferric nitrate has been found to be consistently free from the ferrous salt, and should be substituted for the chloride in the Weigert technique and its variations.

Resorcin-fuchsin method *(Weigert 1898)*

Preparation of Weigert resorcin-fuchsin

To 100 ml of distilled water, add 1 g of basic fuchsin and 2 g of resorcin. Boil. Add 12.5 ml of freshly prepared 30% ferric chloride solution (see previous note on the use of ferric nitrate). Continue boiling for 5 minutes. Cool and filter, discarding the filtrate. Dissolve the whole of the precipitate in 100 ml of 95% ethanol, using a hot plate or water bath for controlled heating, and add 2 ml of concentrated hydrochloric acid.

As an improved solvent, the precipitate may be dissolved in:

2-methoxyethanol	50 ml
Distilled water	50 ml
Concentrated hydrochloric acid	2 ml

Staining time is reduced with this solvent.

Method

1. Deparaffinize sections and take to alcohol.
2. Place in staining solution in a Coplin jar, 1–3 hours at room temperature or 1 hour at 56°C.
3. Rinse in tap water.
4. Remove background staining by treating with 1% acid alcohol.
5. Rinse in tap water.
6. Counterstain as desired (van Gieson, eosin or trichrome methods are applicable).
7. Dehydrate through ascending grades of alcohol.
8. Clear in xylene and mount in permanent mounting medium.

Notes

a. Staining may be carried out after most fixatives. Those containing chromium salts produce less intense and more diffuse staining.
b. Acid alcohol treatment for removal of background staining can be brief, a few seconds, but may be prolonged without harm.
c. Treatment before stage 2, for 5 minutes with 1% potassium permanganate followed by oxalic acid, improves the staining.

Results

Elastic tissue fibers	brown to purple

Modification of the Weigert technique

Hart's modification has been recommended for use after fixatives containing potassium dichromate and is simply prepared by making a dilution of between 5 and 20% of the Weigert solution in 70% alcohol containing 1% hydrochloric acid. Staining time must be increased to overnight. Sheridan's resorcin-crystal violet method uses a solution as for the Weigert, but substituting the basic fuchsin by 1 g of crystal violet and 1 g dextrin. The methyl violet/ethyl violet-resorcin method for elastic fibers (given below) has

replaced the dahlia elastic tissue stain given in earlier editions, this substitution being necessary due to the withdrawal of dahlia from the commercial market.

Methyl violet/ethyl violet-resorcin method for elastic fibers

Preparation of staining solution

Dissolve 0.5 g of methyl violet (CI 42535) and 0.5 g of ethyl violet (CI 42600) in 100 ml of boiling distilled water. Add 2 g of resorcin and 25 ml of 30% ferric nitrate solution; continue boiling for an additional 3 minutes. Cool and filter. Discard the filtrate and dissolve the whole of the precipitate by gentle heating on hot plate or water bath in:

2 methoxyethanol	50 ml
Distilled water	50 ml
Concentrated hydrochloric acid	2 ml

Preparation of staining solution may be speeded by the use of a microwave oven at both heating stages.

Method

The same technique as for the Weigert method is employed, using the potassium permanganate and oxalic acid pretreatment. Staining may be adequate, with formalin-fixed tissues, in 15 minutes at room temperature.

Results

Elastic tissue fibers	blue-black

Mechanism of Weigert elastin staining

It has been shown that acetylation, sulfation, and phosphorylation of tissues induce binding of resorcin-fuchsin to glycogen, basement membranes, reticular fibers, collagen, and other tissue structures containing polysaccharides. These structures are unstained by resorcin-fuchsin without prior treatment, indicating that this binding is due to the introduction of ester groups. Extraction procedures designed to remove dyes bonded by salt or ionic linkages indicate that non-ionic bonds are involved.

Aldehyde fuchsin

Aldehyde fuchsin was first introduced into histology as an elastic tissue stain by Gomori (1950). Coarse and fine fibers are stained adequately with a suitably ripened solution although a number of other tissue components are equally well stained, including beta cell granules of pancreas, and sulfated mucosubstances. With prior oxidation in periodic acid, peracetic acid, or potassium permanganate, other components are demonstrated, such as glycogen and neutral mucosubstances, but with increased intensity of elastic tissue staining.

Aldehyde fuchsin method for elastic fibers

Preparation of staining solution

Dissolve 1 g of basic fuchsin in 100 ml of 70% ethanol; heat may be used to speed the process. After cooling and filtering, add 1 ml of concentrated hydrochloric acid and 2 ml of paraldehyde. Stand at room temperature for 2 days to complete the ripening process, which is indicated by a conversion from red to purple. Ripening time may be reduced by increasing the temperature to 50–60°C. The ripened solution should be refrigerated for storage. Batches of basic fuchsin suitable for the production of Schiff's reagent are usually satisfactory for the preparation of aldehyde fuchsin. Paraldehyde may lose some potency upon storage but this may be partially compensated by the addition of an extra 0.5 ml of this solution. The staining potential of aldehyde fuchsin is greatest at between 2 and 4 days after preparation, but may be adequate for the demonstration of elastic tissue fibers for several weeks if stored at 4°C.

Method

1. Deparaffinize sections and take to water.
2. Oxidize in 1% potassium permanganate, 5 minutes.
3. Rinse in tap water.
4. Remove permanganate staining by treatment with 1% oxalic acid.
5. Rinse in tap water.
6. Rinse in 70% ethanol.
7. Place in sealed container of aldehyde fuchsin for 15 minutes.
8. Rinse well in 70% ethanol.
9. Rinse in tap water.
10. Counterstain as desired (eosin, van Gieson or neutral red are suitable).
11. Dehydrate through ascending grades of alcohol.
12. Clear in xylene and mount in permanent mounting solution.

Results

Elastic tissue fibers   blue-purple

Also stained are beta-cell granules of pancreas, some muco substances, some fungi, cartilage matrix, and mast cell granules. Other tissues, according to counterstain.

Note

Contrast between the collagen and fine elastic tissue fibers may be inadequate following van Gieson counterstain, and a purely nuclear counterstain may be considered more suitable.

The demonstration of reticular fibers

Techniques for the demonstration of reticular fibers may be divided into those using dyes as a means of staining, and the metal impregnation methods. Dye techniques for reticular demonstration cannot be considered completely reliable, the density of stain being insufficient to resolve the fine fibers. Staining techniques do not readily differentiate between collagen and reticular fibers. Metal impregnation techniques provide contrast, enabling even the finest fibers to be resolved (Fig. 11.2).

Metal impregnation techniques

Many techniques for the demonstration of reticular fibers, mainly employing silver salts, have been published. Whilst the composition of these solutions varies widely, all have in common the silver in alkaline solution in a state readily able to precipitate as metallic silver. Reticular fibers have only a low natural affinity for silver salts and require suitable pretreatment in order to enhance the selectivity of the impregnation. Pretreatment baths are frequently heavy metal salt solutions, commonly ferric ammonium sulfate. Treatment with silver solution has a twofold effect: submicroscopic sensitized sites of silver in reduced form are created on the reticular fibers, and a considerable quantity of silver is taken up by tissues in unreduced form. These reactions are both optimized at around pH 9.0 and are quite rapid.

Upon treatment with a reducing agent, silver taken up by the tissue in unreduced form is converted to metallic silver which is deposited at the sensitized sites. Any remaining unreacted silver may be removed by treatment with sodium thiosulfate solution. For a completely permanent preparation, the silver may be partially converted to a gold impregnation by treatment with gold chloride solution, at the same time slightly increasing the contrast. Ammoniacal silver salts, when in the dry state, are potentially dangerous due to their explosive properties; they should be stored, only in solution, in plastic rather than glass bottles.

Preparation of silver solutions

All aqueous silver solutions require the solvent to be glass-distilled or deionized water to prevent precipitation of insoluble silver salts. The literature abounds with formulae for suitable silver solutions but the majority follow the same pattern. To a solution of silver nitrate is added a carbonate or hydroxide solution to produce a precipitate. The precipitate is re-dissolved, usually by the addition of ammonia solution. All of these formulae require great attention to detail: glassware must be perfectly clean and solutions prepared from the purest of reagents with weights and volumes accurately measured. Any excess of ammonia in the solution results in a great loss of sensitivity, giving only weak or complete lack of reticular fiber impregnation. The most reliable procedure is to add rather less ammonia than is needed to dissolve the precipitate, and filter to remove remaining turbidity. Alternatively, back titration with silver nitrate may be employed to react with any excess ammonia.

Sections for reticular fiber silver impregnation

Frozen, cryostat, and celloidin sections may be employed for the demonstration of reticular fibers; most of the published techniques are intended for use with paraffin sections. Impregnation is carried out on tissues after a wide range of fixatives. Fixatives containing the heavy metal salts of mercury or osmium occasionally cause a little non-specific background precipitation of silver. Silver impregnation fluids having sufficient sensitivity for these techniques are mainly alkaline, frequently

causing sections to become detached from the slide. Adhesives, previously mentioned in Chapter 7, may be used, although any excess adhesive may cause unwanted precipitate around and beneath the tissue.

Gordon & Sweets' method for reticular fibers
(Gordon & Sweets 1936)

Preparation of silver solution
To 5 ml of 10% aqueous silver nitrate solution add concentrated ammonia, drop by drop, until the precipitate first formed dissolves, taking care to avoid any excess of ammonia. Add 5 ml of 3% sodium hydroxide solution. Re-dissolve the precipitate by the addition of concentrated ammonia, drop by drop, until the solution retains a trace of opalescence. If at this stage any excess of ammonia is present, indicated by the absence of opalescence, add a few drops of 10% silver nitrate solution, to produce a light precipitate. Make up the volume to 50 ml with distilled water. Filter before use. Store in a dark bottle.

Method
1. Deparaffinize sections and take to water.
2. Treat with 1% potassium permanganate solution, 5 minutes.
3. Rinse in tap water.
4. Bleach in 1% oxalic acid solution.
5. Rinse in tap water.
6. Treat with 2.5% iron alum solution for at least 15 minutes.
7. Wash well in several changes of distilled water.
8. Place in a Coplin jar of silver solution, 2 minutes.
9. Rinse in several changes of distilled water.
10. Reduce in 10% aqueous formalin solution, 2 minutes.
11. Rinse in tap water.
12. Tone in 0.2% gold chloride solution, 3 minutes.
13. Rinse in tap water.
14. Treat with 5% sodium thiosulfate solution, 3 minutes.
15. Rinse in tap water.
16. Counterstain as desired.
17. Dehydrate through ascending grades of alcohol.
18. Clear in xylene and mount in permanent mounting medium.

Results

Reticular fibers	black
Nuclei	black or unstained (see Note a below)
Other	elements according to counterstain

Notes

a. A short treatment with iron alum solution, of less than 5 minutes, gives less staining of nuclei.

b. The use of a Coplin jar for the silver solution greatly reduces the possibility of precipitation on the slide. Sections can be counterstained with eosin, nuclear fast red, tartrazine, or van Gieson.

Gomori's method for reticular fibers
(Gomori 1937)

Preparation of silver solution

To 10 ml of 10% potassium hydroxide solution add 40 ml of 10% silver nitrate solution. Allow the precipitate to settle and decant the supernatant. Wash the precipitate several times with distilled water. Add ammonia drop by drop until the precipitate has just dissolved. Add further 10% silver nitrate solution until a little precipitate remains. Dilute to 100 ml and filter. Store in a dark bottle.

Method

1. Deparaffinize sections and take to water.
2. Treat with 1% potassium permanganate solution, 2 minutes.
3. Rinse in tap water.
4. Bleach in 2% potassium metabisulfate solution.
5. Rinse in tap water.
6. Treat with 2% iron alum, 2 minutes.
7. Wash in several changes of distilled water.
8. Place in Coplin jar of silver solution, 1 minute.
9. Wash in several changes of distilled water.
10. Reduce in 4% aqueous formalin solution, 3 minutes.
11. Rinse in tap water.
12. Tone in 0.2% gold chloride solution, 10 minutes.
13. Rinse in tap water.
14. Treat with 2% potassium metabisulfate solution, 1 minute.
15. Rinse in tap water.
16. Treat with 2% sodium thiosulfate solution, 1 minute.
17. Rinse in tap water.
18. Counterstain as desired (van Gieson or eosin is suitable).
19. Dehydrate through ascending grades of alcohol.
20. Clear in xylene and mount in permanent mounting medium.

Results

Reticular fibers	black
Nuclei	gray
Other tissues	according to counterstain

Russell modification of the Movat pentachrome stain
(Carson 1997)

See Figure 11.5.

Fixation

10% neutral buffered formalin or acetic formalin sublimate (mercuric chloride, 4 g; 37–40% formaldehyde, 20 ml; distilled water, 80 ml; glacial acetic acid, 5 ml).

Sections

5 μm.

Solutions

1% alcian blue solution

Alcian blue, 8 GS	1 g
Distilled water	100 ml
Glacial acetic acid	2 ml

Mix well and store at room temperature.

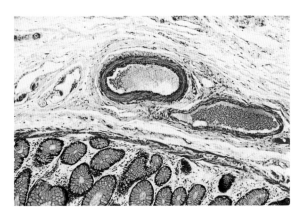

Figure 11.5 Movat pentachrome method demonstrating fibrin, muscle, collagen and muscle in a small intestine section.

Alkaline alcohol
Ammonium hydroxide	10 ml
95% alcohol	90 ml

Iodine solution
Iodine	2 g
Potassium iodide	2 g
Distilled water	100 ml

Add the iodine and potassium iodide to about 25 ml of distilled water and mix until dissolved, and add the remaining water.

10% absolute alcoholic hematoxylin
Hematoxylin	10 g
Absolute alcohol	100 ml

Mix until dissolved. Cap tightly and store at room temperature.

10% ferric chloride
Ferric chloride	10 g
Distilled water	100 ml

Mix until dissolved and store at room temperature.

Hematoxylin solution
10% absolute alcoholic hematoxylin	25 ml
Absolute alcohol	25 ml
10% aqueous ferric chloride	25 ml
Iodine solution	25 ml

Prepare just before use.

2% ferric chloride (for differentiation)
10% ferric chloride	10 ml
Distilled water	40 ml

Prepare just before use.

5% sodium thiosulfate
Sodium thiosulfate	5 g
Distilled water	100 ml

Mix until dissolved and store at room temperature.

Crocein scarlet-acid fuchsin
Solution A (stock)
Crocein scarlet	0.1 g
Distilled water	99.5 ml
Glacial acetic acid	0.5 ml

Mix until dissolved and store at room temperature.

Solution B (stock)
Acid fuchsin	0.1 g
Distilled water	99.5 ml
Glacial acetic acid	0.5 ml

Working solution
Solution A	8 parts
Solution B	2 parts

Prepare just before use.

5% phosphotungstic acid solution
Phosphotungstic acid	5 g
Distilled water	100 ml

Mix until dissolved and store at room temperature.

Alcoholic safran
Safran du Gatinais	6 g
Absolute alcohol	100 ml

Keep tightly closed to prevent hydration.

Method
1. Deparaffinize and take to distilled water.
2. Stain in alcian blue for 20 minutes.
3. Wash in running tap water for 5 minutes.
4. Place slides in alkaline alcohol for 1 hour.
5. Wash in running tap water for 10 minutes.
6. Rinse in distilled water.
7. Stain in hematoxylin solution for 15 minutes.
8. Rinse in several changes of distilled water.
9. Differentiate in 2% aqueous ferric chloride until the elastic fibers contrast sharply with the background.
10. Rinse in distilled water.
11. Place slides in sodium thiosulfate for 1 minute.
12. Wash in running tap water for 5 minutes, and rinse in distilled water.
13. Stain in crocein scarlet-acid fuchsin for 1–5 minutes.
14. Rinse in several changes of distilled water.
15. Rinse in 0.5% acetic acid water.
16. Place slides in 5% aqueous phosphotungstic acid, two changes of 5 minutes each.
17. Rinse in 0.5% acetic acid water.
18. Rinse in three changes of absolute alcohol.
19. Stain in alcoholic safran solution for 15 minutes.
20. Rinse in three changes of absolute alcohol.
21. Clear in two or three changes of xylene and mount with a synthetic resin.

Results
Nuclei and elastic fibers	black
Collagen and reticular fibers	yellow
Ground substance, mucin	blue
Fibrinoid, fibrin	intense red
Muscle	red

Notes

The differentiation of the elastic fibers is usually complete in 2–3 minutes. The complete removal of alkaline alcohol with running water is important. Failure to remove all of the alkaline alcohol will inhibit the subsequent staining steps. This stain may be used to demonstrate *Cryptococcus neoformans*, staining the organism a brilliant blue.

References

Alexander, R.A., Garner, D., 1977. Oxytalan fiber formation in the cornea: a light and electron microscopical study. Histopathology 1, 189.

Bailey, A.J., 1978. Collagen and elastin fibers. Journal of Clinical Pathology 31 (Suppl 12), 49–58.

Baker, J.R., 1958. Principles of biological microtechnique. Methuen, London.

Brinn, N.T., 1983. Rapid metallic histological staining using the microwave oven. Journal of Histotechnology 6, 125.

Carson, F.L., 1997. Histotechnology: a self instruction text, second ed. ASCP Press, Chicago, pp. 151–154.

Cleary, E.G., Gibson, M.A., 1983. Elastin-associated microfibrils and microfibrillar proteins. International review of connective tissue research 10. Academic Press, New York.

Everett, M.M., Miller, W.A., 1974. The role of phosphotungstic and phosphomolybdic acids in connective tissue staining 1. Histochemical studies. Journal of Histochemistry 6, 25.

Fullmer, H.M., Lillie, R.D., 1958. The oxytalan fiber: a previously undescribed connective tissue fiber. Journal of Histochemistry and Cytochemistry 6, 425.

Gawlik, Z., 1965. Morphological and morphochemical properties of the elastic system in the motor organ of man. Folia Histochemistry and Cytochemistry 3, 233.

Goldfischer, S., Coltoff-Schiller, B., Schwartz, E., Blumenfeld, O.O., 1983. Ultrastructure and staining properties of aortic microfibrils (oxytalan). Journal of Histochemistry and Cytochemistry 31, 382–390.

Goldstein, D.G., 1962. Ionic and non-ionic bonds in staining with special reference to the action of urea and sodium chloride on the staining of elastic fibers and glycogen. Quarterly Journal of Microscopical Science 103, 477.

Gomori, G., 1937. Silver impregnation of reticulum in paraffin sections. American Journal of Physiology 13, 993.

Gomori, G., 1950. Aldehyde-fuchsin, a new stain for elastic tissue. American Journal of Clinical Pathology 20, 665.

Gordon, H., Sweets, H.H., 1936. A simple method for the silver impregnation of reticulum. American Journal of Pathology 12, 545.

Horobin, R.W., 1980. Structure–staining relationships in histochemistry and biological staining. I. Journal of Microscopy 119, 345–355.

Horobin, R.W., Flemming, L., 1980. Structure–staining relationships in histochemistry and biological staining. II. Journal of Microscopy 119, 357–372.

Junqueira, L.C.U., Montes, G.S., 1983. Biology of collagen–proteoglycan interaction. Archivum Histologicum Japonicum 46, 589–629.

Laurie, G.W., Leblond, C.P., 1983. What is known of the production of basement membrane components. Journal of Histochemistry and Cytochemistry 31 (Suppl), 159–163.

Lendrum, A.C., Fraser, D.S., Slidders, W., Henderson, R., 1962. Studies on the character and staining of fibrin. Journal of Clinical Pathology 15, 401.

Masson, P., 1929. Some histological methods. Trichrome stainings and their preliminary technique. Bulletin of the International Association of Medicine 12, 75.

Uitto, J., 1979. Biochemistry of the elastic fibers in normal connective tissue and its alterations in diseases. Journal of Investigative Dermatology 72, 1–10.

van Gieson, I., 1889. Laboratory notes of technical methods for the nervous system. New York Medical Journal 50, 57.

Verhöeff, F.H., 1908. Some new staining methods of wide applicability, including a rapid differential stain for elastic tissue. Journal of American Medical Association 50, 876.

Weigert, C., 1898. Über eine Methode zue Färbung elastischer Fasern. Zentralblatt für Allgemeine Pathologie und Pathologische Anatomie 9, 289.

Further reading

Chavrier, C., 1990. Elastic system fibers of healthy human gingiva. Journal de Paradontologie 9, 29–34.

Clemmensen, I., 1984. Significance of plasma fibronectin. Haematologia 17, 101–106.

Courtoy, P.J., Timpl, R., Farquhar, M.G., 1982. Comparative distribution of laminin, type IV collagen and fibronectin in the rat glomerulus. Journal of Histochemistry and Cytochemistry 30, 874–886.

Fleischmajer, R., Jacobs, L., Perlish, J.S., Katchen, B., 1992. Immunochemical analysis of human kidney reticulin. American Journal of Pathology 140, 1225–1235.

Gay, S., Miller, E.J., 1983. What is collagen, what is not: an overview. Ultrastructural Pathology 4, 365–377.

Godfrey, M., Nejezchleb, P.A., Schaefer, G.B., et al., 1993. Elastin and fibrillin mRNA and protein levels in the ontogeny of normal human aorta. Connective Tissue Research 29, 61–69.

Goldstein, R.H., 1991. Control of type I collagen formation in the lung. American Journal of Physiology 261, 29–40.

Horton, W.A., 1984. Histochemistry, a valuable tool in connective tissue research. Collagen Related Research 4, 231–237.

Horton, W.A., Dwyer, C., Goering, R., Dean, D.C., 1983. Immunohistochemistry of types I and II collagen in undecalcified skeletal tissues.

Journal of Histochemistry and Cytochemistry 31, 417–425.

Jackson, D.S., 1978. Collagens. Journal of Clinical Pathology 31 (Suppl 12), 44–48.

Laurie, G.W., Leblond, C.P., 1982a. Intracellular localization of basement membrane precursors in the endodermal cells of the rat parietal yolk sac: I, Ultrastructure and phosphatase activity of endodermal cells. Journal of Histochemistry and Cytochemistry 30, 973–982.

Laurie, G.W., Leblond, C.P., 1982b. Intracellular localization of basement membrane precursors in the endodermal cells of the rat parietal yolk sac: II, Immunostaining for type IV collagen and its precursors. Journal of Histochemistry and Cytochemistry 30, 983–990.

Laurie, G.W., Leblond, C.P., Martin, G.R., Silver, M.H., 1982. Intracellular localization of basement membrane precursors in the endodermal cells of the rat parietal yolk sac: III, Immunostaining for laminin and its precursors. Journal of Histochemistry and Cytochemistry 30, 991–998.

Martinez-Hernandez, A., Chung, A.E., 1984. The ultrastructural localization of two basement membrane components: entactin and laminin in rat tissues. Journal of Histochemistry and Cytochemistry 32, 289–298.

Minor, R.R., 1980. Collagen metabolism: a comparison of diseases of collagen and diseases affecting collagen. American Journal of Pathology 98, 227–271.

Reale, E., Luciano, L., Kühn, K.W., 1983. Ultrastructural architecture of proteoglycans in the glomerular basement membrane: a cytochemical approach. Journal of Histochemistry and Cytochemistry 31, 662–668.

Risteli, J., Melkko, J., Niemi, S., Ristell, L., 1991. Use of a marker of collagen formation in osteoporosis studies. Calcified Tissue International 49 (Suppl), S24–S25.

Robert, L., Jacob, M.P., Frances, C., et al., 1984. Interaction between elastin and elastases and its role in the aging of the arterial wall, skin and other connective tissues: a review. Mechanisms of Aging and Development 28, 155–166.

Rojkind, M., Cordero-Hernandez, J., Ponce, P., 1984. Non-collagenous glycoproteins of the connective tissues and biomatrix. Myelofibrosis and the biology of connective tissue. A.R. Liss, New York, pp. 103–122.

Sternberg, M., Cohen-Forterre, L., Peyroux, J., 1985. Connective tissue in diabetes mellitus: biochemical alterations of the intercellular matrix with special reference to proteoglycans, collagens and basement membranes. Diabète et Métabolisme (Paris) 11, 27–50.

Timpl, R., 1993. Proteoglycans of basement membranes. Experientia 49, 417–428.

Warburton, M.J., Mitchell, D., Ormerod, E.J., Rudland, P., 1982. Distribution of myoepithelial cells in the resting, pregnant, lactating, and involuting rat mammary gland. Journal of Histochemistry and Cytochemistry 30, 667–676.

Carbohydrates 12

Christopher Layton • John D. Bancroft

Introduction

The word 'carbohydrate' is used to encompass a large group of compounds with the general formula $C_n(H_2O)_n$. While the role of carbohydrates in cellular metabolism has been known for many years, carbohydrates have been more recently implicated in a wide range of cellular functions including protein folding, cell adhesion, enzyme activity, and immune recognition (Varki et al. 1999). Histochemical techniques for the detection and characterization of carbohydrates and carbohydrate-containing macromolecules (glycoconjugates) are common practices in the histology laboratory. These techniques often provide invaluable information which may aid the pathologist in diagnosing and characterizing various pathological conditions including neoplasia, inflammation, autoimmune disorders, and infectious diseases.

Classification of carbohydrates

Carbohydrates are broken down into two broad categories: simple carbohydrates or those molecules composed purely of carbohydrates, and glycoconjugates, those molecules composed of carbohydrates and other molecules such as protein or lipid (Table 12.1). The simple carbohydrates are further categorized as monosaccharides, oligosaccharides, or polysaccharides. Glycoconjugates may further be broken down into proteoglycans, mucins, and 'other' glycoproteins. Although lipid-carbohydrate complexes are widely distributed in cells and tissues, these types of molecule are not discussed here, as they are not detectable by the routine histochemical techniques described in this chapter.

Monosaccharide, the basic carbohydrate structure

The most basic or simple form of a carbohydrate is the monosaccharide. Typical monosaccharides are of the empirical formula $(CH_2O)_n$, where n is a value between 3 and 9. The basic monosaccharide is the six-carbon simple carbohydrate glucose (Fig. 12.1). Glucose is not charged or ionized and for this reason is referred to as a neutral sugar. Other neutral sugars include mannose, galactose, and fructose. Monosaccharides contain asymmetric carbons referred to as chiral centers. The letters D or L at the beginning of a name refer to the conformation of one of the chiral carbons within the molecule. This is of little interest to the reader with the exception that monosaccharides of the D conformation predominate in nature.

The high number of hydroxyl (OH) groups present on the monosaccharide renders most of them extremely water soluble. Monosaccharides within a tissue specimen are lost during fixation and tissue processing due to the small size and the water solubility of these molecules. As a result, the monosaccharides are not easily demonstrated by most histochemical techniques. Regardless, readers should familiarize themselves with the basic monosaccharide structures as they represent the building blocks of larger, more complex carbohydrates. The chemical and physical properties or characteristics of

Table 12.1 Basic classification of carbohydrates and glycoconjugates

Simple carbohydrates
Monosaccharides
glucose, mannose, galactose

Oligosaccharides
sucrose, maltose

Polysaccharides
glycogen, starch

Glycoconjugates
Connective tissue glycoconjugates
proteoglycans
hyaluronic acid

Mucins
neutral mucins
sialomucins
sulfomucins

Other glycoproteins
membrane proteins (receptors, cell adhesion molecules)
blood group antigens

Glycolipids
cerebrosides
gangliosides

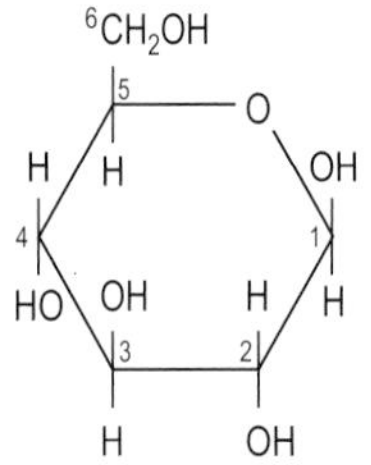

Figure 12.1 Structure of β-D-glucose.

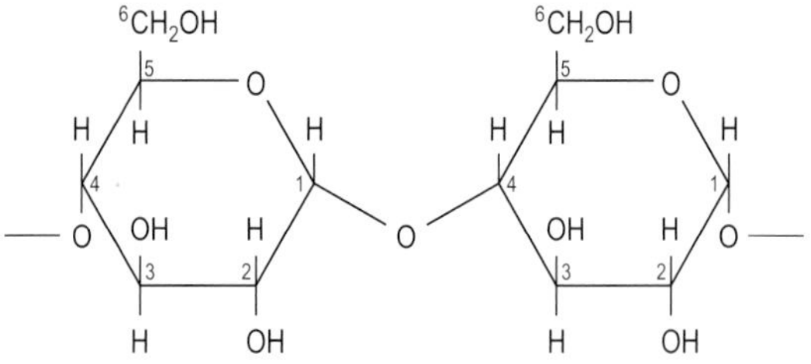

Figure 12.2 Structure of two glucose units joined by an α1–4 glycosidic linkage.

the polysaccharides and glycoconjugates are determined largely by the types of monosaccharide that make up these molecules as well as various reactive groups within the monosaccharides.

Polysaccharides

A polysaccharide is a large macromolecule composed of multiple monosaccharides joined by covalent bonds referred to as glycosidic linkages. Figure 12.2 demonstrates a α1–4 glycosidic linkage connecting molecules of glucose in a large polysaccharide. The α1–4 glycosidic linkage of glucose units is the predominant linkage in the polysaccharides starch and glycogen. In addition, some of the glucose units of these polysaccharides may be involved in more than one glycosidic linkage, thus forming a branching type of structure which may resemble a tree. Both glycogen and starch consist of glucose units with α1–4 as well as α1–6 glycosidic linkages, differing only in size and branching structure. Starch and glycogen are extremely large macromolecules with molecular weights that surpass 1×10^6 daltons.

Glycogen is the only polysaccharide found in animals that frequently is evaluated by histochemical techniques. Glycogen serves as a major form of stored energy reserves in humans. Carbohydrates absorbed following a meal are converted to glycogen by the hepatocytes of the liver. In times of fasting, glycogen is broken down into glucose units that can be used as an immediate source of energy. Glycogen occupies a significant volume of the cytoplasm of hepatocytes and may even form intranuclear inclusions. Skeletal and cardiac muscle cells also store significant quantities of glycogen.

There are a number of disease processes or pathological conditions in which histochemical assessment of glycogen content or accumulation may be of value diagnostically (Table 12.2). There are several well-characterized glycogen storage diseases which are the result of inherited defects of one or more of the enzymes involved in the synthesis or breakdown of glycogen (Cori & Cori 1952; Hers 1963). In most of these disorders, the liver shows massive

Table 12.2 Summary of the different types of carbohydrates and glycoconjugates

Type	Location	Function	Associated pathological condition
Glycogen	Liver, skeletal muscle, cardiac muscle, hair follicles, cervical epithelium, etc.	Storage form of carbohydrate	Found in a wide range of malignancies – Ewing's sarcoma/PNET, rhabdomyosarcoma, seminoma, etc. Abnormal accumulation in tissues of patients with glycogen storage diseases
Proteoglycans and hyaluronic acid	Cartilage, heart valves, blood vessels, tendons, ligaments, extracellular matrices, and ubiquitously expressed on the membranes of many cell types	Support, lubrication, cell adhesion, etc.	Found in certain sarcomas – myxoid chondrosarcomas, myxoid liposarcomas, myxoid fibrous histiocytomas, etc. Abnormal accumulation in tissues of patients with mucopolysaccharidoses
Mucins	Epithelia of the gastrointestinal tract, respiratory tract, reproductive tract	Secreted mucins – lubrication and protection Membrane-bound mucins – cell adhesion and regulation of proliferation	Frequently found in adenocarcinomas of the gastrointestinal tract Aberrant or inappropriate expression of specific mucin types occurs frequently in the neoplastic process
Glycoproteins	Ubiquitously expressed on cell membranes Blood group antigens Secreted products such as peptide hormones and immunoglobulins	Multiple and diverse functions such as cell adhesion, immune recognition, regulation of receptor ligand binding, etc.	Aberrant expression of blood group antigens in various malignancies

accumulation of glycogen. In some diseases, glycogen accumulation is also observed in skeletal and cardiac muscle.

Connective tissue glycoconjugates – the proteoglycans

Proteoglycans also are commonly referred to in the older literature as connective tissue mucins or mucopolysaccharides. These molecules are large glycoconjugate complexes that are found in high concentrations within the extracellular matrix of connective tissues. Proteoglycans are highly glycosylated and, in many cases, 90–95% of the molecular weight of the typical proteoglycan is due to the carbohydrate components.

The carbohydrate components of proteoglycans are known as glycosaminoglycans. Glycosaminoglycans are large polysaccharide polymers that are covalently bound to the protein core of proteoglycans. The typical glycosaminoglycan is a long unbranched polysaccharide composed of repeating disaccharide units each made up of two different monosaccharides. Each disaccharide typically is composed of a carboxylated uronic acid (glucuronic or iduronic acid) and a hexosamine such as N-acetyglucosamine or N-acetylgalactosamine. The hexosamines frequently contain highly acidic sulfate groups. There are six distinct classes of glycosaminoglycans (Table 12.3). The chondroitin sulfates are the most abundant of the glycosaminoglycans in the human. Figure 12.3a illustrates the structure of the repetitive disaccharide unit of chondroitin 4-sulfate.

The glycosaminoglycan chains are covalently bound to a protein core of the proteoglycan via the side chain of the amino acids serine or threonine (O-glycosidic linkage) and to a lesser extent to asparagine (N-glycosidic linkage). The number of glycosaminoglycan chains varies greatly among

Table 12.3	Characterization of glycosaminoglycans	
Glycosaminoglycan	**Disaccharide repeat**	**Location**
Chondroitin sulfate[a]	Glucuronic acid and N-acetylgalactosamine	Cartilage, tendons, ligaments, aorta, cell membranes
Dermatan sulfate	Iduronic acid and N-acetylgalactosamine	Skin, blood vessels, heart valves
Keratan sulfate	Galactose and N-acetylglucosamine	Cartilage, cornea
Heparin sulfate[b]	Glucuronic acid and N-acetylglucosamine or N-sulfate glucosamine	Blood vessels, aorta, cell membranes
Heparin	Glucuronic acid and N-acetylglucosamine or N-sulfate glucosamine	Mast cell granules
Hyaluronic acid	Glucuronic acid and N-acetylglucosamine	Synovial fluid, vitreous humor, loose connective tissues. Small amounts are found in cartilage where it serves as a scaffold for the proteoglycans

[a]Chondroitin sulfates may be subcategorized as chondroitin 4-sulfate or chondroitin 6-sulfate depending upon the position of the sulfate group in the N-acetylgalactosamine.

[b]Heparin and heparin sulfate differ structurally in the degree of sulfation of the glucosamine units. Heparin contains more sulfate and fewer N-acetyl groups in this unit.

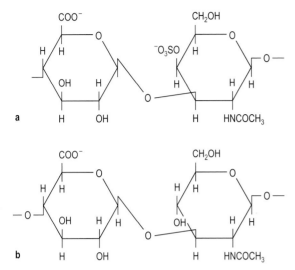

Figure 12.3 The repeating disaccharide units of the glycosaminoglycans, chondroitin 4-sulfate (a) and hyaluronic acid (b).

different proteoglycans. An exception to this structural motif is hyaluronic acid, which does not contain a covalently bound protein core (Mason et al. 1982).

Hyaluronic acid (Fig. 12.3b) is a polymer of repeating N-acetylglucosamine and glucuronic acid disaccharide units (Roden 1980). Hyaluronic acid also differs from the other glycosaminoglycans in the absence of sulfate groups. In spite of these differences, hyaluronic acid is classified as a glycosaminoglycan because of its overall structural similarity to the other glycosaminoglycans.

The negatively charged sulfate and/or carboxyl groups together with numerous hydroxyl groupings render most proteoglycans extremely hydrophilic. This property accounts for the gel-like consistency of the extracellular matrix and connective tissues such as cartilage. The proteoglycans of cartilage in particular contain many glycosaminoglycan chains and thus are capable of binding a large volume of water. Proteoglycans act in stabilizing and supporting fibrous elements of connective tissue. Tissues that contain high concentrations of proteoglycans include cartilage, tendons, ligaments, blood vessels, heart valves, and skin (Table 12.3). Hyaluronic acid is found in high concentrations in synovial fluid and in the ground substance and connective tissue matrices where other proteoglycans are found.

Several pathological conditions involve accumulation of glycosaminoglycans or proteoglycans (Table 12.2). The mucopolysaccharidoses are a group of genetic disorders that result from a deficiency of one or more of the enzymes that are involved in the degradation of heparin sulfate and dermatan sulfate (McKusick & Neufeld 1983). This results in the abnormal accumulation of glycosaminoglycans in connective tissues as well as cell types such as neurons, histiocytes, and macrophages.

Glycosaminoglycans and proteoglycans are expressed by a number of different sarcomas. Hyaluronic acid and chondroitin sulfates in particular may be found in high concentrations in myxoid chondrosarcomas as well as the myxoid variants of liposarcoma and malignant fibrous histiocytoma (Tighe 1963; Kindblom & Angervall 1975; Weiss & Goldblum 2001). In addition, proteoglycans may be observed in the stromal components of sarcomas as well as some carcinomas.

Mucins

Mucins, like the proteoglycans, consist of polysaccharide chains covalently linked to a protein core (Gendler & Spicer 1995). Typically, the carbohydrate component is attached via an O-glycosidic linkage to serine or threonine. The serine and threonine-rich protein core may contain anywhere from several hundred to several thousand amino acids. A defining structure of the epithelial mucins is the presence of tandemly repeated amino acid sequences within the protein core. Mucins are categorized into functionally distinct families (muc1, muc2, muc3, etc.) based in part upon differences in the amino acid sequences within the tandem repeats and the structure of their protein core (Perez-Vilar & Hill 1999).

The carbohydrate content of a mucin may account for up to 90% of its molecular weight. In contrast to the glycosaminoglycans, which are strongly acidic polyanions, the polysaccharide chains of the mucins vary from neutral or weakly acidic to strongly acidic sulfomucins. In addition, mucins demonstrate a

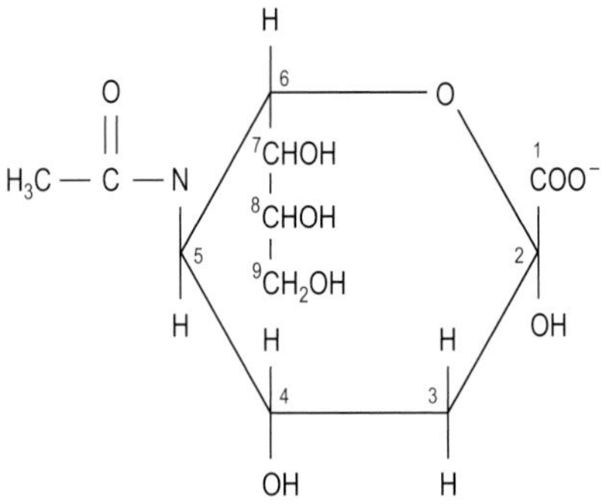

Figure 12.4 Structure of *N*-acetylneuraminic acid, a common sialic acid in humans.

more varied composition of monosaccharide units than the glycosaminoglycans.

The neutral mucins contain a high content of uncharged monosaccharides such as mannose, galactose, and galactosamine. Neutral mucins are found in high concentrations in the surface epithelia of the gastric mucosa, Brunner's glands of the duodenum, and in the prostatic epithelia.

The sialic acids (Fig. 12.4) are a diverse group of nine-carbon monosaccharides that contain a carboxylate group at the carbon in position 1 (Schauer 1982; Varki et al. 1999). The carboxylate group is ionized at a physiological pH and imparts an overall negative charge on the molecule.

The function of the mucins depends in part upon the tissue location of the mucin-producing cell as well as the mucin type. In most cases, the secreted mucins provide lubrication and protection for the secreting cells and/or tissues in the immediate area. The function or role of the membrane-bound mucins is not well understood. These mucins are likely involved in the regulation of cellular functions such as cell proliferation and cell adhesion (Wesseling et al. 1995; Moniaux et al. 1999; Schroeder et al. 2001).

While immunohistochemistry has largely replaced special stains in the differential diagnosis of anaplastic tumors or tumors of unknown origin, detection of mucin in a tumor may be a valuable clue in the identification of a malignancy. Malignancies derived from simple epithelial tissues (carcinomas) frequently contain detectable mucin. In contrast, melanomas, lymphomas, and sarcomas rarely exhibit significant levels of mucins. In addition, determining the type of mucin (i.e. neutral or acidic) may be helpful in evaluating neoplastic changes within a tissue. The detection of acid or sulfomucins within the gastric mucosa may aid in the detection and characterization of intestinal metaplasia, a lesion associated with gastric carcinoma (Turani et al. 1986).

Other glycoproteins

There is a wide range of protein carbohydrate conjugates that are not easily categorized, and fall under the general heading of glycoprotein. This is an extremely varied group of molecules with respect to carbohydrate composition, protein structure, and function. These molecules frequently contain relatively short oligosaccharide or polysaccharide chains attached to a protein core. Common carbohydrate moieties include neutral sugars such as mannose and *N*-acetylglucosamine, and the carboxylated sialic acids also may be present.

Glycoproteins are ubiquitously expressed throughout the cells and tissues of the body. Many of the proteins on the external surface of the cell membrane contain carbohydrates. The cluster of differentiation or CD markers found on the surface of lymphocytes frequently contains numerous glycosylation sites. These glycoproteins are involved in a varied array of cellular functions, including cell adhesion and lymphocyte activation. In addition, many of proteins and peptides secreted from cells contain sites of glycosylation. These include cytokines, growth factors, and hormones.

Fixation

The selection of an appropriate fixative for the histochemical detection of carbohydrates depends largely on the type of carbohydrate to be demonstrated. The fixation of glycogen is somewhat more demanding than that of the glycoconjugates such as the mucins and proteoglycans. Due to the aqueous solubility of glycogen, many of the older studies recommended the avoidance of aqueous-based fixatives such as formalin (Lillie 1954). It is now accepted that glycogen loss during formalin fixation usually does not compromise the ability to detect glycogen with techniques such as the periodic acid-Schiff (PAS) method. This is likely due to the retention of a portion of the cellular glycogen by non-covalent association with adjacent proteins (Manns 1958).

While neutral buffered formalin (NBF) is an acceptable fixative for glycogen, there is agreement that alcoholic formalins are superior fixatives for glycogen preservation (Lillie 1954). Rossman's fluid (alcoholic formalin with picric acid) has also been recommended for glycogen fixation (Bancroft & Cook 1994). Mercuric chloride containing fixatives such as Zenker's-acetic acid or Susa's are not recommended for fixation of glycogen-containing tissues (Manns 1958; Bancroft & Cook 1994).

Regardless of the fixative used, it is essential that tissues intended for glycogen analysis should be placed in a fixative promptly following removal. Glycogen present in many animal tissues is extremely labile to autolytic changes. If immediate fixation is not possible, the tissue should be refrigerated until adequate fixation in possible. When possible, fixation should be carried out at 4°C to minimize the streaming artifact which frequently occurs in fixed tissues (Lillie 1954).

The fixation requirements for the mucins and proteoglycans are less stringent than for glycogen. As these carbohydrates are covalently bound to proteins, the principal effect of fixation occurs on the protein portion of the molecule. In most cases, formalin or alcoholic formalin fixation is adequate for preservation. The carbohydrate deposits of the mucopolysaccharidoses have been reported to be less stable than typical mucins or proteoglycans (Bancroft & Cook 1994). In these cases, fresh or frozen sections are recommended although alcoholic formalin is also satisfactory.

Techniques for the demonstration of carbohydrates

The histochemical techniques used for the demonstration of carbohydrates and glycoconjugates are outlined in (Table 12.4). In the text that follows the potential mechanism(s) for each technique is discussed. Emphasis also is placed on the specificity of the techniques.

The periodic acid-Schiff (PAS) technique

The PAS technique is without question the most versatile and widely used technique for the demonstration of carbohydrates or glycoconjugates. The first histochemical use of this technique was by McManus (1946) for the demonstration of mucin. Subsequently other studies have demonstrated the utility of the PAS technique for demonstration of other carbohydrate-containing molecules, such as glycogen and certain glycoproteins (Lillie 1947, 1951; McManus 1948). The list of PAS-reactive tissues and cell types is long and varied. Table 12.5 is a listing of the PAS-reactive tissues, cells, and cellular structures that are commonly evaluated in the histology laboratory. This listing is not intended to be all-inclusive and the reader is directed to several references (Lillie 1951; Thompson 1966; Bancroft & Cook 1994) for more extensive data.

The PAS technique may aid in the differential diagnosis of tumors through the detection of mucins or glycogen. The reactivity of Schiff reagent with glycoproteins within the basal lamina makes the PAS technique a valuable means of assessing basement membrane thickness (Hennigar 1987). Increased basement membrane thickness, particularly in the glomerular capillaries of the kidney, is indicative of a number of pathological conditions. The PAS technique also is a sensitive and relatively fast means of demonstrating viable fungi in tissue sections. This is due to the presence of periodic acid-reactive polysaccharides in the capsules or walls of many fungal species. Common fungal species that are PAS reactive include *Candida albicans, Histoplasma capsulatum, Cryptococcus,* and *Blastomyces* (Harley 1987).

Mechanism of the PAS technique

As typically employed in the histology laboratory, the PAS technique is based upon the reactivity of free aldehyde groups within carbohydrates with the

Table 12.4 Summary of the specificity of the techniques for the detection of carbohydrates and glycoconjugates

	PAS	PAS-D	Ab 2.5	Ab 1.0	Ab 2.5 /PAS	Muc	Coll	HID	HID Ab 2.5	AF	AF Ab 2.5	Meta
Polysaccharides												
Glycogen	+	−	−	−	+(M)	−	−	−	−	−	−	−
Conn Tiss GC												
Proteoglycans	−	−	+	+	+(B)	V/−	+	+	+(BB)	+	+(P)	+
Hyaluronic acid	−	−	+	−	+(B)	V/−	+	−	+(B)	−	+(B)	+
Mucins												
Neutral	+	+	−	−	+(M)	−	−	−	−	−	−	−
Sialomucin (labile)	+	+	+	−	+(B)	+	+	−	+(B)	−	+(B)	+
Sialomucin (resist)	−	−	+	−	+(B)	+	+	−	+(B)	−	+(B)	+
Sulfomucin	V/−	V/−	+	+	+(B)	+	+	+	+(BB)	+	+(P)	+

PAS = conventional periodic acid–Schiff

D = diastase digestion

Ab 2.5 = alcian blue at pH 2.5

Ab 1.0 = alcian blue at pH 1.0

Muc = mucicarmine

Coll = colloidal iron

HID = high iron diamine

AF = aldehyde fuchsin

Meta = metachromatic techniques

V/− = variable to negative

Conn Tiss GC = connective tissue glycoconjugates

(labile) = digested with neuraminidase

(resist) = resistant to neuraminidase digestion

When two combined stains are used, the letter in parentheses represents the predominant color:

(B) = blue

(BB) = brown/black

(P) = purple

(M) = magenta

Table 12.5 PAS-reactive cells and tissue components

glycogen
starch
mucin (sialomucin, neutral mucin)
basement membranes
α-antitrypsin
reticulin
fungi (capsules)
pancreatic zymogen granules
thyroid colloid
corpora amylacea
Russell bodies

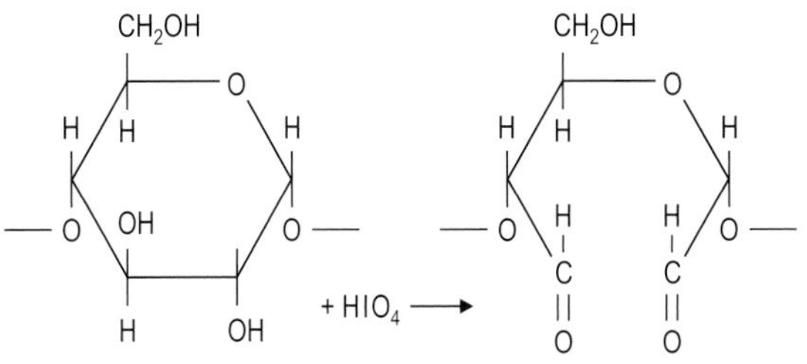

Figure 12.5 Periodic acid (HIO_4) oxidation of a glucose unit within glycogen. Note the cleavage of the bond between carbons 2 and 3 and the formation of aldehyde groups at these carbons.

Schiff reagent to form a bright red/magenta end product. The initial step in the PAS technique is the oxidation of hydroxyl groups attached to adjacent carbon atoms (1,2-glycols) within the carbohydrate. The result is the formation of two free aldehyde groups and the cleavage of the adjoining carbon-to-carbon bond (Fig. 12.5). The oxidation of the 1,2-glycols to form adjacent aldehydes is produced by treatment of the sections with a dilute solution of periodic acid (HIO_4). In most protocols a 0.5–1.0% solution of periodic acid is used for 5–10 minutes. Other oxidants such as chromic acid and potassium permanganate have been used in variations of the technique (Bauer 1933; Thompson 1966). However, these oxidants tend further to oxidize the aldehyde groups to carboxylic groups which are not reactive with Schiff reagent. As a result, the sensitivity of techniques using these oxidants is less than that of the PAS technique.

The intensity of the color that develops following reaction with Schiff reagent is dependent upon the tissue concentrations of reactive glycol structures (Leblond et al. 1957). Monosaccharides that lack 1,2-glycols or contain hydroxyl groups that are involved in an ester or glycosidic linkage are not susceptible to periodic acid oxidation and hence cannot be detected with the PAS technique.

Periodic acid also is known to oxidize substance other than carbohydrates to form reactive aldehydes. The α-amino alcohols of serine and threonine are oxidized by periodic acid but only when present at the end of the protein chain (Thompson 1966). It is also possible for periodic acid to oxidize hydroxylysine regardless of the position in the protein chain. However, it is doubtful whether the reactivity of these amino acids contributes significantly to the PAS reactivity in tissue sections.

Preparation of Schiff reagent

Schiff reagent is prepared from basic fuchsin. Basic fuchsin is not a specific dye but instead represents a mixture of triarylmethane dyes such as pararosaniline, rosaniline, and new fuchsin (Lillie 1977). The individual components of basic fuchsin also provide satisfactory starting points for the preparation of Schiff reagent.

A number of methods for the synthesis of Schiff reagent have been described since Schiff's original report in 1866. All of these methods share a common theme in the production of an aqueous solution of sulfurous acid. The sulfurous acid may be generated from the reaction of sodium metabisulfite ($Na_2S_2O_5$) with a mineral acid such as hydrochloric acid (HCl), or by the reaction of thionyl chloride ($SOCl_2$) with water (Barger & DeLamater 1948; Longley 1952). Sulfur dioxide is the active agent in the production of Schiff reagent and the source of the sulfur dioxide is not critical as long as by-products of the reaction to produce sulfurous acid do not interfere with the reaction of sulfurous acid with basic fuchsin (Barger & DeLamater 1948).

The reaction of sulfur dioxide with basic fuchsin results in the addition of a sulfonic acid group to the central carbon of the triarylmethane molecule.

The magenta or red coloration is lost due to the reduction of the quinoid configuration within the triarylmethane molecule. The free amino groups of the triarylmethane react with additional one or two equivalents of sulfur dioxide to form Schiff reagent (Lillie 1977). As described above, Schiff reagent reacts with the free aldehydes generated from 1,2-glycol groups in periodic acid-treated carbohydrates. The initial monosaccharide-Schiff reagent conjugate is a colorless reaction intermediate. The loosely bound sulfonate of the central carbon is removed in a subsequent aqueous rinse. The re-establishment of the quinoid structure of the triarylmethane molecule results in the deposition of a deep red/magenta coloration in the site of the carbohydrate-Schiff reagent complex (Lillie 1977).

PAS technique (modified McManus 1946)

Periodic acid solution

Periodic acid	1 g
Distilled water	100 ml

Preparation of Schiff reagent

Dissolve 1 g of basic fuchsin and 1.9 g of sodium metabisulfite ($Na_2S_2O_5$) in 100 ml of 0.15 M hydrochloric acid (HCl). Shake the solution at intervals or on a mechanical shaker for 2 hours. The solution should be clear and yellow to light brown in color. Add 500 mg of activated charcoal and shake for 1 to 2 minutes. Filter the solution through a No. 1 Whatman filter into a bottle. The filtered solution should be clear and colorless. If the solution is yellow, repeat the charcoal decolorization using a fresh lot of activated charcoal. Store at 4°C. Solution is stable for several months.

Method

1. Dewax in xylene and rehydrate through graded ethanols to distilled water.
2. Oxidize with periodic acid for 5 minutes.
3. Rinse in several changes of distilled water.
4. Cover the sections with Schiff reagent for 15 minutes.
5. Rinse in running tap water for 5–10 minutes.
6. Stain the nuclei with hematoxylin. Differentiate and blue the sections.
7. Dehydrate in graded ethanols and clear with xylene.
8. Coverslip.

Results

Glycogen, neutral/sialomucins	magenta
Various glycoproteins	magenta
Nuclei	blue

Notes

a. The intensity of stain is dependent to some extent on the length of treatment with the periodic acid and Schiff reagent. For basement membranes, a longer time in periodic acid (10 minutes) and Schiff reagent (20 minutes) may give better results.

b. Earlier descriptions of the PAS procedure frequently recommended post-Schiff bisulfite rinses for the reduction of background. This is not necessary provided the slides are adequately rinsed in tap water.

c. Fixatives containing glutaraldehyde should be avoided if tissues are to be stained with the PAS technique. This is because glutaraldehyde contains two aldehyde groups; tissues fixed in glutaraldehyde contain free aldehyde groups capable of undergoing the Schiff reaction. This results in non-specific background staining.

d. Staining of glycolipids may be detected when frozen sections are used. In addition, staining of unsaturated lipids may occur in some cases due to the oxidation of carbon-to-carbon double bonds to produce Schiff-reactive aldehyde groups. However, glycolipids and unsaturated lipids rarely interfere with interpretation of results obtained from paraffin-embedded tissues as a significant loss of these molecules likely occurs during tissue processing.

Alcian blue

Standard alcian blue technique

Alcian blue is a large conjugated dye molecule that initially was used for the dyeing of textile fibers. It is composed of a central copper-containing phthalocyanine ring linked to four isothiouronium groups via thioether bonds (Scott et al. 1964). The isothiouronium groups are moderately strong bases and account for the cationic nature of alcian blue (Scott et al. 1964). A variety of different alcian blue dyes have been produced in the past that differ in the number of linked isothiouronium groups as well as the components of the diluent (Scott et al. 1964; Horobin & Kiernan 2002). Alcian blue 8GX is the recommended dye for histological techniques (Scott & Mowry 1970).

While the exact mechanisms by which alcian blue stains carbohydrates are unknown, it is widely believed that the cationic isothiouronium groups bond via electrostatic linkages with polyanionic molecules within tissues (Pearse 1960; Quintarelli et al. 1964). The sulfate and carboxylate groups of chondroitin sulfate, dermatan sulfate, heparin sulfate, and hyaluronic acid are ionized at a pH of 2.5 and therefore carry a negative charge. This accounts for the staining of the proteoglycan/hyaluronic acid components of connective tissue and cartilage with alcian blue at a pH of 2.5. Similarly, the acidic epithelial mucins such as the sialomucins and sulfomucins of the large intestine are reactive at pH 2.5. Neutral mucins such as those in the gastric mucosa and Brunner's glands are not reactive with alcian blue.

Alcian blue technique (modified Mowry 1956)

Alcian blue solution

Alcian blue 8GX	1 g
3% acetic acid solution	100 ml

Nuclear fast red

Aluminum sulfate $Al_2(SO_4)_3 \cdot 18H_2O$	5 g
Distilled water	100 ml
Nuclear fast red	0.1 g

Dissolve the aluminum sulfate in the water with heat. Add the nuclear fast red to water while still hot and filter.

Method

1. Dewax in xylene and rehydrate through graded ethanols to distilled water.
2. Stain in the alcian blue solution for 30 minutes.
3. Rinse in running tap water for 5 minutes.
4. Counterstain in nuclear fast red for 10 minutes.
5. Wash in running tap water for 1 minute.
6. Dehydrate in graded ethanols.
7. Clear in xylene and mount in a miscible medium.

Results

Acid mucins (sulfomucins and sialomucins)	blue
Proteoglycans and hyaluronic acid	blue
Nuclei	red

Notes

To selectively identify sulfomucins and proteoglycans a low pH (pH 1) alcian blue solution should be used. Add 1.0 g alcian blue 8GX to 100 ml of 0.1 M hydrochloric acid. The staining procedure and incubation times are the same as those in the alcian blue pH 2.5 protocol.

Low pH alcian blue technique

Varying the pH of the alcian blue solution can be useful in the characterization of the subtypes of acidic mucins and proteoglycans present in a tissue (Spicer 1960; Lev & Spicer 1964; Sorvari & Sorvari 1969). The carboxylated sialomucins and hyaluronic acid do not demonstrate the same magnitude of acidity as the sulfomucins and sulfate-containing proteoglycans and, as a result, these groups are not capable of ionization at a pH of 1 or less. The sialomucins and hyaluronic acid therefore are not charged at this pH. Conversely, the sulfomucins and sulfate-containing proteoglycans are ionized and negatively charged at a pH of 1. It follows that the staining observed following incubation in an alcian blue solution at a pH of 1 is due predominately to sulfate groups among the mucins or proteoglycans. Examples of tissues or cell types that exhibit staining in an alcian blue solution at a pH of 1 include cartilage, goblet cell mucins of the large intestines, and the mucins of the bronchial serous glands.

Combined alcian blue-PAS

The alcian blue and PAS techniques can be combined to differentiate neutral mucins from acidic mucins within a tissue section (Mowry 1963). This technique also is valuable in that it may be used as a broad means of detecting mucins. A lack of staining with the combined alcian blue-PAS technique strongly suggests that the substance in question is not a mucin.

In most protocols, sections are stained with a standard alcian blue (pH 2.5) method followed by PAS.

The alcian blue stains sialomucins, sulfomucins, and proteoglycans blue. Neutral mucins are stained deep red/magenta with the PAS. Tissues and cells that contain both neutral and acidic mucins will stain varying shades of purple due to the binding of alcian blue and the reactivity with Schiff reagent. This is seen in the goblet cells of the small intestine that contain neutral and sialomucins (Spicer 1960).

Combined alcian blue-PAS technique *(Mowry 1956, 1963)*

Alcian blue solution (in 3% acetic acid): see page 225.

Periodic acid solution: see page 224.

Preparation of Schiff reagent: see page 224.

Method

1. Dewax in xylene and rehydrate through graded ethanols to distilled water.
2. Stain in the alcian blue solution for 30 minutes.
3. Rinse in running tap water for 5 minutes and then briefly in distilled water.
4. Oxidize with periodic acid for 5 minutes.
5. Rinse in running tap water for 5 minutes.
6. Cover the sections with Schiff reagent for 15 minutes.
7. Rinse in running tap water for 10 minutes.
8. Stain lightly with hematoxylin.
9. Rinse in running tap water for 5–10 minutes and blue in an appropriate blueing solution.
10. Rinse in tap water for 5 minutes.
11. Dehydrate in graded ethanols, clear with xylene, and mount with a miscible medium.

Results

Glycogen, neutral mucins, various glycoproteins	magenta
Acid mucins (sulfomucins and sialomucins)	blue
Proteoglycans and hyaluronic acid	blue

Cells or tissue that contains neutral mucins and acid mucins may stain various shades of blue-purple to purple.

Notes

a. It is important to stain lightly with hematoxylin in order to avoid cytoplasmic or mucin staining. Such staining could potentially mask the color of the alcian blue.

b. Several studies have shown that the staining sequence of the combined alcian blue/PAS technique can influence the end results (Johannes & Klessen 1984; Yamabayashi 1987). When the PAS technique is applied prior to the alcian blue, neutral mucins and glycogen may stain purple. In contrast, these substances are colored magenta, as would be expected, when stained with the alcian blue-PAS sequence. The reason that neutral carbohydrate moieties acquire an affinity for alcian blue following the PAS procedure is unknown. Although, it has been suggested that the aldehyde groups generated during periodic acid-mediated oxidation may react with sulfite present in the Schiff's solution to form an anionic group that subsequently may bind alcian blue (Johannes & Klessen 1984).

Mucicarmine

This technique is one of the oldest histochemical methods for the visualization of mucins in specimens (Mayer 1896; Southgate 1927). With the subsequent development of methods such as PAS, alcian blue, and colloidal iron the use of the mucicarmine technique has declined somewhat over the past 50 years. The mucicarmine technique, however, remains a valuable means for the demonstration of acidic mucins.

The mucicarmine technique is specific for the mucins of epithelial origin, and like PAS and alcian blue, this technique may be useful for the identification of adenocarcinomas. This is particularly true of adenocarcinomas of the gastrointestinal tract. The capsule of the fungus *Cryptococcus neoformans* also may be detected with the mucicarmine technique.

Mucicarmine technique *(modified Southgate 1927)*

Southgate's mucicarmine stock solution

Carmine (alum lake)	1 g
Aluminum hydroxide	1 g
50% ethanol	100 ml

Add the above reagents and 50% ethanol to a 500 ml Pyrex flask. Shake well and add 0.5 g of anhydrous aluminum chloride. Place the flask in a boiling water bath; bring the solution to a boil. Agitate while boiling for 2.5 to 3 minutes. Cool the flask under running tap water. Filter and store at 4°C. Stable for several months.

Mucicarmine working solution

Southgate's mucicarmine stock solution	10 ml
Distilled water	90 ml

Alcoholic hematoxylin

Hematoxylin	1 g
Ethanol (95%)	100 ml

Acidified ferric chloride stock solution

Ferric chloride ($FeCl_3 \cdot 6H_2O$)	2.48 g
Distilled water	97 ml
Concentrated hydrochloric acid (HCl)	1 ml

Weigert's iron hematoxylin working solution

This solution should be mixed just before use.

Alcoholic hematoxylin	50 ml
Acidified ferric chloride solution	50 ml

Metanil yellow working solution

Metanil yellow	0.25 g
Distilled water	100 ml
Glacial acetic acid	0.25 ml

Mix and store in a brown bottle or a bottle completely wrapped with aluminum foil.

Method

1. Dewax with xylene and rehydrate through graded ethanols to water.
2. Stain in Weigert's iron hematoxylin working solution for 10 minutes.
3. Rinse in running tap water for 10 minutes.
4. Stain in the mucicarmine working solution for 30 minutes.
5. Rinse slides in two changes of distilled water.
6. Stain in the metanil yellow working solution for 30–60 seconds.
7. Rinse quickly in distilled water.
8. Dehydrate in graded ethanols and clear in xylene.
9. Coverslip using a miscible mounting medium.

Results

Acidic epithelial mucins	deep rose to red
Nuclei	black
Other tissue elements	light yellow

Notes

The staining period with the mucicarmine working solution may be increased to 60 minutes if necessary.

Colloidal iron

The colloidal iron technique was initially described by Hale in 1946 as a technique for the detection of acid mucopolysaccharides. Since that time, numerous modifications of the original technique have been reported in the literature (Muller 1946; Rinehart & Abul-Haj 1951; Mowry 1958). However, all of the techniques are based upon the attraction of ferric cations in a colloidal ferric oxide solution for the negatively charged carboxyl and sulfate groups of acid mucins and proteoglycans. The tissue-bound ferric ions subsequently are visualized by treatment with potassium ferrocyanide to form bright blue deposits of ferric ferrocyanide or Prussian blue.

The colloidal iron technique also may be used with a PAS procedure. Sections are incubated with the colloidal iron solution and stained with potassium ferrocyanide prior to periodic acid oxidation. When used in this manner, acid mucins, proteoglycans, and hyaluronic acid stain bright blue with the colloidal iron/potassium ferrocyanide reaction while the neutral mucins and glycogen are colored red/magenta by the Schiff reaction.

Colloidal iron technique (modified Muller 1955; Mowry 1958)

Stock colloidal iron solution

Bring 250 ml of distilled water to a boil and add 4.4 ml of a 29% ferric chloride solution (USP XI). Continue to boil until the solution turns dark red, at which time the solution should be removed from the heat and allowed to cool. This solution is stable for one year.

Colloidal iron working solution

Stock colloidal iron solution	20 ml
Distilled water	15 ml
Glacial acetic acid	5 ml

Prepare just prior to use.

Acetic acid (12%) solution

Glacial acetic acid	24 ml
Distilled water to make	200 ml

Potassium ferrocyanide (5%) solution

Potassium ferrocyanide	5 g
Distilled water	100 ml

Hydrochloric acid (5%) solution

Concentrated hydrochloric acid (HCl)	5 ml
Distilled water	95 ml

Potassium ferrocyanide-hydrochloric acid

5% potassium ferrocyanide solution	50 ml
5% hydrochloric acid solution	50 ml

Mix just prior to use.

Acid fuchsin stock (1%)

Acid fuchsin	1 g
Distilled water	100 ml

van Gieson working solution

1% acid fuchsin stock	5 ml
Saturated picric acid	95 ml

Method

1. Dewax in xylene and rehydrate through graded ethanols to water.
2. Rinse in 12% acetic acid solution for 1 minute.
3. Cover the sections with the colloidal iron working solution for 1 hour.
4. Rinse in four changes of the 12% acetic acid solution (3 minutes each).
5. Place in the potassium ferrocyanide-hydrochloric acid solution for 20 minutes.
6. Rinse in running tap water for 5 minutes.
7. Rinse briefly in distilled water.
8. Cover the specimens with the van Gieson working solution for 5 minutes.
9. Dehydrate the specimens in 95% ethanol and absolute ethanol, three changes each. Clear in xylene.
10. Coverslip using an appropriate mounting medium.

Results

Proteoglycans, hyaluronic acid, and acidic mucins	bright blue
Collagen	red
Muscle and cytoplasm	yellow

Notes

1. The pH of the colloidal iron working solution is critical. At a pH of 2.0 or higher non-specific staining of structures other than acidic carbohydrate groups will occur.
2. Some protocols may recommend dialysis of the stock colloidal iron solution to remove free acid and unhydrolyzed (ionizable) iron salts. To dialyze the solution, transfer the stock colloidal ion solution in 25-ml portions to 41-mm dialysis tubes, suspended in distilled water. Dialyze for 24 hours, changing the water twice during this period. Filter the contents of the dialysis tubes through fine filter paper (Whatman No. 50 or equivalent) to remove any particulate matter (Lillie & Fulmer 1976).
3. Nuclear fast red may be used as an alternative counterstain for this technique.
4. The colloidal iron technique may be performed in conjunction with the PAS protocol. The colloidal iron technique is performed first and after Step 7 of the protocol the section may be subjected to periodic acid oxidation. The remainder of the PAS procedure is performed as described previously.
5. A control slide for each test specimen should be included. This slide should be subjected to the potassium ferrocyanide-hydrochloric acid solution only. This is necessary to exclude the possibility that a positive result of the colloidal iron stain is due to the presence of hemosiderin.
6. If the official iron chloride solution is not available, a solution of 2.73 g of $FeCl_3 \cdot 6H_2O$ in 4.4 ml of distilled water may be used (Lillie & Fulmer 1976).

High iron diamine

The high iron diamine method of Spicer is a useful technique for the detection of the highly acidic sulfomucins. This technique is selective for carbohydrates carrying a high negative charge density due to ionized sulfate groups. Hyaluronic acid and sialomucins are not demonstrated by this technique (Spicer 1965; Gad & Sylven 1969). When combined with the alcian blue protocol the high iron diamine technique facilitates the differentiation of sulfomucins from sialomucins in tissue sections.

When used together with the standard alcian blue procedure, sulfomucins and proteoglycans stain brown to black while sialomucins and hyaluronic acid stain blue. This combined technique is well suited to demonstrate the distribution of sialomucins and sulfomucins in the epithelia of the intestines (Spicer 1965).

Combined high iron diamine and alcian blue technique
(modified Spicer 1965)

High iron diamine solution

N,N-dimethyl-*m*-phenylenediamine (HCl)	120 mg
N,N-dimethyl-*p*-phenylenediamine (HCl)	20 mg

Dissolve the above reagents in 50 ml of distilled water. Pour into a Coplin jar containing 1.4 ml of N.F. 10% ferric chloride (FeCl$_3$).

Alcian blue solution (in 3% acetic acid)

Method

1. Dewax in xylene and rehydrate through graded ethanols to distilled water.
2. Stain the sections in the high iron diamine solution for 18 hours.
3. Rinse in running tap water for 5 minutes.
4. Stain in the alcian blue solution (pH 2.5) for 30 minutes.
5. Rinse in running tap water for 10 minutes.
6. Dehydrate in graded ethanols and clear with xylene.
7. Coverslip with a miscible mounting medium.

Results

Sulfated mucins and proteoglycans	black-brown
Sialomucins and hyaluronic acid	blue

Notes

1. The diamine salts are toxic and handling should be with great care and kept to a minimum.
2. Nuclear fast red may be used to enhance nuclear contrast.
3. The N.F. 10% ferric chloride solution is equivalent to a 62% w/v solution of FeCl$_3$·6H$_2$O (Lillie & Fulmer 1976).

Metachromatic methods

Metachromasia may be defined as the staining of tissue or tissue components such that the color of the tissue-bound dye complex differs significantly from the color of the original dye complex to give a marked contrast in color (Pearse 1960). Typically, there is a shift in the absorption of light by the tissue dye complex toward the shorter wavelengths with an inverse shift in color transmission or emission towards the longer wavelengths. Methylene blue, azure A and toluidine blue are small planar cationic dyes that typically stain tissues blue. Under conditions of metachromasia, these dyes stain tissue components purple-red. The use of such dyes to identify charged mucins and proteoglycans is one of the oldest of the histochemical techniques for carbohydrates.

Metachromasia is believed to result from a specific form of dye aggregation that is characterized by the formation of new intermolecular bonds between adjacent dye molecules (Pearse 1960). The bonds between the dye molecules only occur in situations in which the molecules are brought into close proximity to one another (Sylven 1954; Bergeron & Singer 1958). In cases of acid mucins or proteoglycans, the anionic groups of the carbohydrates act to orient the cationic dye molecules. Simply put, the anionic carbohydrate structure serves as a template to induce the formation of a polymeric dye structure in which the dye molecules likely bind to one another through hydrogen bonds or van der Waals' forces. Integration of water molecules between adjacent dye molecules is believed to be essential for the metachromatic phenomena (Sylven 1954; Bergeron & Singer 1958).

For metachromasia to occur, a certain pattern of distribution and density of repeating anionic structures is necessary (Pearse 1960). The highly anionic proteoglycans with alternating sulfate and carboxylate groups meet these criteria and produce metachromatic stains with dyes such as toluidine blue, methylene blue, and azure. In general, the more strongly acidic or highly sulfated proteolglycans will produce the strongest and most stable metachromasia (Tonna & Cronkite 1959; Thompson 1966).

The post-treatment of sections following staining with metachromasia-producing dyes can have a profound effect on the stability of the metachromasia. Metachromasia may be described as 'alcohol fast' if metachromasia is retained following dehydration, and as 'alcohol labile' if metachromasia is lost in the process (Pearse 1960). For this reason, it has been recommended by some that it is necessary to examine sections first in water prior to placement of the specimens in alcohol. The metachromasia-generating techniques have largely been replaced by techniques such as alcian blue. The reader is directed to older texts such as those of Pearse, Lillie, and Fulmer as well as earlier publications in the literature (Kramer & Windrum 1955; Bergeron & Singer 1958) for more detailed information concerning these techniques.

Azure A technique *(modified Kramer & Windrum 1955)*

Alcoholic azure A solution

Azure A	0.01 g
Ethanol 30%	100 ml

Method

1. Dewax sections in xylene and hydrate through graded ethanols to distilled water.
2. Cover sections with the azure A solution for 10 minutes.
3. Rinse in distilled water.
4. Dehydrate the sections in graded ethanols and clear in xylene.
5. Coverslip using a miscible mounting medium.

Results

Acid mucins and proteoglycans	purple to red
Tissue background	blue

Notes

0.1% azure A solution (0.1 g azure A in 100 ml of 30% ethanol) can be used to demonstrate the weakly metachromatic acid carbohydrate-containing molecules.

Lectins and immunohistochemistry

Lectins

Lectins were initially characterized as proteins isolated from plants that were capable of agglutinating mammalian erythrocytes (Sharon & Lis 1972). Agglutination occurs because the lectin molecule binds multiple glycoprotein molecules on the cell surface and it may cross-link erythrocytes (Sharon & Lis 1972; Goldstein & Hayes 1978). From a histochemical perspective, lectins may be defined as plant or animal proteins which bind specific carbohydrate moieties in tissue specimens. Lectin techniques, however, are

not routinely performed in most histology laboratories. For this reason, the discussion of lectins provided is brief and the reader is directed to the following references for a more thorough discussion and review of lectins (Sharon & Lis 1972; Goldstein & Hayes 1978; Spicer & Schulte 1992).

Lectins have been isolated from a wide range of animal and plant sources. The more commonly used lectins include concanavalin A from the jack bean, peanut agglutinin, and *Ulex europaeus* (gorse). Lectins bind principally to the terminal carbohydrate molecules of the oligosaccharide or polysaccharide chains of glycoproteins (Goldstein & Poretz 1986). However, the affinity of a lectin may be influenced by the monosaccharide unit adjacent to the terminal unit. Concanavalin A binds terminal mannose moieties while peanut agglutinin binds galactose or galactosamine (Hennigar et al. 1987; Spicer & Schulte 1992). *Ulex europaeus* specifically binds L-fucose (Allen et al. 1977).

Lectin molecules can be labeled with fluorochromes such as fluorescein or rhodamine as well as the histochemically detectable enzymes, horseradish peroxidase and alkaline phosphatase (Gonatas & Avrameas 1973). Lectins labeled in this manner have been used for a number of purposes in the histology or diagnostic pathology laboratory. *Ulex europaeus* in particular has been used as a valuable marker of normal and neoplastic endothelial cells (Walker 1985). Nevertheless, the use of *Ulex* in this role, however, has diminished with the emergence of immunohistochemistry and specific antibodies to endothelial markers such as factor VIII, CD31, and CD34.

Immunohistochemistry

Immunohistochemical techniques are rarely used for the routine evaluation of tissue specimens for glycogen or the proteoglycans. In spite of the high sensitivity and specificity of immunohistochemistry, the special stains described in this chapter remain the standard means for the evaluation of these substances. Immunohistochemistry, however, has become an invaluable tool for the detection of a varied number of specific mucins as well as mucin-like molecules that are markers of the neo-plastic process. Examples of these types of molecule include the epithelial membrane antigen (EMA) and the tumor-associated glycoprotein (TAG-72), to mention just two. As the list of mucins, mucin-like molecules, and glycoproteins that are evaluated by immunohistochemistry is long and varied and the discussion of immunohistochemical techniques is outside the scope of this chapter, the reader is referred to the relevant chapters in which the immunohistochemistry of diagnostic pathology is discussed at length.

Enzymatic digestion techniques

Various enzymatic digestion techniques have been applied to increase or verify the specificity of carbohydrate staining techniques. For example, the amylase or diastase techniques for glycogen digestion are commonly utilized in laboratories to enhance the specificity of the PAS technique. The other digestion techniques (neuraminidase, hyaluronidase) described below are not commonly performed in today's histology laboratories. They are more likely to be performed in research laboratories that possess an interest in a specific area of glycobiology.

Diastase digestion

The PAS technique is unique among the procedures described in this chapter in that PAS detects a varied number of mucosubstances such as glycogen, mucins, and glycoproteins. The distinction of mucins from glycogen can be problematic when using the PAS technique. The inclusion of a glycogen digestion step is necessary when the diagnosis requires the correct identification of mucosubstances such as mucin or glycogen. Typically α-amylase may be used in such a situation. Alpha-amylase catalyzes the hydrolysis of the glycosidic bonds of glycogen and the breakdown of the large glycogen molecules to the water-soluble disaccharide known as maltose (Bernfeld 1951). The net result is the removal of glycogen from the tissue section prior to the PAS

technique. Malt diastase, which contains both α- and β-amylases, is frequently used for this purpose (Lillie et al. 1947). Although human saliva is touted as an effective means of digesting glycogen, the use of saliva is discouraged for reasons of safety and the lack of standardization of saliva preparations. Duplicate slides are required when a glycogen digestion procedure is used. Following deparaffinization, one slide is treated with diastase in the appropriate buffer while the other slide is incubated with buffer only. Both slides are then subjected to the PAS procedure. Staining loss following digestion is indicative of glycogen.

Diastase digestion (Lillie & Fulmer 1976)

Phosphate buffer

Sodium phosphate (monobasic)	1.97 g
Sodium phosphate (dibasic)	0.28 g
Distilled water	1000 ml

This solution may be kept in the refrigerator for several months.

Diastase solution

Malt diastase	0.1 g
Phosphate buffer	100 ml

Method
1. Dewax two serial sections in xylene and rehydrate through graded ethanols to water.
2. Place one slide in the diastase solution for 1 hour at 37°C. The other slide is an untreated control and may remain in water for 1 hour.
3. Wash both slides in running tap water for 5–10 minutes.
4. Proceed with the PAS technique.

Results (with PAS procedure)
Glycogen should demonstrate bright red/magenta staining in the untreated slide. Glycogen staining should be absent in the diastase-treated slide.

Notes
1. A known positive control should be included to verify the potency of the enzyme.
2. Commercial batches of diastase or amylase may vary widely in activity and purity. Contaminating enzymes may digest material other than glycogen.
3. Alpha-amylase may be used instead of malt diastase.

Sialidase

The enzyme sialidase or neuraminidase is isolated from the bacterium *Vibrio cholerae* (Kiernan 1999). This enzyme specifically cleaves the terminal sialic acid moieties from sialomucins and glycoproteins (Drzeniek 1973). The loss of PAS or alcian blue staining following sialidase treatment is clearly indicative of the presence of sialic acid in tissue specimens. If the combined alcian blue-PAS protocol is performed following sialidase treatment, sialomucins that normally would stain blue with alcian blue stain red with PAS. Removal of the alcian blue-reactive anionic carboxylate group containing sugars from these mucins renders the mucin reactive with PAS.

By contrast to the scenarios described above, in which staining is lost following treatment, a lack of effect of sialidase is difficult to interpret. While it may indicate a lack of sialic acid in the specimen, such findings do not rule out the possibility of the sialidase-resistant *O*-acetylated sialic acids. These resistant sialic acids can be converted to sialidase labile form by the deacetylation procedure (Ravetto 1968). This technique uses an alkaline (ammonia) alcohol solution to remove the *O*-acetyl groups from the sialic acid. Subsequent treatment with sialidase cleaves the previously enzyme-resistant sialic acids. A comparison of alcian blue (pH 2.5) staining in sections subjected to the deacetylation-sialidase combination to the staining of sections exposed only to sialidase will reveal the presence of *O*-acetyl group-containing sialic acids.

Sialidase digestion (Bancroft & Cook 1994)

Sialidase solution

One unit/ml sialidase (neuraminidase) ex. *V. cholerae* diluted 1 in 5 with 0.2 M acetate buffer, pH 5.5. Add 1% calcium chloride w/v. The activity of the diluted enzyme will persist for a few weeks if stored at 4°C.

Method

1. Dewax two sections from a positive control and two sections from each test specimen. Bring sections to water.

2. Rinse the sections with buffer and treat one positive control section and one section from each test specimen with the sialidase solution for 16–24 hours at 37°C. The remaining slides (one positive control section and one section per test specimen) are incubated in buffer (37°C) alone for the same period of time.

3. Rinse in running tap water for 5 minutes.

4. Proceed to alcian blue or the alcian blue-PAS technique.

Results

Sialidase-labile sialic acids will stain bright blue in the untreated section. This staining is lost following sialidase treatment. Alcian blue-PAS mucins containing sialidase-labile sialic acids will stain bright blue while neutral mucins stain red to magenta in the untreated sections. Following treatment, mucins containing sialidase-labile sialic acids will stain red to magenta secondary to the PAS stain (Spicer & Warren 1959).

Notes

1. Sialic acids containing an *O*-acetyl group usually are resistant to sialidase.

2. A known positive control should be included to verify the potency of the enzyme.

Hyaluronidase

The enzyme hyaluronidase cleaves the glycosidic linkages of hyaluronic acid and, depending upon the source of the enzyme, glycosidic linkages in other glycosaminoglycans. The most commonly used hyaluronidase is isolated from an extract of bull testis. This enzyme removes hyaluronic acid but also attacks the glycosidic linkages of the chondroitin sulfates (Meyer & Rapport 1952). The enzyme may be used as a pretreatment of specimens, prior to staining with alcian blue or colloidal iron. The loss of staining when compared to a non-treated duplicate section is indicative of the presence of hyaluronic acid or the chondroitin sulfates. If there is no effect of the pretreatment, this strongly suggests that the substance is not hyaluronic acid. Thus, in spite of the lack of specificity, a negative response to bull testis hyaluronidase can be used to rule out the possible presence of hyaluronic acid.

A form of hyaluronidase isolated from several bacterial species also has been used for the identification of hyaluronic acid (Meyer & Rapport 1952). These enzymes are more selective than bovine testicular hyaluronidase and have been shown to act specifically on hyaluronic acid.

Hyaluronidase digestion (Gaffney 1992)

Phosphate buffer solution

Sodium chloride	8 g
Sodium phosphate, monobasic	2 g
Sodium phosphate, dibasic	0.3 g
Distilled water	1000 ml

Hyaluronidase solution

Bovine testicular hyaluronidase	50 mg
Phosphate buffer solution	100 ml

Method

1. Dewax two sections from a positive control and two sections from each test specimen. Bring sections to distilled water.
2. Incubate one positive control section and one section from each test specimen with the hyaluronidase solution for 3 hours at 37°C. The remaining slides (one positive control and one section per test specimen) should be treated with buffer alone for 3 hours at 37°C.
3. Wash all slides in running tap water for 5 minutes.
4. Perform staining technique such as alcian blue.

Results

Alcian blue (pH 2.5)

Connective tissue proteoglycans containing chondroitin sulfate and/or hyaluronic acid stain bright blue in sections not treated with hyaluronidase. This staining is lost following hyaluronidase treatment.

Notes

A known positive control is necessary to verify the potency of the enzyme. A good control is umbilical cord, which contains Wharton's jelly rich in hyaluronic acid.

Chemical modification and blocking techniques

There are a number of techniques that have been used to block the reactive groups of carbohydrates such as hydroxyls, carboxyls, and sulfate esters. Blocking these groups prevents the reaction with the reagents used in subsequent histochemical techniques. The blocking techniques, although infrequently used in today's histology laboratory, may be particularly useful for determining the specific types of carbohydrate present in a tissue specimen.

Methylation

There are a number of variations of this technique that have been used to identify the type (carboxyl or sulfate) of acid groups in mucins. However, all of these techniques are based upon the treatment of the specimens with an acidified methanolic solution. In the so-called 'mild' technique, the sections are exposed to the solution for a relatively short period (4 hours) at 37°C (Spicer 1960). Under these conditions, the carboxylate groups of the mucins are converted to methyl esters. The loss of alcian blue (pH 2.5) reactivity within a specimen following this procedure is indicative of a preponderance of carboxylated carbohydrates in the tissue. Conversely, any staining following this procedure is likely due to sulfate-containing carbohydrates.

Treatment of specimens with an acidified methanolic solution for 5 hours or more at 60°C converts carboxylate groups to methyl esters and also removes or hydrolyzes O-sulfate and N-sulfate groups in mucins and proteoglycans. Sections treated in this manner should demonstrate a total loss of alcian blue reactivity. This technique is of little value if performed alone and this frequently is performed with the saponification technique.

Saponification

The alkaline alcoholic solution used in this technique cleaves the linkage of the O-acetyl groups within the enzyme-resistant sialic acids. As with the deacetylation procedure described above, this technique renders the O-acetylated sialic acids sensitive to neuraminidase. The removal of the O-acetyl group and the restoration of the hydroxyl groups on the C7–C9 side chain of sialic acid also restore the PAS reactivity of the sialic acids (Culling et al. 1974).

This technique also is used for the reversal of the effects of methylation. Saponification cleaves the bonds of the methyl esters formed during methylation and restores the carboxylate groups (Spicer & Lillie 1959). Following the methylation protocol, saponification will restore the alcian blue staining of the carboxylated carbohydrates. Sulfate esters that are lost due to the more aggressive methylation protocol are not restored by saponification. The restoration of alcian blue staining following saponification is due to the presence of sialomucins or hyaluronic acid.

Mild methylation technique (Spicer 1960)

Acid methanol solution

Concentrated hydrochloric acid (HCl)	0.8 ml
Methanol	99.2 ml

Method

1. Dewax two sections from a positive control and two sections from each test specimen. Bring sections to distilled water.
2. Place one positive control section and one section from each test specimen in preheated (37°C) acid methanol solution for 4 hours. The remaining slides (one positive control and one slide per test specimen) should be placed in distilled water at 37°C for 4 hours.
3. Wash in running tap water for 5 minutes.
4. Perform alcian blue (pH 2.5) stain.

Results

Alcian blue (pH 2.5)

Sulfated mucins and proteoglycans as well as sialomucins and hyaluronic acid will stain bright blue in the untreated specimen. A diminution of staining following treatment with the acid methanol reflects a loss of stainable sialomucins and/or hyaluronic acid. Any staining that remains following treatment is due to sulfomucins and/or sulfate proteoglycans.

Notes

Treatment beyond 4 hours may result in the hydrolysis of sulfate groups. Positive control slides are necessary to verify the effectiveness of the methylation procedure.

Combined methylation-saponification technique
(Spicer & Lillie 1959)

Acid methanol solution

Same as solution used for mild methylation (see section above).

Saponification solution

Potassium hydroxide	1 g
Ethanol	70 ml
Distilled water	30 ml

Method

1. Dewax three positive control sections and three sections from each test specimen. Bring sections to water.
2. Place two positive controls and two test sections in the acid methanol solution at 60°C for 5 hours. The additional positive control and test specimen should be placed in 60°C distilled water for 5 hours.
3. Wash all sections in running tap water for 5 minutes.
4. Place one each of the positive control sections and test sections that were treated with acid methanol (Step 2) in the saponification solution for 30 minutes at room temperature. Place all other sections in 70% ethanol at room temperature for 30 minutes.
5. Wash for 5 minutes.
6. Stain with alcian blue.

Results

With alcian blue (pH 2.5) stain:

a. Sections without methylation or saponification: sulfated and carboxylated mucins as well as proteoglycans and hyaluronic acid will stain bright blue.
b. Sections treated with acid methanol but not subjected to saponification: there should be little or no alcian blue staining.
c. Sections treated with acid methanol and subjected to saponification: the carboxylated mucins and hyaluronic acid should demonstrate bright blue staining with alcian blue. Any loss of staining when compared to the sections that were not treated with acid methanol or subjected to saponification (group a) is due to the presence of sulfated mucins and/or sulfated proteoglycans.

Notes

1. Silanized slides should be used.
2. Celloidinization of slides has been recommended to reduce tissue loss during the saponification process.

References

Allen, H.J., Johnson, E.A., Matta, K.L., 1977. A comparison of the binding specificities of lectins from *Ulex europaeus* and *Lotus tetragonolobus*. Immunology Communications 6, 585–602.

Bancroft, J.D., Cook, H.C., 1994. Manual of histological techniques and their diagnostic applications. Churchill Livingstone, New York.

Barger, J.D., DeLamater, E.D., 1948. The use of thionyl chloride in the preparation of Schiff's reagent. Science 108, 121–122.

Bauer, H., 1933. Microskopisch-chemischer Natwer's von Glykogen und einigen anderen Polysacharden. Zeitschrift für mikroskopische-anatomische Forschung 33, 143.

Bergeron, J.A., Singer, M., 1958. Metachromasy: an experimental and theoretical re-evaluation. Journal of Biophysical and Biochemical Cytology 4, 433–457.

Bernfeld, P., 1951. Enzymes of starch degradation and synthesis. Advances in Enzymology 12, 379–428.

Cori, G.T., Cori, C.F., 1952. Glucose-6-phosphatase of the liver in glycogen storage disease. Journal of Biological Chemistry 199, 661–667.

Culling, C.F.A., Reid, P.E., Clay, M.G., Dunn, W.L., 1974. The histochemical demonstration of *O*-acylated sialic acid in gastrointerstinal mucin. Their association with the potassium hydroxide-periodic acid-Schiff effect. Journal of Histochemistry and Cytochemistry 22, 826–831.

Drzeniek, R., 1973. Substrate specificity of neuraminidases. Histochemical Journal 5, 271–290.

Gad, A., Sylven, B., 1969. On the nature of the high iron diamine method for sulfomucins. Journal of Histochemistry and Cytochemistry 17, 156–160.

Gaffney, E., 1992. Carbohydrates. In: Prophet, E.B., Mills, B., Arrington, J.B., Sobin, L.H. (Eds.), Armed Forces Institute of Pathology: laboratory methods in histochemistry. American Registry of Pathology, Washington, DC.

Gendler, S.J., Spicer, A.P., 1995. Epithelial mucin genes. Annual Reviews of Physiology 57, 607–634.

Goldstein, I.J., Hayes, C.E., 1978. The lectins: carbohydrate-binding proteins of plants and animals. Advances in Carbohydrate Chemistry and Biochemistry 35, 127–340.

Goldstein, I.J., Poretz, R.D., 1986. Isolation, physiochemical characterization, and carbohydrate-binding specificity of lectins. In: Liener, I.E., Sharon, N., Goldstein, J.J. (Eds.), The lectins: properties, functions and applications in biology and medicine. Academic Press, Orlando, FL, pp. 35–248.

Gonatas, N.K., Avrameas, S., 1973. Detection of plasma membrane carbohydrates with lectin peroxidase conjugates. Journal of Cell Biology 59, 436–443.

Hale, C.W., 1946. Histochemical demonstration of acid mucopolysaccharides in animal tissues. Nature (London) 157, 802.

Harley, R.A., 1987. Histochemical and immunochemical methods of use in pulmonary pathology. In: Spicer, S.S. (Ed.), Histochemistry in pathologic diagnosis. Marcel Dekker, New York.

Hennigar, G.R., 1987. Techniques in nephropathology. In: Spicer, S.S. (Ed.), Histochemistry in pathologic diagnosis. Marcel Dekker, New York.

Hennigar, L.M., Hennigar, R.A., Schulte, B.A., 1987. Histochemical specificity of β-galactose binding lectins from *Arachis hypogaea* (peanut) and *Ricinus communis* (castor bean). Stain Technology 62, 317–325.

Hers, H.G., 1963. Glucosidase deficiency in generalized glycogen storage disease (Pompe's disease). Biochemical Journal 86, 11–16.

Horobin, R.W., Kiernan, J.A., 2002. Conn's biological stains. A handbook of dyes, stains and fluorochromes for use in biology and medicine, tenth ed. BIOS Scientific Publishers, Oxford, UK.

Johannes, M.L., Klessen, C., 1984. Alcian blue/PAS or PAS/alcian blue? Remarks on a classical technique used in carbohydrate histochemistry. Histochemistry 80, 129–132.

Kiernan, J.A., 1999. Histological and histochemical methods: theory and practice, third ed. Butterworth Heinemann, Oxford.

Kindblom, L.G., Angervall, L., 1975. Histochemical characterization of mucosubstances in bone and soft tissue-tumors. Cancer 36, 985–984.

Kramer, H., Windrum, G.M., 1955. The metachromatic staining reaction. Journal of Histochemistry and Cytochemistry 3, 227–237.

Leblond, C.P., Glegg, R.E., Eidinger, D., 1957. Presence of carbohydrates with free 1,2-glycol groups in sites stained by the periodic acid-Schiff technique. Journal of Histochemistry and Cytochemistry 5, 445–458.

Lev, R., Spicer, S.S., 1964. Specific staining of sulfate groups with alcian blue at low pH. Journal of Histochemistry and Cytochemistry 12, 309.

Lillie, R.D., 1947. Reticulum staining with Schiff reagent after oxidation by acidified sodium periodate. Journal of Laboratory and Clinical Medicine 32, 910–912.

Lillie, R.D., 1951. Histochemical comparison of the Casella, Bauer and periodic acid oxidation leucofuchsin techniques. Stain Technology 26, 123–136.

Lillie, R.D., 1954. Histologic technique, second ed. McGraw-Hill, New York.

Lillie, R.D., 1977. H.J. Conn's biological stains. Williams and Wilkins, Baltimore, MD.

Lillie, R.D., Fulmer, H.M., 1976. Histopathologic technique and practical histochemistry, fourth ed. McGraw-Hill, New York.

Lillie, R.D., Laskey, A., Greco, J., Jacquier, H., 1947. Studies on the preservation and histologic demonstration of glycogen. Bulletin of the International Association of Medical Museums 27, 23.

Longley, J.B., 1952. Effectiveness of Schiff variants in the periodic Schiff and Feulgen nucleal technics. Stain Technology 27, 161–169.

McKusick, V., Neufeld, E.F., 1983. The mucodisaccharide storage diseases. In: Stanbury J.B., Wyngaarden J.B., Frederickson D.S., et al. (Eds.), The metabolic basis of inherited disease, fifth ed. McGraw-Hill, New York.

McManus, J.F.A., 1946. Histological demonstration of mucin after periodic acid. Nature (London) 158, 202.

McManus, J.F.A., 1948. The periodic acid routine applied to the kidney. American Journal of Pathology 24, 643–653.

Manns, E., 1958. The preservation and demonstration of glycogen in tissue sections. Journal of Medical Laboratory Technology 15, 1–12.

Mason, R.M., d'Arville, C., Kimura, J.H., Hascoll, V.C., 1982. Absence of covalently linked core protein from newly synthesized hyaluronate. Biochemical Journal 207, 445–457.

Mayer, P., 1896. Uber schleimfarbung. Mitteilungeu aus der Zoologischen Station Zu Neapel 12, 303.

Meyer, K., Rapport, M.M., 1952. Hyaluronidases. Advances in Enzymology 13, 199–236.

Moniaux, N., Nollet, S., Porchet, N., et al., 1999. Complete sequence of the human mucin MUC4: a putative cell membrane-associated mucin. Biochemical Journal 338, 325–333.

Mowry, R.W., 1956. Alcian blue techniques for the histochemical study of acid carbohydrates. Journal of Histochemistry and Cytochemistry 4, 407.

Mowry, R.W., 1958. Improved procedure for the staining of acidic polysaccharides by Muller's colloidal (hydrous) ferric oxide and its combination with the Feulgen and the periodic acid-Schiff reactions. Laboratory Investigation 7, 566–576.

Mowry, R.W., 1963. The special value of methods that color both acidic and vicinal hydroxyl groups in the histochemical study of mucins, with revised directions for the colloidal iron stain, and the use of alcian blue 8GX and their combinations with the periodic acid-Schiff reaction. Annals of the New York Academy of Sciences 106, 402–423.

Muller, G., 1946. Über eine vereinfachung der reaction nach Hale. Acta Histochemie 2, 68–70.

Muller, G., 1955. [Simplification of the reaction after Hale, 1946.] Acta Histochemica 2, 68–70.

Pearse, A.G.E., 1960. Histochemistry, theoretical and applied. Little, Brown, Boston.

Perez-Vilar, J., Hill, R.L., 1999. The structure and assembly of secreted mucins. Journal of Biological Chemistry 274, 31751–31754.

Quintarelli, G., Scott, J.E., Dellovo, M.C., 1964. The chemical and histochemical properties of alcian blue II. Dye binding of tissue polyanions. Histochemie 4, 86–98.

Ravetto, C., 1968. Histochemical identification of N-acetyl-O-diacetylneuraminic acid resistant to neuraminidase. Journal of Histochemistry and Cytochemistry 16, 663.

Rinehart, J.F., Abul-Haj, S.K., 1951. Improved method for histochemical demonstration of acid mucopolysaccharides in tissues. Archives of Pathology 52, 189–194.

Roden, L., 1980. Structure and metabolism of connective tissue proteoglycans. In: Lennarz, W.J. (Ed.), The biochemistry of glycoproteins and proteoglycans. Plenum Press, New York, pp. 267–371.

Schauer, R., 1982. Sialic acids: chemistry, metabolism and function. Cell Biology Monographs, vol. 10. Springer-Verlag, New York.

Schroeder, J.A., Thompson, M.C., Mockenstrum Gardner, M., Gendler, S.J., 2001. Transgenic MUC1 interacts with epidermal growth factor receptor and correlates with mitogen-activated protein kinase activation in the mouse mammary gland. Journal of Biological Chemistry 276, 13057–13064.

Scott, J.E., Mowry, R.W., 1970. Alcian blue: a consumer's guide. Journal of Histochemistry and Cytochemistry 18, 842.

Scott, J.E., Quintarelli, G., Dellovo, M.C., 1964. The chemical and histochemical properties of alcian blue. I. The mechanism of alcian blue staining. Histochemie 4, 73–85.

Sharon, N., Lis, H., 1972. Lectins: cell-agglutinating and sugar-specific proteins. Science 177, 949–959.

Sorvari, T., Sorvari, R.M., 1969. The specificity of alcian blue pH 1.0-alcian yellow pH 2.5 staining in the histochemical differentiation of acid groups in mucosubstances. Journal of Histochemistry and Cytochemistry 17, 291–293.

Southgate, H.W., 1927. Note on preparing mucicarmine. Journal of Pathology and Bacteriology 30, 729.

Spicer, S.S., 1960. A correlative study of the histochemical properties of rodent acid mucopolysaccharides. Journal of Histochemistry and Cytochemistry 8, 18–35.

Spicer, S.S., 1965. Diamine methods for differentiating mucosubstances histochemically. Journal of Histochemistry and Cytochemistry 13, 211–234.

Spicer, S.S., Lillie, R.D., 1959. Saponification as a means of selectively reversing the methylation blockade of tissue basophilia. Journal of Histochemistry and Cytochemistry 7, 123–125.

Spicer, S.S., Schulte, B.A., 1992. Diversity of cell glycoconjugates shown histochemically: a perspective. Journal of Histochemistry and Cytochemistry 40, 1–38.

Spicer, S.S., Warren, L., 1959. The histochemistry of sialic acid mucoproteins. Journal of Histochemistry and Cytochemistry 8, 135–137.

Sylven, B., 1954. Metachromatic dye-substrate interactions. Quarterly Journal of Microbiological Science 95, 327–358.

Thompson, S.W., 1966. Selected histochemical and histopathological methods. Charse C. Thomas, Springfield, IL.

Tighe, J.R., 1963. The histological demonstration of mucopolysaccharides in connective-tissue tumors. Journal of Pathology and Bacteriology 86, 141–149.

Tonna, E.A., Cronkite, E.P., 1959. Histochemical and autoradiographic studies on the effects of aging on the mucopolysaccharides of the periosteum. Journal of Biophyscial and Biochemical Cytology 6, 171–178.

Turani, H., Lurie, B., Chaimoff, C., Kessler, E., 1986. The diagnostic significance of sulfated acid mucin content in gastric intestinal metaplasia with early gastric cancer. American Journal of Gastroenterology 81, 343–345.

Varki, A., Cummings, R., Esko, J., et al. (Eds.), 1999. Essentials of glycobiology. Cold Spring Harbor Laboratory Press, Cold Spring Harbor, NY.

Walker, R.A., 1985. *Ulex europeus* I-peroxidase as a marker of vascular endothelium: its application in routine histopathology. Journal of Pathology 146, 123–127.

Weiss, S.W., Goldblum, J.R., 2001. Enzinger and Weiss's soft tissue tumors, fourth ed. Mosby, St. Louis, MO.

Wesseling, J., van der Valk, S.W., Vos, H.L., Sonnenberg, A., 1995. Episialin (MUC1) overexpression inhibits integrin-mediated cell adhesion to extracellular matrix components. Journal of Cell Biology 129, 255–265.

Yamabayashi, S., 1987. Periodic acid-Schiff-alcian blue: a method for the differential staining of glycoproteins. Histochemical Journal 19, 565–571.

Further reading

Johnson, W.C., Helwig, E.B., 1963. Histochemistry of primary and metastatic mucus-secreting tumors. Annals of the New York Academy of Sciences 106, 794–803.

Pigments and minerals 13

Guy E. Orchard

Introduction

In biology, pigments are defined as substances occurring in living matter that absorb visible light (electromagnetic energy within a narrow band that lies approximately between 400 and 800 nm). The various pigments may greatly differ in origin, chemical constitution and biological significance. They can be either organic or inorganic compounds that remain insoluble in most solvents. Minerals are naturally occurring homogeneous inorganic substances having a definite chemical composition and characteristic crystalline structure, color and hardness. In biology they are necessary for growth and development.

Pigments can be classified under the following headings

1. Endogenous pigments

These substances are produced either within tissues and serve a physiological function, or are by-products of normal metabolic processes. They can be further subdivided into:

- hematogenous (blood-derived) pigments
- non-hematogenous pigments
- endogenous minerals

2. Artifact pigments

These are deposits of artifactually produced material caused by the interactions between certain tissue components and some chemical substances, such as the fixative formalin. Formalin and malaria pigments are sometimes classified as a subdivision of endogenous pigments.

3. Exogenous pigments and minerals

These substances gain access to the body accidentally through a variety of methods (e.g. carbon anthracotic pigment, which is seen in lung and lymph nodes). These pigments and minerals serve no physiological function. Entry is gained either by inhalation into the lungs or by implantation (e.g. tattoos) into the skin. Most exogenous pigments are minerals, few of which are pigmented.

The above classification, although not scientifically precise, is used as a convenient aid in the identification of pigments. It is important to bear in mind that the same pigment may present itself in tissue sections in a variety of ways. Iron, for example, may be present as an endogenous pigment in liver sections in an iron overload condition and as an exogenous pigment in the case of a shrapnel wound/ prosthetic implantation. It is advisable to note a pigment's morphology, tissue site, and relevant clinical data before carrying out the various stains and histochemical reactions available in order that a pigment can be identified.

Endogenous pigments

Hematogenous

This group contains the following blood-derived pigments:

- hemosiderins
- hemoglobin
- bile pigments
- porphyrins

Hemosiderins

These pigments are seen as yellow to brown granules and normally appear intracellularly. They contain iron in the form of ferric hydroxide that is bound to a protein framework and is unmasked by various chemicals. Iron is a vital component of the human body as it is an essential constituent of the oxygen-carrying hemoglobin found in the red cells, where 60% of the body's total iron content resides. It also occurs in myoglobin and certain enzymes, such as cytochrome oxidase and the peroxidases.

Normal and abnormal iron metabolism

Dietary iron is absorbed in the small intestine and attached to a protein molecule for transfer to the sites in the body where it is to be utilized or stored. Approximately 30% is stored within the reticuloendothelial system, especially the bone marrow. The bone marrow is also the main site of iron utilization in the body, where it is incorporated into the hemoglobin molecule during red cell formation. The normal breakdown of worn-out red cells results in the release of iron that is recirculated back into the various areas of iron storage for further utilization. Under normal conditions, this efficient system of recycling usually means that iron deficiency rarely occurs. There is a minimal loss of iron by the way of epithelial desquamation, hair loss, and sweating. The main reason for loss of iron from the body is hemorrhage in the form of either chronic bleeding (e.g. a peptic ulcer, bowel neoplasia), or in the female by menstruation, with approximately 25% of females being iron deficient. The small intestine normally only absorbs sufficient iron from the excess iron in the diet to counteract any losses, but in excessive blood loss the dietary content may be relatively inadequate for the need, and even though the absorption mechanism is working at full efficiency, a state of clinical iron deficiency occurs. In iron deficiency, the iron stores in the bone marrow become depleted, insufficient hemoglobin is produced because of the lack of iron, and anemia develops in which the red cells contain diminished amounts of hemoglobin. The iron deficiency is characteristically demonstrated by the absence of stainable iron in the bone marrow.

There is no active method of iron excretion from the body. Iron excess is a much less common condition, because under normal conditions the intestine will not absorb iron from the diet when there is already a surplus within the body. However, this controlling mechanism may be bypassed when iron is given therapeutically, such as in the form of either iron injections or blood transfusion. If excess iron is given this way, the iron stores may become overloaded, and excessive amounts of hemosiderin may be deposited in the organs with a prominent reticuloendothelial component (e.g., spleen, bone marrow, liver). This condition is called *hemosiderosis*. A rarer cause of iron overload is the genetic disease *hemochromatosis*, in which the controlling mechanism at the small intestine absorption stage becomes impaired, and the iron is absorbed indiscriminately in amounts irrelevant to the state of the body's iron stores. In this disorder, large quantities of hemosiderin are deposited in many of the organs, often interfering with those organs' structure and function.

Demonstration of hemosiderin and iron

In unfixed tissue, hemosiderin is insoluble in alkalis but freely soluble in strong acid solutions; after fixation in formalin, it is slowly soluble in dilute acids, especially oxalic acid. Fixatives that contain acids but no formalin can remove hemosiderin or alter it in such a way that reactions for iron are negative. Certain types of iron found in tissues are not demonstrable using traditional techniques. This is because the iron is tightly bound within a protein complex. Both hemoglobin and myoglobin are examples of such protein complexes and, if treated with hydrogen peroxide (100 vol), the iron is released and can then be demonstrated using Perls' Prussian blue reaction (Fig. 13.1). A similar result is obtained if the

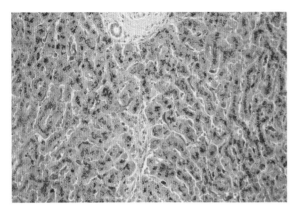

Figure 13.1 A section of liver from a patient with hemochromatosis stained for ferric iron with Perls' method. Ferric iron is stained blue.

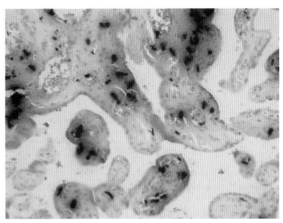

Figure 13.2 A section of placenta treated with ferrous sulfate and stained with Lillie's method for ferrous iron. Ferrous iron is stained dark blue.

acid ferrocyanide solution is heated to 60°C in a water bath, oven, or microwave oven. However, the use of heat will sometimes cause a fine, diffuse, blue precipitate to form on both the tissue section and slide. This precipitate will not occur when the slides are stained at room temperature. Metallic iron deposits, or inert iron oxide seen in tissues because of industrial exposure, are not positive when treated with acid ferrocyanide solutions. As a consequence of the tissue response, various mechanisms release some of the iron in a demonstrable form, and such deposits are almost invariably surrounded by hemosiderin. In almost all the instances where demonstrable iron appears in tissues, it does so in the form of a ferric salt. On those rare occasions that iron appears in its reduced state as the ferrous salt, then Lillie's (1965) method may be used to achieve the Turnbull's blue reaction to visualize its presence in tissue sections (Fig. 13.2).

An interesting and sometimes useful modification of a serum iron technique was introduced by Hukill and Putt (1962) to demonstrate both ferrous and ferric iron in tissue sections. This method was claimed to be a more sensitive demonstration for the detection of both ferric and ferrous salts, but has not succeeded in replacing the more traditional method for the demonstration of iron. The method uses bathophenanthroline and the resultant color of any iron present in tissues is bright red.

Perls' Prussian blue reaction for ferric iron (Perls 1867)

This method is considered to be the first classical histochemical reaction. Treatment with an acid ferrocyanide solution will result in the unmasking of ferric iron in the form of the hydroxide, $Fe(OH)_3$, by dilute hydrochloric acid. The ferric iron then reacts with a dilute potassium ferrocyanide solution to produce an insoluble blue compound, ferric ferrocyanide (Prussian blue).

Fixation
Avoid the use of acid fixatives. Chromates will also interfere with the preservation of iron.

Sections
Works well on all types of section, including resin.

Ferrocyanide solution
1% aqueous potassium ferrocyanide	20 ml
2% aqueous hydrochloric acid	20 ml

Preferably freshly prepared just before use.

Method
1. Take a test and control section to water.
2. Treat sections with the freshly prepared acid ferrocyanide solution for 10–30 minutes (see Note a below).
3. Wash well in distilled water.
4. Lightly stain the nuclei with 0.5% aqueous neutral red or 0.1% nuclear fast red.
5. Wash rapidly in distilled water.
6. Dehydrate, clear, and mount in synthetic resin.

Results

Ferric iron	blue
Nuclei	red

Notes

a. Depending on the amount of ferric iron present, it may be necessary to vary the staining times.

b. Some laboratories keep the two stock solutions made up separately and stored in the refrigerator. The two solutions must not be stored for prolonged periods; this precaution will ensure that the solutions retain their viability.

c. It is essential that a positive control is used with all test sections. The choice of material that is most suitable as a control specimen is important. A useful control would be postmortem lung tissue that contains a reasonable number of iron-positive macrophages (heart failure cells). Freshly formed deposits of iron may be dissolved in the hydrochloric acid.

Lillie's method for ferric and ferrous iron (Lillie & Geer 1965)

Fixation

Avoid the use of acid fixatives. Chromates will also interfere with the preservation of iron.

Sections

Paraffin, frozen, and resin.

Method

1. Take test and control sections to distilled water.
2. Dissolve 400 mg of potassium ferrocyanide in 40 ml of 0.5% hydrochloric acid when testing for ferric iron. For testing ferrous iron substitute, 400 mg of potassium ferricyanide. Prepare just before use. Expose sections for 30 minutes.
3. Wash well in distilled water.
4. Stain nuclei with 0.1% aqueous nuclear fast red for 5 minutes.
5. Rinse in distilled water.
6. Dehydrate, clear, and mount in synthetic resin.

Results

Ferric iron	dark Prussian blue
Ferrous iron	dark Turnbull's blue
Nuclei	red

Hukill and Putt's method for ferrous and ferric iron
(Hukill & Putt 1962)

Fixation

Not critical but avoid prolonged exposure in acid fixatives.

Sections

All types of tissue section may be used including resin.

Solution

Bathophenanthroline (4, 7-diphenyl-1, 10-phenanthroline)	100 mg
3% aqueous acetic acid	100 ml

Place in oven at 60°C for 24 hours, agitating at regular intervals. Cool to room temperature and filter. This solution is stable for about 4 weeks. Before use, add thioglycolic acid to a concentration of 0.5% (this should be replenished each time before use as it rapidly undergoes oxidation on exposure to air).

Method

1. Take test and control sections to distilled water.
2. Stain sections in bathophenanthroline solution for 2 hours at room temperature.
3. Rinse well in distilled water.
4. Counterstain in 0.5% aqueous methylene blue for 2 minutes.
5. Rinse well in distilled water.
6. Stand slides on end until completely dry.
7. Dip slides in xylene and mount in synthetic resin.

Results

Ferrous iron	red
Nuclei	blue

Notes

a. It is important that the bathophenanthroline is completely dissolved prior to use.

b. Dehydration with alcohol will remove the resultant red coloration.

Hemoglobin

Hemoglobin is a basic conjugated protein that is responsible for the transportation of oxygen and carbon dioxide within the bloodstream. It is composed of a colorless protein, globin, and a red pigmented component, heme. Four molecules of heme are attached to each molecule of globin.

Heme is composed of protoporphyrin, a substance built up from pyrrole rings and combined with ferrous iron. Histochemical demonstration of the ferrous iron is possible only if the close binding in the heme molecules is cleaved. This can be achieved by treatment with hydrogen peroxide, but this has no practical use. As hemoglobin appears normally within red blood cells its histological demonstration is not usually necessary. The need to demonstrate the pigment may arise in certain pathological conditions such as casts in the lumen of renal tubules in cases of hemoglobinuria or active glomerulonephritis.

Demonstration of hemoglobin

Two types of demonstration method can be used to stain hemoglobin in tissue sections. The first demonstrates the enzyme, hemoglobin peroxidase, which is reasonably stable and withstands short fixation and paraffin processing. This peroxidase activity was originally demonstrated by the benzidine-nitroprusside methods, but because of the carcinogenicity of benzidine these methods are not recommended and are no longer used. Lison (1938) introduced the patent blue method that was later modified by Dunn and Thompson (1946) (Fig. 13.3). Tinctorial methods have also been used for the demonstration of hemoglobin; the amido black technique (Puchtler & Sweat 1962) and the kiton red-almond green technique (Lendrum 1949) are worth noting.

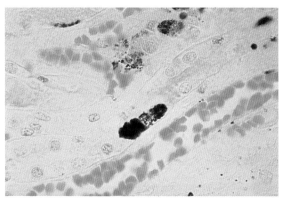

Figure 13.3 A section of kidney from a patient with hemoglobinuria stained for hemoglobin with leuco patent blue V. Hemoglobin is stained blue.

Leuco patent blue V method for hemoglobin
(Dunn & Thompson 1946)

Fixation

Formalin (removed formal mercury due to toxicity?) Poor preservation with Heidenhain's Susa has been noted by Drury and Wallington (1980).

Solutions

Stock solution

1% aqueous patent blue V (CI 42045)	25 ml
Powdered zinc	2.5 g
Glacial acetic acid	0.5 ml

Mix well on a magnetic stirrer. The solution will become pale green-blue. Filter and store in a refrigerator at 3–6°C. The solution is stable for about 1 week.

Working solution

Stock solution	10 ml
Glacial acetic acid	2 ml
3% hydrogen peroxide	1 ml

Prepare immediately before use.

Method

1. Take test and control sections to distilled water.
2. Stain in patent blue solution for 5 minutes at room temperature.
3. Rinse in distilled water.
4. Lightly counterstain in 0.5% aqueous neutral red or 0.1% aqueous nuclear fast red for 1 minute.
5. Rinse in distilled water.
6. Dehydrate, clear, and mount in synthetic resin.

Results

Hemoglobin peroxidase (red blood cells and neutrophils)	dark blue
Nuclei	red

Notes

a. Experience has shown that the hemoglobin demonstrated by this method tends to be more of a green-blue color.
b. In some instances, if the staining solution is left on the section for too long, it may start to decolor a positive reaction.
c. Fixation in excess of 36 hours may give rise to unreliable results.
d. This method demonstrates peroxidase activity, including the peroxidases in other blood cells, particularly in the lysosomes of polymorphonuclear leukocytes and their precursors. Tissue peroxidases are also demonstrated.

Bile pigments

Red blood cells are broken down in the reticuloendothelial system when they have reached the end of their useful life, usually after 120 days. Hemoglobin is released after the red cell membrane has been ruptured. The protein globin and iron components are released for recycling within the body after the hemoglobin has been broken down. After the heme portion has been split from the globin, the tetrapyrrole ring of the heme molecule is cleaved and opened out into a chain composed of four linked pyrrole groups. With the opening out of the tetrapyrrole ring, the iron component is removed to be stored in those tissues that specialize in iron storage. This iron component is now free to be incorporated into the hemoglobin molecule during red cell formation. The opened tetrapyrrole ring, which has had its iron component removed, is known as biliverdin. This residue is formed in the phagocytic cells that populate the reticulo-endothelial system, particularly the bone marrow and spleen. Biliverdin is transported to the liver, where it is reduced to form bilirubin. In this form, the bilirubin is insoluble in water, but after conjugation with glucuronic acid it forms a water-soluble compound, bilirubin-glucuronide. This process takes place in liver hepatocytes due to the activity of the enzyme glucuronyl transferase. The conjugated bilirubin passes from the hepatocytes into the bile canaliculi, and then via the hepatic ducts into the gallbladder, which acts as a reservoir. The bilirubin passes along the common bile duct to be released into the duodenum via the ampulla of Vater.

The term *bile pigments* used by many authors when discussing the various (generic) staining techniques can be applied to all bile pigments. In using this terminology, it is implied that all bile pigments react in an identical manner, but this is not the case. Contained within the group 'bile pigments' are both conjugated and unconjugated bilirubin, biliverdin, and hematoidin, all of which are chemically distinct and show different physical properties, particularly with regard to their solubility in water and alcohol. Microscopic examination of any liver section that contains 'bile pigments' will almost certainly reveal a mixture of biliverdin and both conjugated and unconjugated bilirubin. This is particularly likely when the liver contains an excess of bile pigments, either through bile duct obstruction, e.g., due to a stone or tumor, an abnormality of biliverdin-bilirubin metabolism in the rare congenital enzyme disorders, or where there is extensive liver cell death or degeneration. The non-specific term *bile* will be used to include biliverdin and both conjugated and unconjugated bilirubin in the following text.

In a hematoxylin and eosin (H&E) stained section of liver, bile, if present, is most commonly seen in the hepatocytes in the early stages as small yellow-brown globules and then subsequently within the bile canaliculi as larger, smooth, round-ended rods or globules commonly referred to as *bile thrombi*. The latter, if present, in liver sections is a histopathological indication that the patient has obstructive jaundice due to a blockage in the normal flow of bile from the liver into the gallbladder and subsequently into the bowel, probably because of gallstones or a carcinoma of the head of pancreas. Masses of bile in the canaliculi of liver sections are easily distinguished microscopically because of their characteristic morphology and their situation. Bile in hepatocytes must be distinguished from the lipofuscins that are also commonly seen within these cells and can appear as small yellow-brown globules. The need to distinguish between bile and lipofuscin in hepatocytes is particularly important in liver biopsies taken from liver transplant patients where sepsis is suspected. Bile is difficult to identify in the sections of normal liver. It is important to note that both bile and lipofuscin can be positive with Schmorl's ferric ferricyanide reduction test (Golodetz & Unna 1909). Bile is also seen in H&E-stained sections in the gallbladder where it can appear as amorphous, yellow-brown masses adherent to the mucosa or included as yellow-brown globules within the epithelial-lined Aschoff-Rokitansky sinuses in the gallbladder. Bile is also present, together with cholesterol, in gallstones.

Virchow (1847) first described extracellular yellow-brown crystals and amorphous masses within old hemorrhagic areas, which he called hematoidin. Pearse (1985) reviewed the histochemistry of bile pigments. Microscopically, *hematoidin* frequently appears as a bright yellow pigment in old splenic infarcts, where it contrasts well against the pale gray of the infarcted tissue. Hematoidin can also be found in old hemorrhagic areas in the brain. Bearing in mind the differences discussed above, it is almost certain that hematoidin is related to both bilirubin and biliverdin, even though it differs from them both morphologically and chemically. It is thought that heme has undergone a chemical change within these areas which has led to it being trapped, thus preventing it from being transported to the liver to be processed into bilirubin.

Demonstration of bile pigments and hematoidin

The need to identify bile pigments arises mainly in the histological examination of the liver, where distinguishing bile pigment from lipofuscin may be of significant importance. Both appear yellow-brown in H&E-stained paraffin sections, and it is worth remembering that the green color of biliverdin is often masked by eosin. In such cases, unstained paraffin or frozen sections, lightly counterstained with a suitable hematoxylin (e.g. Mayer), will prove of value. Bile pigments are not autofluorescent and fail to rotate the plane of polarized light (monorefringent), whereas lipofuscin is autofluorescent. The most commonly used routine method for the demonstration of bile pigments is the modified Fouchet technique (Hall 1960), in which the pigment is converted to the green color of biliverdin and blue cholecyanin by the oxidative action of the ferric chloride in the presence of trichloroacetic acid (Fig. 13.4). The Fouchet technique is quick and simple to carry out, and when counterstained with van Gieson's solution the green color is accentuated.

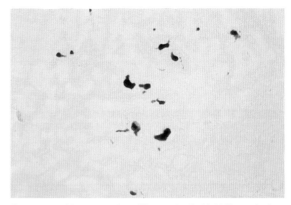

Figure 13.4 Bile in a section of liver stained with Hall's method for bilirubin. Bilirubin is stained emerald green.

Modified Fouchet's technique for liver bile pigments
(Hall 1960)

Fixation

Any fixative appears suitable.

Sections

Any.

Solutions

Fouchet's solution

25% aqueous trichloroacetic acid	36 ml
10% aqueous ferric chloride	4 ml

   Freshly prepared before use.

Van Gieson stain

Dissolve 100 mg of acid fuchsin (CI 42685) in 100 ml of saturated aqueous picric acid (see Note c below).

Method

1. Take test and control sections to distilled water.
2. Treat with the freshly prepared Fouchet's solution for 10 minutes.
3. Wash well in running tap water for 1 minute.
4. Rinse in distilled water.
5. Counterstain with van Gieson solution for 2 minutes.
6. Dehydrate, clear, and mount in synthetic resin.

Results

Bile pigments	emerald to blue-green
Muscle	yellow
Collagen	red

Notes

a. Two control sections are stained with the test section, one stained with Fouchet's reagent and van Gieson, and the other with Fouchet's reagent alone.

b. Although the solutions used in Fouchet's reagent have a reasonable shelf life, experience has shown that a freshly prepared solution gives a more reliable result.

c. Bile that may be present in situations outside the liver such as that seen in the Aschoff-Rokitansky sinuses or in hemorrhagic and infarcted areas is likely to show no color change with this method. This type of pigment can be shown using the Gmelin (see below) or the Stein technique. Sirus Red F3B (CI 35780) may be substituted for acid fuchsin. Bile is a reducing substance and therefore will stain with the Masson-Fontana and Schmorl techniques.

Gmelin technique *(Tiedermann & Gmelin 1826)*

This technique is the only method that shows an identical result with liver bile, gallbladder bile, and hematoidin. The method tends to be messy, capricious, and gives impermanent results. Deparaffinized sections of tissue containing bile pigments are treated with nitric acid, and a changing color spectrum is produced. Because it can be unreliable, it is advisable to repeat the test at least three times before a negative result is acceptable. A popular modification of this technique is that of Lillie and Pizzolato (1967), in which bromine in carbon tetrachloride is used as an oxidant.

Sections
Paraffin.

Method
1. Sections to distilled water and mount in distilled water.
2. Place mounted section under the microscope using an objective with reasonable working distance.
3. Place 2–3 drops of concentrated nitric acid to one side of the coverglass and draw under the coverglass by means of a piece of blotting paper on the opposite side.
4. Remove excess solution and observe pigment for color changes.

Results
Bile pigments will gradually produce the following spectrum of color change:
yellow-green-blue-purple-red.

Notes
a. This method is impermanent, thus preventing storage of sections.
b. The reaction can occur rapidly, but by using a 50–70% solution of nitric acid it can be slowed down.
c. Sulfuric acid can also be used in this method.

Oxidation methods aim to demonstrate bilirubin by converting it to green biliverdin. In practice they fail to produce the bright blue-green color seen in the more popular Fouchet technique and tend to be a dull olive green color. These oxidation methods are of little value in routine surgical pathology and are rarely used. Another group of methods that has been used to demonstrate bile pigments is the diazo methods that are based on a well-known technique previously used in chemical pathology, namely the van den Burgh test for bilirubin in blood. The method is based on the reaction between bilirubin and diazotized sulfanilic acid. Raia (1965, 1967) modified the method for use on cryostat sections but the reagents are complex to make up and section loss may be high; therefore its use is limited.

Porphyrin pigments

These substances normally occur in tissues in only small amounts. They are considered to be precursors of the heme portion of hemoglobin. The porphyrias are rare pathological conditions that are disorders of the biosynthesis of porphyrins and heme.

In erythropoietic protoporphyria, porphyrin pigment can be seen as focal deposits in liver sections. The pigment appears as a dense dark brown pigment and in fresh frozen sections exhibits a brilliant red fluorescence that rapidly fades with exposure to ultraviolet light. The pigment, when seen in paraffin sections and viewed using polarized light, appears bright red in color with a centrally located, dark Maltese cross.

Non-hematogenous endogenous pigments

This group contains the following:

- melanins
- lipofuscins

- chromaffin
- pseudomelanosis (melanosis coli)
- Dubin-Johnson pigment
- ceroid-type lipofuscins
- Hamazaki-Weisenberg bodies

Melanins

Melanins are a group of pigments whose color varies from light brown to black. The pigment is normally found in the skin, eye, substantia nigra of the brain, and hair follicles (a fuller account of these sites is given later.) Under pathological conditions, it is found in benign nevus cell tumors and malignant melanomas. The chemical structure of the melanins is complex and varies from one type to another. Melanin production is not fully understood but the generally accepted view is that melanins are produced from tyrosine by the action of an enzyme tyrosinase (syn. DOPA oxidase). This enzyme acts on the tyrosine slowly to produce the substance known as DOPA (dihydroxyphenylalanine) which is subsequently rapidly acted upon by the same enzyme to produce an intermediate pigment which then polymerizes to produce melanin. The later stages of melanogenesis remain largely speculative, and it is beyond the scope of this chapter to evaluate the many studies relating to melanin biosynthesis that have been carried out recently. Pearse (1985) gives a more detailed account of melanin production.

The melanins are bound to proteins, and these complexes are localized in the cytoplasm of cells within so-called 'melanin granules'. Ghadially (1982) described these granules as the end stage of the development of the melanosome as seen at ultrastructural level.

There are four recognized stages of melanosome maturation:

1. Tyrosine is synthesized in the Golgi lamellae and pinched off into vesicles with no melanin present.
2. The characteristic lattice-like appearance becomes evident at this stage.
3. Melanin deposition is first observed.

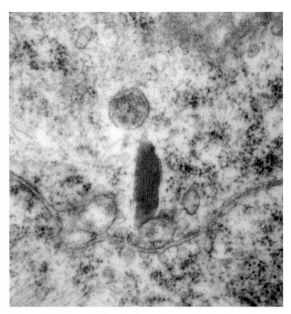

Figure 13.5 Transmission electron micrograph of a stage 3 melanosome, demonstrating the characteristic internal lamellae structure. (Courtesy of Ms Tracey Deharo.)

4. The fully mature granule has its structure obscured by melanin pigment.

Ultrastructurally the lamellar structures become increasingly difficult to see following melanin deposition. By the time the melanosome reaches stage 4 the lamellae structures are completely obscured (Fig. 13.5).

The enzyme tyrosinase cannot be demonstrated in the mature granule.

The most common sites where melanin can be found are

1. *Skin*, where it is produced by cells called melanocytes that are usually scattered within the basal layer of the epidermis. In certain inflammatory skin diseases melanin may also be found in phagocytic cells ('melanophages') in the upper dermis. The melanophages may also phagocytize other material such as lipofuscins and lipoproteins, thus producing a mixture that after denaturation may give unexpected staining results. Pathological deposition of melanin occurs in a benign lesion

called a nevus or 'mole'. The malignant counterpart to the nevus is the malignant melanoma; it is in the diagnosis of this important tumor, and its metastases, that histological demonstration of melanin finds its most important practical application (Fig. 13.5). Melanin is also found in the hair follicles of dark-haired people.

2. *Eye*, where it is found normally in the choroid, ciliary body, and iris. Similar brown-black pigment is found in the retinal epithelium but its identity with melanin is uncertain. Melanomas can occur in the eye but these tumors are rare.

3. *Brain*, where it is found particularly in the substantia nigra, in such quantities that this structure is macroscopically visible as a black streak on both sides of the mesencephalon. In patients with long-standing Parkinson's disease this area is markedly reduced. Black melanin is also found in patches in the arachnoid covering some human brains, and has been described as having a 'sooty' appearance.

A number of methods can be used for the identification of melanin and melanin-producing cells. The most reliable of these are:

1. Reducing methods such as the Masson-Fontana silver technique and Schmorl's ferric-ferricyanide reduction test.
2. Enzyme methods (e.g. DOPA reaction).
3. Solubility and bleaching characteristics.
4. Fluorescent methods.
5. Immunohistochemistry (melanin activation antigens).

Melanin and its precursors are capable of reducing both silver and acid ferricyanide solutions. It also shows the marked physical property of being completely insoluble in most organic solvents, which is almost certainly due to the fact that formed melanin is tightly bound to protein within the melanosome. The other physical characteristic shown by melanin is its ability to be bleached by strong oxidizing agents. This property is particularly useful when trying to identify nuclear detail in heavily pigmented melanocytic tumors. Further reference to these procedures will follow the conventional demonstration techniques for melanin. These two physical characteristics relate to formed melanin and not to melanin precursors.

The enzyme tyrosinase can be demonstrated by the DOPA reaction and is therefore demonstrable in any cell capable of synthesizing melanin. Cells that have produced an abundance of melanin, and in which the melanosomes are filled with pigment, are said no longer to show tyrosinase activity, but some workers have found that tyrosinase is active in most cells, even though melanin may be present in large quantities.

The fluorescent method depends upon the ability of certain biogenic amines, including DOPA and dopamine, to show fluorescence after exposure to formaldehyde (formalin-induced fluorescence). This method therefore demonstrates melanin precursors rather than formed melanin. Recent advances in antibody production have produced a wide range of antibodies which recognize antigens in the melanin synthesis pathway, e.g. tyrosinase or tyrosinase related protein 1 and 2 (TRP 1 and 2), or those recognizing melanocyte activation antigens, e.g. gp100 (HMB 45), Mart-1 (Melan A). The use of enzyme histochemical procedures is now rarely required.

Reducing methods for melanin

Melanin is a powerful reducing agent and this property is used to demonstrate melanin in two ways:

1. The reduction of ammoniacal silver solutions to form metallic silver without the use of an extraneous reducer is known as the argentaffin reaction. Masson's (1914) method (using Fontana's silver solution) and its various modifications, which also rely on melanin's argentaffin properties, are now widely used for routine purposes. Melanins are blackened by acid silver nitrate solutions. Melanin is also argyrophilic, meaning that melanin is colored black by silver impregnation methods that use an extraneous reducer (Fig. 13.6). This is not a property considered to be of diagnostic value.

2. Melanin will reduce ferricyanide to ferrocyanide with the production of Prussian blue in the presence of ferric salts (the Schmorl reaction). This type of reaction (Fig. 13.7) is also seen with certain other pigments (e.g. some lipofuscins, bile, and neuroendocrine cell granules).

3. Other methods for demonstrating melanin are Lillie's ferrous ion uptake (described in Lillie & Fullmer 1976) and Lillie's Nile blue A (1956).

Masson-Fontana method for melanin *(Fontana 1912; Masson 1914)*

Fixation
Formalin is best; chromate and mercuric chloride should be avoided.

Sections
Works on all types of section, although some adjustment may be necessary for resin sections.

Preparation of silver solution *(after Fontana)*
Place 20 ml of a 10% aqueous silver nitrate solution in a glass flask. Using a fine-pointed dropper pipette, add concentrated ammonia drop by drop, constantly agitating the flask until the formed precipitate *almost* dissolves. This titration is critical if the method is to work consistently well. The end point of the titration is seen when a faint opalescence is present, and is best viewed using reflected light against a black background. If too much ammonia is inadvertently added then the addition of a few drops of 10% silver nitrate will restore the opalescence. To this correctly titrated solution add 20 ml triple distilled water and then filter into a dark bottle. Store the solution in the refrigerator and use within 4 weeks.

Note: Ammoniacal silver solutions are potentially explosive if stored incorrectly.

Method
1. Take test and control sections to distilled water.
2. Treat with the ammoniacal silver solution in a Coplin jar that has been covered with aluminum foil, for 30–40 minutes at 56°C or overnight at room temperature.
3. Wash well in several changes of distilled water.
4. Treat sections with 5% aqueous sodium thiosulfate (also known as hypo) for 1 minute.
5. Wash well in running tap water for 2–3 minutes.

6. Lightly counterstain in 0.5% aqueous neutral red or 0.1% aqueous nuclear fast red for 5 minutes.
7. Rinse in distilled water.
8. Dehydrate, clear, and mount in a synthetic resin.

Results
Melanin, argentaffin, chromaffin and some lipofuscins	black
Nuclei	red

Notes
a. Only use thoroughly clean glassware, as the silver solution will react with any residual contaminant left on glassware.
b. Prolonged exposure to 56°C may give rise to a fine deposit over the section.
c. Friable material may need to be coated with celloidin as the ammonia in the silver solution could lead to sections lifting off the slide.

Microwave ammoniacal silver method for argentaffin and melanin *(Churukian 2005)* (Fig. 13.6)

Fixation
10% buffered neutral formalin.

Sections
Paraffin.

Preparation of solutions
Ammoniacal silver
To 10 ml of 2% silver nitrate add 5 ml of 0.8% lithium hydroxide monohydrate. Then add 28% ammonium

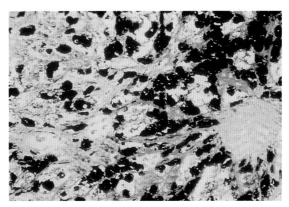

Figure 13.6 A section of liver from a patient with malignant metastatic melanoma stained with Churukian's method for melanin. Melanin is stained black.

hydroxide, drop by drop with constant shaking, until the precipitate almost dissolves. Make up the solution to 200 ml with distilled water and store in a refrigerator at 3–6°C. The solution is stable for at least 1 month.

0.2% aqueous gold chloride
2% aqueous sodium thiosulfate

Method

1. Take slides to distilled water.
2. Place slides in 40 ml of refrigerated cold ammoniacal silver solution in a plastic Coplin jar and microwave at a power setting of 360 W for 35 seconds. Gently agitate the Coplin jar for about 15 seconds. Microwave again at power setting 6 for 35 seconds. Gently agitate the Coplin jar for about 15 seconds. Allow the slides to remain in the hot solution (approximately 80°C) for 2–3 minutes or until the sections appear a light brown.
3. Rinse in four changes of distilled water.
4. Place slides in 0.2% aqueous gold chloride for 1 minute.
5. Rinse in two changes of distilled water.
6. Place slides in 2% aqueous sodium thiosulfate for 1 minute.
7. Rinse in four changes of distilled water.
8. Counterstain with 0.1% aqueous nuclear fast red for 3 minutes.
9. Rinse in three changes of distilled water.
10. Dehydrate, clear, and mount in synthetic resin.

Results

Melanin, argentaffin, chromaffin, lipofuscin and other silver reducing substances	black
Nuclei	red

Notes

The results obtained with this method are similar to those obtained with the Masson-Fontana technique.

a. When preparing the ammoniacal silver solution, care must be taken not to add too much ammonium hydroxide. Add just enough almost to dissolve the precipitate.
b. The microwave oven used in this method had a maximum output of 600 watts with multiple power settings. Microwave ovens of higher or lower wattage may be used for this method by varying the microwave exposure times.

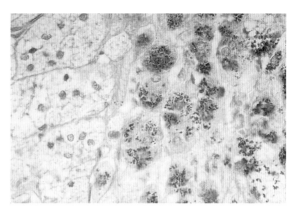

Figure 13.7 A section of adrenal stained with Schmorl's method for reducing substances. Chromaffin is stained blue.

Schmorl's reaction *(taken from Lillie 1954)* (Fig. 13.7)

Fixation

10% buffered neutral formalin.

Solution

Freshly prepared 0.4% aqueous potassium ferricyanide	4 ml
Freshly prepared 1% aqueous ferric chloride (or 1% ferric sulfate)	30 ml

N.B. Use this solution soon after mixing.

Method

1. Take test and control sections to distilled water.
2. Treat sections with the ferric-ferricyanide solution for 5–10 minutes.
3. Wash well in running tap water for several minutes to ensure that all residual ferricyanide is completely removed from the section.
4. Lightly counterstain with 0.5% aqueous neutral red or 0.1% aqueous nuclear fast red for 5 minutes.
5. Dehydrate, clear, and mount in synthetic resin.

Results

Melanin, argentaffin cells, chromaffin, some lipofuscins, thyroid colloid and bile	dark blue
Nuclei	red

Notes

a. This modification is preferred to the more traditional method because it is easier to control and gives less background staining.
b. The time for the reaction to take place depends on the substance to be demonstrated, with melanin

generally reacting faster than lipofuscin. This fact should not be taken as a definitive diagnostic pointer but only as a general guideline.

c. When choosing a control section it is important to remember that melanin reduces the ferric-ferricyanide faster than other reducing substances. Therefore, control sections should always match the test sections so that a lipofuscin control should not be used if the test pigment is thought to be melanin.

Enzyme methods

Cells that are capable of producing melanin can be demonstrated by the DOPA (dihydroxyphenylalanine) method. The enzyme tyrosinase that is localized within these cells will oxidize DOPA to form an insoluble brown-black pigment. The best results are obtained when using post-fixed cryostat sections, although a useful, but less reliable method is that which uses freshly fixed blocks of tissue.

In the past, cells that are capable of producing melanin have been demonstrated by the DOPA-oxidase methods. The enzyme tyrosinase that is located within these cells will oxidize DOPA to form an insoluble brown-black pigment. These methods are those of Bloch (1917) and Laidlaw and Blackberg (1932) for tissue sections, and Bloch (1917) and Rodriguez and McGavran (1969) for tissue blocks. Though previously included in the fifth edition of this book, these methods are currently not in use.

Solubility and bleaching methods

Melanins are insoluble in most organic solvents or in anything that will significantly destroy the tissue that contains them. The insolubility shown by melanin is due to the tight bond it has with its protein component. Use of strong oxidizing agents, such as permanganate, chlorate, chromic acid, peroxide, and peracetic acid, will bleach melanin. The blacker the melanin, the longer the bleach takes to decolor, or bleach, the pigment. Lipofuscin tends to take longer to be bleached from paraffin sections than melanin. The method of choice is peracetic acid, but treatment with 0.25% potassium

permanganate followed by 2% oxalic acid also works well. The difficulty with these procedures is that they can have detrimental effects on the quality of the tissue section following the oxidation steps. In addition, the oxidation can also damage antigenic binding sites for subsequent immunocytochemical investigations. One of the methods of choice is dilute hydrogen peroxide bleaching. Certainly in the investigation of ophthalmic pathology this method has proved popular (Kivela 1995). In cutaneous pathology a method introduced by Orchard (1999, 2007) involving the use of 10% diluted hydrogen peroxide made in a phosphate buffer saline (PBS pH 7.6) and incubated in a water bath or oven at 60°C works very effectively, with complete bleaching being achieved within 1 hour, in the majority of cases. The key benefit of this is that it does not destroy or damage antigenic epitopes and therefore allows an extensive panel of immunocytochemical antibody investigations. Immunocytochemistry is often required in such cases, since the distinction between melanocytes and melanophages (melanin-containing macrophages) is often critical. A good example of this is the need to distinguish between cases of malignant melanoma and dysplastic nevi with extensive dermal melanosis (Figs 13.8a, b and c). This distinction is based on the use of a selective melanocyte antibody, such as HMB 45 (Fig. 13.8d) or Melan A and an antibody that recognizes macrophages for example, CD68 (KP1). This procedure becomes mandatory in cases where melanin deposits are so dense that the nuclear detail of the involved cells is totally obscured. The standard chromogen for immunocytochemical procedures is 3, 3-diaminobenzidine tetrahydrochloride (DAB), which produces a brown reaction product. The use of red chromogens such as alkaline phosphatase may enable clear visualization in some cases, although not often adequate to clearly see the immunocytochemical localization of the antigen to be demonstrated in cases of extensive dermal melanosis. Similarly, stains such as azure B, proposed by Kamino and Tam (1991), which will stain the melanin pigment a green color in an immunocytochemical procedure, can also be employed.

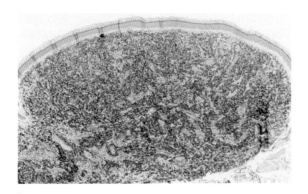

a

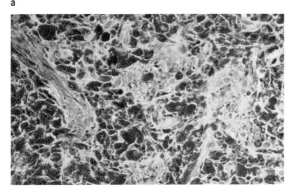

b

Figure 13.8a A section of a dysplastic naevus with extensive dermal melanosis stained with H&E.

Figure 13.8b The same case at higher magnification, showing extensive melanin deposition.

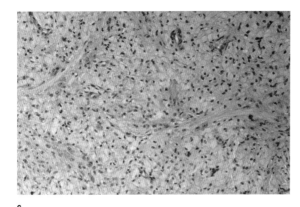

c

Figure 13.8c The same case at the higher magnification bleached prior to H&E staining.

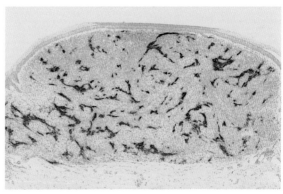

d

Figure 13.8d The same case at lower magnification labeled with HMB 45 following melanin bleaching, demonstrating cords of residual melanocytes remaining following destruction of the lesion by the host immune response. The melanin-containing cells are melanophages. (Courtesy of Ms Tracey Deharo.)

Bleaching melanin pigment using hydrogen peroxide (H_2O_2) *Orchard's method (2007)*

Fixation

10% neutral buffered formalin

Solution

40% H_2O_2	5 ml
Phosphate buffered saline (pH 7.6)	45 ml

(Dissolve PBS tablets according to instructions in 200 ml of distilled water per tablet)

Make the solution fresh and place in a 50 ml Coplin jar.

Method

1. Take test and control sections to distilled water.
2. Prepare the incubating solution fresh and place in a water bath or oven at 60°C for 10 minutes.
3. Place slides into the incubating solution and ensure the Coplin jar lid is securely placed over the jar.
4. Incubate in the jar for 1 hour.
5. Remove slides and wash in running tap water for 3 minutes.
6. Continue with immunocytochemical procedures (heat-mediated or enzyme digestion antigen retrieval techniques).

Notes

a. The melanin bleaching effect can be seen with the naked eye in 1 hour with most cases. In circumstances of excessive melanin deposition slightly longer incubation times may be required. The end point can be determined by removing slides, washing in tap water, and checking under the staining microscope to ensure completeness of the bleaching effect.

b. Heat-mediated antigen retrieval procedures can be performed according to normal immunocytochemical procedures; enzyme digestion techniques may require reductions in the time for digestion (normally half the usual exposure time).

Formalin-induced fluorescence (FIF)

Certain aromatic amines such as 5-hydroxytryptamine, dopamine, epinephrine (adrenaline), norepinephrine (noradrenaline), and histamine, when exposed to formaldehyde, show a yellow primary fluorescence. This is particularly useful when demonstrating amelanotic melanoma, because these tumors can be difficult to diagnose using conventional methods due to their lack of pigment. Any melanin precursors present will form a product of isocarboline derivatives that are dehydrogenated and will show yellow fluorescence. The best results are seen when using tissue that has been freeze-dried (Chapter 7) and then fixed using paraformaldehyde vapor. Formalin-fixed frozen sections will give acceptable results. Paraffin-processed tissue can also be used but shows weak fluorescence that is difficult to visualize.

Formaldehyde-induced fluorescence method for melanin precursor cells *(Eranko 1955)*

Fixation
10% buffered neutral formalin.

Sections
Cryostat, or 5 μm paraffin sections.

Method

1. Deparaffinize sections in xylene. Fix frozen sections in 10% buffered formalin for 5 minutes, dehydrate, and place in xylene.
2. Rinse in fresh xylene.
3. Mount in a medium that is fluorescence free.
4. Examine using a fluorescence microscope with BG38, UG1, and a barrier filter.

Results
Melanin precursor cells   weak yellow fluorescence

Notes

a. A brighter image will be seen if epi-illumination is used.

b. Some commercially produced mountants are unsuitable as they fluoresce and will confuse the result.

c. One of the claims originally made about FIF was that archived paraffin-processed material could be examined to see if there was evidence of melanin precursor cells, but because of the indifferent results it is not widely used.

Ferrous ion uptake reaction for melanin
(Lillie & Fullmer 1976) **(Fig. 13.9)**

Fixation
Formalin is best: avoid all chromate fixatives.

Sections
Paraffin.

Solutions
2.5% ferrous sulfate
1% potassium ferricyanide in 1% acetic acid

Method

1. Take test and control sections to distilled water.
2. Place in 2.5% ferrous sulfate for 1 hour.
3. Wash with six changes of distilled water.
4. Place in 1% potassium ferricyanide in 1% acetic acid for 30 minutes.
5. Wash with four changes of distilled water.
6. Counterstain with 0.5% aqueous neutral red or 0.1% nuclear fast red.
7. Rinse in two changes of distilled water.
8. Dehydrate, clear, and mount in synthetic resin.

Results
Melanins and neuromelanin   dark green
Nuclei   red

Notes

a. According to Lillie, this method is specific for melanin.

b. Ferric iron and lipofuscins do not stain with the method.

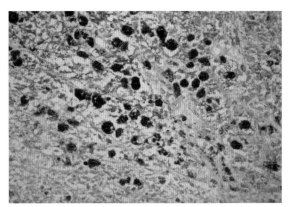

Figure 13.9 A section of liver from a patient with malignant melanoma stained with Lillie's ferrous ion uptake method for melanin. Melanin is stained black.

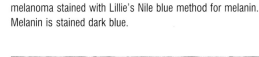

Figure 13.10 A section of liver from a patient with malignant melanoma stained with Lillie's Nile blue method for melanin. Melanin is stained dark blue.

Nile blue method for melanin and lipofuscin (Lillie 1956) (Figs 13.10 and 13.11)

Fixation

10% buffered neutral formalin.

Sections

Paraffin.

Solution

Dissolve 0.05 g Nile blue (CI 51180) in 99 ml of distilled water and then add 1.0 ml of sulfuric acid.

Method

1. Take test and control sections to distilled water.
2. Place in Nile blue solution for 20 minutes.
3. Wash with four changes of distilled water.
4. Mount in an aqueous mountant (e.g. glycerin jelly).

Results

Melanin	dark blue
Lipofuscin	dark blue
Nuclei	blue or unstained

Notes

a. Some samples of Nile blue may not yield satisfactory results with this method.

b. Using frozen sections, this method will stain neutral lipids (triglycerides, cholesterol esters, and steroids) red to pink. Acidic lipids (fatty acids and phospholipids) stain blue.

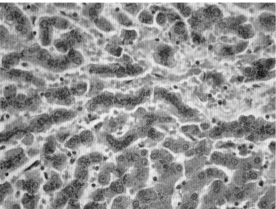

Figure 13.11 A section of liver stained with Lillie's Nile blue method for lipofuscin. Lipofuscin within the hepatocytes is stained dark blue.

Immunohistochemistry

Brief mention should be given to the use of melanocyte selective antibodies to highlight melanocytic lesions. The large majority of these antibodies recognize an antigen associated with melanocyte activation, gp100 (HMB 45) or Mart-1 (Melan A). Other selective antibodies such as tyrosinase are directly linked to antigens associated with melanin synthesis. These antibodies are highly valuable in cases of delineating atypical melanocytic lesions from a host of other tumor types, particularly if the lesions are amelanotic. The histological and morphological appearances of malignant melanomas can be highly variable, with epithelioid, spindle or even small round cell appearances to the tumor cells. There are currently no antibodies that can reliably distinguish between malignant and benign melanocytic lesions for use in routine histopathology. The 'gold standard' antibody remains S100 protein, since it will label the majority of melanocytic lesions. However, this antibody recognizes an antigen expressed in cells derived from the neural crest and, as such, is not specific for melanocytes alone. In difficult cases a panel of antibodies is often applicable (Orchard 2000).

Lipofuscins

These yellow to red-brown pigments occur widely throughout the body and are thought to be produced by an oxidation process of lipids and lipoproteins. The oxidation process occurs slowly and progressively, and therefore the pigments exhibit variable staining reactions, different colors, and variation in shape and size, which appears to be dependent upon their situation. This type of pigment is found in the following sites:

- Hepatocytes, sometimes as a mixture with other types of pigment.
- Cardiac muscle cells, particularly around the nucleus. Large amounts of pigment are found in the small brown hearts of elderly debilitated people, a condition known as 'brown atrophy of the heart'.
- Inner reticular layer of the normal adrenal cortex, where the pigment imparts a brown color and is particularly prominent in patients dying after a long and stressful illness.
- Testis, particularly in the interstitial cells of Leydig; it is responsible for giving testicular tissue its brown color.
- Ovary, in the walls of involuting corpora lutea and in some macrophages around the corpora lutea. Hemosiderin tends to be seen more commonly in this situation.
- Cytoplasmic inclusions in the neurons of the brain, spinal cord, and ganglia.

- The edge of a cerebral hemorrhage or infarct.
- Some lipid storage disorders such as Batten's disease.
- Other tissues such as bone marrow, involuntary muscle, cervix, and kidney.

Demonstration of lipofuscins

It is important to bear in mind that because lipofuscin is formed by a slow progressive oxidation process of lipids and lipoproteins, histochemical reactions will vary according to the degree of oxidation present in the pigment when the demonstration techniques are applied. Therefore, it is advisable to carry out a variety of techniques in order to be sure whether the pigment is lipofuscin. The lipofuscins react with a variety of histochemical and tinctorial staining methods, the most common and useful being:

- Periodic acid-Schiff method
- Schmorl's ferric-ferricyanide reduction test (see above)
- Long Ziehl-Neelsen method (see below)
- Sudan black B method
- Gomori's aldehyde fuchsin technique (Fig. 13.12)
- Masson-Fontana silver method (see above)
- Basophilia, using methyl green
- Churukian's silver method
- Lillie's Nile blue sulfate method.

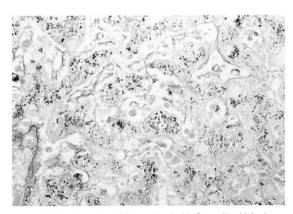

Figure 13.12 A section of liver stained with Gomori's aldehyde fuchsin. Lipofuscin is stained purple.

Long Ziehl-Neelsen method *(Pearse 1953)*

Fixation
Any fixative.

Sections
Works well on all types of tissue section.

Method
1. Slides to distilled water.
2. Stain in a Coplin jar with filtered carbol fuchsin using a 60°C water bath for 3 hours, or overnight at room temperature.
3. Wash well in running water.
4. Differentiate in 1% acid alcohol until the background staining is removed.
5. Wash well in running tap water.
6. Counterstain nuclei with 0.25% aqueous methylene blue in 1% aqueous acetic acid for 1 minute.
7. Dehydrate, clear, and mount in synthetic resin.

Results

Lipofuscin	magenta
Ceroid	magenta
Nuclei	blue
Background	pale magenta to pale blue

Notes
a. Experience has shown that a more reliable result is obtained if the staining is carried out using a thermostatically controlled water bath.
b. A useful variant of this method is cited by Lillie (1954), in which the staining solution is modified so that Victoria blue is substituted for basic fuchsin. It is sometimes difficult to distinguish between the red of the fuchsin and the red-brown of the pigment, whereas the blue color of lipofuscin with the Victoria blue may be more convincing.

Aldehyde fuchsin technique *(Gomori 1950)* (Fig. 13.12)

Fixative
10% buffered neutral formalin.

Sections
Paraffin.

Solutions

Acidified potassium permanganate solution
(0.25% aqueous potassium permanganate in 0.1% sulfuric acid)
2% aqueous oxalic acid

Aldehyde fuchsin
Dissolve 1 g pararosanilin (CI 42500) in 100 ml aqueous 70% ethanol. Add 1 ml concentrated hydrochloric acid and 2 ml paraldehyde or acetylaldehyde, shaking the mixture thoroughly. Stand for 3–5 days at room temperature or preferably longer, near natural light, to allow the solution to blue. Store the solution at 4°C. The solution will remain viable for approximately 2 months. Any increase in the background staining will indicate deterioration of the staining solution.

Method
1. Sections to distilled water.
2. Treat with acidified potassium permanganate solution for 5 minutes.
3. Wash well in distilled water and treat for 2 minutes with oxalic acid solution to bleach section.
4. Wash well in distilled water.
5. Rinse in 70% ethyl alcohol.
6. Stain section in aldehyde fuchsin for 5 minutes. Longer staining times will be needed as the solution ages.
7. Rinse in 70% ethyl alcohol followed by a rinse in three changes of distilled water.
8. Dehydrate, clear, and mount in synthetic resin.

Results

Lipofuscin	purple
Elastic fibers	purple

Notes
a. Paraldehyde should be freshly opened (Moment 1969). It keeps well when stored in the freezing compartment of a refrigerator. If paraldehyde is not available, acetaldehyde may be used and need not be refrigerated.
b. Other tissue constituents, such as beta cells of the pancreas and pituitary, elastin, sulfated mucins, gastric chief cells, and neurosecretory granules, will stain with this method.
c. The basic fuchsins, rosanilin and new fuchsin are closely related to pararosanilin. Only pararosanilin will give satisfactory staining results in this procedure.

Chromaffin

This pigment is normally found in the cells of the adrenal medulla as dark brown, granular material. It may occur in tumors of the adrenal medulla (pheochromocytomas).

Fixation in formalin is not recommended, and fixatives containing alcohol, mercury bichloride, or acetic acid should be avoided. Orth's or other dichromate-containing fixatives are recommended. Chromaffin may be demonstrated by Schmorl's reaction, Lillie's Nile blue A, the Masson-Fontana, Churukian's microwave ammoniacal silver method, and the periodic acid-Schiff (PAS) technique.

Pseudomelanosis pigment (melanosis coli)

This pigment is sometimes seen in macrophages in the lamina propria of the large intestine and appendix. Various theories have been put forward as to its nature. The current view is that it is an endogenous lipopigment whose reactions are those of a typical ceroid-type lipofuscin. It appears to be strongly associated with anthraquinone purgatives ('cascara sagrada'). Its distinction from melanin may occasionally be important. Pseudomelanosis will, in general, stain with those methods that are used to demonstrate lipofuscin, such as Masson-Fontana and Schmorl.

Dubin-Johnson pigment

This pigment is found in the liver of patients with Dubin-Johnson syndrome and is due to defective canalicular transport of bilirubin. It is characterized by the presence of a brownish-black, granular, intracellular pigment situated in the centrilobular hepatocytes. The true nature of the pigment has yet to be established, but histochemically it is similar to lipofuscin, though there are ultrastructural differences.

Ceroid-type lipofuscins

Lillie et al. (1941, 1942) were the first to describe ceroid in the cirrhotic livers of animals maintained on inadequate diets. Lillie thought that ceroid was different from lipofuscin because it failed to stain with the ferric-ferricyanide reaction. Pearse (1985) states that ceroid is in fact a lipofuscin at an early stage of oxidation. Further oxidation would produce lipofuscin proper.

Hamazaki-Weisenberg bodies

These small, yellow-brown, spindle-shaped structures are found mainly in the sinuses of lymph nodes, either lying free or as cytoplasmic inclusions, and their significance is unknown. First described by Hamazaki (1938), they have been described as being present in lymph nodes from patients with sarcoidosis (Weisenberg 1966). Further studies have shown them to be present in a number of conditions (Boyd & Valentine 1970). Hall and Eusebi (1978) have reported their presence in association with melanosis coli. Histochemically they are similar to lipofuscin, and at ultrastructural level have an appearance that suggests that they are probably giant lysosomal residual bodies (Doyle et al. 1973).

Endogenous minerals

Iron is discussed under the heading 'Hematogenous pigments'.

Calcium

Insoluble inorganic calcium salts are a normal constituent of bones and teeth, and their demonstration is well covered in Chapter 16. From a histochemical viewpoint, the free ionic form of calcium, found in the blood, cannot be demonstrated. Abnormal depositions of calcium can be found in necrotic areas of tissue associated with tuberculosis, infarction (Gandy-Gamna bodies), atheroma in blood vessels, and malakoplakia of the bladder (Michaelis-Gutman bodies). The most common forms of calcium salts occurring in these conditions are phosphates and carbonates. Calcium salts are usually monorefringent but calcium oxalate is birefringent (Fig. 13.13). Calcium usually stains purple blue with H&E.

The use of various dyes that act by forming chelate complexes with calcium has been practiced by many workers. These dyes include alizarin red S, purpurin, naphthochrome green B, and nuclear fast red. In

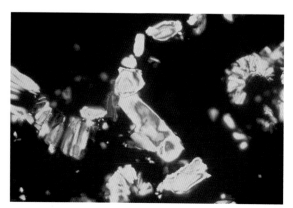

Figure 13.13 A section of kidney with calcium oxalate crystals as seen with polarization microscopy.

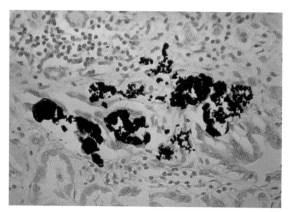

Figure 13.14 A section of kidney stained with von Kossa's silver nitrate method for calcium. An ultraviolet lamp was used to perform the method. Calcium is stained black.

general, these dyes demonstrate medium to large amounts of calcium better than particulate deposits that stain weakly, the exception being alizarin red S, which tends to give more reliable results with small deposits. None of these dyes is specific to calcium salts, although alizarin red S when used at pH 4.2 is so considered. The classic method of von Kossa (1901), which uses silver nitrate, is generally preferred for routine demonstration purposes on paraffin sections (Fig. 13.14).

This method demonstrates only phosphate and carbonate radicals, giving good results with both large and small deposits of calcium. The method is not specific, as melanin will also reduce silver to give a black deposit. As a general rule, fixation of tissue containing calcium deposits is best when using non-acidic fixatives such as buffered neutral formalin, formal alcohol, or alcohol.

Alizarin red S method for calcium (*Dahl 1952; McGee-Russell 1958; Luna 1968*)

Fixation

Buffered neutral formalin, formal alcohol, and alcohol.

Sections

Paraffin or frozen.

Solutions

1% aqueous alizarin red S (CI 58005) adjusted to pH 4.2 or pH 6.3–6.5 (see Note c) with 10% ammonium hydroxide.
0.05% fast green FCF (CI 42053) in 0.2% acetic acid.

Method

1. Sections to 95% alcohol.
2. Stand slides on end and thoroughly air dry.
3. Place sections in a Coplin jar filled with the alizarin red S solution for 5 minutes (see Notes below).
4. Rinse quickly in distilled water.
5. Counterstain with fast green for 1 minute.
6. Rinse in three changes of distilled water.
7. Dehydrate, clear, and mount in synthetic resin.

Results

Calcium deposits	orange-red
Background	green

Notes

a. The staining time is dependent on the amount of calcium present.
b. Calcium deposits are birefringent after staining with alizarin red S.
c. McGee-Russell recommends using the alizarin red S at pH 4.2. Dahl indicated that it be used at pH 6.36 to pH 6.4. Churukian is in agreement with Dahl as to the higher pH and has observed that a pH as high as 7.0 produces good results.
d. This method is particularly useful in the identification and detection of small amounts of calcium like those seen in heterotropic calcification in the kidney (hypercalcinosis). This type of tissue also makes excellent control material (Fig. 13.15).

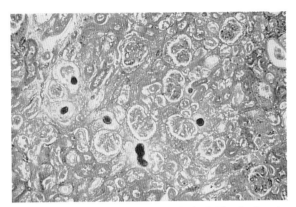

Figure 13.15 A section of kidney stained with Dahl's alizarin red S method at pH 6.4. Calcium is stained orange-red.

Copper

Many enzymes in the body would fail to function without the presence of copper, although copper deficiency is extremely rare. Copper accumulation is associated with Wilson's disease, the most important disorder of copper metabolism. This disease is a rare, inherited, autosomal recessive condition which gives rise to copper deposition in the liver, basal ganglia of the brain, and eyes. In the eye, the Kayser-Fleischer ring, a brown ring of deposited copper, may be seen in the cornea (Descemet's membrane), and is diagnostic of this condition. Copper deposition in the liver is also associated with primary biliary cirrhosis and certain other hepatic disorders.

Copper, like many metallic cations, is capable of forming a blue dye lake using Mallory's unripened hematoxylin. Uzman (1956) modified the Okamoto-Utamura rubeanate method (1938) and obtained excellent results on formalin-fixed tissue. The rhodanine method (Lindquist 1969) has also been used to demonstrate copper and copper-associated protein (CAP). Although the quality of the reagent, dimethylaminobenzylidine rhodanine (DMABR), varies considerably, it is considered to be the method of choice. CAP is also well demonstrated by the Shikata orcein method (Shikata et al. 1974).

Rubeanic acid method for copper *(Okamoto & Utamura 1938; Uzman 1956)*

Fixative

10% buffered neutral formalin.

Solution

0.1% rubeanic acid (dithio-oxamide) in absolute ethyl alcohol	5 ml
10% aqueous sodium acetate	100 ml

Prepare fresh before use.

Method

1. Take the test section, together with a known positive control section, to distilled water.
2. Place sections in a Coplin jar filled with rubeanic-acetate solution for at least 16 hours at 37°C. Times may need to be extended and the method is best carried out in a water bath.
3. Wash in 70% ethyl alcohol.
4. Rinse briefly in distilled water.
5. Drain section and blot dry.
6. Lightly counterstain with 0.5% aqueous neutral red or 0.1% aqueous nuclear fast red for 1 minute.
7. Rinse in distilled water.
8. Dehydrate, clear, and mount in synthetic resin.

Results

Copper	greenish black
Nuclei	pale red

Notes

a. Correct choice of fixative is essential. Buffered neutral formalin is acceptable, but avoid the use of acid formalin and fixatives containing mercury and chromium salts.
b. To demonstrate any copper that is bound to CAP, deparaffinized sections are placed downwards over a beaker of concentrated hydrochloric acid for 15 minutes. The sections are washed well in absolute alcohol and then transferred to the rubeanic-acetate solution.
c. The method is best carried out using a thermostatically controlled water bath.

Modified rhodanine technique *(Lindquist 1969)*

Fixative

10% buffered neutral formalin.

Sections

Paraffin.

Solutions

Rhodanine stock solution

5-*p*-Dimethylaminobenzylidene-rhodanine	0.05 g
Absolute ethanol	25 ml

Prepare fresh and filter prior to use.

Working solution

Take 5 ml of the stock rhodanine solution and add to 45 ml of 2% sodium acetate trihydrate.

Borax solution

Disodium tetraborate	0.5 g
Distilled water	100 ml

Method

1. Take test and control sections to water.
2. Incubate in the rhodanine working solution at 56°C for 3 hours or overnight in a 37°C oven.
3. Rinse in several changes of distilled water for 3 minutes.
4. Stain in acidified Lillie-Mayer or other alum hematoxylin for 10 seconds.
5. Briefly rinse in distilled water and place immediately in borax solution for 15 seconds.
6. Rinse well in distilled water.
7. Mount with Apathy's mounting media.

Results

Copper and copper-associated protein	red to orange-red
Nuclei	blue
Bile	green

Notes

a. Certain synthetic mountants will cause fading of the copper and CAP in archived material. No fading occurs when sections are mounted with Apathy's media. This method will give the most consistent results when in the hands of an experienced practitioner.

c. Results help distinguish between bile and iron pigments (Irons et al. 1977).

d. Analytical grade reagents and triple distilled water are recommended when performing this technique.

e. Control material is best obtained from livers of patients suffering from Wilson's disease, primary biliary cirrhosis, or other forms of chronic cholestasis. Fetal liver of the third trimester (Fig. 13.16) fixed in buffered neutral formalin for not more than 36 hours makes a good positive control.

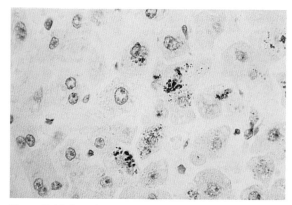

Figure 13.16 A section of fetal liver of the third trimester stained with Lindquist's method for copper. Copper is stained red to orange-red.

Uric acid and urates

Uric acid is a breakdown product of the body's purine (nucleic acid) metabolism, although a small proportion is obtained from the diet. Most, but not all, uric acid is excreted by the kidneys. The uric acid circulating in the blood is in the form of monosodium urate, which in patients with gout may be high, forming a supersaturated solution. These high levels may result in urate depositions, which are water soluble in tissues, causing:

- subcutaneous nodular deposits of urate crystals (known as 'tophi')
- synovitis and arthritis
- renal disease and calculi

Another condition that occasionally can mimic gout is known as *pseudogout* or *chondrocalcinosis*, and is a pyrophosphate arthropathy. This results in calcium pyrophosphate crystals being deposited in joint cartilage. The cause of this deposition is unknown and is more common in the elderly, affecting mainly the large joints, such as the knee. It is important that gout and pseudogout are distinguishable.

To aid the diagnosis, a polarizing microscope fitted with a quartz, first-order, red compensator will prove useful, although sellotape applied in a single strip on a glass slide can occasionally suffice! Whilst pyrophosphate crystals exhibit a positive birefringence (Fig. 13.17a) as small cuboidal/oblong

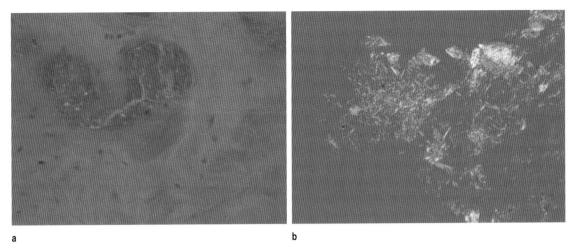

a

b

Figure 13.17 Visualized through a quartz first-order red compensator, small, rather brick-like/oblong pyrophosphate crystals (pseudogout) exhibit a positive birefringence (a), contrasting with the needle-shaped urate crystals (b) which show a negative birefringence.

crystals often within the tissues, urate crystals show a negative birefringence with needle-shaped crystals (Fig. 13.17b). If sections have been prepared from routine formalin-fixed, paraffin-processed material, many crystals may have been leached out. Urates can be extracted by saturated aqueous lithium carbonate solution (Gomori 1951), while pyrophosphate crystals are unaffected. If this extraction sequence is used in combination with Grocott's modification of Gomori's hexamine silver technique, both types of crystal can usually be identified.

Lithium carbonate extraction-hexamine silver technique
(Gomori 1936, 1951; Grocott 1955)

Fixation

Urate crystals are water soluble, therefore fixation in alcohol will give a more specific reaction.

Sections

Paraffin, frozen, or celloidin.

Solutions

Grocott's hexamine silver solution
Saturated aqueous lithium carbonate solution
2% aqueous sodium thiosulfate (hypo)
0.05% aqueous fast green (CI 42053) in 0.2% acetic acid

Method

1. Take two test sections and two control sections to 70% ethyl alcohol.
2. Place one section from each pair in saturated aqueous lithium carbonate solution for 30 minutes.
3. Rinse all sections in distilled water.
4. Place all sections in a Coplin jar filled with hexamine silver solution for 1 hour at 45°C.
5. Wash sections in distilled water.
6. Treat sections with hypo for 30 seconds.
7. Counterstain with fast green solution for 1 minute.
8. Wash in water, dehydrate, clear, and mount in synthetic resin.

Results

Extracted sections	urates only are extracted
Unextracted sections	urates and possibly pyrophosphates are blackened
Background	green

Notes

a. The urates reduce the silver solution due to their argentaffin properties.
b. More accurate control of incubation temperature is achievable using a thermostatically controlled water bath.

Artifact pigments

This group of pigments comprises:

- formalin
- malaria
- schistosome
- mercury
- chromic oxide
- starch

Formalin pigment

This pigment is seen as a brown or brown-black deposit in tissues that have been fixed in acidic formalin. The deposit is usually present in blood-rich tissues such as spleen, hemorrhagic lesions, and large blood vessels filled with blood. The morphology of the pigment can vary but is commonly seen as a microcrystalline deposit that is anisotropic (birefringent). It is related to the acid hematins, but is spectroscopically distinct from hydrochloric acid and acetic acid hematins (Herschberger & Lillie 1947).

One way of removing this pigment from tissue sections is by treating unstained tissue sections with saturated alcoholic picric acid. Alcoholic solutions of both sodium and potassium hydroxide will also remove the pigment but these may have deleterious effects on subsequent staining techniques. Treatment with 10% ammonium hydroxide in 70% alcohol for 5–15 minutes will remove this pigment and is less harmful to tissue sections than the other hydroxides. The use of buffered neutral formalin will help to minimize the problem of formalin pigment deposition. Fixation of large blood-rich organs, such as spleen, for a long period will tend to increase the amount of formalin pigment formed. Under these conditions it is advisable to change the fixative on a regular basis.

Malarial pigment

This pigment is morphologically similar to formalin pigment and occasionally may be identical, even though it is produced in a slightly different manner.

It is formed within, or in the region of, red blood cells that contain the malarial parasites (*Plasmodium malariae*, *ovale*, *vivax* and *falciparum*). In cases of cerebral malaria, due to infection with *Plasmodium falciparum*, malarial pigment can be seen in, or over, the red blood cells within the tiny blood capillaries of the brain. The presence of heavy erythrocyte parasitization areas provides the support for the diagnosis before confirmatory histochemistry. The pigment may, on occasion, be so heavily deposited that it obscures the visualization of the malarial parasite. Malarial pigment may also be present within phagocytic cells that have ingested infected red cells. Therefore one should carefully examine the Kupffer cells of the liver, the sinus lining cells of lymph nodes and spleen, and within phagocytic cells in the bone marrow. Malarial pigment, like formalin pigment, exhibits birefringence and can be removed from tissue sections with saturated alcoholic picric acid, but usually requires 12–24 hours treatment for complete removal.

Much less time is required to remove the pigment by using 10% ammonium hydroxide, as described above.

Extraction method for formalin and malarial pigment

Solutions

10% ammonium hydroxide in 70% ethyl alcohol.

Method

1. Sections to 70% ethyl alcohol.
2. Place sections in a Coplin jar containing ammonium hydroxide alcohol for 5–15 minutes.
3. Wash well in distilled water.
4. Apply staining method desired.

Notes

a. The time necessary for the removal of formalin pigment will vary, depending on the amount of pigment present.
b. Malarial pigment usually requires treatment for at least 15 minutes or longer.

Schistosome pigment

This pigment is occasionally seen in tissue sections where infestation with *Schistosoma* is 'present'. The pigment, which tends to be chunky, shows similar properties to those of both formalin and malaria pigments.

Mercury pigment

This pigment is seen in tissues that have been fixed in mercury-containing fixatives, although it is rarely seen in tissue fixed in Heidenhain's Susa. Mercury pigment varies in its appearance but it is usually seen as a brown-black, extracellular crystal. Although usually seen as monorefringent, occasionally it is birefringent, particularly when formalin-fixed tissue has been secondarily fixed in formal mercury.

A little-known but unusual finding is that prolonged storage of stained sections that contain mercury pigment can bring about a change in the structure of the pigment. The pigment changes from crystalline to a globular form (H.C. Cook, personal communication). The reason for this is unclear but it may be caused by interaction between the pigment and the mounting medium. Furthermore, the globular form exhibits a Maltese cross birefringence.

Treatment of sections with iodine solutions, such as Lugol's iodine, is the classical method of removing the pigment. Subsequent bleaching with a weak sodium thiosulfate (hypo) solution completes the treatment.

It is advisable *not* to remove mercury pigment with iodine solutions prior to staining with Gram's method. The effect is such that connective tissue will take up the crystal violet and then resist acetone color removal. Staining methods such as phosphotungstic acid hematoxylin may be impaired if 'hypo' is used before staining.

Chromic oxide

This pigment is rarely seen in tissue sections and is extremely difficult to produce intentionally. When seen, it presents as a fine yellow-brown particulate deposit in tissues, as a result of not washing in water, tissues that have been fixed in chromic acid or dichromate-containing fixatives. Subsequent treatment of tissues with graded alcohols, as used in tissue processors, may result in the reduction of chrome salts to the chromic oxides, which are

insoluble in alcohol. The pigment is monorefringent and extracellular. It can be removed from sections by treatment with 1% acid alcohol.

Starch

This pigment is introduced by powder from the gloves of surgeons, nurses, or pathologists. It is PAS and Gomori methenamine silver (GMS) positive and can be easily identified by its characteristic appearance. When polarized, it will produce a Maltese cross configuration.

Exogenous pigments and minerals

Although often listed as being exogenous pigments, the majority of the following substances are, in fact, colorless. Some of these substances are inert and unreactive, while other materials can be visualized in tissue sections using various histochemical methods that are often capricious and unreliable. Most routine surgical pathology laboratories rarely see this type of material. Certain types of mineral gain access to the body by inhalation, ingestion, or skin implantation, commonly as a result of industrial exposure. Some minerals, in the form of dye complexes, can be seen in the skin and adjacent lymph nodes as a result of tattooing. Occasionally mineral deposition may occur due to medication or wound dressing. Where there is a need to identify one of these substances, for example with an industrial injury insurance claim, then use of the electron probe micro analyzer (EDAX) will prove to be the most reliable method. This specialized piece of equipment can usually be found in teaching and research laboratories.

The most common minerals seen in tissue sections are carbon, silica, and asbestos. Other less common minerals that may be present in tissues are lead, beryllium, aluminum, mercury, silver, and bismuth.

Tattoo pigment

This is associated with skin and any adjacent lymphoid areas. If viewed using reflected light, the

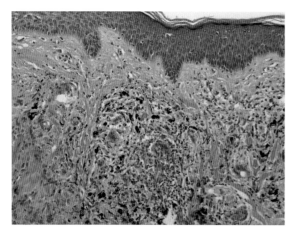

Figure 13.18 A section of skin demonstrating exogenous tattoo pigment in a tattoo granuloma stained with hematoxylin and eosin.

various colors of the dye pigments used to create the tattoo can be seen (Fig. 13.18).

Amalgam tattoo

Brown-black areas of pigmentation in the mouth may result from traumatic introduction of mercury and silver from dental amalgam during dental procedures. Histologically, brown granules are deposited in collagen, basement membranes, nerve sheath, blood vessel walls, and elastic fibers. The pattern of distribution is similar to that seen in the skin in argyria.

Carbon

This exogenous substance is the most commonly seen mineral in tissues and is easily recognized in stained tissue sections. Commonly found in the lung and adjacent lymph nodes of urban dwellers, the main sources of this material are car exhausts and smoke from domestic and industrial pollution. Tobacco smokers also inhale particulate carbon, and also give passers-by a small sample. Inhaled carbon particles generally are trapped by the thin film of mucus in the nose, pharynx, trachea, and bronchi. A small amount can find the way into the alveoli of the lung, where the particulate matter is phagocytosed by alveolar macrophages. Some carbon particles will also find their way into the

peribronchiolar lymphatics and lymph nodes draining the lungs.

Heavy black pigmentation of the lung (anthracosis) may be seen as a result of massive deposition of carbonaceous matter in coal workers. Indeed, the lungs can appear almost black. Whilst not all coal workers will develop lung disease, the lung disorder known as coal workers' pneumoconiosis is caused by the inhalation of silica, coal dust, and many other particulates. The silica and other minerals are found in association with coal and other mined ores. Coal workers are also prone to cuts and abrasions while working, and coal 'tattoos' are fairly common in the skin.

The carbonaceous material is relatively inert and fails to be demonstrated with conventional histological stains and histochemical methods. The site and nature of the carbon deposits make identification relatively easy. In skin tissues it can be confused with melanin deposition, but treatment with bleaching agents will show carbon unaffected, whereas in the case of melanin the color will disappear.

Silica

Silica in the form of silicates is associated with the majority of all mined ores, because they are found in, or near, rocks that contain silica. Mine workers can inhale large quantities of silica, which can give rise to the disease silicosis. This disease may present as a progressive pulmonary fibrotic condition which gives rise to impaired lung capacity and in some cases extreme disability. Silicates are also abundant in stone and sand, and any industrial worker involved in grinding stone, sandblasting or equivalent will be at risk from silicosis. Silica is unreactive, and is thus not demonstrated by histological stains and histochemical methods. It is weakly anisotropic (birefringent) when examined using polarized light, but the coexisting mica absorbed does show as refractile particulate matter. The histology of the scarring, nevertheless, is fairly characteristic.

Asbestos

Asbestos has been used for many years as a fire-resistant and insulating material. There are two

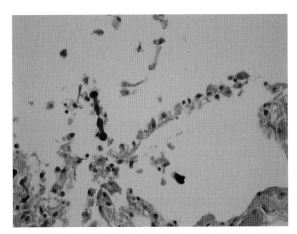

Figure 13.19 A H&E-stained section of lung alveoli demonstrating an amphibole fiber (ferruginous body) coated with hemosiderin pigment in a case of mesothelioma.

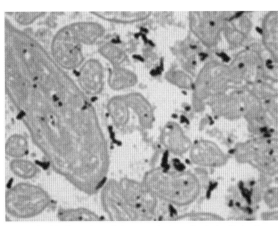

Figure 13.20 A section of placenta that was treated with lead nitrate stained with Lillie's rhodizonate method for lead. Lead is stained black.

groups of asbestos that cause pulmonary disease in humans: serpentine (curly fibers) and amphibole (straight/chain-like fibers). There is one type of serpentine asbestos known as white asbestos (chrysotile). There are many types of amphibole asbestos; the most common are blue asbestos (crocidolite) and brown asbestos (amosite) (Fig. 13.19). Perhaps the most dangerous type is crocidolite (blue asbestos). The fibers are 5–100 μm long and only 0.25–0.5 μm in diameter, and can collect in the alveoli at the periphery of the lung. These fibers are anisotropic but fail to show birefringence when they appear as an asbestos body, because of the protein coat covering the fiber. The characteristic appearance of the asbestos body is as a beaded, yellow-brown, dumb-bell shape in lung sections. The proteinaceous coat contains hemosiderin and is positive with Perls' Prussian blue. Micro-incineration techniques can be used to demonstrate asbestos fibers, as they withstand the high temperatures produced by the oven. In cases where asbestosis is suspected but no asbestos fibers or bodies are readily demonstrable, lung tissue can be digested with 40% sodium hydroxide or ashed. The resultant tissue sludge is then centrifuged and washed in water. Smears from the deposit are made and examined using polarized light or using transition electron

microscopy +/− EDAX. This method has proved to be reliable when detecting/counting asbestos fibers and bodies. Alternatively, thick paraffin sections (20 μm) of lung tissue are mounted on glass slides coated with an adhesive. The sections are dewaxed and mounted unstained, then examined using polarized light.

Lead

Environmental pollution due to lead has greatly reduced in recent decades. Lead pipes that carried much of the domestic water supply have been replaced by alternative materials. Lead in paint, batteries, and gasoline has been reduced by the various manufacturers. Cases of lead poisoning are rare and are usually diagnosed biochemically using the serum from suspected cases. In chronic lead poisoning, excessive amounts can be deposited within many tissues, particularly bone and kidney tubules. For many years various methods have been used to demonstrate lead in tissue sections; the most popular method is the rhodizonate method (Lillie 1954) (Fig. 13.20). Other methods for lead include the sulfide-silver of Timm (1958) and the unripened hematoxylin technique of Mallory and Parker (1939), although neither of these is specific for lead.

Rhodizonate method for lead salts *(Lillie 1954)*

Fixation

Avoid the use of mercury-containing fixatives. Bones containing lead salts can be decalcified in 5–10% sulfuric acid containing 5–10% sodium sulfate. This procedure should convert lead deposits into insoluble lead sulfate.

Sections

Paraffin.

Solutions

Sodium rhodizonate	100 mg
Distilled water	50 ml
Glacial acetic acid	0.5 ml

0.05% fast green FCF (42053) in 0.02% acetic acid

Method

1. Sections to distilled water.
2. Place in rhodizonate solution for 1 hour.
3. Rinse well in distilled water.
4. Counterstain in 0.05% aqueous fast green in 0.2% acetic acid for 1 minute.
5. Rinse in three changes of distilled water.
6. Dehydrate, clear, and mount in synthetic resin.

Results

Lead salts	black
Background	green

Notes

a. This method relies on any lead salts present forming a red chelated compound when treated with the chelating agent sodium rhodizonate.
b. This method can be performed using a microwave oven by heating the solution to 60–65°C and allowing the slides to remain in the heated solution for 5 minutes.

Beryllium and aluminum

The same methods are used to demonstrate both of these metals. It is therefore convenient to consider both together. Beryllium, used in the manufacture of fluorescent light tubes, gains access to the body by inhalation or traumatization of the skin. A foreign body granuloma is formed, often resembling the appearance of sarcoidosis. Conchoidal (shell-like) bodies can also be found, which are typical of, but not specific to, beryllium. These bodies usually give a positive reaction with Perls' Prussian blue.

Aluminum is rarely seen in tissues, but gains access to the body in a similar way to beryllium. It can also be found in bone biopsies from patients with encephalopathy on regular hemodialysis for chronic renal failure. Prolonged dialysis can cause osteodystrophy in the present era. It can develop insidiously and may present with a non-specific ache. The most severe pain occurs with osteomalacia, particularly when it is associated with aluminum deposition (Brenner 2004). Beryllium and aluminum can both be demonstrated by solochrome azurine that forms a deep blue chelate. Aluminum is also positive with the fluorescent Morin method (Pearse 1985), together with other minerals such as calcium, barium, and zirconium. Naphthochrome green can also be used to demonstrate beryllium and aluminum, but is less specific than the solochrome azurine method as other metallic dye lakes can be formed.

Solochrome azurine method for beryllium and aluminum *(Pearse 1957)*

Fixation

Not critical.

Sections

Paraffin or frozen.

Preparation of solutions

a. 0.2% solochrome azurine (syn. Pure blue B).
b. 0.2% solochrome azurine in normal sodium hydroxide.

Method

1. Take two test sections to distilled water.
2. Stain one section in solution a and one in solution b for 20 minutes.
3. Wash in distilled water.
4. Lightly counterstain in 0.5% aqueous neutral red or 0.1% aqueous nuclear fast red for 5 minutes.
5. Wash in distilled water and mount in synthetic resin.

Results

Solution A: aluminum and beryllium	blue
Solution B: beryllium only	blue-black
Nuclei	red

Notes

a. This method is reliable and will give consistent results.

b. Control sections should always be used if readily available.

c. Aluminum will fail to react at an alkaline pH.

d. A modification of this method applicable to resin sections of undecalcified bone is given in Chapter 16 on bone histology.

Aluminon method for aluminum *(Lillie & Fullmer 1976)*

Sections

Undecalcified glycol methacrylate or paraffin sections cut at 5 μm.

Solutions

pH buffer 5.2. Dissolve 40 g ammonium acetate and 28 g ammonium chloride in 210 ml distilled water. Add 27 ml 6 M (50%) hydrochloric acid. Adjust to pH 5.2 with hydrochloric acid or 28% ammonium hydroxide. Store in a refrigerator at 3–6°C.

Aluminon solution

Dissolve 0.8 g aluminon (aurine tricarboxylic acid) in 40 ml pH buffer 5.2 with the aid of heat to 80–85°C. Prepare just before use.

Decolorizing solution

To 22 ml buffer pH 5.2 add 8 ml 1.6 M ammonium carbonate that consists of 15.4 g ammonium carbonate in distilled water to make a total of 100 ml.

Fast green counterstain

Dissolve 0.05 g fast green FCF (CI 42053) in 100 ml 0.2% acetic acid.

Method

1. Sections to distilled water.

2. Pour freshly prepared aluminon solution that is heated to 80–85°C in a plastic Coplin jar. Place slides in this solution.

3. Place Coplin jar in a 600 W microwave oven and microwave at 120 W for 30 seconds (see Notes below). Allow the slides to remain in the solution for 10 minutes.

4. Rinse in three changes of distilled water.

5. Place in freshly prepared decolorizing solution for 5 seconds.

6. Rinse in three changes of distilled water.

7. Counterstain with fast green solution for 3 minutes.

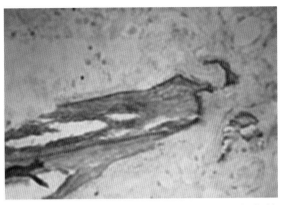

Figure 13.21 An undecalcified plastic section of bone stained with Lillie's aluminon method for aluminum. Aluminum is stained red.

8. Rinse in three changes of distilled water.

9. Stand slides on end and allow slides to air dry.

10. Dip in xylene and mount with synthetic resin.

Results

Aluminum	red
Background	green

Notes

a. Currently available microwave ovens have a maximum wattage of 900–1500 W. Therefore, when using a microwave oven greater than 600 W, the time of exposure to microwaves should be reduced proportionally in Step 3.

b. Another counterstain that may be used in this method is methylene blue, as it contrasts well with the red positive stain (Fig. 13.21), like the fast green.

Silver

Silver is occasionally found in the skin of silver workers as a result of industrial exposure. It is now more commonly seen as a localized change in the mouth (amalgam tattoo, see above) or in association with silver earrings in ineptly pierced lobes. The resultant permanent blue-gray pigmentation is called argyria and is most marked in those areas exposed to sunlight. In unstained and H&E-stained sections the silver appears as fine dark brown or black granules, particularly in basement membranes and sweat glands. The method of Okamoto and Utamura (1938), a metal chelating method that utilizes dimethylaminobenzylidene-rhodanine, will demonstrate silver. The method tends to be capricious and may give rise to the diffusion of chelate complex. The best results are obtained using frozen sections.

Rhodanine method for silver (Okamoto & Utamura 1938)

Fixation

Not critical but avoid the use of mercury-containing fixatives.

Sections

Paraffin; frozen (see Note a below).

Incubating solution

P-Dimethylaminobenzylidene-rhodanine (saturated solution in 90%)	3.5 ml
M nitric acid	3 ml
Distilled water	93.5 ml

Method

1. Paraffin sections to distilled water.
2. Incubate sections in rhodanine solution at 37°C for 24 hours.
3. Wash well in distilled water.
4. Mount in glycerin jelly.

Results

Silver deposits	reddish-brown

Notes

a. Better results are obtained on free-floating frozen sections using a 0.2% rhodanine solution in 0.1% nitric acid for 2 hours at 37°C.
b. The reaction product is not completely insoluble and some diffusion occurs, so sections should be examined immediately. Long incubation times will give poor localization.
c. The exogenous pigments, particularly of the elements, can also be analyzed for tissue density by mass spectrometry.

References

Bloch, B., 1917. Des Problem Pigmentbildung in der Haut. Archives Dermato-Syphiligraphiques 124, 129.

Boyd, J.F., Valentine, J.C., 1970. Unidentified yellow bodies in human lymph-nodes. Journal of Pathology 102, 58–60.

Brenner, B.M. (Ed.), 2004. Brenner and Rector's the kidney, seventh ed. Saunders, Philadelphia.

Churukian, C.J., 2005. Manual of the special stains laboratory, tenth ed. University of Rochester, Rochester, pp. 101, 102.

Dahl, L.K., 1952. A simple and sensitive histochemical method for calcium. Journal of Experimental Medicine 95, 474–479.

Doyle, W.F., Braham, H.D., Burgess, J.H., 1973. The nature of yellow-brown bodies in peritoneal lymph nodes. Histochemical and electron microscopic evaluation of these bodies in a case of sarcoidosis. Archives of Pathology 96, 320–326.

Drury, R.A.B., Wallington, E.A., 1980. Carleton's histological technique, fifth ed. Oxford University Press, Oxford.

Dunn, R.C., Thompson, E.C., 1946. A simplified stain for hemoglobin in tissue and smears using patent blue. Stain Technology 21, 65.

Eranko, O., 1955. Distribution of adrenaline and noradrenaline in the adrenal medulla. Nature 175, 88.

Fontana, A., 1912. Verfahren zur intensiven und raschen Färbung des Treponema pallidum und anderer Spirochaten. Dermatologische Wochenshrift 55, 1003.

Ghadially, F.N., 1982. Ultrastructural pathology of the cell and matrix. Butterworth, London, p. 602.

Golodetz, L., Unna, P.C., 1909. Zur Chemie der Haut III. Das Reduktionsvermogen der histologischen Elemente der Haut. Mh. Prakt. Dermatogie 48, 149.

Gomori, G., 1936. Microchemical demonstration of iron. American Journal of Pathology 13, 655.

Gomori, G., 1950. Aldehyde fuchsin: a new stain for elastic tissues. American Journal of Clinical Pathology 20, 665.

Gomori, G., 1951. Histochemical staining methods. In: Vischer, M.B. (Eds.), Methods in medical research, Vol. 4. Year Book Publishers, Chicago, p. 14.

Grocott, R.G., 1955. A stain for fungi in tissue sections and smears. American Journal of Clinical Pathology 25, 975.

Hall, M., Eusebi, V., 1978. Yellow-brown spindle bodies in mesenteric lymph nodes: a possible relationship with melanosis coli. Histopathology 2, 47–52.

Hall, M.J., 1960. A staining reaction for bilirubin in tissue sections. American Journal of Clinical Pathology 34, 313.

Hamazaki, Y., 1938. Uber eine neues, saurefeste Substanz führendes Spindelkörperchen der menschlichen Lymphdrusen. Virchows Archiv fur Pathologische Anatomie und Physiologie 301, 490–522.

Herschberger, L.R., Lillie, R.D., 1947. Physical properties of acid formalin hematin, or formalin pigment. Journal of Technical Methods and Bulletin of the International Association of Medical Museums 27, 162.

Hukill, P.B., Putt, F.A., 1962. A specific stain for iron using 4,7-diphenyl-1,10-phenanthroline. Journal of Histochemistry 10, 490.

Irons, R.D., Schenk, E.A., Lee, J.C.K., 1977. Cytochemical methods for copper semiquantitation screening procedure for identification of abnormal copper levels in liver. Archives of Pathology and Laboratory Medicine 101, 298.

Kamino, H., Tam, S.T., 1991. Immunoperoxidase technique modified by counterstain with azure B as a diagnostic aid in evaluating heavily pigmented melanocytic neoplasms. Journal of Cutaneous Pathology 18, 436–439

Kivela, T., 1995. Immunohistochemical staining followed by bleaching of melanin: a practical method for ophthalmic pathology. British Journal of Biomedical Science 52, 325.

Laidlaw, G.F., Blackberg, S.N., 1932. Melanoma studies; DOPA reaction in normal histology. American Journal of Pathology 8, 491.

Lendrum, A.C., 1949. Staining of erythrocytes in tissue sections; a new method and observations on some of the modified Mallory connective tissue stains. Journal of Pathology and Bacteriology 61, 443.

Lillie, R.D., 1954. Histopathologic technic and practical histochemistry. Blakiston, New York.

Lillie, R.D., 1956. A Nile blue staining technic for the differentiation of melanin and lipofuscin. Stain Technology 31, 151.

Lillie, R.D., 1965. Histopathologic technic and practical histochemistry, third ed. McGraw-Hill, New York.

Lillie, R.D., Fullmer, H.M., 1976. Histopathologic technic and practical histochemistry, fourth ed. McGraw-Hill, New York, pp. 526–527.

Lillie, R.D., Geer, J.C., 1965. On the relation of enterosiderosis pigments of man and guinea pig, melanosis and pseudomelanosis of colon and villi and the intestinal iron uptake and storage mechanism. American Journal of Pathology 47, 965–1007.

Lillie, R.D., Pizzolato, P., 1967. A stable histochemical Gmelin reaction of bile pigments with dry bromine carbon tetrachloride solution. Journal of Histochemistry and Cytochemistry 15, 600.

Lillie, R.D., Daft, F.S., Sebrell, W.N.J., 1941. Cirrhosis of liver in rats on deficient diet and effect of alcohol. Public Health Reports 56, 1255.

Lillie, R.D., Ashburn, L.L., Sebrell, W.H.J., et al., 1942. Histogenesis and repair of hepatic cirrhosis in rats produced on low protein diets and preventable with choline. Public Health Reports 57, 502.

Lindquist, R.R., 1969. Studies on the pathogenesis of hepatolenticular degeneration. II: Cytochemical methods for the localisation of copper. Archives of Pathology 87, 370.

Lison, L., 1938. Zur Frage der Ausscheidung und Speicherung des Hämoglobins in der Amphibienniere. Beitrage zur Pathologischen Anatomie und zur Allgemeinen Pathologie 101, 94.

Luna, L.G., 1968. Manual of histologic staining methods of the Armed Forces Institute of

Pathology, third ed. McGraw-Hill, New York, pp. 175–176.

McGee-Russell, S.M., 1958. Histochemical methods for calcium. Journal of Histochemistry and Cytochemistry 6, 22.

Mallory, F.B., Parker, F., 1939. Fixing and staining methods for lead and copper in tissues. American Journal of Pathology 16, 517.

Masson, P., 1914. La glande endocrine de l'intestine chez l'homme. Comptes Rendus Hebdomadaires des Séances de l'Académie des Sciences 158, 59.

Moment, G.B., 1969. Deteriorated paraldehyde: an insidious cause of failure in aldehyde fuchsin staining. Stain Technology 44, 52–53.

Okamoto, K., Utamura, M., 1938. Biologische Untersuchen des Kupfers über die histochemische Kupfernachweiss Methode. Acta Scholae Medicinalis Universitatis Imperialis in Kisto 20, 573.

Orchard, G. E., 1999. Heavily pigmented melanocytic neoplasms: comparison of two melanin-bleaching techniques and subsequent immunohistochemical staining. British Journal of Biomedical Science 56, 188–193.

Orchard, G. E., 2000. Comparison of immunohistochemical labeling of melanocyte differentiation antibodies melan-A, tyrosinase and HMB 45 with NKIC3 and S100 protein in the evaluation of benign naevi and malignant melanoma. The Histochemical Journal 32, 475–481.

Orchard, G. E., 2007. Use of heat provides a fast and efficient way to undertake melanin bleaching with dilute hydrogen peroxide. British Journal of Biomedical Science 64, 89–91.

Pearse, A.G.E., 1953. Histochemistry, theoretical and applied. Churchill, London.

Pearse, A.G.E., 1957. Solochrome dyes in histochemistry with particular reference to nuclear staining. Acta Histochimica 4, 95.

Pearse, A.G.E., 1985. Histochemistry: theoretical and applied, Vol. 2. Churchill Livingstone, Edinburgh.

Perls, M., 1867. Nachweis von Eisenoxyd in geweissen Pigmentation. Virchows Archiv für Pathologische Anatomie und Physiologie und für Klinische Medizin 39, 42.

Puchtler, H., Sweat, F., 1962. Amido black as a stain for hemoglobin. Archives of Pathology 73, 245.

Raia, S., 1965. Histochemical demonstration of conjugated and unconjugated bilirubin using a modified diazo-reagent. Nature (London) 205, 304.

Raia, S., 1967. PhD thesis. University of London, London.

Rodriguez, H.A., McGavran, M.H., 1969. A modified DOPA reaction for the diagnosis and investigation of pigment cells. American Journal of Clinical Pathology 52, 219.

Shikata, T., Uzawa, T., Yoshiwara, N., et al., 1974. Staining methods for Australia antigen in paraffin sections – detection of cytoplasmic inclusion bodies. Japanese Journal of Experimental Medicine 44, 25.

Tiedermann, F., Gmelin, L., 1826. Die Verdauung nach Versuchen. Heidelberg, K. Gross 1, 89.

Timm, F., 1958. Zur Histochemie der Schwermetalle; das Sulfid-silberverfahren. Deutsche Zeitschrift für die Gesampte Gerichtliche Medizin 46, 706.

Uzman, L.L., 1956. Histochemical localisation of copper with rubeanic acid. Laboratory Investigations 5, 299.

Virchow, R., 1847. Die pathologischen pigmente. Archiv für Pathologische Anatomie und Physiologie Kinische Medizin 379.

von Kossa, J., 1901. Ueber die im Organismus kuenstlich erzeugbaren Verkakung. Beiträge zur Pathologischen Anatomie und zur Allgemeinen Pathologie 29, 163.

Weisenberg, W., 1966. Über saurefeste 'Spindelkorper Hamazaki' bei Sarkoikose der Lymphknoten und über doppellichtbrechende Zelleinschlusse bei Sarkoidose der Lungen. Archiv für Klinische und Experimentelle Dermatologie 227, 101–107.

Amyloid 14

Janet A. Gilbertson • Toby Hunt

Introduction

History

Amyloidosis is a disorder of protein folding, in which normally soluble proteins accumulate in the tissues as abnormal insoluble fibrils (or filaments), thus disrupting their function. The deposited proteins, generically known as amyloid, damage the structure and function of the tissues and so cause serious disease which is often fatal when it affects major organs.

The term amyloid means 'starch-like' and was first used in botany to describe the starchy cellulose material found in plants. It was identified by a botanical test for carbohydrate through its reaction with iodine. Starch gives a deep blue color when iodine is applied, whereas cellulose gives a violet color. This reaction was adapted by Virchow (1853, 1854) to tissue containing amyloid, which also gives a violet coloration and was often used in early studies of amyloidosis. Amyloid is still, to date, identified by its characteristic histological staining reactions in tissue.

At autopsy the cut surface of amyloid-affected organs may show a 'waxy' texture and was often described by early pathologists as 'waxy degeneration' or 'lardaceous disease' (von Rokitansky 1842). During the nineteenth century this appearance was a frequent post-mortem finding in patients suffering from chronic inflammatory diseases such as tuberculosis (TB), but amyloidosis itself was rarely diagnosed during the patient's lifetime.

Friedrich and Kekule (1859) came to the conclusion that 'amyloid livers and spleen' were of albuminous nature due to the high proportion of nitrogen. Subsequent analyses confirmed that amyloid was predominately of a proteinaceous nature with a variable amount (about 1–5%) of various mucopolysaccharides. Knowledge of the exact composition was at that time hampered by the inability to separate amyloid from the normal extracellular ground substance.

Crystal violet and Congo red dyes were used in early histological techniques for the demonstration of amyloid (Bennhold 1922), but it wasn't until 1925 that the dichroic effect of Congo red stained amyloid was noted (Neubert 1925) when viewed under polarized light. Subsequently, in 1927, the optical activity of Congo red stained amyloid giving the unique 'apple green birefringence' was described (Divery and Florkin 1927). This phrase is still in use today to describe the birefringence and dichroism that amyloid displays when viewed under crossed polarized light, although Howie et al. (2009) suggested the correct phrase should be of 'anomalous colors', which describes all the colors Congo red stained amyloid can show – from yellow to green to blue.

With the arrival of electron microscopy it was observed that amyloid had a unique fibrillary ultrastructure independent of anatomical site, quite different to any other ultrastructural fibrils described before. Eanes and Glenner (1968), using X-ray diffraction, showed that the protein within the fibrils was arranged in an anti-parallel β-pleated sheet (Fig. 14.1).

Since then it has been shown that all amyloid fibrils share a common β-core structure with polypeptides chains running perpendicular to the fibril

Fibril aggregate

A tangled mass of amyloid fibrils of random orientation

Occasional parallel bundles are seen, predominantly extracellular

The amyloid fibril

A double helix of 1000 Å periodicity consisting of two pleated sheet micelles in the form of twin filaments separated by a clear interspace

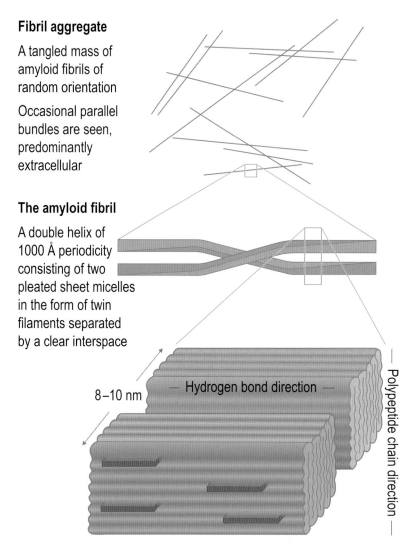

8–10 nm

— Hydrogen bond direction —

— Polypeptide chain direction —

The amyloid filament

Lozenge-shaped Congo red or toluidine blue dye molecules retained in grooved face of β-pleated sheet protein by hydrogen bonds

Figure 14.1 Schematic diagram of amyloid structure.

long axis, regardless of the particular protein from which they are formed (Sunde 1997).

Composition

With the development of techniques for amyloid fibril extraction (Pras et al. 1968; Glenner et al. 1972) it was confirmed that the bulk of amyloid deposits were composed of protein. They also contain up to 15% of a non-fibrillary glycoprotein known as amyloid P component (AP), derived from and identical to the normal circulating plasma protein serum amyloid P component (SAP). SAP is a calcium-dependent, ligand-binding protein that forms a normal component of basement membranes and elastic fibers, and may have a function related to its binding to glycosaminoglycans (GAGs), fibronectin and other cellular components (Pepys & Baltz 1983). It belongs to the pentraxin family and becomes specifically and highly concentrated in amyloid deposits of all types. This binding to amyloid fibrils is used in patients with amyloidosis for radiolabeled SAP scintigraphy, a diagnostic technique that is used for quantitative monitoring of amyloid deposits. (Hawkins 1990). The generic SAP ligand on amyloid fibrils remains uncharacterized (Pepys 1992).

The composition of the GAGs includes various sulfates, heparin, chrondition and dermatan, which may be involved in amyloidogenesis. The presence of the carbohydrate moieties of GAGs provides a possible explanation for the staining reaction in some of the histological methods used for amyloid detection.

Ultrastructure

As mentioned earlier, electron microscopy (EM) played an important role in the identification of the composition of amyloid, showing its unique fibrillary arrangement. To this day, EM is one of the methods for identifying amyloid. Amyloid deposits appear as masses of extracellular, non-branched filaments usually in a random orientation, though occasionally in parallel arrays of a few fibrils. Each fibril consists of two electron-dense filaments 2.5–3.5 nm in diameter, separated by a 2.5 nm space, giving a total diameter of 8–10 nm, with variable length of up to several microns (μm) (Cohen & Calkins 1959; Glenner 1981) (Fig. 14.2a, b).

Classification

There have been many attempts to identify and classify amyloid proteins in order to collate the endless variety of clinical manifestations, histopathological appearances and associated pathology. Until 1980, the main classification used for amyloid was that of Reimann et al. (1935), who divided amyloid types into four categories:

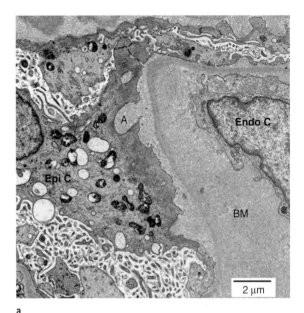

a

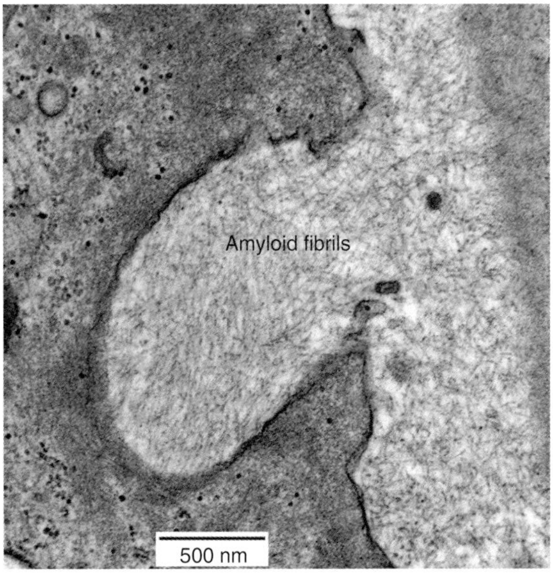

b

Figure 14.2a An electron micrograph of kidney from a case of amyloidosis with renal involvement showing amyloid (A), epithelial cytoplasm (Epi C), basement membrane (BM) and an endothelial cell (Endo C).
Figure 14.2b A higher magnification of Figure 14.2a where amyloid fibrils can be clearly seen.

1. Primary amyloid occurring spontaneously in the absence of an apparent predisposing illness. It affects organs and tissues such as heart, muscle, skin, and tongue.
2. Secondary amyloid occurring in patients with chronic infective disease, such as syphilis and TB. Later, inflammatory diseases such as rheumatoid arthritis were also included in this group.
3. Tumor-associated amyloid.
4. Myeloma-associated amyloid.

As more and more amyloid-forming proteins were identified, this classification became obsolete and Husby et al. (1990) proposed guidelines for a better classification based on the identity of the amyloid fibril protein, which was adopted by the World Health Organization-International Union of Immununological Societies (WHO-IUIS) and forms the currently accepted classification of amyloid.

Today there are about 25 different unrelated amyloid-forming proteins (Table 14.1). Amyloidosis nomenclature uses the letter A to designate amyloid followed by an abbreviation of the name of the fibril protein.

Pathogenesis

The process that causes proteins to become involved in amyloid formation, converting them from normal functioning proteins into inert amyloid deposits is the focus of much research. There is little to connect the different types of proteins involved (Merlini 2003). In certain amyloid types, only a limited portion of the amyloid protein precursor forms the fibril – as is the case in Alzheimer's disease; several amyloid proteins are rich in β-pleated sheet conformation in their native form; prion protein contains no β-pleated sheet and it is the formation of β-pleated sheets *de novo* that is the pathological event of the prion diseases. In some amyloidosis, the whole precursor protein may be involved, or there may be proteolysis of the precursor protein with liberation of a smaller amyloidogenic fragment as with AβPP. In transthyretin (TTR) amyloidosis, the circulating protein is a tetramer and a vital pathological event appears to be release of the monomer. The pathogenesis of amyloid has been recently reviewed (Sipe 2005).

Amyloidosis is considered to belong to the category of conformational diseases, because the pathological protein aggregation is due to the reduced stability and a strong propensity to acquire more than one conformation. It is thought that such a grouping helps to provide an understanding of the etiology or episodic onset of these diseases, and opens the prospect for common approaches to therapeutic stratagems in the same way that recognition of bacteria as the causative agents of many infections allowed the idea of antibiotics being useful in all such conditions, or of steroid therapy being of potential use for all inflammatory conditions (Carrell & Lomas 1997; Carrell & Gooptu 1998). In this context it is interesting to note the development of 'designer' peptides that bind to Aβ and to prion protein, preventing, and even reversing, the conformational change responsible for the respective disease processes (Soto et al. 2000). This concept is becoming increasingly accepted, and it is becoming evident that amyloid is but one, albeit definable, subgroup within a larger group of misfolded or altered protein deposits which are associated with human disease (Table 14.2).

Amyloidosis

In AL amyloidosis, previously known as 'primary amyloidosis', abnormal proteins, monoclonal light chains, are produced by plasma cells or B-cells and form amyloid deposits in the tissues. These can be either of kappa (κ) or lambda (λ) isotypes. Systemic AL amyloidosis is the most common form of clinical amyloid disease in developed countries and causes the most fatalities. In systemic amyloidosis, deposits can be present in any or all of the viscera, connective tissue and blood vessels walls, although intracerebral amyloid deposits are never found (Pepys 2006).

AL amyloidosis can also be localized when it is restricted to a particular organ or tissue, and usually has a benign prognosis. In the skin, the deposits

Table 14.1 Unrelated amyloid-forming proteins

Abbreviation	Protein precursor	Dominant tissues affected	Amyloid type
AA[‡]	Serum amyloid A protein	Spleen, gut	Reactive systemic AA amyloidosis
AL (κ & λ)[‡]	Immunoglobulin light chain	Any tissue except the brain parenchyma	Systemic AL amyloidosis or localized AL amyloidosis
AH[‡]	Immunoglobulin heavy chain	Renal	Systemic AL amyloidosis or localized AL amyloidosis
ATTR[‡]	Variant transthyretin (prealbumin)	Peripheral and/or autonomic nerves, cardiac, gastro-intestinal	Familial amyloid polyneuropathy (FAP), familial amyloid cardiomyopathy (FAC)
STTR[‡]	Wild-type transthyretin (prealbumin)	Cardiac	Senile TTR
AapoAI[‡]	Variant apolipoprotein AI	Kidney, liver	Hereditary systemic amyloidodsis
AapoAII[‡]	Apolipoprotein AII	Kidney, liver	Hereditary
AapoAIV[‡]	Apolipoprotein AIV	Kidney, liver	Sporadic aging amyloidosis
AGel[‡]	Gelsolin	Kidney	Hereditary
ACys[‡]	Cystatin C	Brain	Hereditary
AβPP	Amyloid β-protein precursor	Brain	Alzheimer's disease, Down's syndrome, cerebral amyloid angiopathy
$A\beta_2M$[‡]	β_2-Microglobulin	Kidney, prostate	Dialysis-associated amyloid, corpora amyleacea
APrP	Prion protein	Brain	CJD, prion disease
ACal	Calcitonin	Thyroid	Medullary carcinoma of thyroid-associated disease
AANF	Atrial natriuretic factor	Heart	Senile cardiac amyloid
AIAPP	Amylin	Pancreas	Type II diabetes amyloid, insulinoma
AFib[‡]	Fibrinogen A α-chain	Kidney	Hereditary
ALys[‡]	Lysozyme	Kidney	Hereditary
APro	Prolactin	Pituitary	Aging amyloid
AIns	Insulin	Skin	Injection sites
ABri	ABriPP	Brain	Familial dementia (British)
ADan	A Dan PP	Brain	Familial dementia (Danish)
AMed	Lactadherin	Arteries	Aging amyloid in arteries
ALac	Lactoferrin	Cornea	Corneal amyloidosis
AKer	Kerato-epitheliun	Eyes	Familial corneal amyloidosis
ALect2[‡]	Leukocyte common antigen 2	Kidney, liver	LECT 2 amyloidosis

[‡]One of the 14 forms of amyloid proteins that can give rise to systemic disease.

Table 14.2 Protein conformation diseases		
Conditions	**Affected proteins**	**Associated diseases**
Amyloidosis	25 known in humans – see Table 14.1	
Serpinopathies	α_1-Antitrypsin	α_1-Antitrypsin storage disease
	neuroserpin	
Hemoglobinopathies	Hemoglobulin	Sickle cell anemia
		Drug and aging induced inclusion body hemolysis
Lewy body diseases	α-Synuclein	Parkinson's disease
Neuronal inclusion bodies	Tau	Alzheimer's disease
		Pick's disease
		Progressive supranuclear palsy
	Superoxide dismutase	Motor neuron disease, AML
	Ferritin	Familial neurodegenerative disorder
Hirano bodies	Actin	Alzheimer's disease
Polyglutamine repeats	Huntingtin	Huntington's disease
	Ataxin	Spinocerebellar ataxias
	Androgen receptor	Spinomuscular atrophies
Prion diseases	Prion protein	Creutzfeldt-Jacob disease (CJD)
		Variant CJD
		Gerstmann-Straussler-Scheinker
		Kuru
		Fatal familial insomnia
		Japanese CAA

cause benign lumps and can be excised or left untreated, but localized amyloid deposits are also common in the bladder and in pulmonary tissue, often causing obstruction which can lead to complications.

There are five possible types of heavy chain amyloidosis (AH); G, A, D, E and M – these are rare but not unknown.

AA amyloidosis, previously known as 'secondary amyloidosis', is an occasional complication of chronic infection and inflammatory conditions, characterized by an acute phase response in which production of serum amyloid A protein (SAA) is increased. SAA is an apolipoprotein produced in the liver and is an acute phase protein which is synthesized at increased levels in patients with diseases such as rheumatoid arthritis, TB, Crohn's disease, familial Mediterranean fever (FMF) and other hereditary periodic fevers. Chronically high levels of SAA are a prerequisite for development of AA amyloidosis.

Hereditary systemic amyloidosis is a rare disorder that is difficult to treat and often fatal. This group of disorders occurs in small clusters around the world and has an autosomal dominant pattern of inheritance. Its most common cause is a mutation in the TTR (prealbumin) gene, which affects about 10,000 individuals worldwide. Over 100 mutations, most of which are amyloidogenic, are known in TTR. The major features of hereditary TTR amyloidosis include severe and ultimately fatal peripheral and/or autonomic neuropathy (familial amyloid polyneuropathy, FAP); cardiac involvement is also common. Other mutations associated with the disorder are those in the genes encoding apolipoproteins AI and AII, fibrinogen A α-chain, gelsolin, lysozyme, cystatin C and β-protein. In all these forms the variant protein is deposited as amyloid fibrils predominantly in the abdominal viscera, although cardiac and nerve involvement can occur.

All amyloidogenic mutations are dominant, but can display both variable penetrance and expressivity. Thus there may be marked differences in age of onset, amyloid deposition and clinical presentation, not only between families but also within families with the same mutation. In contrast to AA amyloidosis, where the concentration of the amyloid fibril protein SAA is raised but of normal structure, AL and hereditary amyloidosis are associated with abnormal protein which is inclined to refold as a β-pleated sheet, resulting in amyloidosis.

LECT2 amyloidosis was discovered while studying proteins with leukocyte chemotactic activity (Yamagoe 1996). The pathogenesis of LECT2 remains to be understood, but there is no evidence that LECT2 is an inherited condition though the first cases reported were Hispanic patients (Larsen et al. 2010).

Other diseases in which amyloid occurs

As outlined by Pepys in 2006, amyloid is a histological feature of Alzheimer's disease and type 2 diabetes mellitus but, unlike systemic amyloidosis, it is not known whether the amyloid causes these diseases. In Alzheimer's there is an abundance of intracerebral amyloid deposits composed of β-protein, though there is poor correlation between the quantity of amyloid and the cognitive impairment. However, mutations that result in abundant deposition of β-protein as amyloid may result in early-onset Alzheimer's disease.

In patients with type 2 diabetes, amyloid is frequently found in the pancreatic islets of Langerhans, though this is not universal in all islets or in all patients with type 2 diabetes. As well as this, in diabetic patients amyloid can also be found at the site of insulin injection as a result of the injected insulin adopting a fibillary conformation *in vitro* (when subjected to certain physical or chemical stimuli such as heat or acidity), causing a localized cutaneous lump (Lonsdale-Eccles et al. 2009).

It is also frequently cited that transmissible spongiform encephalopathy (TSE) is an example of amyloidosis, although in fact amyloid has never been determined histopathologically in brains of patients with the disease, nor in cows with bovine spongiform encephalopathy (BSE).

There are other protein misfolding diseases that are not amyloid or amyloidosis; these diseases produce abnormal aggregates of proteins, for example Lewy bodies in Parkinson's disease and polyglutamine repeats present in Huntington's disease. However, it is unclear whether the removal of these aggregates alters the disease process.

Another protein deposition disease which is often confused with amyloid is light chain deposition disease (LCDD) which has a similar histological appearance. However LCDD deposits lack the affinity for Congo red stain and do not produce the characteristic green birefringence of amyloid under cross-polarized light. Under EM, LCDD deposits are granular, which aides the distinction (Gibbs et al. 2011).

Diagnosis

There is an increased awareness of amyloidosis nowadays and more patients are being recognized. However some patients are still overlooked. The diagnosis requires presence of amyloid in a tissue, and the gold standard technique is Congo red histology although EM may aid diagnosis. Biopsies are usually taken to investigate organ dysfunction, for example of the kidneys in nephrotic patients or of sural nerves in familial polyneuropathies. Amyloid is present in up to 90% of rectal and/or subcutaneous fat biopsies in systemic AA or AL amyloidosis; so much so that rectal biopsies or fine needle aspirates of subcutaneous tissue used to be the main method of screening (Westermark & Senkvist 1973; Pepys 1992). Nowadays techniques have improved greatly such that cardiac biopsies, after a suggestive echocardiogram, are becoming more popular. It must be noted that a negative biopsy does not exclude the possibility of amyloidosis due to sample selection and site. In rectal biopsies, amyloid is usually found in the walls of submucosal vessels, so if the full thickness of the muscularis is not obtained the deposits will go undetected.

The use of SAP scintigraphy allows *in vivo* diagnosis as well as the monitoring of progression and regression of the amyloid deposits with treatment (Hawkins et al. 1993; Hawkins 1994). Unfortunately SAP scintigraphy is unable to visualize amyloid within cardiac tissue because the heart is a moving organ. The bone scanning method DPD scintigraphy (^{99m}Tc-3,3-diphosphono-1,2-propanodicarboxylic acid) was serendipitously discovered to have high affinity for cardiac TTR amyloid, and is currently under evaluation at the National Amyloidosis Centre as a method for visualizing cardiac involvement.

Differentiation between different amyloid types

With the recognition that different proteins form amyloid and are associated with different clinical syndromes came the need to identify particular fibril types histologically. Furthermore, treatment of amyloidosis is entirely type-specific; hence the correct identification of the fibril type is indispensable in clinical practice.

Methods of section pretreatment using trypsin or potassium permanganate before Congo red staining were devised (Wright et al. 1976, 1977). After such pretreatment some amyloids lose their affinity for Congo red, most notably AA amyloid, whereas AL amyloid is resistant. These methods were always equivocal in practice and have been rendered obsolete by the use of immunohistochemistry and other techniques to identify the particular amyloid fibril protein specifically and reliably.

It is vitally important to discriminate between AL, hereditary amyloidosis and AA amyloidosis, as their treatments are entirely different. AL treatment is aimed at ablating the B-cell clone responsible for the amyloidogenic free light chain production using cytotoxic drugs. Hereditary amyloidosis treatment sometimes involves organ transplantation. Therapy for patients with AA amyloidosis involves measures to reduce SAA production by treating the cause of the underlying inflammation.

The tools available today to differentiate the amyloid type include direct assessment of the fibril type by immunohistochemistry, proteomics and, occasionally, fibril sequencing. Indirect, but very helpful, investigations include searches for monoclonal immunoglobulins using conventional electrophoresis and immunoassays of serum and urine, the serum free light chain assay, assessment of the hepatic acute phase response by measuring SAA and CRP and, where indicated, genetic sequencing of genes known to be associated with hereditary amyloidosis or the periodic fever syndromes. All these techniques are frequently employed for a patient with amyloidosis.

Demonstration

In hematoxylin and eosin (H&E) stained sections amyloid appears as an amorphous, eosinophilic, extracellular, faintly refractive substance that sometimes displays green birefringence under polarized light. However, it should be noted that collagen also has this appearance under polarized light in a H&E-stained section. Amyloid can also be weakly birefringent using a powerful light source when stained with periodic acid-Schiff. Whilst large deposits of amyloid can be observed with a H&E-stained section, the small deposits, for example in vessels in rectal or bone marrow samples, may be missed.

Dyes used for the demonstration of amyloid are compounds developed by the textile industry. This includes Congo red, which was developed as the first direct cotton dye in 1884 and has been 're-invented' many times in the search for a differential method for the detection of amyloid (Puchtler et al. 1964). As in all histopathological methods, they are often performed on tissues that have been formalin fixed and processed in to paraffin wax. Sometimes the samples can be left standing in fixative for long periods of time, which may make the staining less sensitive and intense. Control sections must be used in all staining methods, and in the demonstration of amyloid they should be cut as they are needed as they can lose their reactivity if stored for long periods.

Congo red

The molecular formula for Congo red is $C_{32}H_{22}N_6Na_2O_6S_2$ (Fig. 14.3).

Congo red is a symmetrical sulfonated azo dye containing a hydrophobic center with two phenyl groups bound by a diphenyl bond to give a linear molecule that is largely hydrophobic (Turnell & Finch 1992). Congo red is also a fluorescent dye (Puchtler 1965), although is not specific for amyloid. Two factors are important to the Congo red-amyloid reaction: the linearity of the dye molecule and the β-pleated sheet configuration. If the spatial configuration of either is altered, even though the chemical groupings are left intact, the reaction fails. Furthermore, the Congo red-mediated positive birefringence of amyloid implies that the dye molecules are arranged in a parallel fashion (Romhányi 1971). Recent work confirms the long-held belief that the Congo red molecule intercalates between two protein moieties at the interface between two adjacent antiparallel β-pleated sheets by disrupting the hydrogen bonds that are responsible for maintaining the β-sheet polymer, yet allowing maintenance of the integrity of the structure by the formation of new hydrogen bonds between protein and dye (Carter & Chou 1998).

Since its introduction on tissue sections by Bennhold (1992), Congo red staining for amyloid and

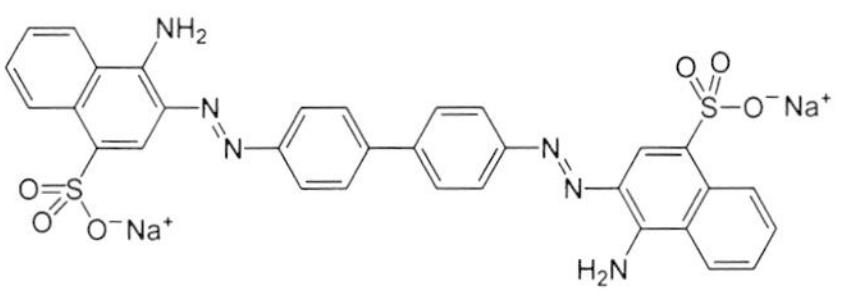

Figure 14.3 Chemical structure of Congo red dye.

its subsequent green birefringence when viewed by polarized light has become the gold standard. Although it was many years before the exact staining mechanism was understood, it is now well established that staining of amyloid by Congo red is due to hydrogen bonding between the Congo red dye and the β-pleated sheet in a highly orientated linear and parallel manner on the amyloid fibrils (Glenner et al. 1980). Any tissue component that binds Congo red in a linear way also exhibits green birefringence in polarized light. As well as amyloid, dense collagen fibers can also bind Congo red dye in this fashion, often meaning that formalin-fixed tissue gives false positives. By using an alkaline Congo red method this phenomenon is reduced (Puchtler et al. 1962). However Romhányi (1971) used 1% aqueous Congo red and claimed that if the tissue sections were mounted in gum arabic this problem is overcome. Bély et al. (2006) adapted Romhányi's original method, using a long deparaffinization step of up to 5 days, together with a longer incubation in Congo red. This technique has shown that the amyloid has a stronger affinity to Congo red and therefore can be seen as more sensitive and selective. Many different tissue structures will also stain with 1% aqueous Congo red, and so it must be used under strict controlled conditions using known amyloid-positive sections in conjunction.

The specificity of Congo red staining of amyloid can also be increased by using an alcoholic method combined with high ion strength and high pH. Puchtler et al. (1962) combines all these aspects, giving a superior method to demonstrate amyloid and green birefringence under polarized light.

Recent comparison of several Congo red staining methods made during a run of the UK NEQUAS histology external quality control scheme found that Highman's method gave the highest scores. At the referral center quoted above, they get a number of biopsies that are either false positive or false negative. Consequently, they recommend the Putchler method since the lack of a differentiation step means there is less intervention by the operator. It should be noted that false positives and false negatives can be caused by other factors even in this technique; for example, in very thin tissue sections.

Highman's Congo red technique *(Highman 1946)*

This simple method has found wide application. The solutions are relatively stable and the method affords a high degree of selectivity in practiced hands.

Fixation

Not critical; formal saline gives satisfactory results.

Solutions

Immerse in alkaline sodium chloride solution for 20 minutes.

0.5% Congo red in 50% alcohol
0.2% potassium hydroxide in 80% alcohol

Method

1. Sections to water, removing pigment where necessary.
2. Stain in Congo red solution, 5 minutes.
3. Differentiate with the alcoholic potassium hydroxide solution, 3–10 seconds.
4. Wash in water, stain nuclei in alum hematoxylin, differentiate, and blue.
5. Dehydrate, clear, and mount.

Results

Amyloid, elastic fibers, eosinophil granules	red
Nuclei	blue

Note

Differentiation in Step 3 can be arrested in water and resumed if necessary. Over-differentiation can occur.

Alkaline Congo red technique *(Puchtler et al. 1962)*

The method obviates the need for a differentiation step by the inclusion of a high concentration of sodium chloride. This reduces background electrochemical staining whilst enhancing hydrogen bonding of Congo red to amyloid, resulting in a progressive and highly selective technique. The solutions should be freshly made.

Fixation

Not critical.

Stock solutions

Stock solution A

Saturated sodium chloride in 80% ethanol.

Stock solution B

Saturated Congo red in 80% ethanol saturated with sodium chloride.

1% aqueous sodium hydroxide.

Working solutions

To 100 ml of stock solution A add 1 ml of 1% aqueous sodium hydroxide and filter.

To 100 ml of stock solution B add 1 ml of 1% aqueous sodium hydroxide and filter.

Method

1. Sections to water, removing pigment where necessary.
2. Stain nuclei in alum hematoxylin, differentiate, and blue.
3. Transfer directly to the alkaline Congo red solution for 20 minutes.
4. Rinse briefly in alcohol, clear, and mount.

Results (Fig. 14.4)

Amyloid, elastic fibers, eosinophil granules	red
Nuclei	blue

Note

Although the stock solutions are stable for a couple of months, the working solutions do not keep and should be used within 20 minutes of preparation.

Congo red technique *(Stokes 1976)*

In this method there is no differentiation step as Congo red is applied in an alkaline alcoholic solution. Harris's hematoxylin was originally used as a counterstain but any alum hematoxylin will suffice.

Fixation

Not critical.

Preparation of solutions

Staining solution

Dissolve 0.5 g potassium hydroxide in 50 ml distilled water, add 200 ml absolute alcohol and add Congo red until saturated (about 3 g). Stand overnight before use and discard after 3 months.

Method

1. Sections to water, removing pigment where necessary.
2. Stain in filtered Congo red solution, 25 minutes.
3. Wash in distilled water, then running tap water, 5 minutes
4. Counterstain nuclei in Harris's hematoxylin, 1 minute.
5. Blue, differentiate, hematoxylin if necessary, blue.
6. Dehydrate, clear, and mount.

Results

Amyloid, elastic tissue, eosinophil granules	red
Nuclei	blue

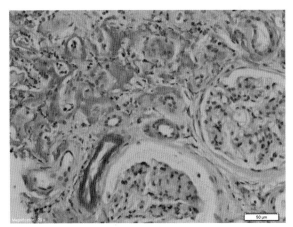

Figure 14.4 A Congo red stained section of kidney demonstrating amyloid deposition.

Sirius red

Sirius red F3B (direct red 80), is similar to Congo red and has been proposed to give a more intense staining reaction which is valuable for photographic purposes. Sirius red stained amyloid, like Congo red, also gives green birefringence with polarized light. However, as described by Brigger (1975), Sirius red does not display fluorescence.

Sirius red technique *(Llewellyn 1970)*

Llewellyn's method is a modification of Sweat's and uses the cotton dye Sirius red F3B – not to be confused with Sirius red 4B, which does not stain amyloid. Although this method is considerably simpler than the original technique, the staining solution does not keep well and tends to precipitate out.

Fixation

Not critical.

Preparation of solution

Dissolve 0.5 g Sirius red F3B in 45 ml distilled water. Add 50 ml absolute alcohol and 1 ml 1% sodium hydroxide. Stirring the solution vigorously, slowly add just sufficient 20% sodium chloride (above 4 ml) to produce a fine precipitate when viewed against strong backlighting. Leave to stand overnight and filter.

Method

1. Sections to water, removing pigment where necessary.

2. Stain nuclei in alum hematoxylin, differentiate, and blue.
3. Rinse in water and then 70% ethanol.
4. Treat with Sirius red solution for 1 hour.
5. Wash in tap water for 10 minutes.
6. Dehydrate, clear, and mount.

Results

Amyloid, elastic, eosinophil, and Paneth cell granules	red
Nuclei	blue

Note

The staining solution is liable to precipitation, especially if excess 20% sodium chloride is added during preparation.

Metachromatic techniques for amyloid

As we move into the next generation of technology in the modern histopathology laboratory, metachromatic techniques are very rarely used for the identification of tissue components and will only be mentioned briefly.

Methyl violet

Methyl violet was the first synthetic dye used for the demonstration of amyloid (Cornil 1875), but the rationale of the staining reaction remains unexplained. It was thought that the mucopolysaccharide content of amyloid was responsible for the reaction, though this is now thought to be unlikely. The staining reaction of amyloid produces a red/purple coloration. This coloration is also seen by other tissue components, especially mucins found in rectal biopsies, so is not selective for amyloid. Methyl violet is a mixture of tetra-, penta-, and hexa-parasaniline, so the red/purple coloration of amyloid is probably a polychromatic reaction (Windrum & Kramer 1957). Methyl stained sections have to be mounted using an aqueous mountant, since dehydration destroys the staining reaction. The amyloid from some primary amyloidosis may fail to give a positive reaction. Due to the low sensitivity and lack of specificity, this method is not now recommended for amyloid detection and diagnosis (Westermark et al. 1999).

Crystal violet method (Hucker & Conn 1928)

This method uses ammonium oxalate, which accentuates the polychromatic effect. Formic acid can also be used as an accentuator of the polychromic effect (Fernando 1961).

Methyl green (Bancroft 1963)

This method is slightly more selective, in that tissue sections are stained with methyl violet and then differentiated and counterstained simultaneously with methyl green, which replaces the former dye in tissue components other than amyloid.

Polarizing microscopy

As discussed earlier, when viewed using polarized light and an analyzing polarizing filter, Congo redstained amyloid exhibits a characteristic bright green birefringence, usually termed 'apple-green birefringence' or 'anomalous colors' (Fig. 14.5). This property is shared by other β-pleated sheet proteins and appears to be specific to that conformation.

Birefringence and dichroism are optical properties of anisotropic substances, i.e., substances that have different physical properties in different directions.

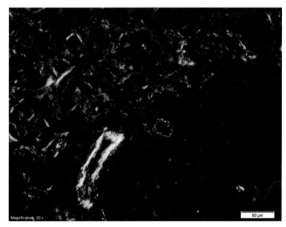

Figure 14.5 Same field as Figure 14.4 viewed by polarized light (crossed polarizer and analyzer). The characteristic 'green birefringence' is clearly seen against the dark background.

This property is observed in crystals, and is widely used in mineralogy as a qualitative test for the identification of various minerals. Birefringence is exhibited when an optically active substance has two differing refractive indices (RI), so that two rays of light vibrating in perpendicular planes will travel at different velocities through the substance, producing a faster and a slower ray. The substance is said to show positive birefringence if the plane of vibration of the slow ray (greater RI) is parallel to the length of the fiber or crystal, or negative if the plane of vibration of the slow ray is perpendicular to the length of the fiber. Normally birefringent substances appear colorless (white) against a dark background when viewed through crossed polarizing filters, but where the thickness of the crystal or fiber is uniform, interference colors may be produced when the two rays are reunited in the analyzer. Such colors are characteristic of, and can thus be used to identify, the substance being viewed. Practical details of polarizing microscopy and birefringence are given in Chapter 3.

Dichroism is due to light-absorbing differences along different planes of an asymmetrical substance. The spatial arrangement of light-absorbing bands is such that either light of a definite wavelength is selectively absorbed, or a change in intensity of white light occurs when light passes through the substance in certain planes. The dichroism of Congo red stained amyloid is that of the dye molecule, whose linear molecules are bound by hydrogen bonds along the parallel folds in the β-pleated sheet protein, producing different light-absorbing characteristics along certain planes of the fibril (Wolman 1965, 1971). The different amounts of absorption of light may be seen as different colors or different intensity of a color (Born & Wolf 1999).

Amyloid in unstained sections can be seen to be weakly birefringent when using a strong light source; weak birefringence may also often be seen following methyl violet, toluidine blue, and eosin staining. Such birefringence is usually faint, unreliable and non-specific, and is therefore of little diagnostic use. By contrast, the bright apple-green birefringence of amyloid following Congo red staining is easily visualized, highly selective, and thought by many to be the most reliable diagnostic characteristic of amyloid in current use (Missmahl & Hartwig 1953; Cohen 1967; Pearse 1968). This green birefringence, first noticed by Divery and Florkin (1927), is an intrinsic property of the amyloid fibril-Congo red complex. The thickness of the section is critical; 8–10 μm is ideal (Wolman & Bubis 1965). Sections which are too thin may show faint red colors, while yellow birefringent colors can be seen if the section is too thick, if there is strain birefringence in the optical system, or if the direction of the fibrils is oblique to the direction of the polarizer.

The use of a good microscope of high optical quality with color-corrected optics is essential to visualize faint birefringence. A revolving stage and subdued background lighting are also advisable. The strongest possible light source should be used. Many laboratory microscopes do not have strong enough light sources, and sections should preferentially be viewed using a modern photomicroscope, most of which are equipped both with essentially perfect optics and with powerful lamps. Only by using such a setup can the smallest of amyloid deposits be appreciated.

Apple-green birefringence is also given by certain other filamentous structures, most notably the neurofibrillary tangles characteristic of Alzheimer's disease and certain other degenerative brain diseases, as well as the intracellular inclusions seen in adrenal cortical cells (Eriksson & Westermark 1990). Whilst these structures fulfill many of the characteristics of amyloid, they are not currently considered so to be, although the matter remains under debate (Westermark et al. 2005). Green birefringence is also given by cellulose and chitin, both of which avidly bind Congo red. They are easily distinguished from amyloid on morphological grounds. Occasionally other structures may appear to give green birefringence: most commonly, dense collagen. This can usually be distinguished from amyloid by its whiter color, and the difference can be emphasized by the use of sections cut at the recommended thickness.

As mentioned previously, Congo red is a fluorescent dye, and provided that sections have been mounted in a non-fluorescent mountant this property can be used to detect small amyloid deposits. The fluorescence should not be considered as specific for amyloid as is the apple-green birefringence seen with polarizing microscopy (Puchtler & Sweat 1965; Westermark et al. 1999).

Acquired fluorescence methods

The ability of amyloid to fluoresce following treatment with fluorochromic dyes was discovered by Chiari (1947), although little use was made of this property until Vassar and Culling (1959) recommended the basic fluorochrome dye thioflavine T. The method has the advantage of not requiring microscopic differentiation and, save for staining of renal tubular myeloma casts and mast cell granules, specificity for amyloid was claimed.

Thioflavine T staining has enjoyed considerable popularity as a screening method for amyloid, as the intensity of fluorescence allows good visualization of minimal deposits. It has become evident that the specificity originally claimed for the method was overstated and that many other tissue components, including fibrinoid, arteriolar hyaline, keratin, intestinal muciphages, Paneth cells, and zymogen granules, also have an affinity for the dye. The addition of 0.4 M magnesium chloride to a 0.1% thioflavine T solution at pH 5.7 is claimed to improve selectivity by competitive ionic inhibition (Mowry & Scott 1967). Similar results are obtained by using thioflavine T at pH 1.4, favoring the reaction of the blue fluorescing dye component responsible for fluorescence of amyloid (Burns et al. 1967). The mechanism of binding of thioflavine T to amyloid is not known but *in vitro* studies of binding to purified amyloid fibrils and synthetic amyloids show that the dye interacts with the quaternary structure of the β-pleated sheet rather than with protein moieties, and so the binding is not dependent on any amino acid sequence (LeVine 1995).

A related fluorochrome, thioflavine S, has been widely used for the demonstration of amyloid (Schwartz 1970). However, it is considered to be non-specific and is not recommended (Puchtler et al. 1985).

Thioflavine T method *(Vassar & Culling 1959)*

Fixation

Not critical.

Preparation of solution

1% aqueous thioflavine T.

Method

1. Sections to water, removing pigment where necessary.
2. Treat with alum hematoxylin solution, 2 minutes.
3. Wash in water and stain in thioflavine T solution, 3 minutes.
4. Rinse in water and differentiate excess fluorochrome from background in 1% acetic acid, 20 minutes.
5. Wash well in water, dehydrate, clear, and mount in a non-fluorescent mountant.

Results

Using a UV light source (mercury vapor lamp), UG1 Exciter filter, BG38 red suppression filter, and K430 barrier filter: amyloid, elastic tissue, etc. – silver-blue fluorescence.

Using blue light fluorescence quartz-iodine or mercury vapor lamp with BG12 exciter filter and K530 barrier filter: amyloid, elastic tissue, etc. – yellow fluorescence.

Notes

a. Step 2 quenches nuclear autofluorescence.
b. The mountant must be non-fluorescent such as glycerine-saline (1 : 9 parts) or DPX. Avoid Canada balsam, which autofluoresces.
c. Thioflavine T deteriorates, especially if kept in sunlight, as do the stained sections on prolonged storage.

pH 1.4 Thioflavine T *(Burns et al. 1967)*

Acid pH increases the selectivity by favoring the fluorochromic fraction binding to amyloid while depressing non-amyloid fluorochrome staining.

Method

As above but use a freshly prepared solution of 0.5% thioflavine T in 0.1 M hydrochloric acid.

Results

Amyloid, Paneth cells, and oxyntic cells – silver-blue or yellow fluorescence according to filters used.

Miscellaneous methods

Many dyes, notably alcian blue and toluidine blue, commonly used for the identification of mucopolysaccharides, have been used on amyloid-containing tissue sections to substantiate histochemically the mucopolysaccharides frequently found in biochemical assays of amyloid tissue extracts. In most instances the results have been disappointing. Uptake of these dyes is poor and variable. Differing electrolyte concentrations (Mowry & Scott 1967) and partial pepsin digestion (Windrum & Kramer 1957) may enhance alcian blue uptake and toluidine blue metachromasia, respectively, but staining is never strong and interpretation difficult. The variable periodic acid Schiff's staining of amyloid, which is often intense, was thought to indicate the presence of carbohydrate within amyloid fibrils, but this has been disproved. The glycoprotein AP component is now thought to be the origin of this positivity. Alcian blue borax, with a celestine blue hemalum and van Gieson counterstain, elegantly demonstrates some amyloid, but the method is not specific (Lendrum et al. 1972).

There are several silver impregnation methods that have been used for the demonstration of amyloid, such as that of King (1948). There are several silver methods used on central nervous system tissue for the detection of amyloid-containing plaques (and neurofibrillary tangles) in Alzheimer's disease. There have been several reviews of these methods (Lamy et al. 1989; Wisniewski et al. 1989; Wilcock et al. 1990; Vallet et al. 1992), and the methenamine silver method of Haga is given in Chapter 17 on the nervous system.

Fibril extraction

Fibril extraction is a tool that utilizes small amounts of unfixed tissue to identify the amyloid fibril type and is especially useful when no other material is available. Briefly, small amounts of unfixed tissue are washed in a series of buffers and homogenized in saline, centrifuged and washed several times, leaving a suspension and a pellet of fibrils. These are then subjected to drying in layers for Congo red staining and immunohistochemistry, the optical density of the suspension is measured and SDS-PAGE, immunoblotting and SAP electroimmunoassays are carried out. Polypeptide analysis of the fibril isolates by *N*-terminal amino acid sequencing is also performed when necessary (Tennent 1999).

Immunohistochemistry for amyloid

Immunohistochemistry is a widely used method in histopathology for identification of tissue disease and can be used to determine the amyloid fibril type in most cases (Fig. 14.6). Due to the distinct protein nature of amyloid, antibodies can recognize specific epitopes on amyloid fibrils and on associated components, like amyloid P (AP) and proteoglycans. Some of the amyloid proteins can be masked by fixation of the tissue due to the cross-linking of the amino acid side groups which mask the antigenic site. These authors find that antigen retrieval is of little, if any, use for the detection of amyloid. It is thought that the β-pleated conformation of the amyloid can 'hide' some antigenic sites and for identification of amyloid of transthyretin (TTR) type, oxidation and high molarity guanidine treatment (Costa et al. 1986) are needed.

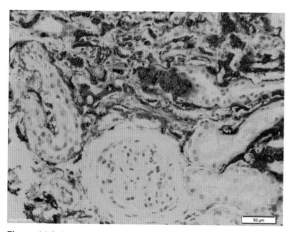

Figure 14.6 Immunoperoxidase-DAB stained section of the same field as Figure 14.4 using antiserum to LECT2 antibody.

AP is found in variable proportion of all amyloid fibrils. It is a non-fibrillar component that does not have a β-pleated conformation, so antisera raised against AP can be used to demonstrate amyloid. However, SAP is also found naturally in basement membranes and other tissue components and so will also bind antiserum raised against AP, and this is not a definitive marker. In early attempts using immunohistochemistry to identify all the fibril types, various antigen retrieval methods were used with varied success. Nowadays retrieval methods are commonplace in most laboratories and, since each antibody differs in the epitope that it recognizes, it is important to try the whole range of available antigen recovery methods for each antiserum tried. As well as testing all the retrieval methods, the correct way to evaluate the specificity of immunoreactions is to absorb antiserum with its specific antibody (Westermark et al. 1999). Antiserum to all known amyloid-forming protein is commercially available, and most are reliable in identifying the different fibrils.

Differentiation between AA and AL amyloid is clinically important, and both conditions are likely to occur at one time or another at most hospitals. Identification of the polyneuropathy-related amyloid types, ATTR, AApoAI and AGel, as well as other hereditary types such as ALys, and AFib, may be reasonably expected to be done only at specialist centers. The context or clinical presentation of the patient and disease should be considered when trying to type the amyloid by immunohistochemistry so that informed choices regarding sites of tissue biopsies and use of relevant antisera can be made.

In AL amyloidosis, about 70% of kappa and lambda types are identifiable, leaving 30% of 'probable' AL type, regardless of methods or retrieval recoveries used. This is due to the amyloid fibrils being formed from the variable light chain fragment of the immunoglobulin molecule. Patients with AL amyloidosis may have very high concentrations of free light chains in the serum, which may cause high background staining with kappa and lambda antisera, making interpretation difficult (Pepys 1992).

It is exceptionally rare, although not completely unknown, for a patient to have two types of amyloid.

When there is staining of amyloid deposits with two amyloid fibril antisera by immunohistochemistry, we would suggest that proteomics should be undertaken to determine the fibril type.

The demonstration of prion-derived amyloid deposits, APrP, is difficult and most cases are referred to the Creutzfeldt-Jakob Disease Surveillance Unit, who have vigorous immunohistochemical criteria and obtain consistently good results (Bell et al. 1997). It is important to follow these criteria so as to avoid false-positive interference from normal prion protein, and it should be noted that the proteins within all amyloid deposits differ from the normal precursor proteins largely by alteration of conformation rather than any antigenically determinable character.

Laser microdissection-proteomics: a new tool for typing amyloid

Proteomics is a high sensitivity, mass spectrometric method for identifying proteins. Laser capture microdissection (LCMD) allows one to precisely remove an area of interest from a tissue section. This can now be coupled with a proteomics approach to offer histologists a powerful tool for identifying proteins in both freshly prepared and formalin-fixed, paraffin embedded tissues. Although slides specifically made for LCMD can be obtained, it is also possible to extract material from previously cut unstained sections (archived as a matter of routine), which allows work to be carried out retrospectively to type amyloid. This approach was pioneered at the Mayo Clinic, USA, and is now being developed at a number of centers, including the National Amyloid Centre in London. A simplified laser microdissection-proteomics procedure is outlined below.

A tissue sample is mounted onto a slide, dewaxed and stained with Congo red. The amyloid is visualized by its characteristic, apple-green birefringence and with the use of the fluorescent properties of the Congo red dye and using a fluorescent laser capture microscope. Congo red positive material is excised and collected into a 0.5 ml tube, where it is reduced and carbamidomethylated to protect cysteines. The tissue sample is then digested with the proteolytic enzyme trypsin. This generates a complex mixture of peptides arising from each of the proteins in the tissue. The mixture is chromatographed on a reverse phase high-performance liquid chromatography (HPLC) column to separate the tryptic peptides, which are then analyzed directly by electrospray mass spectrometry (MS). MS generates information about the molecular mass and sequence for each of the peptides in the mixture. These MS-derived data are then collated and compared against a database of all proteins using a search engine such as MASCOT, which identifies the protein(s) present in tissue by using a probability-based algorithm. This LCMD-proteomics approach can not only identify the class of proteins in tissues, allowing us to type the amyloid (e.g. TTR or AL), but also can identify novel amyloidogenic proteins (cf. Lec-2) as well as protein variants found in TTR such as M30V or V122I.

Although LCMD-proteomics requires a substantial investment both in terms of equipment and staff, it is rapidly becoming the method of choice for typing amyloid tissue and for the identification of novel amyloidogenic proteins. Within 10 years, this approach will be common in leading specialist centers for the typing of amyloid fibrils.

Evaluation of methods

The 'gold standard' for amyloid demonstration remains the use of Congo red staining with 'apple green' birefringence. The preferred method for paraffin-embedded material remains that of Puchtler et al. (1962). Thioflavine T and other fluorescent dyes may offer an alternative to Congo red, but they may be less selective, as other hyaline and fibrinoid fibers also give positive results (Cooper 1969).

Positive immunohistochemistry with antisera to amyloid P component may be useful when used in conjunction with Congo red staining, though it must be remembered that elastin and collagen fibers will also stain positively. It is of value to identify the type of amyloid present using immunohistochemistry, as the success of treatment may well depend on such identification.

The future

New treatments are constantly being investigated for the treatment of amyloidosis. At the National Amyloidosis Centre a bis-D-proline compound, CPHPC, which depletes circulating SAP, when combined with a treatment using antibodies to human SAP, triggers a potent, complement-dependent, macrophage-derived giant cell reaction that swiftly removes massive murine visceral amyloid deposits without adverse effect (Bodin 2010). The unprecedented capacity of this novel combined therapy to eliminate amyloid deposits may be applicable to all forms of systemic and localized amylodoidosis in the future.

LCMD-proteomics is proving to be a valuable technique and is becoming more popular in leading specialist laboratories and could possibly be the technique of the future.

Acknowledgments

We thank Dr Julian Gillmore for his advice and comments. Special thanks to our friends and colleagues at the National Amyloidosis Centre for their support and encouragement.

References

Bancroft, J.D., 1963. Methyl green as a differentiator and counterstain in the methyl violet technique for the demonstration of amyloid. Stain Technology 38, 336.

Bell, J.E., Gentleman, S.M., Ironside, J.W., et al., 1997. Prion protein immunocytochemistry – UK five center consensus report. Neuropathology and Applied Neurobiology 23 (1), 26–35.

Bély, M., Makovitzky, J., 2006. Sensitivity and specificity of Congo red staining according to Romhányi. Comparison with Puchtler's or Bennhold's methods. Acta Histochem 108 (3), 175–180.

Bennhold, H., 1922. Eine specifische amyloid-färbung mit kangorot. Münchener Medizinische Wochenschrift 33, 1537–1541.

Bodin, K., Ellmerich, S., Kahan, M.C., et al., 2010. Antibodies to human serum amyloid P component eliminate visceral amyloid deposits. Nature 468, 760–767.

Born, M., Wolf, E., 1999. Principles of optics. Electomagnetic theory of propagation interference and diffraction of light, seventh ed. Cambridge University Press, Cambridge, pp. 12, 49, 95–103, 820–823, 843.

Brigger, D., Muckle, T.J., 1975. Comparison of Sirius red and Congo red as a stain for amyloid in animal tissues. Journal of Histochemistry and Cytochemistry 23, 84.

Burns, J., Pennock, C.A., Stoward, P.J., 1967. The specificity of the staining of amyloid deposits with thioflavine T. Journal of Pathology and Bacteriology 94, 337–344.

Carrell, R.W., Gooptu, B., 1998. Conformational changes and disease – serpins, prions and Alzheimer's. Current Opinion in Structural Biology 8 (6), 799–809.

Carrell, R.W., Lomas, D.A., 1997. Conformational disease. Lancet 350 (9071), 134–138.

Carter, D.B., Chou, K.C., 1998. A model for structure-dependent binding of Congo red to Alzheimer beta-amyloid fibrils. Neurobiology of Aging 19 (1), 37–40.

Chiari, H., 1947. Ein Beitrag zue sekundaren fluorezenzdesogen localen Amyloids. Mikroscopie 2, 79.

Cohen, A.S., 1967. Amyloidosis. New England Journal of Medicine 277, 522–530.

Cohen, A.S., Calkins, E., 1959. Electron microscopic observations on a fibrous component in amyloid of diverse origins. Nature 183, 1202–1203.

Cooper, J.H., 1969. An evaluation of current methods for the diagnostic histochemistry of amyloid. Journal of Clinical Pathology 22 (4), 410–413.

Cornil, V., 1875. Cited by Cohen A.S., 1965. CR (Paris) 80, 1288.

Costa, P.P., Jacobsson, B., Collin, V.P., et al., 1986. Unmasking antigen determinants in amyloid.

Journal of Histochemistry and Cytochemistry 34 (12), 1683–1685.

Divery, P., Florkin, M., 1927. Sur les propriétés optiques de l'amyloide. Comptes Rendus des Séances de la Société de Biologie et des Filiales 97, 1808–1810.

Eanes, E.D., Glenner, G.G., 1968. X-ray diffraction studies on amyloid filaments. Journal of Histochemistry and Cytochemistry 16, 673–677.

Eriksson, L., Westermark, P., 1990. Age-related accumulation of amyloid inclusions in adrenal cortical cells. American Journal of Pathology 136 (2), 461–466.

Fernando, J.C., 1961. A durable method of demonstrating amyloid in paraffin sections. Journal of the Institute of Science Technology 7, 40.

Friedrich, N., Kékulé, A., 1859. Zur Amyloidfrage. Virchows Archiv für Pathologische Anatomie und Physiologie und für Klinische Medizin 16, 50.

Gibbs, S.D.J., Hawkins, P.N., 2011. Amyloidosis. In: Hoffbrand, A,V., Catovsky, D., Tuddenham, E.G.D., et al. (Eds.), Postgraduate haematology, sixth ed. Wiley-Blackwell, Oxford.

Glenner, G.G., 1980. Amyloid deposits and amyloidosis. The beta-fibrilloses (in 2 parts). New England Journal of Medicine 302, 1283–1333.

Glenner, G.G., 1981. The bases of the staining of amyloid fibers: their physico-chemical nature and the mechanism of their dye-substrate interaction. Progress in Histochemistry and Cytochemistry 13 (3), 1–37.

Glenner, G.G., Harada, M., Isersky, C., 1972. The purification of amyloid fibril proteins. Preparative Biochemistry 2 (1), 39–51.

Hawkins, P.N., 1994. Studies with radiolabelled serum amyloid P component provide evidence for turnover and regression of amyloid deposits in vivo. Clinical Science (Colch) 87 (3), 289–295.

Hawkins, P.N., Lavender, J.P., Pepys, M.B., 1990. Evaluation of systemic amyloidosis by scintigraphy with ^{123}I-labeled serum amyloid P component. New England Journal of Medicine 323 (8), 508–513.

Hawkins, P.N., Richardson, S., Vigushin, D.M., et al., 1993. Serum amyloid P component scintigraphy and turnover studies for diagnosis and quantitative monitoring of AA amyloidosis in juvenile rheumatoid arthritis. Arthritis and Rheumatism 36 (6), 842–851.

Highman, B., 1946. Improved methods for demonstrating amyloid in paraffin sections. Archives of Pathology 41, 559.

Howie, A.J., Brewer, D.B., 2009. Review – optical properties of amyloid stained by Congo red: History and mechanisms. Micron 40, 285–301

Hucker, G.J., Conn, H.J., 1928. Gram stain. I. A quick method for staining Gram-positive organisms in the tissues. Archives of Pathology 5, 828.

Husby, G., Araki, S., Benditt, E.P., et al., 1990. The 1990 guidelines for the nomenclature and classification of amyloid and amyloidosis. In: Natvig, J., Forre, O., Husby, G. (Eds.), Amyloid and amyloidosis. Kluwer Academic Publishers, Dordrecht, pp. 7–11.

King, L.S., 1948. Atypical amyloid disease, with observations on a new silver stain for amyloid. 45th Annual Meeting of the American Association of Pathologists and Bacteriologists. Philadelphia, AAPB.

Lamy, C., Duyckaerts, C., Delaere, P., et al., 1989. Comparison of seven staining methods for senile plaques and neurofibrillary tangles in a prospective series of 15 elderly patients. Neuropathology and Applied Neurobiology 15 (6), 563–578.

Larsen, C.P., Walker, P.D., Weiss, D.T., et al., 2010. Prevalence and morphology of leukocyte chemotactic factor 2-associated amyloid in renal biopsies. Kidney Int 77, 816–819.

Lendrum, A.C., Slidders, W., Fraser, D.S., 1972. Renal hyaline. A study of amyloidosis and diabetic vasculosis with new staining methods. Journal of Clinical Pathology 25, 373.

LeVine, H.I., 1995. Thioflavin T interaction with amyloid β-sheet structures. Amyloid 2 (7), 6.

Llewellyn, B.D., 1970. An improved Sirius red method for amyloid. Journal of Medical Laboratory Technology 27, 308.

Lonsdale-Eccles, A.A., Gonda, P., Gilbertson, J.A., et al., 2009. Localized cutaneous amyloid at insulin injection site. Clin Exp Dermatol 34 (8), 1027–1028.

Merlini, G., Bellotti, V., 2003. Molecular mechanisms of Amyloidosis. Review Article. New England Journal of Medicine 349, 6.

Missmahl, H.P., Hartwig, H., 1953. Polarisation-optische untersuchungen an der amyloidsubstanz. Virchows Archiv für Pathologische Anatomie und Physiologie und für Klinische Medizin 324, 489.

Mowry, R.W., Scott, J.E., 1967. Observations on the basophilia of amyloids. Histochemie 10, 8.

Neubert, H., 1925. Über Doppelbrechung und Dichroismus gefärbter Gele (on the birefringence and dichroism of colored gels). Kolloidchem. Beiheft Supp 20, 244–272.

Pearse, A.G.E., 1968. Histochemistry: theoretical and applied. Churchill Livingstone, Edinburgh.

Pepys, M.B., 1992. Amyloid P component and the diagnosis of amyloidosis. Journal of International Medical Research 232 (6), 519–521.

Pepys, M.B., 2006. Amyloidosis. Annu Rev Med 57, 223–241.

Pepys, M.B., Baltz, M.L., 1983. Acute phase proteins with special reference to C-reactive protein and related proteins (pentaxins) and serum amyloid A protein. Advances in Immunology 34, 141.

Pras, M., Schubert, M., Zucker-Franklin, D., et al., 1968. The characterization of soluble amyloid prepared in water. Journal of Clinical Investigation 47 (4), 924–933.

Puchtler, H., Sweat, F., 1965. Congo red as a stain for fluorescence microscopy of amyloid. Journal of Histochemistry and Cytochemistry 13 (8), 693–694.

Puchtler, H., Sweat, F., Levine, M., 1962. On the binding of Congo red by amyloid. Journal of Histochemistry and Cytochemistry 10, 355.

Puchtler, H., Sweat, F., Kuhns, J.G., 1964. On the binding of direct cotton dyes by amyloid. Journal of Histochemistry and Cytochemistry 12, 900.

Puchtler, H., Sweat Waldrop, F., Meloan, S.N., 1985. A review of light, polarization and fluorescence microscopic methods for amyloid. Applied Pathology 3 (1–2), 5–17.

Reimann, H.A., Koucky, R.F., Eklund, C.M., 1935. Primary amyloidosis limited to tissue of mesodermal origin. American Journal of Pathology 11, 977.

Romhányi, G., 1971. Selective differentiation between amyloid and connective tissue structures based on the collagen specific topo-optical staining reaction with Congo red. Virchows Archiv. A: Pathology. Pathologische Anatomie 354 (3), 209–222.

Schwartz, P., 1970. Amyloidosis: cause and manifestation of senile deterioration. Charles C. Thomas, Springfield, IL.

Sipe, J.D. (Ed.), 2005. Amyloid proteins. The beta sheet conformation and disease. Wiley-VCH, Weinheim.

Soto, C., Kascsak, R.J., Saborio, G.P., et al., 2000. Reversion of prion protein conformational changes by synthetic beta-sheet breaker peptides. Lancet 355 (9199), 192–197.

Stokes, G., 1976. An improved Congo red method for amyloid. Medical Laboratory Sciences 33, 79.

Sunde, M., Serpell, L.C., Bartlam, M., et al., 1997. Common core structure of amyloid fibrils by synchrotron X-ray diffraction. Journal of Molecular Biology 273 (3), 729–739.

Tennent, G.A., 1999. Isolation and characterization of amyloid fibrils from tissue. Methods in Enzymology 309, 26–47.

Turnell, W.G., Finch, J.T., 1992. Binding of the dye Congo red to the amyloid protein pig insulin reveals a novel homology amongst amyloid-forming peptide sequences. Journal of Molecular Biology 227 (4), 1205–1223.

Vallet, P.G., Guntern, R., Hof, P.R., et al., 1992. A comparative study of histological and immunohistochemical methods for neurofibrillary tangles and senile plaques in Alzheimer's disease. Acta Neuropathologica 83 (2), 170–178.

Vassar, P.S., Culling, F.A., 1959. Fluorescent stains with special reference to amyloid and connective tissue. Archives of Pathology 68, 487.

Virchow, R., 1853. Weitere mittheilungen über das vorkommen der planzlichen cellulose beim menschen. Virchows Archiv für Pathologische Anatomie und Physiologie und für Klinische Medizin 6 (246).

Virchow, R., 1854. Zur Cellulose-Frage. Virchows Archiv für Klinische Medizine 8, 140.

Von Rokitansky, C.F., 1842. On the abnormalities of the liver. Braumuller Seidel, Vienna.

Westermark, G.T., Johnson, K.H., Westermark, P., 1999. Staining methods for identification of amyloid in tissue. Methods in Enzymology 309, 3–25.

Westermark, P., Stenkvist, B., 1973. A new method for the diagnosis of systemic amyloidosis. Archives of Internal Medicine 132 (4), 522–523.

Westermark, P., Benson, M.D., Buxbaum, J.N., et al., 2005. Amyloid: towards terminology clarification. Report from the Nomenclature Committee of the International Society of Amyloidosis. Amyloid 12 (1), 1–4.

Wilcock, G.K., Matthews, S.M., Moss, T., 1990. Comparison of three silver stains for demonstrating neurofibrillary tangles and neuritic plaques in brain tissue stored for long periods. Acta Neuropathologica 79 (5), 566–568.

Windrum, G.M., Kramer, H., 1957. Fluorescence microscopy of amyloid. Archives of Pathology 63, 373.

Wisniewski, H.M., Wen, G.Y., Kim, K.S., 1989. Comparison of four staining methods on the detection of neuritic plaques. Acta Neuropathologica 78 (1), 22–27.

Wolman, M., 1971. Amyloid, its nature and its molecular structure: Comparison of a new toluidine blue polarized light method with traditional procedures. Laboratory Investigations 25, 104

Wolman, M., Bubis, J.J., 1965. The cause of the green polarization color of amyloid stained with Congo red. Histochemie 4 (5), 351–356.

Wright, J.R., Humphrey, R.L., Calkins, E., et al., 1976. Different molecular forms of amyloid histologically distinguished by susceptibility or resistance to trypsin digestion. Amyloidosis: Proceedings of the Fifth Sigrid Fuselius Foundation Symposium. Academic Press, London.

Wright, J.R., Calkins, E., Humphrey, R.L., 1977. Potassium permanganate reaction in amyloidosis. A histologic method to assist in differentiating forms of this disease. Laboratory Investigation 36 (3), 274–281.

Yamagoe, S., Yamaka, Y., Matsuo, Y., et al., 1996. Purification and primary amino acid sequence of a novel neutrophil chemotactic factor LECT2. Immunol Lett 52, 9–13.

Microorganisms 15

Jeanine H. Bartlett

Introduction

We have all heard the expression, 'The world is getting smaller'. Nowhere is that statement truer than in the world of microorganisms. Microorganisms (also called microbes) are organisms which share the property of being only individually seen by microscopy. Most do not normally cause disease in humans, existing in a state of commensalism, where there is little or no benefit to the person, or mutualism, where there is some benefit to both parties. Pathogens are agents that cause disease. These fall into five main groups:

- Viruses
- Bacteria
- Fungi
- Protozoa
- Helminths

With the advent of new and more powerful antibiotics, improved environmental hygiene, and advances in microbiological techniques it was widely expected that the need for diagnosis of infectious agents in tissue would diminish in importance. This assumption underestimated the infinite capacity of infectious agents for genomic variation, enabling them to exploit new opportunities to spread infections that are created when host defenses become compromised. The following are currently the most important factors influencing the presentation of infectious diseases:

- The increased mobility of the world's population through tourism, immigration, and international commerce has distorted natural geographic boundaries to infection, exposing weaknesses in host defenses, and in knowledge. Some agents, such as Ebola, have been around for many years but the first human outbreaks were not recorded until 1976. Previous outbreaks would flare up and then burn themselves out, undetected and confined, before deforestation and the like altered this state.

- Immunodeficiency states occurring either as part of a natural disease, such as acquired immune deficiency syndrome (AIDS), or as an iatrogenic disease. As treatment becomes more aggressive, depression of the host's immunity often occurs, enabling organisms of low virulence to become life-threatening, and allows latent infections, accrued throughout life, to reactivate and spread unchecked.

- Emerging, re-emerging, and antibiotic-resistant organisms such as the tubercle bacillus and staphylococcus are a constant concern.

- Adaptive mutation occurring in microorganisms, which allows them to jump species barriers and exploit new physical environments, thus evading host defenses, and resisting agents of treatment.

- Bioterrorism has become an increasing concern. The world's public health systems and primary healthcare providers must be prepared to address varied biological agents, including pathogens that are rarely seen in developed countries. High-priority agents include organisms that pose a risk to national security because they:

- Can be easily disseminated or transmitted from person to person
- Cause high mortality, with potential for a major public health impact
- Might cause public panic and social disruption, and require special action for public health preparedness.

The following are listed by the Centers for Disease Control and Prevention (CDC) in the United States as high-risk biological agents:

- Anthrax
- Smallpox
- Botulism
- Tularemia
- Viral hemorrhagic fever (various).

These factors, acting singly or together, provide an ever-changing picture of infectious disease where clinical presentation may involve multiple pathological processes, unfamiliar organisms, and modification of the host response by a diminished immune status.

Size

The term 'microorganism' has been interpreted liberally in this chapter. Space limitation precludes a comprehensive approach to the subject, and the reader is referred to additional texts such as that of von Lichtenberg (1991) for greater depth. The organisms in Table 15.1 are discussed, and techniques for their demonstration are described.

Table 15.1 Size of organisms

Organisms	Size
Viruses	20–300 nm
Mycoplasmas	125–350 nm
Chlamydia	200–1000 nm
Rickettsia	300–1200 nm
Bacteria	1–14 μm
Fungi	2–200 μm
Protozoa	1–50 μm
Metazoans	3–10 mm

Safety

Most infectious agents are rendered harmless by direct exposure to formal saline. Standard fixation procedures should be sufficient to kill microorganisms, one exception being material from patients with Creutzfeldt-Jakob disease (CJD). It has been shown that well-fixed tissue, paraffin-processed blocks, and stained slides from CJD remain infectious when introduced into susceptible animals. Treatment of fixed tissue or slides in 96% formic acid for 1 hour followed by copious washing inactivates this infectious agent without adversely affecting section quality (Brown et al. 1990). Laboratory safety protocols should cover infection containment in all laboratory areas and the mortuary, or necropsy area, where handling unfixed material is unavoidable. When available, unfixed tissue samples should be sent for microbiological culture as this offers the best chance for rapid and specific identification of etiological agents, even when heavy bacterial contamination may have occurred.

General principles of detection and identification

The diagnosis of illness from infectious disease starts with clinical presentation of the patient, and in most cases a diagnosis is made without a tissue sample being taken. Specimens submitted to the laboratory range from autopsy specimens, where material maybe plentiful and sampling error presents little problem, to cytology samples where cellular material is often scarce and lesions may easily be missed. A full clinical history is always important, especially details of the patient's ethnic origin, immune status, any recent history of foreign travel, and current medication.

The macroscopic appearance of tissue, such as abscesses and pus formation, cavitations, hyperkeratosis, demyelination, pseudo-membrane or fibrin formation, focal necrosis, and granulomas can provide evidence of infection. These appearances are often non-specific but occasionally in hydatid cyst disease or some helminth infestations the appearances are diagnostic. The microscopic appearance of routine stains at low-power magnification often reveals indirect evidence of the presence of infection, such as neutrophil or lymphocytic infiltrates, granuloma formation, micro-abscesses, eosinophilic aggregates, Charcot-Leyden crystals and caseous necrosis. Some of these appearances may be sufficiently reliable to provide an initial, or provisional, diagnosis and allow treatment to be started even if the precise nature of the suspect organism is never identified, particularly in the case of tuberculosis.

At the cellular level, the presence of giant cells, (such as Warthin-Finkeldy or Langhans' type) may indicate measles or tuberculosis. Other cellular changes include intra-cytoplasmic edema of koilocytes, acantholysis, spongiform degeneration of brain, margination of chromatin, syncytial nuclear appearance, 'ground-glass' changes in the nucleus or cytoplasm, or inclusion bodies, and can indicate infectious etiology. At some stage in these processes, suspect organisms may be visualized. A well-performed hematoxylin and eosin (H&E) method will stain many organisms. Papanicolaou stain and Romanowsky stains, such as Giemsa, will also stain many organisms together with their cellular environment. Other infectious agents are poorly visualized by routine stains and require special techniques to demonstrate their presence. This may be due to the small size of the organism, as in the case of viruses, where electron microscopy is needed. Alternatively, the organism may be hydrophobic, or weakly charged, as with mycobacteria, spirochetes, and cryptococci, in which case the use of specific histochemical methods is required for their detection. When organisms are few in number, fluorochromes may be used to increase microscopic sensitivity of a technique. Finally, there are two techniques that offer the possibility of specific identification of microorganisms that extend to the appropriate strain level.

Immunohistochemistry

Immunohistochemistry is now a routine and invaluable procedure in the histopathology lab for the detection of many microorganisms. There are many commercially available antibodies for viral, bacterial, and parasitic organisms. Most methods today utilize (strept)avidin-biotin technologies. These are based on the high affinity that (strept)avidin (*Streptomyces avidinii*) and avidin (chicken egg) have for biotin. Both possess four binding sites for biotin, but due to the molecular orientation of the binding sites fewer than four molecules of biotin will actually bind. The basic sequence of reagent application consists of primary antibody, biotinylated secondary antibody, followed by either the preformed (strept)avidin-biotin enzyme complex of the avidin-biotin complex (ABC) technique or by the enzyme-labeled streptavidin. Both conclude with the substrate solution. Horseradish peroxidase and alkaline phosphatases are the most commonly used enzyme labels (see later chapters).

In situ hybridization, the polymerase chain reaction

In situ hybridization (ISH) has even greater potential for microorganism detection. The use of single-stranded nucleic acid probes offers even greater possibilities by identifying latent viral genomic footprints in cells, which may have relevance to extending our knowledge of disease. Acquired immunodeficiency syndrome (AIDS) and human immunodeficiency virus (HIV) are good examples. The polymerase chain reaction (PCR) can also be a very useful technique to obtain diagnoses of microbial infections from autopsy tissues and surgical specimens. While fresh/frozen tissues provide the best-quality nucleic acids for analysis, DNA and RNA extracted from formalin-fixed, paraffin-embedded (FFPE) tissues can be used quite successfully in both PCR and reverse-transcriptase PCR (Tatti et al. 2006; Bhatnagar et al. 2007; Guarner et al. 2007; Shieh et al. 2009). Since formalin cross-links proteins and nucleic acids, resulting in significant degradation, it is critical to design PCR assays targeting small amplicons, typically 500 base pairs or fewer in length (Srinivasan et al. 2002). To this end, it is essential to begin processing of specimens as quickly as possible, ensuring that a 10% concentration of formalin is used for fixation, and making certain that fixation times are kept to no longer than 48 hours (von Ahlfen et al. 2007; Chung et al. 2008).

Table 15.2 A simplified classification of important bacteria

Gram-positive bacteria		Gram-negative bacteria		
Cocci	Bacilli	Cocci	Bacilli	Coccobacilli
Staphylococcus sp.	Bacillus	Neisseria	Escherichia	Brucella
	Clostridium		Klebsiella	Bordetella
Streptococcus sp.	Corynebacterium		Salmonella	Haemophilus
(inc. Pneumococcus)	Mycobacteria (weak+)		Shigella	
	Lactobacillus (commensal)		Proteus	
	Listeria		Pseudomonas	
			Vibrio	
			Pasteurella	

Furthermore, the use of real-time PCR technology, which often requires small amplicons for successful detection of products, is ideally suited for use with nucleic acid extracts from FFPE tissues (Denison et al. 2011). (Thanks are due to Amy M. Denison, PhD, for her assistance with this information.)

While modern advances in technique are important, emphasis is also placed upon the ability of the microscopist to interpret suspicious signs from a good H&E stain. The growing number of patients whose immune status is compromised, and who can mount only a minimal or inappropriate response to infection, further complicates the picture, justifying speculative use of special stains such as those for mycobacteria and fungi on tissue from AIDS patients. It should be remembered that, for a variety of reasons, negative results for the identification of an infectious agent do not exclude its presence. In particular, administration of antibiotics to the patient before a biopsy is often the reason for failure to detect a microorganism in tissue.

Detection and identification of bacteria

When bacteria are present in large numbers, in an abscess or in vegetation on a heart valve, they appear as blue-gray granular masses with an H&E stain. However, organisms are often invisible or obscured by cellular debris. The reaction of pyogenic bacteria to the Gram stain, together with their morphological appearance (i.e. cocci or bacilli) provides the basis for a simple historical classification (Table 15.2).

Use of control sections

The use of known positive control sections with all special stain methods for demonstrating microorganisms is essential. Results are unsafe in the absence of positive controls, and should not be considered valid. The control section should be appropriate, where possible, for the suspected organism. A pneumocystis containing control, for instance, should be used for demonstrating *Pneumocystis jiroveci* (previously called *carinii*). A Gram control should contain both Gram-positive and Gram-negative organisms. Post-mortem tissues have previously been a good source of control material, although medico-legal issues have now limited this in some countries. Alternatively, a suspension of Gram-positive and Gram-negative organisms can be injected into the thigh muscle of a rat shortly before it is sacrificed for some other purpose. Gram-positive and Gram-negative organisms can also be harvested from microbiological plates, suspended in 10% neutral buffered formalin (NBF), centrifuged, and small amounts mixed with minced normal kidney, then chemically processed along with other tissue blocks (Swisher & Nicholson 1989).

The Gram stain

In spite of more than a century having passed since Gram described his technique in 1884, its chemical rationale is still obscure. It is probably due to a mixture of factors, the most important being increased thickness, chemical composition, and the functional integrity of cell walls of Gram-positive bacteria. When these bacteria die, they become Gram negative. The following procedure is only suitable for the demonstration of bacteria in smears of pus and sputum. It may be of value to the pathologist in the necropsy room where a quick technique such as this may enable rapid identification of the organism causing a lung abscess, wound infection, septicemic abscess or meningitis.

Gram method for bacteria in smears *(Gram 1884)*

Method

1. Fix dry film by passing it three times through a flame or placing on a heat block.
2. Stain for 15 seconds in 1% crystal violet or methyl violet, and then pour off excess.
3. Flood for 30 seconds with Lugol's iodine, pour off excess.
4. Flood with acetone for not more than 2–5 seconds, wash with water immediately.
5. Alternatively decolorize with alcohol until no more stain comes out. Wash with water.
6. Counterstain for 20 seconds with dilute carbol fuchsin, or freshly filtered neutral red for 1–2 minutes.
7. Wash with water and carefully blot section until it is dry.

Results

Gram-positive organisms	blue-black
Gram-negative organisms	red

Modified Brown-Brenn method for Gram-positive and Gram-negative bacteria in paraffin sections *(Churukian & Schenk 1982)*

Sections

Formalin-fixed, 4–5 μm, paraffin-embedded sections.

Solutions

Crystal violet solution (commercially available)

Crystal violet, 10% alcoholic	2 ml
Distilled water	18 ml
Ammonium oxalate, 1%	80 ml

Mix and store; always filter before use.

Modified Gram's iodine commercially available, or

Iodine	2 g
Potassium iodide	4 g
Distilled water	400 ml

Dissolve potassium iodide in a small amount of the distilled water, add iodine and dissolve; add remainder of distilled water.

Ethyl alcohol-acetone solution

Ethyl alcohol, absolute	50 ml
Acetone	50 ml

0.5% basic fuchsin solution (stock) commercially available, or

Basic fuchsin or pararosaniline	0.5 g
Distilled water	100 ml

Dissolve with aid of heat and a magnetic stirrer.

Basic fuchsin solution (working)

Basic fuchsin solution (stock)	10 ml
Distilled water	40 ml

Picric acid-acetone

Picric acid	0.1 g
Acetone	100 ml

Note

With concerns over the explosiveness of dry picric acid in the lab, it is recommended that you purchase the picric acid-acetone solution pre-made. It is available through most histology suppliers.

Acetone-xylene solution

Acetone	50 ml
Xylene	50 ml

Staining method

1. Deparaffinize and rehydrate through graded alcohols to distilled water.
2. Stain with filtered crystal violet solution, 1 minute.
3. Rinse well in distilled water.
4. Iodine solution, 1 minute.
5. Rinse in distilled water, blot slide but NOT the tissue section.
6. Decolorize by dipping in alcohol-acetone solution until the blue color stops running. (One to two dips only!)

7. Counterstain in working basic fuchsin for 1 minute. Be sure to agitate the slides well in the basic fuchsin before starting the timer.
8. Rinse in distilled water and blot slide but not section.
9. Dip in acetone, one dip.
10. Dip in picric acid-acetone until the sections have a yellowish-pink color.
11. Dip several times in acetone-xylene solution. At this point, check the control for proper differentiation. (Go back to picric acid-acetone if you need more differentiation.)
12. Clear in xylene and mount.

Results

Gram-positive organisms, fibrin, some fungi, Paneth cell granules, keratohyalin, and keratin	blue
Gram-negative organisms	red
Nuclei	red
Other tissue elements	yellow

Be sure you do not allow the tissue sections to dry at any point in the staining process. If this occurs after treatment with iodine, decolorization will be difficult and uneven.

Gram-Twort stain (Twort 1924; Ollett 1947)

Sections

Formalin fixed, paraffin.

Solutions

Crystal violet solution (see previous method)

Gram's iodine (see previous solution)

Twort's stain

1% neutral red in ethanol	9 ml
0.2% fast green in ethanol	1 ml
Distilled water	30 ml

Mix immediately before use.

Method

1. Deparaffinize and rehydrate through graded alcohols to distilled water.
2. Stain in crystal violet solution, 3 minutes.
3. Rinse in gently running tap water.
4. Treat with Gram's iodine, 3 minutes.
5. Rinse in tap water, blot dry, and complete drying in a warm place.

6. Differentiate in preheated acetic alcohol until no more color washes out (2% acetic acid in absolute alcohol, preheated to 56°C). This may take 15–20 minutes; the section should be light brown or straw colored.
7. Rinse briefly in distilled water.
8. Stain in Twort's, 5 minutes.
9. Wash in distilled water.
10. Rinse in acetic alcohol until no more red runs out of the section; this takes only a few seconds.
11. Rinse in fresh absolute alcohol, clear, and mount.

Results

Gram-positive organisms	blue-black
Gram-negative organisms	pink-red
Nuclei	red
Red blood cells and most cytoplasmic structures	green
Elastic fibers	black

Techniques for mycobacteria

These organisms are difficult to demonstrate by the Gram technique as they possess a capsule containing a long-chain fatty acid (mycolic acid) that makes them hydrophobic. The fatty capsule influences the penetration and resistance to removal of the stain by acid and alcohol (acid- and alcohol-fastness), and is variably robust between the various species that make up this group. Phenolic acid, and frequently heat, are used to reduce surface tension and increase porosity, thus forcing dyes to penetrate this capsule. The speed with which the primary dye is removed by differentiation with acid alcohol is proportional to the extent of the fatty coat. The avoidance of defatting agents, or solvents, such as alcohol and xylene, in methods for *Mycobacterium leprae*, is an attempt to conserve this fragile fatty capsule.

Mycobacteria are PAS positive due to the carbohydrate content of their cell walls. However, this positivity is evident only when large concentrations of the microorganisms are present. When these organisms die, they lose their fatty capsule and consequently their carbol fuchsin positivity. The carbohydrate can still be demonstrated by Grocott's methenamine silver reaction, which may prove useful when acid-fast procedures fail, particularly if the patient is already receiving therapy for tuberculosis.

A possible source of acid-fast contamination may be found growing in viscous material sometimes lining water taps and any rubber tubing connected to them. These organisms are acid- and alcohol-fast but are usually easily identified as contaminants by their appearance as clumps, or floaters, above the microscopic focal plane of the section.

Ziehl-Neelsen (ZN) stain for *Mycobacterium* bacilli
(Kinyoun 1915)

Sections
Formalin or fixative other than Carnoy's, paraffin.

Solutions
Carbol fuchsin commercially available, or

Basic fuchsin	0.5 g
Absolute alcohol	5 ml
5% aqueous phenol	100 ml

Mix well and filter before use.

Acid alcohol

Hydrochloric acid	10 ml
70% alcohol	1000 ml

Methylene blue solution (stock) commercially available, or

Methylene blue	1.4 g
95% alcohol	100 ml

Methylene blue solution (working)

Methylene blue (stock)	10 ml
Tap water	90 ml

Method
1. Deparaffinize and rehydrate through graded alcohols to distilled water.
2. Carbol fuchsin solution, 30 minutes.
3. Wash well in tap water.
4. Differentiate in acid alcohol until solutions are pale pink. (This usually only takes 2–5 dips.)
5. Wash in tap water for 8 minutes, then dip in distilled water.
6. Counterstain in working methylene blue solution until sections are pale blue.
7. Rinse in tap water, then dip in distilled water.
8. Dehydrate, clear, and mount.

Results

Mycobacteria, hair shafts, Russell bodies, Splendore-Hoeppli immunoglobulins around actinomyces, and some fungal organisms	red
Background	pale blue

Notes
a. The blue counterstain may be patchy if extensive caseation is present. Care should be taken to avoid over-counterstaining as scant organisms can easily be obscured.
b. Decalcification using strong acids can destroy acid-fastness; formic acid is recommended.
c. Victoria blue can be substituted for carbol fuchsin and picric acid for the counterstain if color blindness causes a recognition problem.

Fluorescent method for *Mycobacterium* bacilli
(Kuper & May 1960)

Sections
Formalin fixed, paraffin.

Solution

Auramine O	1.5 g
Rhodamine B	0.75 g
Glycerol	75 ml
Phenol crystals (liquefied at 50°C)	10 ml
Distilled water	50 ml

Method
1. Deparaffinize (1 part groundnut oil and 2 parts xylene for *M. leprae*).
2. Pour on preheated (60°C), filtered staining solution, 10 minutes.
3. Wash in tap water.
4. Differentiate in 0.5% hydrochloric acid in alcohol for *M. tuberculosis*, or 0.5% aqueous hydrochloric acid for *M. leprae*.
5. Wash in tap water, 2 minutes.
6. Eliminate background fluorescence in 0.5% potassium permanganate, 2 minutes.
7. Wash in tap water and blot dry.
8. Dehydrate (not for *M. leprae*), clear, and mount in a fluorescence-free mountant.

Results

Mycobacteria	golden yellow (using blue light fluorescence below 530 nm)
Background	dark green

Notes

The advantage of increased sensitivity of this technique is offset by the inconvenience of setting up the fluorescence microscope. Preparations fade over time, as a result of their exposure to UV light.

Modified Fite method for *M. leprae* and *Nocardia*

Fixation

10% neutral buffered formalin (NBF).

Sections

Paraffin sections at 4–5 μm.

Solutions

Carbol fuchsin solution commercially available, or 0.5 g basic fuchsin dissolved in 5 ml of absolute alcohol; add 100 ml of 5% aqueous phenol. Mix well and filter before use. Filter before each use with #1 filter paper.

5% sulfuric acid in 25% alcohol

25% ethanol	95 ml
Sulfuric acid, concentrated	5 ml

Methylene blue (stock) commercially available, or

Methylene blue	1.4 g
95% alcohol	100 ml

Methylene blue, working

Stock methylene blue	5 ml
Tap water	45 ml
Xylene-peanut oil	1 part oil: 2 parts xylene

Method

1. Deparaffinize in two changes of xylene-peanut oil, 6 minutes each.
2. Drain slides vertically on paper towel and wash in warm, running tap water for 3 minutes. (The residual oil preserves the sections and helps accentuate the acid fastness of the bacilli.)
3. Stain in carbol fuchsin at room temperature for 25 minutes. (Solution may be poured back into bottle and reused).
4. Wash in warm, running tap water for 3 minutes.
5. Drain excess water from slides vertically on paper towel.
6. Decolorize with 5% sulfuric acid in 25% alcohol, two changes of 90 seconds each. (Sections should be pale pink.)
7. Wash in warm, running tap water for 5 minutes.
8. Counterstain in working methylene blue, one quick dip. (Sections should be pale blue.)
9. Wash in warm, running tap water for 5 minutes.
10. Blot sections and dry in 50–55°C oven for 5 minutes.
11. Once dry, one quick dip in xylene.
12. Mount with permanent mountant.

Results See Figure 15.1

Acid-fast bacilli including *M. leprae*	bright red
Nuclei and other tissue elements	pale blue

Quality control/notes

Be careful not to overstain with methylene blue and do not allow sections to dry between carbol fuchsin and acid alcohol.

Cresyl violet acetate method for *Helicobacter* sp.

Sections

Formalin fixed, paraffin.

Method

1. Deparaffinize and rehydrate through graded alcohols to distilled water.
2. Filter 0.1% cresyl violet acetate onto slide or into Coplin jar, 5 minutes.
3. Rinse in distilled water.
4. Blot, dehydrate rapidly in alcohol, clear, and mount.

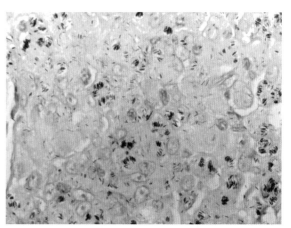

Figure 15.1 The modified Fite's procedure is necessary to demonstrate *Mycobacterium leprae* due to the organism's fragile, fatty capsule.

Results

Helicobacter and nuclei	blue-violet
Background	shades of blue-violet

Notes

This simple method allows for good differentiation of *Helicobacter* sp. from other organisms.

Gimenez method for *Helicobacter pylori* (Gimenez 1964; McMullen et al. 1987)

Sections

Formalin fixed, paraffin.

Solutions

Buffer solution (phosphate buffer at pH 7.5, or 0.1 M)

0.1 M sodium dihydrogen orthophosphate	3.5 ml
0.1 M disodium hydrogen orthophosphate	15.5 ml

Stock carbol fuchsin

Commercial cold acid-fast bacilli stain, or basic fuchsin	1 g
Absolute alcohol	10 ml
5% aqueous phenol	10 ml

Filter before use.

Working carbol fuchsin

Phosphate buffer	10 ml
Stock carbol fuchsin	4 ml

Filter before use.

Malachite green

Malachite green	0.8 g
Distilled water	100 ml

Method

1. Deparaffinize and rehydrate through graded alcohols to distilled water.
2. Stain in working carbol fuchsin solution, 2 minutes.
3. Wash well in tap water.
4. Stain in malachite green, 15–20 seconds.
5. Wash thoroughly in distilled water.
6. Repeat steps 4 and 5 until section is blue-green to the naked eye.
7. Blot sections dry, and complete drying in air.
8. Clear and mount.

Results

Helicobacter	red-magenta
Background	blue-green

Notes

The greatest problem with this method is overstaining or irregularity of staining, with Malachite green. It is valuable in demonstrating the *Legionella* bacillus in postmortem lung smears.

Toluidine blue in Sorenson's buffer for *Helicobacter*

Sections

Formalin fixed, paraffin.

Solutions

Toluidine blue in pH 6.8 phosphate buffer

Sorenson's phosphate buffer, pH 6.8	50 ml
1% aqueous toluidine blue	1 ml

Method

1. Deparaffinize and rehydrate through graded alcohols to distilled water.
2. Stain in buffered toluidine blue, 20 minutes.
3. Wash well in distilled water.
4. Dehydrate, clear, and mount.

Results

Helicobacter	dark blue against a variably blue background

Warthin-Starry method for spirochetes (Warthin & Starry 1920)

Sections

Formalin fixed, paraffin.

Solutions

Acetate buffer, pH 3.6

Sodium acetate	4.1 g
Acetic acid	6.25 ml
Distilled water	500 ml

1% silver nitrate in pH 3.6 acetate buffer

Developer

Dissolve 3 g of hydroquinone in 10 ml pH 3.6 buffer, and mix 1 ml of this solution and 15 ml of warmed 5% Scotch glue or gelatin; keep at 40°C. Take 3 ml of 2% silver nitrate in pH 3.6 buffer solution and keep at 55°C. Mix these two solutions immediately before use.

Method

1. Deparaffinize and rehydrate through graded alcohols to distilled water.

2. Celloidinize in 0.5% celloidin, drain, and harden in distilled water, 1 minute.
3. Impregnate in preheated 55–60°C silver solution (b), 90–105 minutes.
4. Prepare and preheat developer in a water bath.
5. Treat with developer (solution c) for $3\frac{1}{2}$ minutes at 55°C. Sections should be golden-brown at this point.
6. Remove from developer and rinse in tap water for several minutes at 55–60°C, then in buffer at room temperature.
7. Tone in 0.2% gold chloride.
8. Dehydrate, clear, and mount.

Results

| Spirochetes | black |
| Background | golden-yellow |

Notes

It is wise to take a few slides through at various incubation times to ensure optimum impregnation.

Modified Steiner for filamentous and non-filamentous bacteria (Steiner & Steiner 1944; Modified Swisher 1987)

Sections

Formalin fixed, paraffin.

Solutions

1.0% uranyl nitrate commercially available, or

| Uranyl nitrate | 1 g |
| Distilled water | 100 ml |

1% silver nitrate

| Silver nitrate | 1 g |
| Distilled water | 100 ml |

Make fresh each time and filter with #1 or #2 filter paper before use.

0.04% silver nitrate

| Silver nitrate | 0.04 g |
| Distilled water | 100 ml |

Refrigerate and use for only 1 month.

2.5% gum mastic commercially available, or

| Gum mastic | 2.5 g |
| Absolute alcohol | 100 ml |

Allow to dissolve for 24 hours, then filter until clear yellow before use. Refrigerate unused portion for reuse.

2% hydroquinone

| Hydroquinone | 1 g |
| Distilled water | 25 ml |

Make fresh solution for each use.

Reducing solution

Mix 10 ml of 2.5% gum mastic, 25 ml of 2.0% hydroquinone, and 5 ml absolute alcohol. Make just prior to use and filter with #4 filter paper; add 2.5 ml of 0.04% silver nitrate. Do not filter this solution. When the gum mastic is added, the solution will take on a milky appearance.

Method

1. Deparaffinize and rehydrate through graded alcohols to distilled water.
2. Sensitize sections in 1% aqueous uranyl nitrate at room temperature, and place in microwave oven until solution is just at boiling point, approx. 20–30 seconds; do not boil. *Alternatively*, place in preheated 1% uranyl nitrate at 60°C in a water bath for 15 minutes, or in microwave oven and bring to boiling point – do not boil; 2% zinc sulfate in 3.7% formalin may be substituted.
3. Rinse in distilled water at room temperature until uranyl nitrate residue is eliminated.
4. Place in 1% silver nitrate at room temperature and microwave *until* boiling point is just reached. Do not boil. Remove from oven, loosely cover jar, and allow to stand in hot silver nitrate, 6–7 minutes; *alternatively*, preheat silver nitrate for 20–30 minutes in a 60°C water bath, add slides, and allow to impregnate for $1\frac{1}{2}$ hours.
5. Rinse in three changes of distilled water.
6. Dehydrate in two changes, each of 95% alcohol and absolute alcohol.
7. Treat with 2.5% gum mastic, 5 minutes.
8. Allow to air dry, 5 minutes.
9. Rinse in two changes of distilled water. Slides may stand here while reducing solution is being prepared.
10. Reduce in preheated reducing solution at 45°C in a water bath for 10–25 minutes, or until sections have developed satisfactorily with black microorganisms against a light yellow background. Avoid intensely stained background.
11. Rinse in distilled water to stop reaction.
12. Dehydrate, clear, and mount.

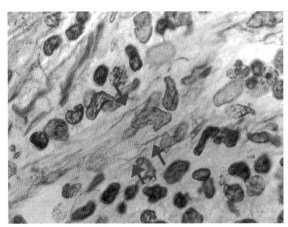

Figure 15.2 Syphilis *Treponema pallidum*, bacilli (arrowed), seen with the modified Steiner technique. The resistance to coloration is shared by *Helicobacter*, spirochetes, and *Legionella*.

Results See Figure 15.2

Spirochetes, cat-scratch organisms, Donovan bodies, non-filamentous bacteria of *L. pneumophila*	dark brown-black
Background	bright yellow to golden yellow

Notes

Bring all solutions to room temperature before using. All glassware making contact with silver nitrate should be chemically cleaned. Avoid the use of metal forceps in silver solutions. When doing a bacterial screen, Gram controls should be run along with diagnostic slides. As spirochetes take longer to develop, Gram controls should be used in addition to spirochete controls. When Gram controls have a yellow appearance, remove them to distilled water, and check on microscope for microorganisms. Return to silver solution if they are not ready, and repeat, realizing that spirochetes will take longer. Most solutions can be made in large quantities and kept in the refrigerator.

Some important bacteria

Staphylococcus aureus is perhaps the most important pathogen of this group. It causes boils, wound and burn infections, and a form of cavitating pneumonia in children and adults. Septicemic states and the formation of multiple scattered abscesses sometimes occur. Staphylococci tend to form clusters. Multi-resistance to antibiotics is sometimes encountered.

Neisseria meningitidis (meningococcus) is a common cause of meningitis, and may produce a fulminating septicemia. Organisms can be seen in histological sections of meningococcal meningitis, but are difficult to identify because they are usually within neutrophil cytoplasm.

Neisseria gonorrhoeae (gonococcus) is the cause of gonorrhea. Organisms may be seen within polymorphs in sections of cervix, endometrium, or Fallopian tubes in cases of gonorrhea but, again, are difficult to find. Members of the *Neisseria* family are generally difficult to see in histological sections, although easily detectable in smears of fresh pus or cerebrospinal fluid (CSF), characteristically in pairs. They are easier to detect using the Gram-Twort method.

Lactobacillus acidophilus (Döderlein's bacillus) is a normal inhabitant of the human vagina and is seen in cervical smears taken in the secretory phase of the cycle.

Corynebacterium vaginale is a short Gram-negative bacillus which may cause cervicitis, and is present in about 6% of women of childbearing age. It may be seen in cervical smears where it accumulates as blue-stained masses on the surface of squamous cells stained by Papanicolaou's method, with these cells being known as 'clue cells'.

Helicobacter pylori is frequently seen in gastric biopsies. A spiral vibrio organism is heavily implicated as the organism causing many cases of chronic gastritis. It is seen as small, weakly hematoxyphilic organisms (usually in clumps) in the lumina of gastric glands, often adherent to the luminal surface of the epithelial cells. With practice, these can be identified from an H&E stain. However, Warthin-Starry, Steiner, Gimenez, toluidine blue, or cresyl violet acetate methods demonstrate them more clearly. A commercial specific antiserum has recently become available for their demonstration.

Clostridium difficile causes pseudomembranous colitis, an inflammation of the large bowel. This arises following the administration of broad-spectrum antibiotics; the balance of the normal anaerobic gut microflora is disturbed, allowing the organism to proliferate unchecked. *C. difficile* is difficult to stain but the 'volcano lesions' of purulent necrosis are a good indicator.

Listeria monocytogenes is the cause of a rare form of meningitis and may cause septicemia in humans. Focal necrosis with macrophages that contain tiny intracellular rods arranged in a 'Chinese letter' formation, and staining variably with the Gram stain, are the hallmark of this disease.

Mycobacterium tuberculosis remains a significant pathogen in developed countries where the familiar caseating granulomatous lesion and its associated 1–2 µm, blunt-ended, acid- and alcohol-fast bacilli can still be seen. In Africa and other countries, this organism has developed an opportunistic relationship with AIDS, where it is a major cause of death.

Mycobacterium avium/intracellulare are representatives of a group of intracellular opportunistic mycobacteria that are frequently present in the later stages of immunosuppression, particularly that associated with AIDS. They frequently persist in spite of treatment, and are often lethal. The lesions produced are non-caseating and consist of collections of vacuolated macrophages that often contain vast numbers of organisms. On occasion, there is little evidence of a cellular reaction on an H&E-stained section, and the organism is detected only by routinely performing an acid-fast stain, such as the ZN, on all tissue from AIDS patients. This group also includes *M. kansasii*.

Mycobacterium leprae is an obligate intracellular, neurotrophic mycobacterium that attacks and destroys nerves, especially in the skin. The tissue reaction to leprosy depends on the immune status of the host. It can be minimal with a few macrophages packed with crescentic, pointed, intracytoplasmic bacilli (lepromatous leprosy), or may contain scanty organisms and show florid granulomatous response (tuberculoid leprosy). *M. leprae* is only acid-fast and can often be demonstrated with a standard ZN technique.

Legionella pneumophila was first identified in 1977 as the cause of a sporadic type of pneumonia of high mortality. The small Gram-positive coccobacillus is generally spread in aerosols from stagnant water reservoirs, usually in air-conditioning units. The bacterium may be difficult to stain except with the Dieterle and modified Steiner silver stains, and specific antiserum.

Treponema pallidum is the organism causing syphilis, and is infrequently seen in biopsy specimens as the primary lesion or 'chancre' is diagnosed clinically. The spirochete is quite obvious using darkground microscopy, as an 8–13 µm corkscrew shaped microorganism that often kinks in the center. Dieterle, Warthin-Starry, or modified Steiner methods may demonstrate the organism. In addition, specific antiserum is also available.

Leptospira interrogans is the organism causing leptospirosis or Weil's disease. It is a disease characterized by spirochetes, and is spread in the urine of rats and dogs, causing fever, profound jaundice, and sometimes death. Spirochetes can be seen in the acute stages of the disease where they appear in Warthin-Starry and modified Steiner techniques as tightly wound 13 µm microorganisms with curled ends resembling a shepherd's crook.

Intestinal spirochetosis appears as a massive infestation on the luminal border of the colon by spirochete *Brachyspira aalborgi* (Tomkins et al. 1986). It measures 2–6 µm long, is tightly coiled, and arranged perpendicularly to the luminal surface of the gut, giving it a fuzzy hematoxyphilic coat in an H&E stain. There is no cellular response to the presence of this spirochete. It is seen well with the Warthin-Starry and the modified Steiner techniques.

Cat-scratch disease presents as a self-limiting, local, single lymphadenopathy appearing about 2 weeks after a cat scratch or bite. Histologically the node shows focal necrosis or micro-abscesses. Two Gram-negative bacteria (*Afipia felis* and *Bartonella henselae*) have been implicated. Because of the timing or maturation factor of the bacterium, it is difficult to demonstrate on paraffin sections, but the modified Steiner and the Warthin-Starry methods are valuable techniques for demonstrating this organism.

Fungal infections

Fungi are widespread in nature, and humans are regularly exposed to the spores from many species, yet the most commonly encountered diseases are the superficial mycoses that affect the subcutaneous or horny layers of the skin or hair shafts, and cause conditions such as athlete's foot or ringworm. These dermatophytic fungi belong to the *Microsporum* and *Trichophyton* groups and may appear as yeasts or mycelial forms within the keratin. They are seen fairly well in the H&E stain, but are demonstrated well with the Grocott and PAS stains. As with other infections, the increase in the number of patients with diminished or compromised immune systems has increased the incidence of *systemic mycoses*, allowing opportunistic attacks by fungi, often of low virulence, but sometimes resulting in death.

When fungi grow in tissue they may display primitive asexual (imperfect) forms that appear as either spherical *yeast* or *spore* forms. Some may produce vegetative growth that appears as tubular *hyphae* that may be septate and branching; these features are important morphologically for identifying different types of fungi. A mass of interwoven hyphae is called a fungal *mycelium*. Only rarely, when the fungus reaches an open cavity, the body surface, or a luminal surface such as the bronchus, are the spore-forming fruiting bodies called *sporangia*, or *conidia*, produced.

Identification of fungi

Some fungi may elicit a range of host reactions from exudative, necrotizing, to granulomatous; other fungi produce little cellular response to indicate their presence. Fortunately, most fungi are relatively large and their cell walls are rich in polysaccharides, which can be converted by oxidation to dialdehydes and thus detected with Schiff's reagent or hexamine-silver solutions. Fungi are often weakly hematoxyphilic and can be suspected on H&E stains. Some fungi, such as sporothrix, may be surrounded by a stellate, strongly eosinophilic, refractile Splendore-Hoeppli precipitates of host immunoglobulin and degraded eosinophils.

Fluorochrome-labeled specific antibodies to many fungi are available, and are in use in mycology laboratories for the identification of fungi on fresh and paraffin sections. These antibodies have not found widespread use, however, on fixed tissue where identification still relies primarily on traditional staining methods.

An H&E stain, a Grocott methenamine (hexamine)-silver (GMS), a mounted unstained section to look for pigmentation, and a good color atlas (Chandler et al. 1980) when experience fails permit most fungal infections to be identified to levels sufficient for diagnoses. However, there is no substitute for microbiological culture.

Grocott methenamine (hexamine)-silver for fungi and *Pneumocystis* spp. organisms (Gomori 1946; Grocott 1955; Swisher & Chandler 1982)

Sections
Formalin fixed, paraffin.

Solutions

4% chromic acid commercially available, or
Chromic acid	4.0 g
Distilled water	100 ml

1% sodium bisulfite
Sodium bisulfite	1 g
Distilled water	100 ml

5% sodium thiosulfate
Sodium thiosulfate	5.0 g
Distilled water	100 ml

(A) 0.21% silver nitrate (stock)
Silver nitrate	2.1 g
Distilled water	1000 ml

Refrigerate for up to 3 months.

(B) Methenamine-sodium borate solution (stock)
Methenamine	27 g
Sodium borate decahydrate (borax)	3.8 g
Distilled water	1000 ml

Refrigerate for up to 3 months.

Methenamine-silver sodium borate solution (working)
Equal parts of solutions A and B. Make fresh each time and filter before use.

0.2% light green (stock)
Light green	0.2 g
Distilled water	100 ml
Glacial acetic acid	0.2 ml

Light green (working)

Stock light green	10 ml
Distilled water	50 ml

Prepare working solution fresh before each use.

Method

1. Deparaffinize and rehydrate through graded alcohols to distilled water.
2. Oxidize in 4% aqueous chromic acid (chromium trioxide), 30 minutes.
3. Wash briefly in distilled water.
4. Dip briefly in 1% sodium bisulfite.
5. Wash well in distilled water
6. Place in preheated (56–60°C water bath) working silver solution for 15–20 minutes. Check control after 15 minutes. If section is 'paper bag brown' then rinse in distilled water and check under microscope. If it is not ready, dip again in distilled water and return to silver. Elastin should not be black. Check every 2 minutes from that point onwards. (See Note a.)
7. Rinse well in distilled water.
8. Tone in 0.1% gold chloride, 5 seconds. Rinse in distilled water.
9. Place in 5% sodium thiosulfate, 5 seconds.
10. Rinse well in running tap water.
11. Counterstain in working light green solution until a medium green (usually 5–15 seconds).
12. Dehydrate, clear, and mount.

Results

Fungi, pneumocystis, melanin	black
Hyphae and yeast-form cells	sharply delineated in black of fungi
Mucins and glycogen	taupe to dark gray/brown
Background	pale green

Notes

a. Incubation time is variable and depends on the type and duration of fixation, and organism being demonstrated. Impregnation is controlled microscopically until fungi are dark brown. Background is colorless at this point. Over-incubation produces intense staining of elastin and fungi that may obscure fine internal detail of the hyphal septa. This detail is essential for critical identification, and is best seen on under-impregnated sections. To avoid excess glycogen impregnation in liver sections, section may be digested prior to incubation. A water bath may be used effectively to insure an even incubation temperature.
b. Borax insures an alkaline pH.
c. Sodium bisulfite removes excess chromic acid.
d. Some workers prefer a light H&E counterstain. This is especially useful when a consulting case is sent with only one slide, providing morphological detail for the pathologist.
e. Solutions A and B need to be made and stored in chemically clean glassware (20% nitric acid), as does the working solution. This includes graduates and Coplin jars. Do not use metal forceps.
f. Allow all refrigerated solutions to reach room temperature before using.

McManus' PAS method for glycogen and fungal cell walls

Fixation
10% NBF.

Sections
3–5-μm paraffin sections.

Solutions

Schiff's reagent, also commercially available
0.5% periodic acid solution

Periodic acid	0.5 g
Distilled water	100 ml

0.2% light green (stock)

Light green	0.2 g
Distilled water	100 ml
Glacial acetic acid	0.2 ml

This is the same stock solution used in the GMS.

Light green (working)

Stock light green	10 ml
Distilled water	50 ml

Make fresh before each use.

Method

1. Deparaffinize and hydrate slides to distilled water.
2. Oxidize in periodic acid solution for 5 minutes.
3. Rinse in distilled water.
4. Place in Schiff's reagent for 15 minutes.
5. Wash in running tap water for 10 minutes to allow pink color to develop.
6. Counterstain for a few seconds in working light green solution.

7. Dehydrate in 95% alcohol, absolute alcohol, and clear in xylene.

8. Mount in resin-based mountant.

Results

Fungal cell walls and glycogen	magenta to red
Background	pale green

Quality control/notes

A solution of 5% aqueous sodium hypochlorite reduces overstaining by Schiff's.

A selection of the more important fungi and actinomycetes

Actinomyces israelii is a colonial bacterium which can be found as a commensal in the mouth and tonsillar crypts. It can cause a chronic suppurative infection, actinomycosis, which is characterized by multiple abscesses drained by sinus tracts. Actinomycotic abscesses can be found in liver, appendix, lung, and neck. The individual organisms are Gram-positive, hematoxyphilic, non-acid-fast, branching filaments 1 μm in diameter. They become coated in 'clubs' of Splendore-Hoeppli protein when the organism is invasive. These clubs are eosinophilic, acid-fast, 1–15 μm wide, and up to 100 μm long, and stain polyclonally for immunoglobulins. This arrangement of a clump of actinomyces or fungal hyphae, which measures 30–3000 μm, surrounded by eosinophilic protein, is called a 'sulfur' granule and is an important identification marker for certain fungal groups. These granules may be macroscopically visible and their yellow color is an important diagnostic aid.

Nocardia asteroides is another actinomycete. It is filamentous and may be visible in an H&E stain, but is Grocott positive and variably acid-fast using the modified ZN for leprosy. However, it is difficult to demonstrate even with the acid-fast bacillus. Its pathology is similar to that of actinomycosis, but its organisms are generally more disseminated than those of actinomycosis.

Candida albicans is a common fungus, but with immunosuppression can become systemic. It infects the mouth as thrush, the esophagus, the vagina as vaginal moniliasis, the skin and nails, and may be found in heart-valve vegetations. It is seen as both ovoid budding yeast-form cells of 3–4 μm, and more commonly as slender 3–5 μm, sparsely septate, non-branching hyphae and pseudo-hyphae. While difficult to see on H&E, this organism is strongly Gram positive, and is obvious with the Grocott and PAS techniques.

Aspergillus fumigatus is a soil saprophyte and a commensal in the bronchial tree. It may infect old lung cavities (Fig. 15.3) or become systemic in immunosuppressed patients. The fungus has broad, 3–6 μm, parallel-sided, septate hyphae showing dichotomous (45 degrees) branching. It may be associated with Splendore-Hoeppli protein and sometimes forms fungal balls within tissue. This fungus may be seen in an H&E stain and is demonstrated well with a PAS or Grocott. When it grows exposed to air, the conidophoric fruiting body may be seen as *Aspergillus niger*, a black species that can cause infection of the ear.

Zygomycosis is an infrequently seen disease caused by a group of hyphated fungi belonging mainly to the genera *Mucor* and *Rhizopus*. They have thin-walled hyphae (infrequently septate) with non-parallel sides, ranging from 3 to 25 μm in diameter, branch irregularly, and often show empty bulbous hyphal swelling. Grocott and PAS are the staining methods of choice (Figs 15.4 and 15.5).

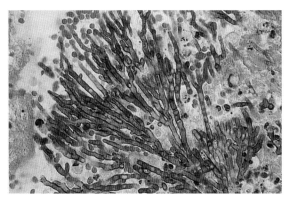

Figure 15.3 A strong hematoxylin (Ehrlich's and eosin stain) will show the fine detail of many infectious agents. The hyphal structure identifies this as *Aspergillus* which was colonizing an old tuberculosis cavity in the lung.

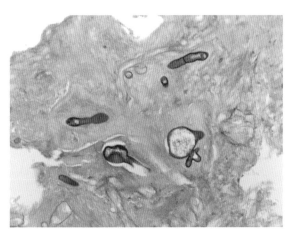

Figure 15.4 *Rhizomucor* spp. (a cosmopolitan, filamentous fungus) is well demonstrated by this PAS stain with light green counterstain.

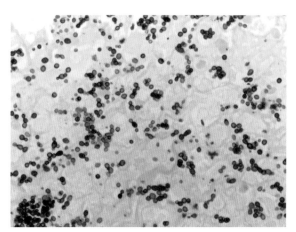

Figure 15.6 Grocott's methenamine-silver stains a wide variety of infectious agents. Here seen with light green counterstain is the method of choice for *Histoplasma capsulatum*, a dimorphic endemic fungus.

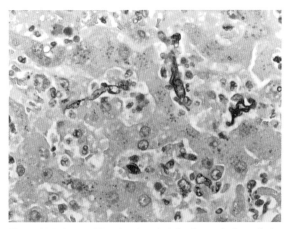

Figure 15.5 Immunohistochemistry is being increasingly applied to the demonstration of microorganisms using labeled specific antibody. This figure demonstrates *Zygomycetes*, a fast-growing fungus, with fast red chromogen.

Cryptococcus neoformans exists solely in yeast-form cells, is variable in diameter (2–20 μm) with ovoid, elliptical, and crescentic forms frequently seen. There is an extensive mucopolysaccharide coat around the yeasts that is mostly dissolved during processing, but, when present, appears as a halo around the organism and is visible with special stains such as Mayer's or Southgate's mucicarmine procedures. Yeasts may be free form or within the cytoplasm of giant cells, staining faintly with

an H&E stain. The PAS and Grocott procedures demonstrate these cells well. Infection is found in the lungs and in the brain within the parenchyma or in the leptomeninges. Often, these patients are immunosuppressed.

Histoplasma capsulatum is another soil-dwelling yeast that can cause a systemic infection in humans called histoplasmosis. It is especially common along the southern border of the United States, and where there are large bird populations. The organism is usually seen within the cytoplasm of macrophages that appear stuffed with small, regular, 2–5 μm yeast-form cells that have a thin halo around them in H&E and Giemsa stains. Langhans' giant cells forming non-caseating granulomas may be present. PAS and Grocott stains demonstrate this fungus well (Fig. 15.6).

Pneumocystis jiroveci. There is still some debate over the taxonomy of this organism, although recent analysis of its ribosomal RNA has placed it nearer to a fungal than a protozoan classification (Edman et al. 1988). It came to prominence as a pathogen following immunosuppressive therapies associated with renal transplants in the 1960s, and has become a life-threatening complication of AIDS. It most frequently causes pneumonia, where the lung alveoli are progressively filled with amphophilic, foamy plugs of parasites and cellular debris. It is found rarely in other sites such as intestines and lymph nodes. The cysts are invisible in an H&E stain, and can barely be seen in a Papanicolaou stain, as they appear refractile when the microscope condenser is racked down. Specific immunohistology is available to use; otherwise, Grocott methenamine-silver is recommended.

Only electron microscopy or an H&E stain on a resin-embedded thin section will show their internal structure. The cysts are 4–6 μm in diameter and contain 5–8 dot-like intracystic bodies. The cysts rupture and collapse, liberating the trophozoites which can be seen as small hematoxyphilic dots in a good H&E and Giemsa stain; these attach to the alveolar epithelium by surface philopodia.

The demonstration of rickettsia

Rickettsial organisms, such as those causing Q fever, Rocky Mountain spotted fever, or typhus, rarely need to be demonstrated in tissue sections. They can sometimes be seen with a Giemsa stain, or by using the Macchiavello technique which also demonstrates some viral inclusion bodies (Fig. 15.7).

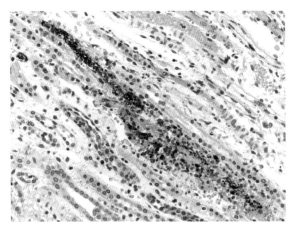

Figure 15.7 Immunohistochemical method demonstrating Rocky Mountain spotted fever in kidney. It is caused by the bacterium *Rickettsia rickettsii*, which is carried by ticks.

Macchiavello's stain for rickettsia and viral inclusions, modified *(Culling 1974)*

Sections

Formalin fixed, paraffin.

Method

1. Deparaffinize and rehydrate through graded alcohols to distilled water.
2. Stain in 0.25% basic fuchsin, 30 minutes.
3. Differentiate in 0.5% citric acid, 3 seconds.
4. Wash in tap water, 2 minutes.
5. Counterstain in 1% methylene blue, 15–30 seconds.
6. Rinse in tap water.
7. Dehydrate, clear, and mount.

Results

Rickettsia and some viral inclusions	red
Background	blue

The detection and identification of viruses

While the cytopathic effects of viruses can often be seen in a good H&E stain, and may be characteristic of a single viral group, the individual viral particles are too small to be seen with the light microscope, thus requiring the electron microscope to reveal their structure. This may allow a rapid and accurate diagnosis in viral infections; an outline of the value of electron microscopy in the diagnosis of viral lesions is given in Chapter 22. Some viruses aggregate within cells to produce *viral inclusion bodies*, which may be intranuclear, intracytoplasmic, or both. These inclusion bodies may be acidophilic and usually intranuclear, or can be basophilic and cytoplasmic. Most special staining methods are modified trichromes, using contrasting acid and basic dyes to exploit these differences in charges on the inclusion body and the host cell. These methods include Mann's methyl blue-eosin stain for the Negri bodies of rabies, Macchiavello's method, and more recently the elegant Lendrum's phloxine-tartrazine stain. Unfortunately, the need for optical differentiation in these methods increases the chance of technical error.

The introduction of commercially available monoclonal immunohistology to viruses, which are either class or species specific, has revolutionized the tissue detection of viruses. Hepatitis B virus is a good example of the diagnostic value of this technique where the surface antigen (also known as HBs or Australia antigen) and the core antigen (HBc) can be specifically detected immunohistochemically, providing clinically important information about the stage of this disease. More recently, nucleic acid hybridization probes have become available and can be used to detect genomically inserted viral nucleic acid *in situ*, in cells and tissues that are frozen or formalin fixed. It should be remembered, however, that the detection of microorganisms using nucleic acid probes, unlike specific biotinylated antiserum, does not necessarily mean active disease.

Phloxine-tartrazine technique for viral inclusions
(Lendrum 1947)

Sections
Formalin fixed, paraffin.

Solutions
Phloxine

Phloxine	0.5 g
Calcium chloride	0.5 g
Distilled water	100 ml

Tartrazine
A saturated solution of tartrazine in 2-ethoxyethanol, or cellosolve.

Method
1. Deparaffinize and rehydrate through graded alcohols to distilled water.
2. Stain nuclei in alum hematoxylin (Carazzi's or Harris's), 10 minutes.
3. Wash in running tap water, 5 minutes.
4. Stain in phloxine solution, 20 minutes.
5. Rinse in tap water and blot dry.
6. Controlling with the microscope, stain in tartrazine until only the viral inclusions remain strongly red, 5–10 minutes on average.
7. Rinse in 95% alcohol.
8. Dehydrate, clear, and mount.

Results

Viral inclusions	bright red
Red blood cells	variably orange-red
Nuclei	blue-gray
Background	yellow

Notes
All tissue is stained red with phloxine, which is then differentiated by displacement with the counterstain tartrazine. The red color is first removed from muscle, then other connective tissues. Paneth cells, Russell bodies, and keratin can be almost as dye retentive as viral inclusions, and can occasionally be a source of confusion.

Shikata's orcein method for hepatitis B surface antigen
(modified Shikata et al. 1974)

Sections
Formalin fixed, paraffin.

Solutions
Acid permanganate

0.25% potassium permanganate	95 ml
3% aqueous sulfuric acid	5 ml

Orcein

Orcein (synthetic)	1 g
70% alcohol	100 ml
Concentrated hydrochloric acid (gives a pH of 1–2)	1 ml

Saturated tartrazine in cellosolve (2-ethoxyethanol).

Method
1. Deparaffinize and rehydrate through graded alcohols to distilled water.
2. Treat with acid permanganate solution, 5 minutes.
3. Bleach until colorless with 1.5% aqueous oxalic acid, 30 seconds.
4. Wash in distilled water, 5 minutes, then in 70% alcohol.
5. Stain in orcein solution at room temperature, 4 hours, or in a Coplin jar of 37°C preheated orcein, 90 minutes.
6. Rinse in distilled alcohol and examine microscopically to determine desired staining intensity.
7. Rinse in cellosolve, stain in tartrazine, 2 minutes.
8. Rinse in cellosolve, clear, and mount.

Results

Hepatitis B infected cells, elastic and some mucins	brown-black
Background	yellow

Notes

The success of this method largely depends on the particular batch of orcein used, and on freshly prepared solutions. This method relies on permanganate oxidizing of sulfur-containing proteins to sulfonate residues that react with orcein. Results compare well with those obtained using labeled antibodies, but the selectivity is inferior.

Viral infections

Whilst not exhaustive, this brief summary reflects some viruses that are encountered in surgical and post-mortem histopathology (Table 15.3).

Viral hepatitis. To date, five hepatitis viruses have been reported, hepatitis viruses (HV) A, B, C, D, and E, that show great biological diversity, and three of which are incompletely characterized. The liver is the target organ and damage varies with the viral strain, ranging from massive acute necrosis to chronic 'piecemeal necrosis' of liver cells, leading to cirrhosis. An eosinophilic 'ground glass' appearance is seen in the cytoplasm of some hepatocytes, due to dilated smooth endoplasmic reticulum that contains tubular HB surface antigen. It is this component that can be demonstrated using Shikata's orcein method, or by specific immunohistochemistry.

Herpes viruses are usually acquired subclinically during early life and enter a latent phase, to be reactivated during times of immunological stress. These viruses cause blistering or ulceration of the skin and mucous membranes, but can cause systemic diseases, including encephalitis, in immunosuppressed or malnourished individuals. The cytopathic effects of the herpes virus are well seen in Tzanck smears of blister fluid, and include the margination of chromatin along nuclear membranes, Cowdry type A ('owl's eye') inclusion bodies, and syncytial or 'grape-like' nuclei within giant cells. *Cytomegalovirus* (CMV) is sometimes seen as a systemic opportunistic infection in AIDS patients. It is seen in the

Table 15.3 Viral infections seen in histopathology

Virus	Family	Genome	Disease
Measles	Paramyxo	SS RNA	Measles
Varicella-zoster	Herpes	DS DNA	Chickenpox, shingles
Herpes simplex	Herpes	DS DNA	Cold sores, genital herpes
Cytomegalovirus (CMV)	Herpes	DS DNA	Cytomegalic inclusion disease
Epstein-Barr virus	Herpes	DS DNA	Glandular fever, African Burkitt's lymphoma
Human T-cell leukemia virus (HTLV-1)	Retro	SS RNA	Adult T-cell leukemia
Human immunodeficiency virus (HIV)	Retro	SS RNA	AIDS
Human papilloma virus (HPV)	Papova	DS DNA	Human wart viruses
JC virus	Papova	DS DNA	Progressive multifocal leukoencephalopathy
Poliovirus	Picorna	SS DNA	Poliomyelitis
Molluscum virus	Pox	DS DNA	Molluscum contagiosum
Lyssavirus	Rhabdo	SS RNA	Rabies

DS = double-stranded; SS = single-stranded.

endothelial cells, forming prominent intranuclear inclusions that spill into the cytoplasm where they form granular hematoxyphilic clusters. The CMV virus causes obvious cytomegaly in the cells it infects. All herpes viruses have an identical electron microscopic appearance of spherical, 120 nm, membrane-coated particles.

Papilloma viruses are a family of about 50 wart viruses that cause raised verrucous or papillomatous skin warts, or flat condylomatous genital warts. Cytologically, evidence of hyperkeratosis may be present together with koilocytosis (irregular nuclear enlargement and cytoplasmic vacuolation forming perinuclear halos). Skin verrucas are associated with HPV 1–4 strains, genital condylomas with HPV 6, 11, 16, and 18, and cervical cancer with HPV 16 and 18. These uncoated viruses measure 55 nm, are mainly intranuclear, and can be detected using electron microscopy, or immunoperoxidase and gene probes on paraffin sections.

JC virus is a papovavirus that causes progressive multifocal leukoencephalopathy, a demyelinating disease, in AIDS and other immunosuppressed patients. Intranuclear hematoxyphilic inclusions may be seen within swollen oligodendrocytes.

Molluscum virus produces a contagious wart in children and young adults called molluscum contagiosum. Large eosinophilic, intracytoplasmic inclusion bodies can be seen in maturing keratinocytes on routine H&E sections, and are seen well with phloxine-tartrazine. The large 1 μm viral particles have a typical pox virus structure: brick-shaped with a superimposed figure-of-eight nucleic acid sequence.

Rabies virus. This neurotrophic rhabdovirus forms intracytoplasmic eosinophilic inclusions best seen in the axonal hillocks of hippocampal neurons of the brain. Macchiavello, phloxine-tartrazine, Mann's methyl blue-eosin, or PAS stains are recommended. Note: given the pathogenicity of these agents, if suspected, the case should be passed to a relevant diagnostic center rather than a routine laboratory.

Human immunodeficiency virus (HIV) consists of at least two retrovirus strains. The virus is best seen in cultured lymphocytes and is rarely seen in tissues from AIDS patients. It produces a distinctive neuropathological lesion in AIDS encephalitis consisting of microglial nodules, or stars, containing collections of giant cells, microglia, and astrocytes. Synthetic nucleic acid probes have been prepared to HIV genomes.

Influenza virus (flu) is a contagious respiratory illness caused by influenza viruses (Fig. 15.8). It can cause mild to severe illness, and at times can lead to death. According to the Centers for Disease Control (CDC), every year in the United States, on average, 5–20% of the population suffers from the flu, more than 200,000 people are hospitalized from flu complications and about 36,000 people die from flu. More recently, concern about the influenza A H5N1 strain of bird flu has emerged. Some people, such as older people, young children, and people with certain health conditions, are at high risk for serious flu complications.

SARS (severe acute respiratory syndrome) is a viral respiratory illness caused by a coronavirus called SARS-associated coronavirus (SARS-CoV) (Fig. 15.9). SARS was first reported in Asia in February 2003. Over the next few months, the illness spread to more than two dozen countries in North America, South America, Europe, and Asia before the SARS global outbreak of 2003 was contained.

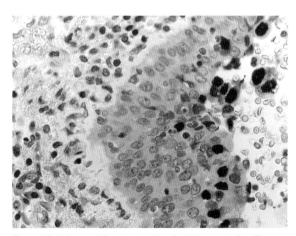

Figure 15.8 Immunohistochemical method demonstrating Flu A virus infected cells in the bronchus.

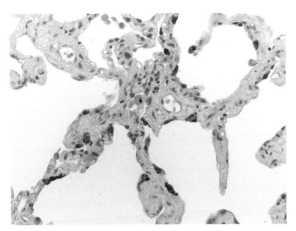

Figure 15.9 Immunohistochemical method demonstrating the previously unrecognized SARS-associated coronavirus which is responsible for severe acute respiratory syndrome (SARS).

Association of Neuropathologists. Visit their website (http://www.cjdsurveillance.com) for details on how to submit specimens for testing; they perform these tests at no charge for laboratories in the USA. In addition, both CDC and the World Health Organization (WHO) also offer guidelines regarding the handling of suspected and known cases of prion disease. Visit http://www.cdc.gov and search for CJD for a fact sheet and other relevant information. WHO offers a manual in pdf form for downloading. It gives information about what to do should you find yourself with a suspected or known positive case in your lab: http://who.int/bloodproducts/TSE-manual2003.pdf. Remember that these types of cases should never knowingly be handled in a routine histology lab. Contact your local health department for additional guidelines.

Prion disease

To date, more than eight transmissible neurodegenerative diseases have been described affecting the central nervous system (CNS). The diseases caused by prions include Creutzfeldt-Jakob disease (CJD) and variant CJD (vCJD), Germann-Straussler-Shienker disease, fatal familial insomnia, and kuru in humans, bovine spongiform encephalopathy (BSE, also known as 'mad cow disease'), scrapie (in goats and sheep), and chronic wasting disease (CWD) (in mule deer and elk). Prions are not microbes in the usual sense because they are not alive, but the illness they cause can be transmitted from one animal to another. All usually produce a characteristic spongiform change, neuronal death, and astrocytosis in affected brains. The infectious agent is a prion, a small peptide, free of nucleic acid and part of a normal transmembrane glycoprotein which is not, strictly speaking, a virus. Antibodies have been prepared from prion protein that strongly mark accumulated abnormal protein in these diseases (Lantos 1992).

The CJD Surveillance Center in the USA is an invaluable source for monitoring and testing human prion disease in the United States. The Center is supported by the CDC and by the American

The demonstration of protozoa and other organisms

The identification of protozoa is most often made on morphological appearance using H&E and, particularly, Giemsa stains. The availability of antisera against organisms such as entamoeba, toxoplasma, and leishmania has made diagnosis much easier in difficult cases (Fig. 15.10a and b).

Giemsa stain for parasites

Sections
Fixative is not critical, but B5 or Zenker's is preferred; thin (3 µm) paraffin sections. (If Zenker's is not used, post-mordant in Zenker's in a 60°C oven for 1 hour before staining.)

Solutions
Giemsa stock (commercially available) or

Giemsa stain powder	4 g
Glycerol	250 ml
Methanol	250 ml

Dissolve powder in glycerol at 60°C with regular shaking. Add methanol, shake the mixture, and allow to stand for 7 days. Filter before use.

Working Giemsa for parasites

Giemsa stock	4 ml
Acetate buffered distilled water, pH 6.8	96 ml

Method

1. Deparaffinize and rehydrate through graded alcohols to water.
2. Rinse in pH 6.8 buffered distilled water.
3. Stain in working Giemsa, overnight.
4. Rinse in distilled water.
5. Rinse in 0.5% aqueous acetic acid until section is pink.
6. Wash in tap water.
7. Blot until almost dry.
8. Dehydrate rapidly through alcohols, clear, and mount.

Results

Protozoa and some other microorganisms	dark blue
Background	pink-pale blue
Nuclei	blue

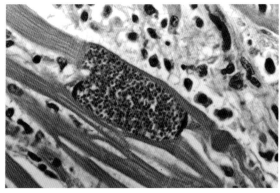

a

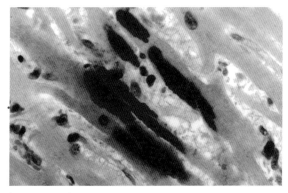

b

Figure 15.10 (a) H&E and (b) immunohistochemical methods demonstrating the single-celled parasite *Toxoplasma gondii* in heart.

Protozoa

Entamoeba histolytica, the organism causing amebic colitis or dysentery, can be found in ulcers that occur in infected colon and in amebic liver abscesses. The trophozoite (adult form) measures 15–50 μm, contains a small nucleus, and has a foamy cytoplasm containing ingested red cells and white cell debris. They may be seen in granulation tissue within ulcers on routine H&E staining, or in the luminal mucus overlying normal-appearing mucosa. They are PAS positive; brief counterstaining in 1% aqueous metanil yellow emphasizes the ingested red cells.

Toxoplasma gondii, a commonly encountered organism that is spread in cat litter, causes an acute lymphadenopathy which is often subclinical. Affected nodes show non-specific changes and no organisms. In AIDS and other immunosuppressed patients this protozoon causes systemic diseases, including meningoencephalitis where encysted bradyzoites and free tachyzoites can be seen in necrotic brain tissue. Cysts also occur in other tissues such as cardiac muscle, and measure up to 40 μm with tachyzoites 4–6 μm, which can be seen on H&E. A Giemsa stain can also be used, but the use of labeled specific antiserum is recommended.

Leishmania tropica is transmitted by sandfly bite and causes a chronic inflammatory disease of the skin sometimes called cutaneous leishmaniasis. The injected parasite forms (2 μm), or amastigotes, are found in large numbers within the cytoplasm of multiple swollen histiocytes that congregate in early lesions in the dermis. A related organism, *L. donovani*, causes a systemic visceral infection, kala azar, in which the organisms are seen within histiocytes in spleen, lymph nodes, liver, and bone marrow. The organisms are hematoxyphilic and can be emphasized with a Giemsa stain.

Giardia duodenalis (lamblia) is a flagellate protozoon that is ingested in cyst form from drinking water with fecal contamination; the trophozoites migrate to the duodenum where they may cause severe diarrhea and malabsorption. These organisms can been seen on an H&E stain, where they appear as eosinophilic, sickle-shaped flakes with indistinct nuclei resting on intestinal mucosa that may show little evidence of inflammation. When seen in a fresh Giemsa-stained duodenal aspirate, they appear kite-shaped, 11–18 μm in size, binucleate, and have faint terminal flagella.

Trichomonas vaginalis is a similar flagellate protozoon most frequently seen in a Papanicolaou stain. Inflammatory cells and mildly dysplastic squamous cells often accompany this parasite as it causes cervicitis in the female, and urethritis in both sexes.

Cryptosporidium is one of a group of protozoa (including *Isospora* and *Microsporidium*) that causes severe and relentless outbreaks of diarrhea among AIDS patients. Cryptosporidial gametes are seen on H&E stain as blue dots arranged along the mucosal surface. Mature cysts are shed into feces and are acid fast in a ZN stain of fecal smears.

Worms

Schistosoma species cause the disease schistosomiasis or 'bilharzia'. Various manifestations of the disease differ according to the particular *Schistosoma* species involved, but granulomata containing schistosome ova are found in the liver, bowel, and bladder mucosa, and sometimes in the lungs. The ova have thick, refractile, eosinophilic walls and are easily detected in H&E-stained sections. The PAS, Grocott, and ZN techniques are positive for these ova. Where the plane of section allows, the presence of a terminal spine to the ovum indicates *S. haematobium*, whereas *S. mansoni* and *S. japonicum* have lateral spines. Any good trichrome procedure will demonstrate worm development.

Echinococcosis. Echinococcus granulosus is a tapeworm found in dogs, but humans and sheep may become intermediate hosts and develop hydatid cyst disease. These cysts form in many organs, particularly liver and lung. The walls of the daughter cysts are faintly eosinophilic, characteristically laminated, and produced by the worm, not by its host. The walls are PAS positive and Congo red positive, showing green birefringence. The scolicial hooklets survive inside old, burnt-out cysts, are of diagnostic shape, and stain brilliant yellow with picric acid.

Acknowledgments

The author would like to acknowledge Amy M. Denison for assistance with the PCR section in this chapter.

References

Bhatnagar, J., Guarner, J., Paddock, C.D., et al., 2007. Detection of West Nile virus in formalin-fixed, paraffin-embedded human tissues by RT-PCR: a useful adjunct to conventional tissue-based diagnostic methods. Journal of Clinical Virology 38 (2), 106–111.

Brown, P., Wolff, A., Gajdusek, D.C., 1990. A simple and effective method for inactivating virus infectivity in formalin-fixed samples from patients with Creutzfeldt-Jakob diseases. Neuropathology 40, 887.

Chandler, F.W., Kaplan, W., Ajello, L., 1980. A colour atlas and textbook of the histopathology of mycotic diseases. Wolfe Medical, London, pp. 109–111.

Chung, J.Y., Braunschweig, T., Williams, R., et al., 2008. Factors in tissue handling and processing that impact RNA obtained from formalin-fixed, paraffin-embedded tissue. Journal of Histochemistry and Cytochemistry 56, 1033–1042.

Churukian, C.J., Schenk, E.A., 1982. A method for demonstrating Gram-positive and Gram-negative bacteria. Journal of Histotechnology 5 (3), 127.

Culling, C.F.A., 1974. Handbook of histopathological and histochemical techniques, third ed. Butterworths, London.

Denison, A.M., Blau, D.M., Jost, H.A. et al., 2011. Diagnosis of influenza from respiratory autopsy tissues: detection of virus by real-time reverse transcriptase-PCR in 222 cases. Journal of Molecular Diagnostics 13 (2), 123–128.

Edman, J.C., Kovacs, J.A., Masur, H., et al., 1988. Ribosomal RNA sequence shows *Pneumocystis carinii* to be a member of the fungi. Nature 334, 519.

Gimenez, D.F., 1964. Staining rickettsia in yolk sac cultures. Stain Technology 39, 135–140.

Gomori, G., 1946. A new histochemical test for glycogen and mucin. American Journal of Clinical Pathology 16, 177.

Gram, C., 1884. Ueber die isolierte Farbung der Schizomyceten in Schnitt und Trocnenpraparaten. Fortsch Med 2, 185.

Grocott, R.G., 1955. A stain for fungi in tissue sections and smears. American Journal of Clinical Pathology 25, 975.

Guarner, J., Bhatnagar, J., Shieh, W.J. et al., 2007. Histopathologic, immunohistochemical, and polymerase chain reaction assays in the study of cases with fatal sporadic myocarditis. Human Pathology 38, 1412–1419.

Kinyoun, J.J., 1915. A note on Uhlenhuth's method for sputum examination for tubercle bacilli. American Journal of Public Health 5, 867–870.

Kuper, S.W.A., May, J.R., 1960. Detection of acid-fast organisms in tissue sections by fluorescence microscopy. Journal of Pathology and Bacteriology 79, 59.

Lantos, P.L., 1992. From slow virus to prion; a review of the transmissible spongioform encephalopathies. Histopathology 20, 1.

Lendrum, A.C., 1947. The phloxine-tartrazine method as a general histological stain for the demonstration of inclusion bodies. Journal of Pathology and Bacteriology 59, 399.

McMullen, L., Walker, M.M., Bain, L.A., et al., 1987. Histological identification of campylobacter using Gimenez technique in gastric antral mucosa. Journal of Clinical Pathology 464–465.

Ollett, W.S., 1947. A method for staining both Gram positive and Gram negative bacteria in sections. Journal of Pathology and Bacteriology 59, 357.

Shieh, W.J., Blau, D.M., Denison, A.M., et al., 2010. 2009 pandemic influenza A (H1N1): pathology and pathogenesis of 100 fatal cases in the United States. American Journal of Pathology 177 (1), 166–175.

Shikata, T., Uzawa, T., Yoshiwara, N., et al., 1974. Staining methods of Australia antigen in paraffin section – detection of cytoplasmic inclusion bodies. Japanese Journal of Experimental Medicine 44, 25.

Srinivasan, M., Sedmak, D., Jewell, S., 2002. Effect of fixatives and tissue processing on the content and integrity of nucleic acids. American Journal of Pathology 161 (6), 1961–1971.

Steiner, G., Steiner, G., 1944. New simple silver stain for demonstration of bacteria, spirochetes, and fungi in sections of paraffin embedded tissue blocks. Journal of Laboratory and Clinical Medicine 29, 868–871.

Swisher, B.L., 1987. Modified Steiner procedure for microwave staining of spirochetes and nonfilamentous bacteria. Journal of Histotechnology 10, 241–243.

Swisher, B.L., Chandler, F.W., 1982. Grocott methenamine silver method for detecting fungi: practical considerations. Laboratory Medicine 13, 568–570.

Swisher, B.L., Nicholson, M.A., 1989. Development of staining controls for *Campylobacter pylori*. Journal of Histotechnology 12, 299–301.

Tatti, K.M., Wu, K.H., Sanden, G.N. et al., 2006. Molecular diagnosis of Bordetella pertussis infection by evaluation of formalin-fixed tissue specimens. Journal of Clinical Microbiology 44 (3), 1074–1076.

Tomkins, D.S., Foulkes, S.F., Goodwin, P.G.R., West, A.P., 1986. Isolation and characterization of intestinal spirochetes. Journal of Clinical Pathology 39, 535.

Twort, F.W., 1924. An improved neutral red, light green double stain for staining animal parasites, microorganisms and tissues. Journal of State Medicine 32, 351.

von Ahlfen, S., Missel, A., Bendrat, K., et al., 2007. Determinants of RNA quality from FFPE samples. PLoS One 2, e1261.

von Lichtenberg, F., 1991. Pathology of infectious diseases. Raven Press, New York.

Warthin, A.S., Starry, A.C., 1920. A more rapid and improved method of demonstrating spirochetes in tissues. American Journal of Syphilis, Gonorrhea, and Venereal Diseases 4, 97.

Website

'Man and Microbes'. Microbiology at Leicester. Available: http://www.microbiologybytes.com/iandi/1a.html

Further reading

Boenisch, T. (Ed.), 2001. Immunochemical staining methods handbook, third ed. DAKO Corporation, Carpinteria, CA.

Luna, L. (Ed.), 1968. Manual of histologic staining methods of the Armed Forces Institute of Pathology, third ed. McGraw-Hill, New York, pp. 158–159.

Neelsen, F., 1883. Ein Casuistischer Beitrag zur Lehre von Tuberkulose. Zentralblatt für die Medizinischen Wissenschaften 21, 497.

Ziehl, F., 1882. Zur Farbung des Tuberkelbacillus. Deutsche Medizinische Wochenschrift 8, 451.

Bone 16

Diane L. Sterchi

Introduction

Bone is considered the most important supporting tissue in the body. It is composed of cells, organic extracellular matrix and inorganic salts. Bone tissue is mineralized in layers which provide great strength and flexibility to the skeletal system. It varies in formation, depending on its function, across the body. These functional/formation differences are also based on the proportion of the different inorganic and organic processes incorporated or produced in the formation of a bone. The most common mineral in bone is hydroxyapatite which consists of collagen, proteins and carbonate ions. The main bulk of bone is approximately 70% mineral and 30% organic components by weight. Bone cells, as opposed to marrow cells, are relatively sparse. This chapter will review bone morphology and its organic and inorganic components, as well as considering methods on preparing sections of bone for analysis that can be used in clinical and research histology laboratories.

Normal bone

Two types of bone can be recognized macroscopically in the adult human skeleton. They are cortical or compact bone and trabecular, cancellous, or spongy bone. Compact bone is the solid, hard, and immensely strong bone that forms the shafts of long bones (e.g. femur and tibia) and exterior surfaces of the flat bones (e.g. ribs and skull). Trabecular bone is found in the diaphysis, epiphysis, and marrow cavities of long bones, vertebrae, and centers of flat bones. It is a mesh of bone strands each about 1 mm thick. Although it looks less solid than cortical bone, this arrangement of trabeculae, particularly in the femoral head and vertebrae where it forms an almost ideal weight-bearing structure, is very strong.

The major components of bone are mineral, cells and an organic extracellular matrix of collagen fibers and ground substance. These are dynamic components as the processes of cell replacement, repair and remodeling of bone, and the erosion and reformation of collagen and mineral occur continually throughout adult life.

Bone collagen

The collagen found in bone differs from other collagen in the body in that it becomes mineralized and is laid down in bands or lamellae roughly parallel to one another. The collagen fibers within each lamella tend to lie next each other but at an angle to the fibers in adjacent lamellae. A cement of proteoglycan ground substance outlining these fibers is seen in sections only at the cement lines. The organization of collagen lamellae is responsible for the distinctive micro-anatomical patterns of bone which are easily seen with polarized light microscopy (Fig. 16.1).

The simplest pattern occurs on the periosteal and endosteal surfaces of compact bone as circumferential lamellae, and in trabecular or non-Haversian bone where lamellae are roughly parallel to the surface. Cortical bone is composed of Haversian systems or osteons in which concentric lamellae surround channels (Volkmann's canals) containing one

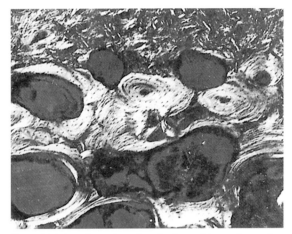

Figure 16.1 Lamellar and non-lamellar (woven) bone of normal rib from child aged 2½ years. Celloidin section; polarized light.

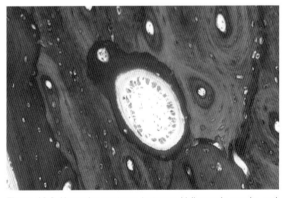

Figure 16.2 Haversian systems (osteons, Volkmann's canals, and bone cells) in ground section of undecalcified bone in methyl methacrylate, acid etched/surfaced stained with McNeal's/toluidine blue stain.

or more blood vessels. These tubular structures run longitudinally in the bone and are packed closely together with irregular interstices filled by the remnants of older osteons (Fig. 16.2). Cement lines outline the boundaries of osteons, and some trabecular and circumferential lamellae.

Another collagen fiber arrangement forms non-lamellar or woven bone and is found in immature bone and some pathological conditions. This collagen is not deposited in the lamellae but in thick, short, randomly oriented bundles. When viewed with polarized light, these appear as coarse fibers resembling a woven fabric.

Unmineralized collagen or osteoid forms a border, or seam, on surfaces of newly formed bone, and after osteoid is deposited there is a lag before it becomes mineralized. Osteoid is normally around 15 μm thick, covering only a small proportion of the surfaces. In some diseases, such as rickets or osteomalacia, it is much thicker and widespread.

On inactive surfaces the osteoid is very thin, difficult to see, and is completely absent where resorption is taking place. This process is called remodeling and consists of resorption and deposition taking place in equilibrium so that the volume and shape of bones stays more or less constant. In later life, remodeling slows down, and deposition may not keep up with resorption, causing increased bone porosity and brittleness, and, in extreme cases, the disease osteoporosis.

Bone mineral

The main mineral content of bone is calcium and phosphate combined with hydroxyl ions to form hydroxyapatite crystals. The mineral is approximately 38% calcium and thought to be deposited as amorphous calcium phosphate in the initial mineralization phase. This transforms to hydroxyapatite by addition of hydroxyl ions to form a crystal lattice into which carbonate, citrate, and fluoride ions as well as magnesium, potassium, and strontium can be substituted or included. Carbonate is present in large quantities but probably only in the hydration shell and on crystal surfaces.

The hydroxyapatite forms needle-like crystals about 22 nm in length, resulting in an enormous total crystal surface area. Thus, the mineral fulfills the obvious function of giving strength and rigidity while approximately 20% remains in the amorphous form to provide a readily available buffer for maintaining total body chemical equilibrium (e.g. pH and enzyme system regulation).

Bone cells

There are three types of bone cell other than the marrow cells belonging to the hemopoietic system.

Osteoblasts

Osteoblasts are fully differentiated to carry out the primary function of bone formation by producing and laying down osteoid. They are seen on surfaces of actively forming bone as plump cells with basophilic cytoplasm and eccentric nuclei distal to the bone surface. The cytoplasm is basophilic due to ribonucleic acid, and before becoming fully differentiated frequently contains glycogen. Acid phosphatase is found in osteoblasts and the surrounding tissues, but decreases at onset of calcification. Upon completion of bone formation, most osteoblasts revert to a quiescent (small undifferentiated cell) state and reside among the heterogeneous cell population.

Osteocytes

In one respect osteoblasts do represent immature cells, as some are trapped in the osteoid matrix they lay down, and become mature osteocytes residing in tiny spaces or lacunae within the bone. Lacunae are connected to each other and to the vascular spaces by canaliculi – tiny channels into which osteocyte processes project for the purpose of passing fluids and dissolved substances necessary for cell metabolism (Fig. 16.3).

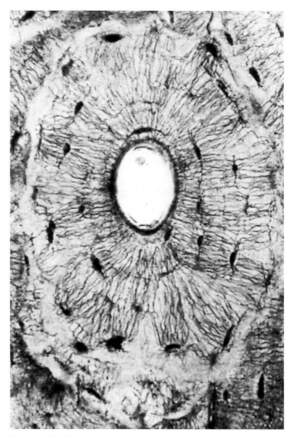

Figure 16.3 Schmorl's picro-thionin stain showing bone canaliculi. Celloidin section of normal femoral shaft.

Osteoclasts

These are the cells responsible for bone resorption or erosion. Osteoclasts are large multinucleated (giant) cells whose cytoplasm contains numerous mitochondria and alkaline phosphatase. They occur in small clusters or singly on bone surfaces undergoing resorption and are often seen in the depressions (Howship's lacunae) they are actively creating by erosion. These surfaces have an irregular outline and lack osteoid (Fig. 16.4). The direction of resorption is random, with no relationship to lamellar structure. Osteoclasts respond to altered mechanical stresses on the skeleton and to growth, and their activity contributes to remodeling. They also respond to hormones that can either stimulate or inhibit their activity. When resorption halts, the process of bone formation resumes (osteoid,

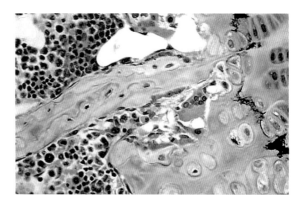

Figure 16.4 Osteoclasts lining trabecular bone. Undecalcified rat knee in GMA microtomed at 2 μm. Hematoxylin and eosin stain.

mineralization, etc.). Cement lines will occur at the junction between old and newly formed bone.

Development and growth

Bone develops in two different ways according to the site and shape of the bone. It begins early in the embryo and is not complete until approximately 15 years of age.

Intramembranous ossification

This occurs in flat bones, e.g. skull, sternum, pelvic bones. A fibrous membrane first develops at the bone formation site in which mesenchymal cells differentiate into osteoblasts that begin the bone formation process by laying down osteoid. This starts in small islets that gradually unite to become trabeculated and finally form an external layer of compact bone.

Endochondral ossification

This occurs in long bones and major parts of the skeleton. This type of bone development begins with differentiation of mesenchymal cells at sites where bone will be formed, but this bone is laid down in a cartilage model that resembles the final shape of the bone. This cartilage model becomes covered with a connective tissue sheath or perichondrium and grows by both apposition and interstitially. Appositional growth or the laying down of more cartilage begins towards the exterior and is mainly responsible for increased diameter; interstitial growth is by cells dividing within the model and mainly occurs towards the extremities, resulting in increased length.

In the central part of the model, cells continue to differentiate, cartilage begins to calcify, blood vessels invade, and the cartilage is broken up into strands. Ossification, by differentiation of perichondrial cells into osteoblasts, begins around the exterior of the primary ossification site at the center of the model. Osteoblasts invade the strands of calcified cartilage and deposit osteoid that soon becomes calcified. This process continues and secondary ossification sites appear at each end of the model, separated from the new bony shaft by cartilage growth or epiphyseal plates capable of interstitial growth. Once bone has ossified, it can only grow by apposition. Remodeling is continuous. In some places deposition exceeds resorption, whereas in others this is reversed and results in the characteristic shape of the bone. When bone is fully grown, the three ossification sites unite and the cartilage growth plates disappear.

Techniques for analyzing bone

Techniques for the demonstration of bone and its components are possibly more varied and difficult than for any other tissue. They include:

- Decalcified bone for frozen, paraffin, and transmission electron microscopy (TEM).
- Mineralized bone for frozen, plastic (microtomed or sawn/ground sections), transmission or scanning EM samples.

The technique chosen for examination of bone is influenced by the initial clinical diagnosis, case urgency, and the extent of investigation required. Specimens arriving in the laboratory can vary in size from a needle biopsy a few millimeters long to whole appendages, e.g. amputation. Mineralized sections are used for microradiographic and histomorphometric studies as well as polarized and fluorescent light microscopy.

Biopsies

Biopsies are used for diagnosis of several diseases such as cancers, hemopoietic disorders, and infections. These specimens are usually small enough to treat much like soft tissue, except that a bone biopsy usually needs decalcification. This is particularly neccesary if it contains a piece of the cortical bone in order to produce paraffin sections. A bone marrow biopsy is usually removed with a Jamshidi needle for diagnosis of metabolic bone disease. Metabolic bone diseases are diagnosed using trabecular bone (Byers & Smith 1967) taken from the iliac crest which is an accessible bone site representative of skeletal bone as a whole.

Sections that are requisite to assess the relationship between mineralized and unmineralized bone (osteoid) are best processed and embedded into a plastic, such as methyl methacrylate (MMA), glycolmethacrylate or a epon-like plastic. The preferred method used for metabolic bone disease research and diagnosis is MMA plastic. Plastic is not a common embedding medium in clinical laboratories but is useful in research and clinical laboratories that are connected with research. It is also possible to produce frozen sections from an undecalcified bone biopsy. There are silver stains that demonstrate bone and osteoid in a decalcified, paraffin-embedded bone section (Tripp & McKay 1972) but many researchers choose the MMA-embedded section.

It is not practical to bisect (half for paraffin/half for plastics) an iliac crest trephine biopsy if both paraffin and plastic embedding methods are employed in the laboratory. Metabolic bone disease laboratories usually prefer a whole trephine bone core for plastic embedding. Needle biopsies should remain whole for paraffin or plastic methods.

Amputation specimens

Large amputation specimens are usually taken as a result of tumor, chronic osteomyelitis, and gangrene. These specimens are often delivered to the laboratory immediately after removal. They often are not in any sealed container and without fixative, and must be dealt with as soon as possible (either in the mortuary or laboratory). The majority of the limb is usually discarded or saved/fixed (if requested by patient) and the area or lesion with actual or suspected involvement in the disease process is retained for final evaluation. Skin, excess muscle, and connective tissue should be cut away from the lesion if possible. Excess bone or a joint disarticulated above and below the lesion should be performed so that fixation is adequate. The relevant portions should be immersed into a large volume of fixative to insure complete fixation. If it is not possible to inspect the specimen for several hours after receipt, it should be refrigerated at 4°C or it can be placed in fixative as a whole and kept at 4°C. Placing it in fixative prior to trimming helps in managing the trimming and prevents autolysis of the outer layers of the specimen. The mortuary/morgue area has a dual advantage for both limb storage and subsequent sample preparation on an available autopsy table. Whenever possible, specimen radiography of large bone specimens helps select the lesion/diseased area for trimming to a smaller sample size for processing.

Resection/replacement specimens

Benign or low-grade malignant tumors and arthritic femoral heads resemble large biopsy specimens, frequently have an established diagnosis and are often considered less urgent. In femoral head or knee replacement surgeries, the bone specimen removed from the patient is usually received in the laboratory whole. Either prior to or after some fixation, a wedge-shaped sample is cut from the whole specimen using a Stryker bone saw or a heavy-duty X-ACTO knife. This wedge-shaped sample is placed back into fixative for 24–48 hours and then decalcified, processed and sectioned for pathology evaluation.

Fixation

Unless immediate diagnosis is needed using cryomicrotomy, all bone specimens must be totally fixed before subjecting them to any decalcification and processing procedures. Complete fixation helps protect bone and surrounding soft tissue from the damaging effects of acid decalcification. Ten percent neutral buffered formalin (NBF) is suitable for both paraffin and non-tetracycline labeled bone. It should be noted that fixation proceeds faster by reducing the size of the bone, opening the bone, and removing excess skin and soft tissue surrounding the lesion. Large specimens can be bisected or reduced in size by sawing into multiple slabs, and immersed into fixative immediately, or no longer than 48 hours after initial fixation. Once cut into smaller pieces, the samples should be placed into fresh fixative.

For MMA embedding, 10% NBF is generally used for fixation. Alcoholic formalin or 70% ethanol fixation is the fixative of choice for tetracycline-labeled bone. Alcohol-based fixatives are not recommended for bone destined for acid decalcification as alcohol can slow or prevent decalcification. Fixatives containing chloroform (Carnoy's) and mercury (B5, Zenker's, Susa), including substitutes of them, should be avoided for specimens to be radiographed since those fixatives tend to make bone radio-opaque and unsuitable for specimen interpretation.

Sawing

Good saws are an essential piece of equipment in a bone histology laboratory. Other than surgical saws, there are a range of hobby shop or handyman's bench saws that are designed to cut through stones, plastic, and some thin metals. These saws cut through cortical bone slowly with cuts no deeper than 7.5 cm. Dry saws may need slight modifications to prevent blade slippage when cutting wet, fatty bone. Water-cooled saws prevent heat damage to bone due to high-speed sawing, and are capable of full-length cuts through long bones and appendages, e.g. femur and tibia. Buehler Isomet Low Speed Saws (Buehler Ltd, USA) are used for trimming specimens, plus cutting bones embedded in plastics. This type of saw has a thin diamond-impregnated blade with a water-cooling bath and is ideal for bisecting biopsies (only when required) and larger bones (depending on the bone specimen diameter). It can make precise, debris-free cuts through 8 mm thick bone cores, other cortical or trabecular and MMA-embedded bone specimens. Scalpel blades, fretted wire or jewelers' saws have been used to cut biopsies with damaging results. These cutting devices can crush or fracture fine trabeculae, creating 'fracture artifact', and force bone fragments into marrow spaces, spoiling the bone histology.

Suitable blade specifications on small saws are 0.5 cm width and 12 to 16 teeth per inch (tpi), making finer, cleaner cuts than a larger saw blade 1.25 cm wide with 6 tpi. Blades in specifications needed are available from tool companies.

Soft tissues and dense connective tissue, e.g. tendons, should be removed before sawing or the sample will drag through the blade. The first cut is made through the mid-plane, then approximately 3–5 mm thick slabs are cut parallel to the first cut. A saw guide plate or wood block held against the first cut edge ensures an even slice. It is safer for workers to hold thinner bones between two wood blocks that will not ruin blades. Sawing should be at a slow even rate to match speed of blade cutting into the bone. Pushing the bone produces uneven cuts, and may jam or break a blade.

Bone slabs should be fixed for an additional 24–48 hours, especially if they appear pinkish-red or partially fixed. After sawing, any bone dust or debris adhering to slab surfaces can be cleaned away using a slow stream of water and a wet paper towel to brush off the debris. Care must be taken not to push debris into marrow spaces or to wash slabs excessively before the bone is totally fixed.

Fine-detail specimen radiography

Radiographs of bone slabs, blocks, or fragments are useful for four main purposes:

1. To examine the nature and extent of a lesion.
2. To provide a diagram of a lesion prior to block selection for processing.
3. To check progress of decalcification, i.e. decalcification endpoint test.
4. To confirm the presence of foreign materials, e.g. prosthetic devices, metal or glass fragments implanted by trauma.

Thin bone slices give sharper-image radiographs than a whole specimen or clinical radiographs. When using film and not digital images, the use of 'soft' X-rays (of low kV) and high-contrast X-ray film provides finer detail and clarity (Fornasier 1975).

Many non-specialist departments of pathology use their in-house radiology department. However, there is the 'Faxitron' (Faxitron Inc., USA) cabinet X-ray system which can be used for specimen X-rays of bone in clinical and research settings. It comes in a free-standing and a tabletop unit. The energy output is 10–110 kV with 3 mA tube current. In addition to the manual exposure capability, the unit should be equipped with its automatic exposure timer with 5-second to 60-minute setting at 1-second intervals. The cabinet has adjustable shelf levels for film-to-source distances of 31–61 mm and is fully lead lined to shield the operator from X-rays. A special door interlock safety device automatically turns off the X-ray beam if the door is opened during operation. This is an instrument that uses X-ray film (Kodak X-OMAT 2, Ready Pak; Kodak Ltd) but newer units produce digital and real-time images. When using a Faxitron for decalcification checks, a bone slab should be first radiographed using the automatic exposure timer, and then exposure time, kV, and mA is recorded. This eliminates guesswork for a first exposure and provides the correct exposure time and kV for a repeat radiograph or for subsequent manual exposures of adjacent bone slabs of the same thickness.

An example of manual exposure requirements is as follows:

- bone slab 3–5 mm thick on polyethylene sheet (moisture barrier)
- Kodak X-OMAT 2, Ready Pak (Kodak Ltd)
- film-to-source distance (FTSD), 50 cm (lowest shelf level)
- settings, 30 kV (3 mA)
- exposure time approximately 1 minute.

Exposure time is dependent on specimen thickness (thicker slabs require longer exposures), film-to-source distance (longer distance requires more time), and type of film used. Large, whole bones, e.g. proximal end of femur with metal prosthesis, can be radiographed using X-OMAT 2, FTSD (upper shelf), longer exposure time (approx. 8 minutes), and higher kV (70 kV). Soft tissues, cartilage, and tumor are more easily seen in underexposed radiographs, useful for evaluating surrounding soft tissue involvement by a bone tumor, e.g. osteosarcoma. The X-ray film can be developed quickly in a radiology department and viewed without delay.

Area selection for embedding

In urgent cases of suspected tumor or infection, an attempt should be made to select a sample with the least mineralization in order to provide the quickest possible diagnosis. These pieces can be fixed, rapidly decalcified, and processed to meet urgent clinical requirements.

The ideal thickness of larger bone pieces is 3–5 mm. If bone slabs are too thick, both decalcification and processing are prolonged while overly thin bone slabs (less than 2 mm) tend to become brittle and bend during processing and embedding which may cause the tissue to pop out of the paraffin block during sectioning. The dense collagen matrix tends to prevent adequate paraffin wax penetration and thin pieces are not held firmly in the softer paraffin embedding media during microtomy.

An addition, an aid in area selection of a specimen is radiography when available, a diagram or 'map' of the lesion can be made from the X-ray to locate area of interest for processing.

Decalcification

In order to obtain satisfactory paraffin sections of bone, inorganic calcium must be removed from the organic collagen matrix, calcified cartilage, and surrounding tissues. This is called decalcification and is carried out by chemical agents, either acids to form soluble calcium salts, or chelating agents that bind to calcium ions. Even after decalcification, the dense collagen of cortical bone is remarkably tough and tends to harden more after paraffin processing. Occasionally, small foci of calcifications in paraffin-embedded or frozen tissues can be sectioned without much noticeable damage to the knife or disruption of surrounding tissue. After hematoxylin staining, these foci usually appear cracked and as dark purple granular masses with lighter purple halos.

The choice of decalcifier is influenced by four inter-dependent factors: urgency of the case, degree of mineralization, extent of the investigation, and staining techniques required.

Any acid, however well buffered, has some damaging effects on tissue stain-aridity. This problem increases with acidity of solutions, i.e. lower pH, and length of decalcification period. Consequently, the rapid decalcifiers are more likely to adversely affect any subsequent staining, especially if not fixed completely. This is most noticeable in cell nuclei with the failure of nuclear chromatin to take up hematoxylin and other basic dyes as readily as soft tissues never exposed to acid solutions. The staining using acid dyes is also less affected, but eosin (an acid dye) can stain tissue a deep, unpleasant, brick red without the preferred three differential shades. These effects on H&E staining can be reduced by doing the decalcification endpoint test, post-decalcification acid removal, and adjustment of the stain procedure.

Decalcifying agents

As noted previously there are two major types of decalcifying agent, i.e. acids and chelating agents, although Gray (1954) lists over 50 different mixtures. Many of these mixtures were developed for special purposes with one used as a fixing and dehydrating agent. Other mixtures contain reagents, e.g. buffer salts, chromic acid, formalin, or ethanol, intended to counteract the undesirable swelling effects that acids have on tissues. Many popular mixtures used today are from the original formulae developed many years ago (Evans & Krajian 1930; Kristensen 1948; Clayden 1952). For most practical purposes, today's laboratories seem to prefer simpler solutions for routine work. Provided the bone is totally fixed and treated with a decalcifier suitable for removal of the amount of mineral present, the simple mixtures work as well or better than more complex mixtures.

Acid decalcifiers

Acid decalcifiers can be divided into two groups: strong (inorganic) and weak (organic) acids. As Brain (1966) suggested, many laboratories keep an acid from each group available for either rapid diagnostic or slower, routine work.

Proprietary decalcifiers

The components in proprietary decalcifying solutions are often trade secrets. Manufacturers provide Material Safety Data Sheets (MSDS) that frequently indicate the type and concentration of acid. Their product data sheets usually indicate if a solution is rapid or slow, and give decalcification instructions and warnings against prolonged use. Rapid proprietary solutions usually contain hydrochloric acid (HCl), whereas slow proprietary mixtures contain buffered formic acid or formalin/formic acid. A study (Callis & Sterchi 1998) found that dilution of a proprietary HCl solution was not deleterious for effective decalcification or staining, and this is an option if a strong mixture is considered too concentrated. Chelating reagents such as EDTA mixtures are also available pre-mixed. Although proprietary mixtures have no obvious advantages over solutions prepared in laboratories, their use is increasingly popular in busy laboratories because they are reliable, time and cost-effective while addressing some safety issues by eliminating handling and storage of concentrated acids.

Strong inorganic acids, e.g. nitric, hydrochloric

These may be used as simple aqueous solutions with recommended concentrations of 5–10%. They decalcify rapidly, cause tissue swelling, and can seriously damage tissue stainability if used longer than 24–48 hours. Old nitric acid is particularly damaging, and should be replaced with fresh stock. Strong acids, however, tend to be more damaging to tissue antigens for immunohistochemical staining, and enzymes may be totally lost.

Strong acids are used for needle and small biopsy specimens to permit rapid diagnosis within 24 hours or less. They can be used for large or heavily mineralized cortical bone specimens with decalcification progress carefully monitored by a decalcification endpoint test (Callis & Sterchi 1998). The following is a list of strong acid decalcifying solutions. The formulae and preparations are available in Bancroft & Gamble, sixth ed. (2008).

1. Aqueous nitric acid, 5–10% (Clayden 1952)
2. Perenyi's fluid (Perenyi 1882)
3. Formalin-nitric acid (use inside a fume hood)

Weak, organic acids, e.g. formic, acetic, picric

Of these, formic is the only weak acid used extensively as a primary decalcifier. Acetic and picric acids cause tissue swelling and are not used alone as decalcifiers but are found as components in Carnoy's, Bouin's, and Zenker's fixatives. These fixatives will act as incidental, although weak, decalcifiers and could be used in urgent cases with only minimal calcification. Formic acid solutions can be aqueous (5–10%), buffered or combined with formalin. The formalin–10% formic acid mixture simultaneously fixes and decalcifies, and is recommended for very small bone pieces or needle biopsies. However, it is still advisable to have complete fixation before any acid decalcifier is used. The salts, sodium formate (Kristensen 1948) or sodium citrate (Evans & Krajian 1930), are added to formic acid solutions making 'acidic' buffers. Buffering is used to counteract the injurious effects of the acid. However, in addition to low 4–5% formic acid concentration, increased time is needed for complete decalcification. Formic acid is gentler and slower than HCl or nitric acids, and is suitable for most routine surgical specimens, particularly when immunohistochemical staining is needed. Formic acid can still damage tissue, antigens, and enzyme staining, and should be endpoint tested. Decalcification is usually complete in 1–10 days, depending on the size, type of bone, and acid concentration. Dense cortical or large bones have been effectively decalcified with 15% aqueous formic acid and a 4% hydrochloric acid–4% formic acid mixture (Callis & Sterchi 1998). The following is a list of weak acid decalcifying solutions. The formulae and preparations are available in Bancroft & Gamble, sixth ed. (2008).

1. Aqueous formic acid
2. Formic acid-formalin (after Gooding & Stewart 1932)
3. Buffered formic acid (Evans & Krajian 1930)

Chelating agents

The chelating agent generally used for decalcification is ethylenediaminetetraacetic acid (EDTA). Although EDTA is nominally 'acidic', it does not act like inorganic or organic acids but binds metallic ions, notably calcium and magnesium. EDTA will not bind to calcium below pH 3 and is faster at pH 7–7.4; even though pH 8 and above gives optimal binding, the higher pH may damage alkali-sensitive protein linkages (Callis & Sterchi 1998). EDTA binds to ionized calcium on the outside of the apatite crystal and as this layer becomes depleted more calcium ions reform from within; the crystal becomes progressively smaller during decalcification. This is a very slow process that does not damage tissues or their stainability. When time permits, EDTA is an excellent bone decalcifier for enzyme staining, and electron microscopy. Enzymes require specific pH conditions in order to maintain activity, and EDTA solutions can be adjusted to a specific pH for enzyme staining. EDTA does inactivate alkaline phosphatase but activity can be restored by addition of magnesium chloride.

EDTA and EDTA disodium salt (10%) or EDTA tetrasodium salt (14%) are approaching saturation and can be simple aqueous or buffered solutions at a neutral pH of 7–7.4, or added to formalin. EDTA tetrasodium solution is alkaline, and the pH should be adjusted to 7.4 using concentrated acetic acid. The time required to totally decalcify dense cortical bone may be 6–8 weeks or longer, although small bone spicules may be decalcified in less than a week. Formulae and preparations are available in Bancroft & Gamble, sixth ed. (2008).

1. Formalin-EDTA (Hillemann & Lee 1953)
2. EDTA (aqueous), pH 7.0–7.4

Factors influencing the rate of decalcification

Several factors influence the rate of decalcification, and there are ways to speed up or slow down this process. The concentration and volume of the active reagent, including the temperature at which the reaction takes place, are important at all times. Other factors that contribute to how fast bone decalcifies are the age of the patient, type of bone, size of specimen, and solution agitation. Mature cortical bone decalcifies slower than immature, developing cortical or trabecular bone. Another factor of mature bone is that the marrow may contain more adipose cells than a young bone. This requires diligent attention to make sure specimens stay immersed in decalcification solution. Of all the above factors, the effectiveness of agitation is still open to debate.

Concentration of decalcifying agent

Generally, more concentrated acid solutions decalcify bone more rapidly but are more harmful to the tissue. This is particularly true of aqueous acid solutions, as various additives, e.g. alcohol or buffers, which protect tissues, may slow down the decalcification rate. Remembering that 1 N and 1 M solutions of HCl, nitric, or formic acid are equivalent, Brain (1966) found that 4 M formic acid decalcified twice as fast as a 1 M solution without harming tissue staining, and felt it was advantageous to use the concentrated formic acid mixture. With combination fixative-acid decalcifying solutions, the decalcification rate cannot exceed the fixation rate or the acid will damage or macerate the tissue before fixation is complete. Consequently, decalcifying mixtures should be compromises that balance the desirable effects (e.g. speed) with the undesirable effects (e.g. maceration, impaired staining).

In all cases, total depletion of an acid or chelator by their reaction with calcium must be avoided. This is accomplished by using a large volume of fluid compared with the volume of tissue (20:1 is recommended), and by changing the fluid several times during the decalcification process. Brain, however, pointed out that if a sufficiently large volume of fluid is used (100 ml per g of tissue) it is not necessary to renew the decalcifying agent because depletion is less apparent in a larger volume. Small number and similar-sized specimens in one container is preferred.

Ideally, acid solutions should be endpoint tested and changed daily to ensure the decalcifying agent is renewed and that tissues are not left in acids too long or overexposed to acids (i.e. 'over-decalcification').

Temperature

Increased temperature accelerates many chemical reactions, including decalcification, but it also increases the damaging effects which acids have on tissue so that, at 60°C, the bone, soft tissues, and cells may become completely macerated almost as soon as they are decalcified.

The optimal temperature for acid decalcification has not been determined, although Smith (1962) suggested 25°C as the standard temperature, but in practice a room temperature (RT) range of 18–30°C is acceptable. Conversely, lower temperature decreases reaction rates and Wallington (1972) suggested that tissues not completely decalcified at the end of a working week could be left in acid at 4°C over a weekend. This practice may result in 'over-decalcification' of tissues, even with formic acid. A better recommendation is to interrupt decalcification by briefly rinsing acid off bone, immersing it in NBF, removing from fixative, rinsing off the fixative, and resuming decalcification on the next working day. Microwave, sonication, and electrolytic methods produce heat, and must be carefully monitored to prevent excessive temperatures that damage tissue (Callis & Sterchi 1998).

Increased temperature also accelerates EDTA decalcification without the risk of maceration. However, it may not be acceptable for preservation of heat-sensitive antigens, enzymes, or electron microscopy work. Brain (1966) saw no objection to decalcifying with EDTA at 60°C if the bone was well fixed.

Agitation

The effect of agitation on decalcification remains controversial even though it is generally accepted that mechanical agitation influences fluid exchange within as well as around tissues with other reagents. Therefore, it would be a logical assumption that agitation speeds up decalcification, and studies have been done which attempt to confirm this theory. Russell (1963) used a tissue processor motor rotating at one revolution per minute and reported the decalcification period was reduced from 5 days to 1 day. Others, including Clayden (1952), Brain (1966), and Drury and Wallington (1980), repeated or performed similar experiments and failed to find any time reduction. The sonication method vigorously agitates both specimen and fluid, and one study noted cellular debris found on the floor of a container after sonication could possibly be important tissue shaken from the specimen (Callis & Sterchi 1998). Gentle fluid agitation is achieved by low-speed rotation, rocking, stirring, or bubbling air into the solution. Even though findings from various studies are unresolved, agitation is a matter of preference and not harmful as long as tissue components remain intact.

Suspension

The decalcifying fluid should be able to make contact with all surfaces of a specimen and flat bone slabs should not touch each other or the bottom of a container, as this is enough to prevent good fluid access between the flat surfaces. Bone samples can be separated and suspended in the fluid with a thread or placed inside cloth bags tied with thread or preferably in a cassette. The cassette will provide identification without having to prepare tags for bag suspension. Some workers have cleverly devised perforated plastic platforms to raise samples above a container bottom to permit fluid access to samples.

Completion of decalcification

Ideally, bone should be taken from the acid solution as soon as all calcium has been removed from it. It is still possible that the outer parts of a sample will be overexposed to the acid, although these parts usually stain no differently from inner portions, which are the last to be decalcified. Tissues decalcified in acids for long time periods or in high acid concentrations are more likely to show the effects of over-decalcification, whether or not all mineral has been removed.

Consequently, it is important for a laboratory to control a decalcification procedure by using a decalcification endpoint test to know when calcium removal is complete and, if incomplete, renew the decalcifying agent. If laboratories do not perform endpoint testing, it is recommended they should do so. When using formic, HCl or nitric acids, daily testing is recommended unless near the endpoint; then test every 3–5 hours when possible. With EDTA, weekly tests are sufficient unless solution changes are more frequent. It is recommended that EDTA be changed often at first, since the reaction with calcium is initially quicker and then slows down as the calcium in the tissue is depleted. Minimally calcified tissues and needle biopsies decalcified by a strong acid may be tested only once. It is wise practice for a laboratory that performs a high number of bone biopsy specimens to establish a time range (that depends on the amount of cortical bone present) for ideal decalcification time for bone biopsies. Once the process is established it would eliminate guessing, testing, and handling of those delicate samples. Biopsy decalcification is fairly consistent on multiple-sized biopsies within an hour or two of acid exposure. Wrapping a bone needle biopsy in tissue paper and leaving it wrapped until embedding prevents any loss of cells or tissue during the washing or decalcification process. Sponges sometimes pull cells from a sample when washing and decalcifying. Often these may be urgent cases where a shorter decalcification time is allowed, but the sample must be carefully treated and incomplete decalcification is still possible. If tissue is still slightly under-decalcified after paraffin embedment and sectioning, surface decalcification can be done. Problem blocks should be identified as such so that proper treatment is given should further microtomy be requested.

Decalcification endpoint test

There are several methods for testing the completion of decalcification, with two considered to be the most reliable. These are specimen radiography, using an X-ray unit and the chemical method to test acids and EDTA solutions. Another method first used to test nitric acid is a weight loss, weight gain procedure that provides relatively good, quick results with all acids and EDTA (Mawhinney et al. 1984; Sanderson et al. 1995). Although still used, 'physical' tests are considered inaccurate and damaging to tissues. Probing, 'needling', slicing, bending, or squeezing tissue can create artifacts, e.g. needle tracks, disrupt soft tumor from bone, or cause false-positive microfractures of fine trabeculae, a potential misdiagnosis. The 'bubble' test is subjective and dependent on worker interpretation.

Methods for chemical testing of acid decalcifying fluids detect the presence of calcium released from bone. When no calcium is found or the result is negative, decalcification is said to be complete and may entail using one extra change of decalcifier after actual completion. EDTA can be chemically end-point tested by acidifying the used solution; this forces EDTA to release calcium for precipitation by ammonium oxalate (Rosen 1981).

Calcium oxalate test (Clayden 1952)

This method involves the detection of calcium in acid solutions by precipitation of insoluble calcium hydroxide or calcium oxalate, but is unsuitable for solutions containing over 10% acid even though these could be diluted and result in a less sensitive test.

Solutions

Ammonium hydroxide, concentrated.

Saturated aqueous ammonium oxalate.

Method

1. Take 5 ml of used decalcifying fluid, add a piece of litmus paper or use a pH meter with magnetic stirrer.
2. Add ammonium hydroxide drop by drop, shaking after each drop, until litmus indicates solution is neutral (pH 7).
3. Add 5 ml of saturated ammonium oxalate and shake well.
4. Allow solution to stand for 30 minutes.

Result

If a white precipitate (calcium hydroxide) forms immediately after adding the ammonium hydroxide, a large quantity of calcium is present, making it unnecessary to proceed further to step 3 which would also be positive. Testing can be stopped and a change to fresh decalcifying solution made at this point. If step 2 is negative or clear after adding ammonium hydroxide, then proceed to step 3 to add ammonium oxalate. If precipitation occurs after adding the ammonium oxalate, less calcium is present. When a smaller amount of calcium is present, it takes longer to form a precipitate in the fluid, so, if the fluid remains clear after 30 minutes, it is safe to assume decalcification is complete.

'Bubble' test. Acids react with calcium carbonate in bone to produce carbon dioxide, seen as a layer of bubbles on the bone surface. The bubbles disperse with agitation or shaking but reform, becoming smaller as less calcium carbonate is reduced. As an endpoint test, a bubble test is subjective and unreliable, but can be used as a guide to check the progress of decalcification, i.e. tiny bubbles indicate less calcium present.

Radiography. This is the most sensitive test for detecting calcium in bone or tissue calcification. The method is the same as specimen radiography using a FAXITRON with a manual exposure setting of approximately 1 minute, 30 kV, and Kodak X-OMAT X-ray film on the bottom shelf. It is possible to expose several specimens at the same time. The method is to rinse acid from the sample, carefully place identified bones on waterproof polyethylene sheet on top of the X-ray film, expose according to directions, and leave bones in place until the film is developed and examined for calcifications. Bones with irregular shapes and variable thickness can occasionally mislead workers on interpretation of results. This problem is resolved by comparing the test radiograph to the pre-decalcification specimen radiograph and correlate suspected calcified areas with specimen variations. Areas of mineralization are easily identified, although tiny calcifications are best viewed using a hand-held magnifier. Metal dust particles from saw blades are radio-opaque, sharply delineated fragments that never change in size. These are unaffected by decalcification, appearing as gray specks on the bone surface and can be easily removed. Spicules of metal, metallic paint, or glass forced deep into tissue by a traumatic injury are also sharply delineated but cannot be removed without damaging the tissue. Radiography only indicates the presence of deeper foreign objects, and care must be taken during microtomy to not damage the knife (Fig. 16.5).

Treatment following decalcification

Acids can be removed from tissues or neutralized chemically after decalcification is complete. Chemical neutralization is accomplished by immersing

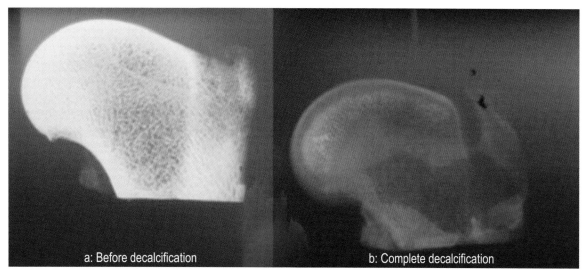

Figure 16.5 An example of a FAXITRON X-ray (a) before decalcification (b) after decalcification is completed. The bright white in the sample is calcium. As the calcium is removed, the bone becomes opaque.

decalcified bone into either saturated lithium carbonate solution or 5–10% aqueous sodium bicarbonate solution for several hours. Many laboratories simply rinse the specimens with running tap water for a period of time. Culling (1974) recommended washing in two changes of 70% alcohol for 12–18 hours before continuing with dehydration in processing, a way to avoid contamination of dehydration solvents even though the dehydration process would remove the acid along with the water.

Adequate water rinsing can generally be done in 30 minutes for small samples and larger bones in 1–4 hours in order to not delay processing. Samples needing immediate processing, e.g. needle biopsies, can be blotted or quickly rinsed to remove acid from surfaces before proceeding to the first dehydrating fluid. It is important to avoid contaminating the first dehydrating fluid with acids, and washing bones even for a short time is good practice particularly with large bone slabs.

Acid-decalcified tissues for cryomicrotomy must be thoroughly washed in water or stored in formal saline containing minimal amounts of sucrose (3–10%), or PBS with 3–10% sucrose, at 4°C before freezing. This helps avoid any residual acid in the tissue from corroding the metal knife. Caution:

higher percentages of sucrose may prevent the tissue from fully freezing or freezing unevenly, causing soft spots in the tissue which will create thick-thin appearing sections or the tissue will fall out due to improper freezing.

Tissues decalcified in EDTA solutions should not be placed directly into 70% alcohol, as this causes residual EDTA to precipitate in the alcohol and within the tissue. The precipitate does not appear to affect tissue staining since EDTA is washed out during these procedures, but may be noticeable during microtomy or storage when a crystalline crust forms on the block surface. A water rinse after decalcification or overnight storage in formal saline, NBF, or PBS should prevent this.

Surface decalcification

Surface decalcification is needed when partially decalcified bone or unsuspected mineral deposits in soft tissue are found during paraffin sectioning. This technique is done to prevent knife damage and torn tissue sections. After finding a calcification, the exposed tissue surface in a paraffin block is placed face down in 1% HCl, 10% formic, or a proprietary acid solution for 15–60 minutes, rinsed with water to remove corrosive acids, and re-sectioned. The acid removes a few micrometers of calcium from the tissue surface, permitting only a few sections to be cut after careful block re-orientation in the microtome to avoid wasting this thin surface decalcified layer.

Processing decalcified bone

In today's laboratories, automated computerized processors with vacuum and pressure options have improved the efficiency and quality of tissue processing, particularly bone. Solvents used for dehydration (ethanol, isopropanol, reagent and proprietary alcohol mixtures) and clearing (xylene, xylene substitutes) will work well for bone and soft tissue processing. Paraffin waxes developed in recent years have been improved by the addition of plastic polymers and other chemicals that allow better wax penetration and sectioning. Decalcified bone sectioning is made easier after infiltration and embedding in a harder paraffin wax. Often bone infiltrated with routine paraffin for all tissues can be embedded in harder paraffin to give firmer support of bone during sectioning. Small bone and needle biopsies containing little cortical bone can be processed with soft tissues.

Oversized, thick bone slabs require an extended processing schedule in order to obtain adequate dehydration, clearing, and paraffin infiltration. Some laboratories specialized in orthopedic work find it advantageous to dedicate one processor to extended processing schedules for bone and not interfere with routine daily soft tissue processing. With an enclosed automatic processor, time in each dehydrating, clearing solvent, and paraffin may vary from 2 to 4 hours, with larger bone slabs needing the longest time. If a bone sample has been endpoint tested for completed decalcification, but still appears chalky, mushy, and crumbles out of the block during sectioning, then dehydration, clearing, or paraffin infiltration may be incomplete. Blocks can be melted down and re-infiltrated with paraffin for up to 8 hours to see if this improves sectioning. Another possibility is reversing processing by

melting paraffin from bone and going back through two changes of xylene, two changes of 100% alcohol to remove residual water, and then reprocessing back into paraffin. The later is not recommended and is not always reliable, especially if the tissue was not well fixed.

Modern embedding methods using metal molds with plastic tissue cassettes have all but eliminated the necessity to mount the paraffin-embedded tissues on wood, hard rubber blocks, or metal chucks. A labeled cassette contains the tissue throughout processing and, after embedding, the plastic back of a block fits into a microtome cassette clamp. Macro-cassette systems including larger cassettes, molds, and a special block holder are available for sledge microtomes. Specimen size is the limiting factor for embedding with cassettes, and with a little creativeness the oversized bone can be embedded in a paraffin-filled metal pan or similar container, a warm hardwood block placed directly on top of bone, with all allowed to harden in place. This results in a hard back, embedded directly in the block, which can be clamped tightly in the microtome, avoiding holding onto softer paraffin, which can crack under excessive clamping pressure.

Microtomes and knives

Bone biopsies and smaller primarily cancellous bone blocks can be cut on any properly maintained microtome. Many newer microtomes are more powerful, heavier, and automated, making them capable of sectioning both paraffin and plastic bone blocks. Oversized and exceptionally hard, dense bone samples too difficult to cut on a smaller microtome are easier to section on a large sledge or heavy duty motorized sliding microtome (Polycut, Leica, USA).

There is a wide choice of good microtome blades including heavy 'c' profile steel and the popular disposable blades. The disposable knives are convenient, extremely sharp, single-use blades capable of sectioning properly decalcified and processed paraffin-embedded bones. Newer microtomes come equipped with disposable blade holders, or disposable blade holder inserts can be purchased for older model microtomes. High-profile disposable blades are slightly thicker and wider than the low-profile blades, and tend to 'chatter' or vibrate less when cutting denser bones. Heavier steel knives range in size from 16 to 18 cm for small microtomes and from 200 to 300 cm for base sledge microtomes with specially designed blades for the Polycut. Because steel knives need frequent sharpening, an automatic knife sharpener is a cost-effective, time-saving device when these knives are used routinely. An automatic knife sharpener is a rare find but a multiple plate type one can also sharpen tungsten carbide knives which are used for undecalcified bone cryotomy and plastic embedded tissues. Sharpening a tungsten carbide knife frequently can be expensive, and a knife sharpener can save time and money. Unlike steel knives, tungsten carbide knives need to be reconditioned after multiple sharpenings.

Microtomy

Small bone samples and biopsies usually section well with knife angles set for routine soft tissue microtomy. Generally, disposable blades work well at the manufacturer's recommended angle settings for their high- or low-profile blades. Slight adjustment of a knife angle can be attempted if dense cortical bone sectioning is not working with the routine soft tissue knife angle, and can be increased or decreased at a microtomist's discretion. Knives must be changed frequently, sometimes after cutting one ribbon or a few sections of cortical bone. When sectioning any bone sample, a sharp knife is necessary in order to get flat, uncompressed, wrinkle-free sections, along with patience and good microtomy skills by the operator.

Longitudinal sections of cortical bone may section better when the knife cuts 'along the grain' or the length of the bone oriented at right angles to the knife. A bone of somewhat rectangular shape can be embedded or oriented in a block holder so that a smaller corner of sample is cut first with the wider area cut last. This helps reduce knife vibration and potential gouging of bone out of the paraffin block. When cartilage is present, it should be located

near the top of a block or angled in a way to avoid compression of the softer cartilage and paraffin into the denser bone, creating wrinkles. Generally, hard tissues cut more easily if cooled by a melting ice block to allow water penetration into the tissue surface. Extensive soaking causes visible tissue swelling away from the block face and, even though the tissue cuts more easily, the sections fall apart on the water bath. A flat ice block made with water-filled polyethylene storage bags keeps blocks dry during cooling, or paraffin bone blocks can be cooled in a −20°C freezer for a short time. Larger blocks can be cut at room temperature as long as the room is not overly warm or humid. If using a tape method to obtain a difficult section, the blocks must be at room temperature and dry so that the tape adheres to the block.

An optimal thickness for bone sections is the same as that for soft tissues, 4–5 μm, and cut routinely from adequately processed blocks. Bone marrow biopsies should be cut at 2–3 μm for marrow cell identification, and sliding microtome sections may vary from approximately 5 to 8 μm.

Flattening and adhesion

Bone sections adhere to slides well when glass surfaces are coated with some type of adhesive. Slides come in all types of coating with different levels of tissue-adhering properties. All work well but a strong charge or coating is preferred when working with bone. The most common is a silanized Plus Charge® (Erie Scientific, NH) or poly-L-lysine-coated (PLL) slides. If only plain, uncoated slides are available there is a simple coating method one can use. Wash slides in soap and water, rinse soap off completely, then dip in a gelatin and potassium dichromate 'subbing' solution, air dry, and store slides in a clean dry box until needed (Drury & Wallington 1980). When sectioning numerous bone blocks, 10 ml of the chrome subbing solution can be added to a 2-liter water bath or simply add a few gelatin granules to the water as it is heating. If some sections are persistently non-adherent, a solution containing amylopectin, a starch (Steedman 1960), or a high molecular weight 225 bloom gelatin in the chrome subbing mixture may be more successful. Gelatin should be used sparingly or an excess coating is stained by hematoxylin giving an unsightly blue background underneath and around sections.

While floating on water, cartilage and bone sections can expand more than the paraffin or other tissue components, and small folds may form as the sections dry. When this occurs, the water bath temperature should be lowered to 10–15°C below the paraffin melting point. Flattening a section by mounting a section in excess water on the slide, then holding the slide against a hot plate to melt the wax and evaporate the water must be used with caution. Bone sections may 'explode' apart, displacing cortical bone from trabecular bone and ruining the gross morphology. Reducing the surface tension of water by floating a section on RT 10% ethanol, picking up the section on a slide, then immediately but slowly lowering the section into a warm water bath allows a section to flatten gently. If cartilage curling is a problem, drying sections flat at 37°C overnight or longer may solve this problem. Most bone sections flatten and dry without problems or special treatment provided the tissue has been properly processed and sectioned with a sharp knife.

Staining methods for decalcified bone sections

Most routine soft tissue staining methods can be used without modification for staining decalcified bone sections. Acid decalcification, particularly when prolonged or used with a heat producing method, e.g. microwave, sonication, or electrolytic, can adversely affect the H&E and some special stains. When the temperature exceeds 37°C during decalcification, Giemsa staining may be too pink and the historical Feulgen stain for DNA will be negative because of excessive protein hydrolysis. Staining is successful after EDTA treatment, but the slower decalcification rate usually rules it out in favor of faster acid methods. H&E is still the primary stain used for most final diagnoses with the aid of special stains. Immunohistochemical staining is now

an important aspect in disease diagnosis, and is used frequently on decalcified bone tumors, bone marrow, and cartilage. Most special stains used with bone sections are available pre-mixed and are more convenient to use than mixing your own. However, it is better to see the original ingredients/formulae in references to understand the mechanism and to help identify proper staining.

Hematoxylin and eosin (H&E)

When staining sections of properly decalcified tissue no modifications to the standard H&E techniques are required. There are several ways to counteract weak nuclear staining damaged by acids and make the hematoxylin stain darker. Freshly prepared hematoxylin, particularly mixtures that lose strength over time, e.g. Harris's, Gill II and III, often stain darker than solutions near an expiration date. Preference in hematoxylin is using a progressive hematoxylin since it does not require differentiation steps that a regressive hematoxylin does. Restoration of basophilic staining can be attempted by immersing a hydrated section in 4–5% aqueous sodium bicarbonate for 10 minutes to 2 hours, rinsing well with water, and staining with hematoxylin. If using a regressive hematoxylin, the acid differentiation step can either be shortened to one or two fast dips in 0.5% acid alcohol or this step can be eliminated entirely. When using a progressive hematoxylin, blueing solutions should be mild bases, e.g. Scott's tap water substitute or saturated lithium carbonate, to avoid bone section loss caused by ammonia water blueing. If poor hematoxylin staining is a persistent problem, it is recommended that the decalcification method be evaluated and appropriate changes made to avoid damage to staining. Alcoholic eosin solutions, 0.5–1%, often stain bone and surrounding tissues overly red, and staining time can be shortened from 1 minute to 30 seconds, or even 10–20 rapid dips. Another excellent counterstain for differential staining of bone components is eosin Y-phloxine B.

In general, most hematoxylin solutions work well for staining bone, including mercury-free Harris's, Ehrlich's, Mayer's, Cole's, Gill II or III, and many

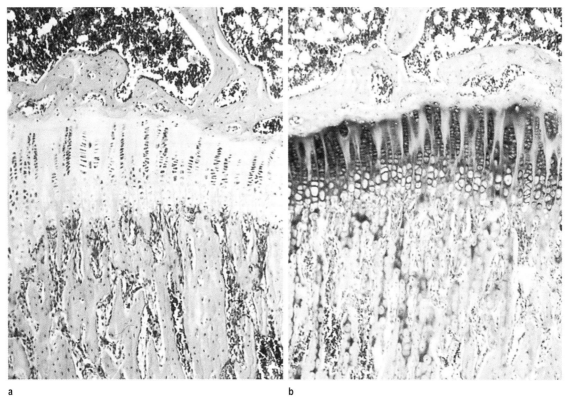

a   b

Figure 16.6 (a) Mayer's hematoxylin and eosin. (b) Ehrlich's hematoxylin and eosin. Epiphyseal growth plate from proximal femur of an 11-week-old rat.

proprietary mixtures. Some workers prefer Ehrlich's hematoxylin to a more specific nuclear stain, e.g. Mayer's (Fig. 16.6) for its ability to stain articular and growth plate cartilages a deeper blue to purple in contrast to the pink collagen and other tissues. In general, a hematoxylin solution can stain decalcified bone to show cement lines in Paget's diseased bone, new bone, and rapidly formed or remodeled bone provided the hematoxylin stains darkly enough. A good H&E stain can stain all cells and bone components including osteoid as long as care is taken to adjust the staining procedure to achieve optimal results.

Collagen stains

Collagen stains can be used to demonstrate mature and finer immature fibers in certain tumors and a fracture callus. van Gieson (VG) picro-fuchsin stains immature fibers a very pale orange compared to the deeper red mature fibers. A trichrome stain (i.e. Masson's) remains a standard, popular method to demonstrate collagen fibers in contrast to bone, cells, and other soft tissues. The immature collagen fibers stain distinctly but are a paler blue or green compared with darker-stained mature fibers. Trichrome-stained adult or mature bone often shows areas of blue or green staining with some bright red areas that frequently have no relationship to bone structure. Osteoid is usually stained with the aniline blue or light green fiber stains.

Polarized light microscopy may be more useful for positive identification of collagen than these stains since the finest fibers do not show distinct colors with routine light microscopy. Sirius red, which is commonly used for amyloid, is an excellent stain to visualize collagen fibers under polarized light. A toluidine blue stain demonstrates collagen fibers.

Cartilage and acid mucopolysaccharides

Cartilage can be stained to demonstrate mucopoly-saccharides using various metachromatic staining methods or the azure method by Hughesdon (1949), recommended for its selectivity and stability.

The critical electrolyte concentration method of Scott and Dorling (1965) provides a more precise identification of acid mucopolysaccharides in cartilage. They used 0.05% 8GX alcian blue in pH 5.8 acetate buffer containing 0.4–0.5 M magnesium chloride to stain these strongly sulfated mucopoly-saccharides blue. Another method useful for showing articular cartilage degradation of ground substances in arthritic and other diseases is safranin O-fast green (Rosenberg 1971), which stains the cartilage varying shades of red. Toluidine blue O, 0.1–1% aqueous solution, is also commonly used to stain NBF-fixed cartilage (Fig. 16.7). Workers should be aware that EDTA, as well as some fixatives and acid decalcifiers, extract proteoglycans and can result in weak cartilage staining by safranin O and possible false-negative quantitative results (Callis & Sterchi 1998).

The positive red periodic acid-Schiff (PAS) reaction demonstrates mucopolysaccharides in new bone, calcifying cartilage, and glycogen in some early osteoblasts. PAS assists in diagnosis of some mucinous metastatic tumors and primary tumors with glycogen with a diastase digestion of glycogen to help make more precise identification of a poorly differentiated primary tumor. The PAS reaction is not affected by decalcification but prolonged treatment with strong acids should be avoided. Reticulin staining, the silver impregnation of reticulin fibers, helps in diagnosis of bone tumors, tumor metastasis to bone, and myelofibrosis. Reticulin staining is not affected by decalcifying agents although the ammoniacal solutions can cause a section to release from the slide, necessitating the use of a stronger section adhesive.

Bone canaliculi

Osteocytes and their lacunae are large enough to be easily identified in most preparations, including H&E-stained paraffin sections of decalcified bone. Fine canaliculi radiating from lacunae are not easily seen in H&E-stained sections, but are well demonstrated with a modified Holmes' silver impregnation method on buffered, formic acid-decalcified, paraffin-embedded bone sections (Taylor et al. 1993).

The major problem in demonstrating canaliculi is the attempt to show spaces too fine for identification by routine staining of surrounding bone, so it is necessary to fill the spaces with a substance that appears dark against a lighter or unstained background. The simple 'air injection' method (Gatenby & Painter 1934) is done with undecalcified ground sections dried, and mounted in hot, melted Canada balsam to trap air inside the canaliculi. These look like black threads against the unstained bone and the balsam but, if sections are too thin or the balsam too fluid, the air will be displaced.

The picro-thionin method (Schmorl 1934) depends on deposition of a thionin precipitate within the lacunae and canaliculi (Fig. 16.3), although frozen or, historically, celloidin sections were recommended. Drury and Wallington (1980) indicated there is less channel shrinkage in such sections as compared to paraffin sections and the dye precipitate could penetrate readily. When frozen sections are not routinely used, one of the staining methods for decalcified bone paraffin sections developed by either Taylor et al. (1993) or Tornero et al. (1991) could provide workers with better options to fit into routine paraffin work. Tornero's group used a

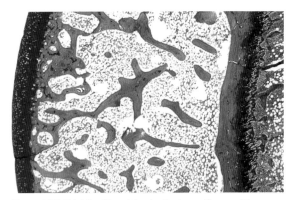

Figure 16.7 Toluidine blue-stained articular cartilage and bone. Formic acid-decalcified rat femur. Paraffin section.

microwave picro-thionin procedure and felt it gave more accurate, uniform staining of canaliculi as compared to Schmorl's method.

A later reference by Schmorl recommended aqueous 0.125% thionin and noted an alkaline solution accelerated and intensified staining by adding one or two drops of concentrated ammonia to approximately 10 ml staining solution just before use. Culling (1974) stated the pH of the thionin solution was critical, with successful staining results dependent on the amount of ammonia added, and recommended one drop of ammonia in 100 ml solution. Drury and Wallington (1980) indicated that thionin dye batches vary considerably, making it necessary to adjust the ammonia content of staining solutions made from different lots in order to obtain suitable staining, and that other dyes may be used with good results, notably azure A.

Schmorl's picro-thionin method *(Schmorl 1934)*

Fixation

Any fixative, but avoid mercuric chloride.

Decalcification

Any decalcifying solution.

Sections

Frozen or celloidin freshly cut.

Solutions

Stock solution

0.25 % aqueous thionin.

Working solution

0.125% thionin: filter 50 ml stock solution and dilute with 50 ml distilled water. Add 1 or 2 drops of concentrated ammonia immediately before use.

Saturated aqueous picric acid

Method

1. Wash sections in distilled water, 10 minutes.
2. Stain in thionin solution, 5–20 minutes or longer.
3. Wash in distilled water.
4. Immerse sections in picric acid solution, 30–60 seconds.
5. Wash in distilled water.
6. Differentiate in 70% alcohol until the bluish-green clouds of stain cease to form, 5–10 minutes or longer.
7. Dehydrate rapidly, clear in xylene, and mount in permanent mounting media.

Results

Lacunae and canaliculi	dark brown-black
Bone matrix	yellow or brownish-yellow
Cells	red

Notes

a. Agitate sections gently during steps 3–6. This is particularly important in step 6, and change 70% alcohol frequently.
b. If bone matrix is decolorized during differentiation (step 6), restore yellow color by returning the section to the picric acid solution for a few seconds before proceeding with dehydration.

Schmorl's modified method with 0.125% thionin solution replaced the picric acid with either phosphotungstic or phosphomolybdic acid and was preferred when staining children's bones. Culling (1974) used the modified method and recommended extended time in the alkaline thionin solution, then a few seconds' treatment in the acid, followed by fixation of the dye with dilute ammonia. This method results in blue-black canaliculi and lacunae on a sky-blue background.

Immunohistochemistry (IHC)

Diagnostic immunohistochemical staining is frequently done on decalcified bone sections embedded in paraffin (e.g. bone marrow biopsies, tumors, cartilage) and uses the same staining methods and materials as for soft tissue immunohistochemistry. Care must be taken to fix bone specimens properly and decalcify with the least damaging agent in the shortest time possible in order to protect antigens from damaging effects of acids. Immunostaining is possible on 2 μm thick methyl methacrylate sections after complete removal of the plastic with warm xylene and a pressure cooker antigen retrieval method (Hand & Church 1998). Glycol methacrylate (GMA) cannot be removed and may inhibit adequate antibody or immunoglobulin penetration to the antigenic sites, so it is suggested that the bone be stained using DAB chromagen after fixation and before GMA embedding. Counterstains work well after microtomy when processed in this manner and it does not diminish or wash out the chromagen.

Preparation of mineralized bone

Sections demonstrating bone mineral and its relationship to the unmineralized components of bone must be prepared by methods that do not interfere with the mineral substance, i.e. undecalcified bone sections. Mineralized bone must be cut with tungsten carbide-tipped knives and needs special, hard support to avoid cracked or crumbling tissue sections. Paraffin is too soft and fails to match the hardness of bone or provide strong, solid support needed to prevent the fragmented mineralized sections.

Acrylic resins and plastics are now widely used and the preferred embedding media for undecalcified bone and their use has revolutionized how this bone is examined. Frozen sections provide some support of cancellous bone, but the bone itself tends to look damaged and somewhat fragmented even though a diagnosis could be made from the soft tissue components.

Adhesive tape methods

Adhesive tape methods or tape transfer methods have been used to maintain the intact sections of undecalcified double-embedded bone sections during microtomy. Two methods, one for undecalcifed bone embedded in MMA (Hardt 1986) and the other for decalcified, paraffin-embedded bone (Eurell & Sterchi 1994), are used for sectioning difficult blocks. Clear adhesive packaging tape is rolled onto the trimmed block face and the cut section sticks to the tape during and after sectioning. The tape-section combination is then attached to an adhesive coated slide and either dried on a hot plate or clamped firmly between sheets of polyethylene or wood inside a 60°C oven overnight. During the staining process, the tape releases in xylene, leaving the section 'transferred' onto the slide for subsequent staining. Plastic sections can be either transferred to a slide or stained directly on the tape. A special tape transfer system is also available for bone frozen sections.

Block impregnation for osteoid demonstration

This method is used solely for the negative demonstration of osteoid in which the calcium in mineralized bone is replaced by silver before decalcification and paraffin sectioning. Block impregnation techniques suffer from inherent defects of peripheral or over-impregnation near the surface with an incomplete reaction deeper in the tissues. As long as these artifacts are recognized in a finished preparation, the osteoid seams counterstained reds are clearly delineated next to the blackened mineralized bone. The deeper, centrally located trabeculae are pale with only the outlines of lacunae and some blackened canaliculi. The advantage of this method is that good-quality paraffin sections are easily prepared.

Silver staining of bone prior to decalcification
(Tripp & Mackay 1972)

Fixation
99% ethyl alcohol.

Tissue
1–2 mm thick bone pieces.

Solutions

2% aqueous silver nitrate
Reducer

Sodium hypophosphite	5 g
0.1 M sodium hydroxide	0.2 ml
Distilled water	100 ml

5% aqueous sodium thiosulfate (anhydrous)
Decalcifier
10% aqueous formic acid

van Gieson's picro-fuchsin
Method
1. Wash in several changes of distilled water, 4 hours.
2. Place in 2% silver nitrate, 48 hours in complete darkness.

3. Rinse in three changes of distilled water, 15–20 seconds each.
4. Wash in running tap water, 4 hours.
5. Place in reducer, 48 hours.
6. Wash in running tap water, 1 hour.
7. Place in sodium thiosulfate solution, 24 hours.
8. Wash in running tap water, 1 hour.
9. Decalcify in 10% formic acid.
10. Process to paraffin wax, cut, and mount.
11. Dewax and bring sections to water.
12. Stain with van Gieson's stain, 2 minutes.
13. Dehydrate, clear, and mount.

Results

Edges of mineralized bone	black
Bone	brown to yellow
Osteoid	red

Notes

a. For cellular detail, an adjacent NBF-fixed, non-impregnated block should be processed.
b. Radiographic decalcification endpoint test cannot be used with the radio-opaque silver deposits.
c. Nitric and hydrochloric acid decalcifiers may attack the silver deposits.
d. NBF-fixed bone may be used provided formaldehyde is completely removed by distilled water washes before impregnation.

Frozen sections

Using a modern cryostat, patience, a slow steady cutting speed, and a tungsten carbide-tipped steel knife, frozen sections from trephine and needle biopsies of cortical and trabecular bone can be cut with ease and minimal section damage. A knife with a tungsten carbide edge is much harder than a steel edge and cuts calcified bone without fragmenting a section or damage to the edge. For demonstration of bone marrow cells, tumor, and calcified bone components, the hematoxylin stains cell nuclei and mineralized bone intensely blue and eosin stains osteoid and other soft tissues shades of red. Some bone with metabolic diseases, such as Paget's, renal osteodystrophy, and hyperparathyroidism showing advanced changes or diseased bone with moderate to severe osteomalacia, can be rapidly diagnosed on an H&E stained frozen section. Other stains can be done on bone frozen sections, including a modified Romanowsky method for patterns in bone remodeling and cartilage development (Dodds & Gowen 1994), enzyme and immunohistochemical methods. Unstained sections can be examined with polarized light to see woven and lamellar patterns in bone.

Laboratories not using MMA embedding techniques may find bone cryotomy a valuable addition to their facility. Frozen sections permit rapid diagnosis on some bone diseases. Rapid or 'snap' freezing bone samples in liquid nitrogen-cooled 2-methylbutane (isopentane) must be used carefully as some bones can shatter in the extremely cold (–120°C) temperature. A dry ice/isopentane bath (–70°C) snap freezes bone coated with 4% aqueous polyvinyl alcohol (PVA, water soluble, 124,000 MW) or embedded in optimum cutting temperature compound (OCT), gently and without shattering. Hexane can be substituted for isopentane (Dodds & Gowen, 1994). In brief, the technique is:

1. Mount bone on cork or embed in a cryomold with OCT.
2. Snap freeze carefully in 'syrupy' (thawing) isopentane cooled by liquid nitrogen (–120°C) or with dry ice/isopentane (–70°C).
3. Place bone in cryostat at –30 to –35°C. Remount frozen bone onto a metal chuck with OCT to provide maximum stability during sectioning.
4. Cut section at 5–7 µm, pick up section on slide, and fix with fixative of choice. Post-fixation in 95% alcohol, 5 minutes, removes fat.
5. Stain in Harris, Gill II or Gill III for 1 minute or longer or desired intensity.
6. Rinse with water or a blueing reagent to 'blue' section; avoid ammonia water.
7. 1% alcoholic eosin approximately 10–30 seconds or desired intensity.
8. Dehydrate, clear, and mount in permanent mounting medium.

a. Formalin-fixed biopsies can be rinsed, immersed in 5–20% sucrose for 1–8 hours at 4°C to replace water before freezing and improve sectioning, being known as cryoprotection. Higher concentrations of sucrose for cryoprotection may delay freezing and cause uneven freezing. Optimization and practice should be used to determine the amount of sucrose that is used.

b. Fresh frozen sections can be fixed, rinsed, and then decalcified in 10% EDTA before immunostaining.

c. Enzyme staining can be done on fixed or unfixed sections.

d. A special tape transfer system (Cryojane; Leica, Inc.) is available for cryomicrotomy of undecalcified bone and other difficult tissues, keeping sections intact and adhered to special polymer-coated slides (Schiller 1999).

e. Any hematoxylin can be used with staining intensity optimized for worker preference.

Plastic embedding

Mineralized bone sections are best studied when the embedding medium matches bone hardness to permit intact sections necessary to examine bone density or defects in mineralized components in relation to the bone cells, cartilage, osteoid, and other soft tissues. Synthetic resins for both EM (Epon) and light microscopy plastics (GMA, MMA) work well for these purposes. Epoxy EM resins are suitable only for ultra-thin sectioning of tiny bone pieces; their hydrophobicity causes poor stain penetration into tissues.

Methacrylates were used for specimen whole-mount displays in museums before use as support media for sections. Although Woodruff and Norris (1955) favored an *n*-butyl/ethyl methacrylate mixture, methyl methacrylate (MMA) is now the preferred plastic for undecalcified bone work. MMA mixed with polyethylene glycol (Boellaard & von Hirsch 1959) or dibutylphthlate is softer and more elastic. Glycol methacrylate, a softer plastic than MMA, used with bone biopsies results in 'laddered' bone sections cut with glass knives. Mineralized

bone specimens require extended time in dehydration, clearing, and MMA infiltration compared to decalcified bone paraffin processing.

Although some workers 'wash' the polymerization inhibitor from the monomer (Difford 1974), many now use an unwashed monomer method suitable for microtomed or sawn ground sections.

Enclosed automatic processors should not be used with toxic MMA monomers, although bone laboratories use these processors for alcohol and xylene steps but finish MMA infiltration steps with hand processing. Approximate time per change in solvents for all processing steps depends on bone size: small, 24–30 hours; medium (3–5 mm), 48 hours or more; large, 2–4 days.

Procedures for MMA processing and embedding developed by Sterchi (1996) are similar to those in Chapter 8. Sterchi used two changes each of 95% and 100% ethanol: xylene or (1:1) MMA monomer/100% ethanol. MMA infiltration times are the same as processing times. Sterchi's infiltration mixtures vary from those in Chapter 8 by using 100 ml monomer and adding to: Mixture #1, 1 g benzoyl peroxide (BPO) only; Mixture #2, 5 ml dibutylphthlate 1 g BPO, 15 g poly methyl methacrylate powder (996,000 MW; Aldrich, MO); Mixture #3 (same as #2) but 1.5 g BPO. Embed in fresh Mixture #3, polymerize at RT or in a 37°C water bath (small bone), cure blocks for 4–6 hours at 60°C, then freeze blocks for 2 hours to remove polypropylene containers.

Sectioning methacrylate-embedded bone

Bone embedded in MMA can be sectioned by either microtomy (1–20 µm) or sawing and grinding for thick sections (150 µm to 1 mm). Thick ground sections are necessary for microradiography, bone containing metal or other implant material, and extremely large bones that cannot be sectioned. An ultra-miller on a large sliding microtome (Polycut E; Leica, USA) can precisely mill a perfectly flat 15–20 µm section. Ultra-milling and grinding wastes bone and must be used carefully. Thin bone sections cut more easily with a motorized microtome designed for plastic work.

Sawing

Hand sawing and grinding can be done by clamping a block in a vice, cutting a slab with a fretted wire saw, and then grinding the slab to produce a section thin enough for staining and microscopic examination. Hand preparations result in thick, uneven slices with deep scratches requiring extra grinding to obtain a smooth section. This is time consuming and wastes more specimen even though adequate sections are possible with practice and careful sawing/grinding techniques.

Saws designed for cutting metallurgy samples are recommended for obtaining precise, flat, thin sections. A Micro-Grinding System (EXAKT Technologies, Oklahoma, USA) specifically developed for bone work by Donath (1988a, 1988b) is complete with plastic embedding media, plastic slides, special saws, and a grinder/polisher. Low- or high-speed metallurgical saws (Isomet, Buehler Ltd, IL, USA) cut easily through bone blocks with or without metal implants using diamond-impregnated cut-off blades, and produce sections in need of less grinding. These machines cut wafers down to 100 μm thick and, by resetting the micrometer, accurate serial sectioning is possible. These saws are water cooled to disperse heat produced by cutting while continuously cleaning the blade and block face for debris-free sections.

The blade thickness (kerf) increases with larger blade diameters and each cut with a blade wastes only as much tissue as its own thickness (kerf loss). It is advisable to use a smaller-diameter blade with the thinnest kerf whenever possible. Larger blocks generally need sturdier, large-diameter blades for proper clearance through a block and no flexing of blade while cutting even though the kerf loss will be greater.

Milling cutters and precision cutting machines (Malvern Microslice, UK) can cut sections to approximately 150 μm. Sawn sections are ground and polished to produce the final thickness and remove scratches while ultra-milled sections need no further grinding or polishing. The MMA-embedded slab section is glued to white or clear plastic slides with cyano-acrylate glue to endure the stress of grinding and polishing.

Grinding and polishing

Motorized metallurgical grinder/polishers are ideal for final finishing of MMA-embedded bone wafers to a required thickness for microscopic examination and microradiography. These machines have variable speed adjustments, rotating base plates to hold self-adhesive grinding papers or polishing cloths, running water for removing debris, and even have special adapters to hold a specimen during the grinding process. Grinding papers remove scratches with progressively coarser to finer grit papers (360, 400, 600 grits), followed by polishing with an aqueous 1 μm alumina for a mirror-smooth surface. Residual fine scratches produce unsightly patterns in microradiographs and surface stained sections. A dial caliper can be used to check section thickness throughout the grinding process. Hand grinding is inexpensive, simple, and with practice will produce adequate sections but automated grinders have the advantages of speed and producing multiple and flatter sections. It is not recommended to grind unembedded cortical bone between abrasive glass plates (historical method) without support of the plastic. It may fracture the bone; grind away fine trabeculae, cells and soft tissues without complete removal of scratches.

Microtome sections of undecalcified bone

Automated microtomes (Leica 2165, Leica USA, or Olympus Cut 4060E, Triangle Biomedical Systems, NC) and a D profile tungsten carbide-tipped steel knife section, both MMA and GMA. Tungsten carbide knives help avoid the 'laddered' bone sections seen after cutting with glass knives. Large blocks need to be sectioned on a larger, sliding motorized microtome (Leica Polycut E or S) with special tungsten carbide knives.

Staining methyl methacrylate-embedded bone

Methacrylate bone sections can be stained in two ways depending on the type of section available. Sections, 4–8 μm thick, attached to an adhesive-coated glass slide can be stained after either softening or removing the plastic. When section loss is a problem, sections can be stained by 'free-floating' in a dish or attached to adhesive tape. Ultra-milled or ground sections, 20–200 μm thick, glued to plastic slides, can be 'surface' stained, a unique, effective method for examination of mineralized bone and its components.

Unstained thin sections examined with polarized light demonstrate collagen patterns within the bone. There are many staining methods for MMA bone sections, including methods necessary to distinguish the osteoid from the mineralized components. Micro-radiographic evaluation can be done on 100 μm thick sections followed by surface staining of the same section for microscopic examination and correlation of two methods. Paraffin staining methods often do not stain MMA sections well, and must be adapted for these sections by longer staining times, or plastic removal ('deplasticize') or softening with solvents ('etching') to permit stain penetration.

Stains for calcium are of prime importance and include hematoxylin, solochrome cyanin, and the von Kossa silver nitrate methods. Trichrome stains will distinguish calcified bone stained with some hematoxylin and the fiber stain from the osteoid stained with the cytoplasmic stain. Thus, a Masson's trichrome stains bone blue and osteoid red. A modi-fication of this method by Goldner (1937) results in clear, brilliantly detailed staining of osteoclasts, osteoblasts, fibroblasts, and cells from marrow or tumors. Some workers feel the modified MacNeal's tetrachrome and Movat's pentachrome methods give superior staining results for differentiating osteoid from mineralized bone (Schenk et al. 1984).

Various toluidine blue methods with pH ranges of 7–9 are routinely used to specifically stain trabecular mineralization fronts, cartilage, and other bone components.

Detection of tetracycline fluorescence in bone can be done on either unstained sections or sections stained with Villanueva's mineralized bone stain (Sanderson 1997).

Surface staining methods for 20–200 μm thick pol-ished bone MMA sections mounted on white plastic slides are helpful for examining oversized bone sec-tions or sections containing metal implants. This staining technique provides surprisingly excellent cellular detail, and is commonly used to study the interface of the bone with a metal implant. Surface staining can be done by mildly decalcifying (acid 'etching') the exposed bone surface with 1% formic acid for 1 minute to remove a few micrometers of calcium from the section to permit better dye pene-tration into the bone, thereby enhancing staining of bone. MMA is very hydrophobic and only certain low molecular weight dyes actually penetrate MMA for suitable staining of softer tissue compo-nents with the aid of heat or alkaline stain solutions (pH 7–9). Some methods used for surface staining include methylene blue-basic fuchsin, potassium permanganate-oxidized methylene blue (Sander-son's Rapid Bone Stain, Surgipath, USA), modified MacNeal's tetrachrome (Schenk et al. 1984), and 0.75% toluidine blue in phosphate buffer, pH 7–8 (Eurell & Sterchi 1994). These methods stain calcified bone and its components distinctly, i.e. osteoid, cal-cification fronts, lacunae, canaliculi, osteons, osteo-clasts, osteoblasts, marrow cells, collagen, and other soft tissues, various shades of dark to light blue or blue-green, and cartilage shades of deep purple to violet. Basic fuchsin, light green, and van Gieson's are used as counterstains with these methods.

Mounting after staining

Deplasticized stained sections on glass slides are mounted in the same way as paraffin sections using alcohol dehydration, xylene clearing, and mounting with a synthetic mounting medium. Free-floating sections tend to wrinkle and, while in clearing agent, can be flattened with a brush or rolled between pieces of smooth filter paper, then mounted with synthetic resin with a weight placed on top of the cover glass to keep the section flat until the medium dries. Strong clamping devices maintain flat sections briefly but cause the mounting media to retract during storage.

Surface-stained sections in MMA cannot be dehy-drated, cleared, or mounted. Methyl methacrylate is softened by alcohols, and is soluble in xylene and other mounting media solvents. Their use results in ugly cracking of plastic in and around a section. Surface-stained sections are usually not perma-nently coverslipped. To examine surface-stained sections, place a cover glass on top of the dry section or a drop of immersion oil to aid the resolution of the section under the scope. Examine with the brightest light setting on the microscope. If using the immersion oil, wipe the oil off after removing the temporary coverslip. The slide will feel oily but do not use any solvents to clean the oil off since it will not alter the stain after long-term storage whereas the solvent will.

Hematoxylin and eosin for MMA-embedded tissue

These methods are useful for diagnosis of suspected osteomalacia and distinguish mineralized bone from osteoid, with nuclei and other soft tissues stained similarly to decalcified bone paraffin sections.

Hematoxylin and eosin-like stain (Eurell & Sterchi, 1994)

Modified toluidine blue/basic fuchsin (TB/BF) for MMA sections (Fig. 16.8)

Solutions

1% stock toluidine blue O

Toluidine blue O	1.0 g
Distilled water	100 ml

1% stock basic fuchsin

Basic fuchsin	1.0 g
Distilled water	100 ml

Phosphate buffer solution, pH 8.0

Buffer solution A:	0.2 M disodium hydrogen orthophosphate (28.39*g Na_2HPO_4 in 1 L H_2O)
Buffer solution B:	0.2 M sodium dihydrogen orthophosphate (27.60*g NaH_2PO_4 in 1 L H_2O)

Buffer solution A	94.7 ml	47.35 ml	23.67 ml
Buffer solution B	5.3 ml	2.65 ml	1.33 ml
Distilled water	100.0 ml	50.0 ml	25.0 ml
	200.0 ml	100.0 ml	50.0 ml

*Check the molecular weight of the dry chemical to refigure the molarity of the solution when making new stock solution.

Working toluidine blue O solution

Phosphate buffer, pH 8.0	40 ml
1% toluidine blue stock	3 ml

Working basic fuchsin solution

Phosphate buffer, pH 8.0	40 ml
1% basic fuchsin stock	1 ml

1% formic acid**

Formic acid (88%)	1 ml
Distilled water	99 ml

**Or use premixed formic decalcifying solution.

Method

1. Place slides into 1% formic acid, 30 seconds with slight agitation.
2. Rinse slides thoroughly in running tap water.
3. Blot slide with gauze or paper towel to dry.
4. Mix working toluidine blue staining solution.
5. Preheat toluidine blue staining solution to 57–60°C in microwave.
6. Place slides into preheated toluidine blue, cover and let stain for 5 minutes.
7. Rinse in running tap water.
8. Blot slides to drain off excess water.
9. Mix working basic fuchsin staining solution.
10. Preheat basic fuchsin staining solution to 57°C in microwave.
11. Place slides into preheated basic fuchsin, cover and let stain for 3–5 minutes. depending on the staining intensity preferred.
12. Rinse in running tap water.
13. Dry completely, then coverslip.

Note: Do not let slides dry completely during any step of staining procedure except before coverslipping.

Results

Calcified bone	Pink to purple
Osteoid	Dark pink
Cell cytoplasm	Pink
Nuclei	Blue to blue purple
Cartilage	Violet

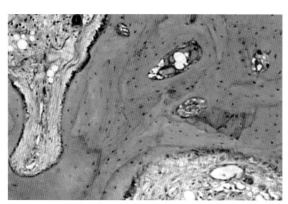

Figure 16.8 Example of the hematoxylin and eosin-like stain. A 4 μm section of rabbit TMJ embedded in methyl metacrylate.

Reagents

Cole's hematoxylin

1% aqueous eosin

Method

1. Deplasticize with xylene and hydrate sections to distilled water.
2. Stain in freshly filtered Cole's hematoxylin, 60 minutes with occasional agitation.
3. Wash well in alkaline tap water.
4. Stain in eosin solution, 30 minutes.
5. Wash in tap water.
6. Dehydrate, clear, and mount.

Results

Osteoid	pink
Calcified bone	purple brown
Nuclei	blue

Solochrome cyanine

The solochrome cyanine stain differentiates osteoid from newly laid down bone and older bone (Fig. 16.9). The following method gives stronger sharper staining compared to 1% solochrome cyanine R in 2% acetic acid (Matrajt & Hioco 1966) but the procedures are essentially the same.

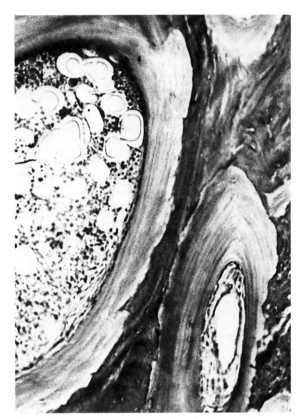

Figure 16.9 Solochrome cyanine method showing osteoid and mineralized bone. Undecalcified section of methacrylate-embedded iliac crest biopsy from a patient with osteomalacia.

Solochrome cyanine *(Hyman & Poulding 1961)*

Solution

Solochrome cyanine R	1 g
Concentrated sulfuric acid	2.5 ml

Mix well until dye incorporates into the resulting 'sludge'. Add 500 ml of 0.5% aqueous iron alum (ferric ammonium sulfate).

Mix and filter.

Method

1. Deplasticize with xylene and hydrate sections to distilled water.
2. Stain in solochrome cyanine solution, 60 minutes.
3. Using a microscope, differentiate in warm (30°C) alkaline tap water until mineralized areas appear blue and other areas light red. Over-differentiation causes all parts to become blue.
4. Dehydrate, clear, and mount.

Results

Mineralized bone	light blue
Calcification front	dark blue
Osteoid	light red-orange
Wide osteoid and orange bands	light red-orange with pale blue
Nuclei	blue

Staining for bone mineral

The classic von Kossa (1901) silver method is used to stain the mineral component (calcium phosphate) in bone, and is a negative stain for osteoid with the calcium component blackened by silver deposition. Osteoid is counterstained red by either the van Gieson's or safranin O (Figs 16.10 and 16.11). This can also be used as a ground section surface stain but without the acid 'etching' removal of calcium.

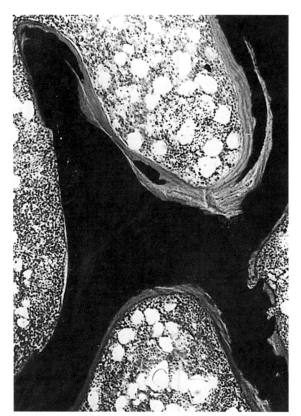

Figure 16.10 Von Kossa's silver deposition method giving a negative demonstration of osteoid, counterstained with safranin O. Undecalcified section of methacrylate-embedded iliac crest biopsy from a patient with osteomalacia. Ground section.

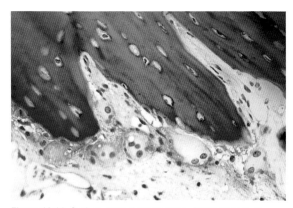

Figure 16.11 Surface-stained canine bone. Rapid bone stain counterstained with van Gieson's. Bone (red), osteocytes and giant osteoclasts (blue). Undecalcified methyl methacrylate-embedded ground section.

Von Kossa method *(modified Von Kossa 1901)*

Solutions

1% aqueous silver nitrate

2.5% sodium thiosulfate

1% safranin O or van Gieson's picro-fuchsin

Method

1. Deplasticize with xylene, and hydrate sections to distilled water.
2. Place in silver nitrate solution, expose to strong light for 10–60 minutes and watch the mineralized bone turn dark brown to black, indicating a completed reaction.
3. Wash in three changes of distilled water.
4. Treat with sodium thiosulfate, 5 minutes.
5. Wash well in distilled water.
6. Counterstain as desired.
7. Dehydrate, clear, and mount.

Results

| Mineralized bone | black |
| Osteoid | red |

Notes

1. Long-wavelength UV light from sunlight or a quartz halogen microscope lamp is preferable to a tungsten filament light bulb, and accelerates the reaction.
2. van Gieson's picro-fuchsin counterstaining may interfere with birefringence of osteoid.

Goldner's trichrome method

This staining technique can be more valuable than the von Kossa method in investigations of metabolic diseases, e.g. Paget's, renal osteodystrophy, and hyperparathyroidism, because of excellent staining of cells. Osteoblast and osteoclast activity is easily assessed, an important factor for both diagnosis and evaluating the effects of treatment in these disorders by repeated bone biopsies. An additional advantage is that metastatic tumor cells in bone marrow are easily identified.

Solutions

Weigert's iron hematoxylin

Ponceau-fuchsin-azophloxin stock solutions

Ponceau de xylidine solution

Ponceau de xylidine	0.75 g
Acid fuchsin	0.25 g
Acetic acid	1 ml
Mix, and add to distilled water	100 ml

Azophloxin solution

Azophloxin	0.5 g
Acetic acid	0.6 ml
Mix, and add to distilled water	100 ml

Final working stain solution

Ponceau-fuchsin solution	5–10 ml
Azophloxin	2 ml
0.2% acetic acid solution	88 ml

Light green solution

Light green	1 g
Acetic acid	1 ml
Mix, and add to distilled water	500 ml

Phosphomolybdic acid-orange G solution

Phosphomolybdic acid	3 g
Orange G	2 g

Dissolve in 500 ml of distilled water, and add a crystal of thymol.

Method

1. Deplasticize with xylene and hydrate sections to water.
2. Immerse sections in alkaline alcohol solution (90 ml of 80% ethanol and 10 ml of 25% ammonia), 1 hour.
3. Rinse in water, 15 minutes.
4. Stain in Weigert's hematoxylin, 1 hour.
5. Rinse in tap water, 10 minutes.
6. Rinse in distilled water, 5 minutes.
7. Stain in final Ponceau-fuchsin-azophloxin solution, 5 minutes.
8. Rinse in 1% acetic acid, 15 seconds.
9. Stain in phosphomolybdic acid-orange G solution, 20 minutes.
10. Rinse in 1% acetic acid, 15 seconds.
11. Stain with light green, 5 minutes.
12. Rinse in three changes of 1% acetic acid.
13. Rinse in distilled water, blot dry, and mount.

Results

Mineralized bone	green
Osteoid	orange-red
Nuclei	blue-gray
Cartilage	purple

Demonstration of aluminum

Patients receiving hemodialysis for chronic renal failure may deposit aluminum at the mineralization sites in bone, producing an osteomalacia-like pattern. Aluminum can be demonstrated by either the aluminon or solochrome azurine method, with the latter considered the most reliable. Two newer methods eliminated staining of free-floating sections (see method below) and used sections attached to glass slides. One is a modified acidic solochrome azurine method for GMA-embedded bone sections (Huffer et al. 1996), and the other is an aluminon method for the study of uremic bone fixed with NBF instead of absolute ethanol and embedded in MMA (Maloney et al. 1982).

Solochrome azurine method for aluminum in bone biopsies (modified from Denton et al. 1984)

Sections
Undecalcified bone embedded in MMA.

Solutions
Stock solution
1% aqueous solochrome azurine (CI 143830). Stable for a long period of time.

Working solution
Adjust pH of 1% solochrome azurine stock solution to pH 5 with 25% acetic acid. This forms an important precipitate needed for staining; do not filter this solution. Prepare working solution immediately before use and discard after use.

Method

1. Free-floating MMA sections to distilled water. Use a small Petri dish to contain all solutions for free-floating sections throughout the procedure.
2. Stain sections in working stain solution (pH 5.0) at RT for 18 hours or overnight.
3. Wash gently in distilled water for 20–30 seconds.
4. Counterstain with 1% neutral red.
5. Wash in distilled water.
6. Blot dry and leave in drying oven overnight.
7. Mount in synthetic mounting medium.

Results

Aluminum	dark blue-purple
Nuclei and background	shades of red

Aluminon method *(after Irwin 1955)*

Fixation

Fix bone in absolute ethanol.

Sections

MMA, free-floating sections.

Solutions

Buffer solution

5 M ammonium chloride	60 ml
5 M ammonium acetate	60 ml
6 M HCl	10 ml

Mix, and check pH (should be approx. pH 5.2).

Working stain solution

Aurinetricarboxylic acid ('aluminon')	2 g
Buffer solution, as above	100 ml

Dissolve aluminon in a few milliliters of buffer, and bring final volume to 100 ml with remaining buffer. Heat to 60°C. Filter immediately before use.

Differentiating solution

Buffer solution, as above	50 ml
1.6 M ammonium carbonate	22 ml

Check pH; should be approx. 7.2.

Method

1. Bring sections to water.
2. Stain for 5–10 minutes at 60°C; use freshly filtered stain, preheated to 60°C (see Notes a and b).
3. Rinse in distilled water.
4. Differentiating solution for 3–5 seconds.
5. Wash in distilled water.
6. Counterstain in 1% aqueous methylene blue for 1 minute.
7. Rinse in distilled water.
8. Dehydrate in alcohols and mount in synthetic resin medium.

Results

Sites of aluminum	bright red
Background	blue

Notes

a. Sections embedded in MMA and other acrylics, e.g. LR White, may detach from glass slides in this 60°C solution.
b. Free-floating MMA sections often wrinkle in the 60°C solution. Multiple sections and careful handling are recommended.

Microradiography

Microradiographs are high-resolution, fine-detail contact X-rays of thinner ground sections for microscopic examination and evaluation of bone mineral density and distribution. The denser, highly mineralized areas appear almost white as fewer X-rays penetrate them, and less dense, non-mineralized areas show shades of yellowish-gray grading to black against the black background of the exposed film (Fig. 16.12).

The requirements for microradiography, even though similar to those for fine-detail specimen radiography, are even more stringent: a fairly powerful, controllable source of 'soft' X-rays (low kV), even overall section thickness, and high-resolution

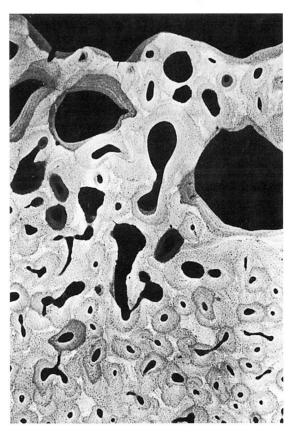

Figure 16.12 Microradiograph of normal femoral shaft showing different densities of mineralization. The lightest areas indicate the heaviest mineral deposition.

film or photographic plates are necessary for this procedure.

Mineralized bone sections embedded in MMA are preferred and must be perfectly flat, measure approximately 70–130 μm thick, and be free of debris and scratches. Thicker sections create blurred images and thinner sections transmit too many X-rays. Sections must be in tight, close contact with the film or plate and developed under controlled conditions for comparative work.

Microradiography has been done with X-ray crystallography units, and, although not called microradiography, even greater resolution work is accomplished with the BSEM or backscatter electron imaging scanning electron microscope (Bloebaum et al. 1990). The Faxitron X-ray unit produces satisfactory results, and Dunn et al. (1974) described a standard procedure with this unit using 20 kV, 20 cm film to source distance (FTSD) for 75 minutes with 5 × 5 cm glass Kodak High Resolution Plates, Type 1A. Unfortunately, photographic plates and films suitable for microradiography are frequently discontinued. Workers should locate replacement film with a resolving power of 2000 lines/mm or higher and high-contrast, fine-grain emulsions, properties that help reduce long exposure times (Boivin & Baud 1984). Some workers are finding success using mammography film (Kodak MIN R 2000; Kodak, Rochester, NY) at higher kV, longer FTSD, and short exposure time (L. Jenkins, personal communication). Using the example below as a guideline, workers should be able to optimize settings needed for any new film or photographic plates.

An example of microradiography using mammography film in Faxitron (L. Jenkins, personal communication, 2000)

Bone section, approximately 100 μm thick, pressed tightly against film inside a vacuum cassette.
A Kodak MIN R 2000 mammography film.
Film-to-source distance (FTSD) 50 cm (lowest shelf level).
Tube, 55 kV.
Tube current, 3 mA.
Exposure time is approximately 5 seconds.

After exposure, the mammography film or plates must be developed exactly according to manufacturer instructions, using solutions and temperatures specified for these products, then dried. The dried film is cut to fit on a larger glass slide mounted under a larger cover glass and secured at the edges by cellophane tape. An exposed area on a photographic plate is mounted under a cover glass with Eukitt's or an equivalent medium. Examination should be made using a 10x objective on light microscope in a dark room.

Fluorescent labeling

Tetracycline antibiotics form fluorescent complexes with calcium at the sites of bone mineral deposition (Milch et al. 1957, 1958) and provide an effective *in vivo* tracer of bone formation in these areas. The drug localizes rapidly in newly mineralized sites of bone or teeth and appears as a bright fluorescent line under UV light. Two or more doses administered to patients at known intervals provide a method for estimating the rate of bone remodeling (Frost 1983a). The measurable distances between parallel uptake lines indicate the amount of bone deposited at each time interval between doses (Fig. 16.13). In order to retain tetracycline labeling, mineralized bone is fixed in 70% ethanol or alcoholic formalin, embedded in MMA, sectioned, mounted unstained and

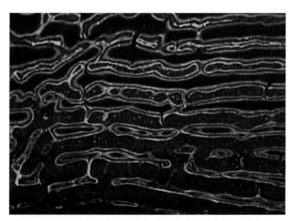

Figure 16.13 Tetracyline-labeled cortical bone from a young horse. Two doses were given at 3 weeks. Specimen was alcohol-fixed, undecalcified, methacrylate-embedded section illuminated with 480 nm wavelength UV light.

viewed with a UV light microscope at approximately 360–480 nm wavelength. After UV light evaluation, sections can be stained with toluidine blue for further microscopic examination.

Morphometry of bone

The general principles and methods of morphometry are outlined in Chapter 23 of this book. This section very briefly deals with some application of techniques for evaluating bone disorders, particularly in metabolic bone disease (MBD).

Normal bone containing trabeculae undergoes constant remodeling or resorption by the osteoclasts and formation by osteoblasts. In disease, remodeling can be disturbed and cause either too much or too little of one of these dynamic processes to occur in the bone.

Assessment of relative amounts of bone trabecular tissue, osteoid, resorption and deposition (apposition) can be made by a subjective microscopic examination of the section. This is adequate where changes are obvious, but subtle alterations may require accurate measurements to detect an abnormality. In metabolic bone disease, tetracycline is administered at specific times prior to biopsy to help determine the amount of active mineralization in bone (Fig. 16.12), followed by an iliac crest biopsy and subsequent MMA embedment. Briefly, bone histomorphometry can be used for detection and assessment of disease severity or effects of treatments of MBD, e.g. post-menopausal osteoporosis. Recker (1990) listed eight metabolic bone diseases with tentative indications for bone biopsy, although this list is anticipated to expand with acquisition of more knowledge and treatment of MBD.

Histomorphometric analysis can be done with manual, semi-automated, or automated methods. A manual method could include a standard microscope with eyepiece reticules, digitized tablets (image display), image storage, and a computer for data storage and output. Increasingly, modern automated computerized image analysis systems with a video camera, a screen with screen grid for area counting, and software designed specifically for

bone work are being used to reduce the time needed for measurements and calculations of final results.

A standardized, generally universal system of nomenclature, symbols, and units for bone histomorphometry was summarized by Parfitt (1988) and it is recommended that workers be familiar with and use this system. This is a terminology list of primary measurements for volume, surface, thickness, mineralization rate, formation rate, and so on. Basic measurements are confined to trabecular bone and are:

(a) trabecular bone volume and surface

(b) eroded (resorption) surface

(c) osteoid surface

(d) mineralized surface

(e) osteoid thickness

(f) wall thickness (of new bone layers at formation site)

(g) mineral apposition rate (calcification rate) (Recker 1983)

Calculations are made from collected data (Parfitt et al. 1987), and results correlated to the various diseases. Chapter 23 explains how area measurements are numerically equated with volume measurements. The derivation of some of these values is shown below:

Bone volume (%)

$$\text{Osteoid volume (\%)} = \frac{\text{area of osteoid}}{\text{area of trabeculae and marrow space}}$$

$$\text{Osteoid surface (\%)} = \frac{\text{length of trabecular surface covered by osteoid}}{\text{total length of trabecular surface}}$$

$$\text{Osteoid index (\%)} = \frac{\text{osteoid volume}}{\text{osteoid surface}}$$

$$\text{Resorption surface (\%)} = \frac{\text{length of trabecular surface occupied by lacunae}}{\text{total length of trabecular surface}}$$

There are many other derived parameters used to describe bone dynamics described by Frost (1983b).

Histomorphometric values for normal males and females with relation to age, and values for the various diseases compared to age and sex-matched normal controls have been published, and are useful as reference guidelines (Melsen et al. 1983). It is important to be aware of pitfalls in techniques for bone morphometry; these are well discussed in Recker's book (1983). An example of a problem is with serial biopsy evaluation of a severe disease, for example Paget's, where known variations occur from site to site and even within the same bone. It is important that each laboratory establish its own set of normal values, along with careful standard operating procedures (SOPs) for sample preparation, staining techniques, and microscopy used for bone morphometry. If standardized stains or magnification are not used, measurements made using different stains can result in different values for the same biopsy. A standardized magnification must be used to estimate surface values, otherwise higher values are produced with increased magnification as finer surface convolutions are resolved. Detailed discussions of bone morphometry can be found in *Bone Histomorphometry: Techniques and Interpretation* (Recker 1983); *Proceedings of the International Workshop on Bone Histomorphometry* (Jee & Parfitt 1980); and a useful review by Revell (1986).

Micro computed tomography (CT)

Micro computed tomography (aka MicroCT) is a tool that allows the micron analysis of bone and tissue without destruction of the sample. MicroCT works on the same principles as clinical CT. A radiation source releases X-rays through a sample; the X-rays that make it through the sample are collected on the detector. In many MicroCT units the sample rotates while projection images are collected at various angles. Generally up to a thousand projections are taken greater than 190 degrees around the sample. Reconstruction then takes the planar projections and compiles them into a three-dimensional image. This 3D image can then be manipulated in all three orthogonal planes. Changing the distance of the sample from the X-ray source and detector or the number of projections can influence the resolution of the scan (Hsieh 2003).

Different tissue types block or 'attenuate' X-ray radiation at varying degrees. This attenuation property of tissue of differing densities is what creates the contrast in the image. Bone has a higher density than tissue, hence its ease of visualization with CT. With a 3D image one can perform geometric analysis and quantify trabecular size, number thickness, spacing and connectivity, along with bone mineral density and content (Abe et al. 2000). The use of contrast agents can allow for 'virtual histology' of tissue (Johnson et al. 2006) (Fig. 16.14).

Acknowledgments

The author would like to thank the following for their contributions to this chapter: Gayle Callis, for writing the previous version; and Chris Bull, for his expertise in CT and providing Figure 16.14.

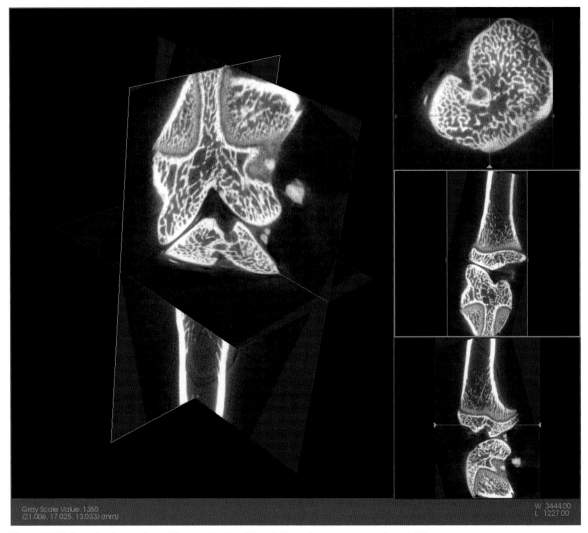

Figure 16.14 Example of a specimen CT scan showing different dimensional measurement capabilities.

References

Abe, S., Watanabe, H., Hirayama, A., et al., 2000. Morphological study of the femur in osteopetrotic (op/op) mice using microcomputed tomography. Br J Radiol 73, 1078–1082.

Bancroft, J.D., Gamble, M., 2008. Theory and practice of histological techniques, sixth ed. Churchill Livingstone Elsevier, Philadelphia, PA, Ch. 18.

Bloebaum, R.D., Bachus, K.N., Boyce, T.M., 1990. Backscattered electron imaging: the role in calcified tissue and implant analysis. Journal of Biomaterial Applications 5, 56–85.

Boellaard, J.W., von Hirsch, T., 1959. Die Herstellung histologischer Schnitte von nichtenkalkten Knochenmittles Einbettung, Methacrylsäure ester. Mikroskopie 13, 386.

Boivin, G., Baud, C.-A., 1984. Microradiographic methods for calcified tissues. In: Dickson, G. (Ed.), Methods of calcified tissue preparation. Elsevier, New York, Ch. 11, p. 403.

Brain, E.B., 1966. The preparation of decalcified sections. C.C. Thomas, Springfield, IL, pp. 86–89.

Byers, P.D., Smith, R., 1967. New appliances: trephine for full-thickness iliac-crest biopsy. British Medical Journal 1, 682.

Callis, G.M., Sterchi, D.L., 1998. Decalcification of bone: literature review and practical study of various decalcifying agents, methods and their effects on bone histology. Journal of Histotechnology 21 (1), 49–58.

Clayden, E.C., 1952. A discussion on the preparation of bone sections by the paraffin wax method with special reference to the control of decalcification. Journal of Medical Laboratory Technology 10, 103.

Culling, C.F., 1974. Handbook of histopathological and histochemical techniques, third ed. Butterworths, London, p. 65.

Denton, J., Freemont, A.J., Ball, J., 1984. Detection and distribution of aluminium in bone. Journal of Clinical Pathology 37, 136–142.

Difford, J., 1974. A simplified method for the preparation of methyl methacrylate embedding medium for undecalcified bone. Medical Laboratory Technology 31, 79–81.

Dodds, R.A., Gowen, M., 1994. The growing osteophyte: a model system for the study of human bone development and remodeling in situ. Journal of Histotechnology 17 (1), 37–45.

Donath, K., 1988a. Preparation of histologic sections by a cutting-grinding technique for hard tissue and other material not suitable to be sectioned by routine methods, second ed. EXAKT-Kulzer Publication, Norderstedt, pp. 1–16.

Donath, K., 1988b. Die Trenn-Dünnschliff-Technik zur Herstellun hisologische Präparate von nicht schniebaren Geweben und Materialien. Der Präpauator 34, 197–206. German report, translated and published by EXAKT-Kulzer Publication.

Drury, R.A.B., Wallington, E.A., 1980. Carelton's histological technique, fifth ed. OxfordUniversity Press, London, pp. 199–220.

Dunn, E.G., Bowes, D.N., Rothert, S.W., Greer, R.B. III, 1974. An inexpensive X-ray source for the microradiography of bone. Calcified Tissue Research 15, 329.

Eurell, J., Sterchi, D.L., 1994. Microwaveable toluidine blue stain for surface staining of undecalcified bone sections. Journal of Histotechnology 17 (4), 357–359.

Evans, N., Krajian, A., 1930. A new method of decalcification. Archives of Pathology 10, 447.

Fornasier, V.L., 1975. Fine detail radiography in the examination of tissue. Human Pathology 6 (5), 623–631.

Frost, H.M., 1983a. Choice of marking agent and labelling schedule. In: Recker, R.R. (Ed.), Bone histomorphometry: techniques and interpretation. CRC Press, Florida, pp. 37–52.

Frost, H.M., 1983b. Bone histomorphometry: analysis of trabecular bone dynamics. In: Recker, R.R. (Ed.), Bone histomorphometry: techniques and interpretation. CRC Press, Florida, pp. 109–132.

Gatenby, J.B., Painter, T., 1934. In: The microtomist's Vade Mecum, tenth ed. Churchill, London, p. 427.

Goldner, J., 1937. A modification of the Masson trichrome technique for routine laboratory purposes. American Journal of Clinical Pathology 20, 237–243.

Gooding, H., Stewart, D., 1932. A comparative study of histological preparations of bone which have been treated with different combinations of fixatives and decalcifying fluids. Laboratory Journal 7, 55.

Gray, P., 1954. The microtomist's formulary and guide. Constable, London, pp. 256–260.

Hand, N.M., Church, R.J., 1998. Superheating using pressure cooking: its use and application in unmasking antigens embedded in methyl methacrylate. Journal of Histotechnology 21 (3), 233.

Hardt, A.B., 1986. Modification of the tape transfer technique: reduced shattering and distortion of hard tissue sections. Journal of Histotechnology 13 (3), 125–126.

Hillemann, H.H., Lee, C.H., 1953. Organic chelating agents for decalcification of bone and teeth. Stain Technology 28, 285.

Hsieh, J., 2003. Computed tomography: principles, design, artifacts, and recent advances, SPIE Press, Bellingham, WA.

Huffer, W.E., Zhu, J.M., Ruegg, P., 1996. Modified acidic solochrome azurine stain for video image analysis of aluminum lines in bone biopsies. Journal of Histotechnology 19 (2), 115–119.

Hughesdon, P.E., 1949. Two uses of uranyl nitrate. Journal of the Royal Microscopical Society 69, 1.

Hyman, J.M., Poulding, R.H., 1961. Solochrome cyanin-iron alum for rapid staining of frozen sections. Journal of Medical Laboratory Technology 18, 107.

Irwin, D.A., 1955. The demonstration of aluminum in human tissues. American Medical Association Archives of Industrial Health 12, 218–220.

Jee, W.S.S., Parfitt, A.M. (Eds.), 1980. Bone histomorphometry, 3rd International Workshop. Metabolic Bone Disease and Related Research 2 (Suppl).

Johnson, J.T., Hansen, M.S., Wu, I., et al., 2006. Virtual histology of transgenic mouse embryos for high-throughput phenotyping. PLoS Genetics 2 (4), 471–477.

Kristensen, H.K., 1948. An improved method of decalcification. Stain Technology 23, 151.

Maloney, N.A., Ott, S.M., Alfrey, A.C., et al., 1982. Histological quantification of aluminium in iliac bone from patients with renal failure. Journal of Laboratory and Clinical Medicine 99, 206–216.

Matrajt, H., Hioco, D., 1966. Solochrome cyanine R as an indicator dye of bone morphology. Stain Technology 41, 97.

Mawhinney, W.H., Richardson, E., Malcolm, A.J., 1984. Control of rapid nitric acid decalcification. Journal of Clinical Pathology 37, 1409–1415.

Melsen, F., Mosekilde, L., Kragstrup, J., 1983. Metabolic bone diseases as evaluated by bone histomorphometry. In: Recker, R.R. (Ed.), Bone histomorphometry: techniques and interpretation. CRC Press, Florida, pp. 265–285.

Milch, R.A., Rall, D.P., Tobie, J.E., 1957. Bone localization of the tetracyclines. Journal of the National Cancer Institute 19, 87.

Milch, R.A., Rall, D.P., Tobie, J.E., 1958. Fluorescence of tetracycline antibiotics in bone. Journal of Bone and Joint Surgery 40A, 897.

Parfitt, A.M., 1988. Bone histomorphometry: standardization of nomenclature, symbols and units (summary of proposed system). Bone 99, 67–69.

Parfitt, A.M., Drezner, M.K., Glorieux, F.H., et al., 1987. Bone histomorphometry: standardization of nomenclature, symbols, and units. Journal of Bone and Mineral Research 2, 595–610.

Perenyi, J., 1882. Übereineneue Erhärtungsflussigkeit. Zoologischer Anzeiger 5, 459.

Recker, R.R., 1983. Bone histomorphometry: techniques and interpretation. CRC Press, Florida.

Recker, R.R., 1990. Bone biopsy and histomorphometry in clinical practice. In: Clinical evaluation of bone and mineral disorders, primer on the metabolic diseases and disorder of mineral metabolism, first ed. American Society for Bone and Mineral Research, William Byrd Press, Virginia, pp. 101–104.

Revell, P., 1986. Quantitative methods in bone biopsy examination. In: Pathology of bone. Springer, Heidelberg.

Rosen, A.D., 1981. End-point determination in EDTA decalcification using ammonium oxalate. Stain Technology 56, 48–49.

Rosenberg, L., 1971. Chemical basis for the histological use of safranin O in the study of articular cartilage. Journal of Bone and Joint Surgery 53A, 69–82.

Russell, N.L., 1963. A rapid method for decalcification of bone for histological examination using the 'Histette'. Journal of Medical Laboratory Technology 20, 299.

Sanderson, C., 1997. Entering the realm of mineralized bone processing: a review of the literature and techniques. Journal of Histotechnology 20 (3), 259–266.

Sanderson, C., Radley, K., Mayton, L., 1995. Ethylenediaminetetraacetic acid in ammonium hydroxide for reducing decalcification time. Biotechnics and Histochemistry 70, 18.

Schenk, R.K., Olah, A.J., Herrmann, W., 1984. Preparation of calcified tissues for light microscopy. In: Dickson, G. (Ed.), Methods of calcified tissue preparation. Elsevier, Amsterdam, pp. 1–56.

Schiller, B., 1999. A cost-effective system for paraffin-quality frozen sections. American Clinical Laboratory 18, 8.

Schmorl, G., 1934. Die Pathologisch-Histologisch en Untersuchungsmethoden. Vogel, Berlin, p. 259.

Scott, J.E., Dorling, J., 1965. Differential staining of acid glycosaminoglycans (mucopolysaccharides) by Alcian Blue in salt solutions. Histochemie 5, 221.

Smith, A., 1962. The use of frozen sections in oral histology Part I. Journal of Medical Laboratory Technology 19, 26.

Steedman, H.F., 1960. Section cutting in microscopy. Blackwell, Oxford.

Sterchi, D.L., 1996. Kodak methylmethacrylate replacement (Letter). Journal of Histotechnology 19 (1), 88.

Taylor, R.L., Flechtenmacher, J., Dedrick, D.K., 1993. Variation of the Holmes method for histologic staining of bone canaliculi. Journal of Histotechnology 16 (4), 355–357.

Tornero, G., Latta, L.L., Godoy, G., 1991. Use of microwave radiation for the histological study of bone canaliculi. Journal of Histotechnology 14 (1), 27–30.

Tripp, E.J., Mackay, E.H., 1972. Silver staining of bone prior to decalcification for quantitative determination of osteoid in sections. Stain Technology 47, 129.

von Kossa, J., 1901. Nachweis von Kalk. Beitrage zur pathologischen Anatomie und zur allgemeinen. Pathologie 29, 163.

Wallington, E.A., 1972. Histological methods for bone. Butterworths, London.

Woodruff, L.A., Norris, W.P., 1955. Sectioning of undecalcified bone with special reference to radiautographic applications. Stain Technology 30, 174.

Further reading

Chappard, D., Blouin, S., Libouban, H., et al., 2005. Microcomputed tomography of hard tissues and bone biomaterials. Microscopy and Analysis 19 (3), 23–25(AM).

Chevrier, A., Rossomacha, E., Buschmann, M.D., Hoemann, C.D., 2005. Optimization of histoprocessing methods to detect glycosaminoglycan, collagen Type II and collagen Type I in decalcified rabbit osteochondral sections. Journal of Histotechnology 28 (3), 165–175.

Dotti, L.B., Paparo, G.B., Clarke, B.E., 1951. The use of ion exchange resin in decalcification of bone. American Journal of Clinical Pathology 21, 475.

Fornasier, V.L., Ho, C.L., 2003. Radiological examination of calcified tissues with emphasis on bone. In: An, Y.H., Martin, K.L. (Eds.), Handbook of histology methods for bone and cartilage. Humana, Totowana, NJ, pp. 531–535.

Frost, H.M., 1976. Histomorphometry of trabecular bone 1. Theoretical correction of appositional rate measurements. In: Meunier, P.J. (Ed.), Bone histomorphometry, second international workshop. Société de la Nouvelle Imprimerie Fournie, Toulouse, pp. 361–370.

Mawhinney, W.H., Richardson, E., Malcolm, A.J., 1984. Control of rapid nitric acid decalcification. Journal of Clinical Pathology 37, 1409–1415.

Rittman, B.R.J., 2000. Teeth and their associated tissues. Microscopy Today 00–1, 18–20.

Sobel, A.E., Hanok, A., 1951. Rapid method for determination of ultramicro quantities of calcium and magnesium. Archives of Pathology 44, 92–95.

SudhakerRao, D., 1983. Practical approach to obtaining a bone biopsy. In: Recker, R.R. (Ed.), Bone histomorphometry: techniques and interpretation. CRC Press, Florida, pp. 3–11.

Thomas, C.B., Jenkins, L., Kellen, J.F., Burg, J.L., 2003. Endpoint verification of bone demineralization for tissue engineering applications. Tissue Engineered Medical Products (TEMPs), ASTM STP 1452, Picciolo, G.L.

Villanueva, A.R., 1980. Bone, Part II. Basic preparation and staining in decalcified bone. In: Sheehan, D.C., Hrapchak, B.B. (Eds.), Theory and practice of histotechnology. C.V. Mosby, London, pp. 96–98.

Techniques in neuropathology 17

J. Robin Highley • Nicky Sullivan

Introduction

Neuropathology has classically been seen as something of a dark art by general histologists because of the tradition of using a large number of obscure and often capricious stains. However, with the ascendancy of molecular pathology, many of the more unreliable stains are being replaced by immunohistochemistry. As such, many of the preparations that have been described in previous editions of this volume have been omitted from this chapter as they are no longer in use. Nonetheless, a number of reliable and useful tinctorial and metal-based stains remain in common usage. These are described in this chapter together with some preparations that are still employed, albeit less frequently. Finally, in neuropathology as in most other areas of histological practice, hematoxylin and eosin (H&E) remains the most useful and commonly used stain, as it demonstrates most cell types well and with good detail.

The components of the normal nervous system

The nervous system can be subdivided into the central, peripheral and autonomic nervous systems. This chapter will concern itself principally with the central nervous system and secondarily with the peripheral nervous systems. The principal components of the central nervous system are:

- Neurons
- Glial cells
- Meninges
- Blood vessels

The neuron is an excitable cell that is responsible for processing and transmitting information. Neurons communicate with each other via intercellular interfaces called synapses. At the synapse, an electrical impulse in the presynaptic neuron causes it to release a chemical transmitter that diffuses across a narrow gap to influence the electrical activity of the postsynaptic target neuron. Neurons have several components (Fig. 17.1):

- The cell body (or 'soma'), which contains various subcellular organelles responsible for the metabolic upkeep of the cell.
- The axon, an elongated fibrous process that transmits electrical impulses away from the soma to synapses with either other neurons or muscle fibers. This may be a meter or more in length in the case of the lower motor neurons that reside in the lower (lumbar) spinal cord and innervate muscles of the lower leg.
- The dendritic tree, a plexus of cell process responsible for receiving synaptic inputs from other neurons.
- The nucleus, which resides in the cell body and is the site of storage of the cell's genetic code in DNA.

Two naturally occurring pigments may be observed to accumulate in the brain with age: lipofuscin and neuromelanin. Both are generally believed to represent cellular waste products. Lipofuscin is a yellow-brown, autoflourescent, granular substance composed of peroxidized protein and

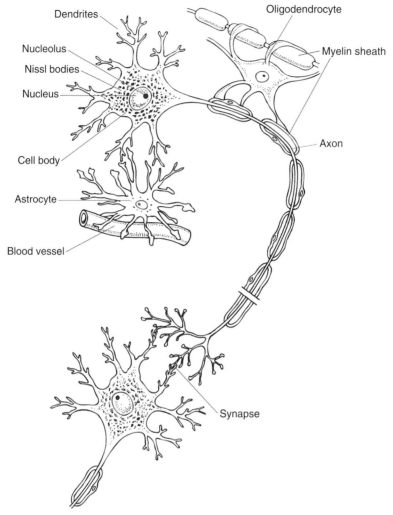

Figure 17.1 Diagram showing a neuron with its component parts together with other cells of the central nervous system. (Courtesy of Patrick Elliott of the Medical Illustration Department, Royal Hallamshire Hospital, Sheffield, UK.)

lipids. It is seen in larger neurons, such as the lower motor neurons of the spinal cord and pyramidal cells of the hippocampus in the context of Alzheimer pathology. Large amounts of lipofuscin-like pigment accumulate in the context of inherited neuronal ceroid lipofuscinoses, of which Batten's disease is the most common (Goebel & Wisniewski 2004). Neuromelanin is most commonly seen in the cytoplasm of neurons of the substantia nigra and the locus ceruleus. It is the cause of the macroscopic pigmentation of these structures. Under the microscope, it is a dark brown, granular material that is believed to be the by-product of

oxidative metabolism of catecholamines (Sulzer et al. 2008).

Glial cells are the support cells of the nervous system. They are diverse in nature, the principal types being:

• Astrocytes, which have a number of functions. They maintain the extracellular ion and neurotransmitter balance. They are involved in repair and scarring responses to brain damage and also form part of the blood–brain barrier, which protects the brain from harmful blood-borne substances.

- Oligodendroglia, which form myelin, a phospholipid sheath around nerve axons that enhances the speed of conduction of impulses.
- Ependymal cells, which line the ventricles of the brain and central canal of the spinal cord.

Neuropil is a term used to denote the feltwork of neuronal processes in which neuron cell bodies reside. Central nervous system tissue is classically subdivided into gray matter, which contains the majority of neuronal cell bodies and little myelin, and white matter, which is predominantly formed of myelinated axons and few neurons.

The meninges form three layers of protective covering over the brain. The outer layer, beneath the skull, is formed by the dura mater. It is a tough, fibrous membrane. The arachnoid mater is a more delicate, fibrillary covering that lies inside the dura mater and is more closely adherent to the brain surface, but it does not invaginate into the surface infoldings of the brain (or sulci). The pia mater is the most delicate covering. It is closely apposed to the brain surface, following its contours down into the depths of sulci.

Techniques for staining neurons

Tinctorial stains for Nissl substance

Hematoxylin and eosin (H&E) preparations demonstrate most important features of neurons. However, Nissl preparations are also popular for examining the basic architecture of neural tissue and its components. These are often combined with the luxol fast blue myelin stain. Granules of Nissl substance are found in the cell body (Fig. 17.1) and correspond to rough endoplasmic reticulum. They are basophilic due to the associated nucleic acid (Palay & Palade 1955). Many basic dyes (e.g. neutral red, methylene blue, azur, pyronin, thionin, toluidine blue and cresyl fast violet) stain Nissl substance. Variation in the stain used, pH and degree of differentiation allow preparations to label either Nissl substance alone, or Nissl substance in combination with cell nuclei.

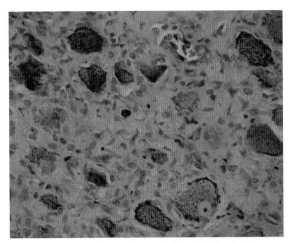

Figure 17.2 Anterior horn cells in spinal cord. Notice their large size and the prominent nucleolus. Paraffin section, stained with toluidine blue. Similar results can be obtained with cresyl fast violet.

Motor neurons generally have very coarse ('tigroid') Nissl substance, and regions such as the anterior horns of the spinal cord, where these cells are abundant, are good tissues to use when learning these stains (Fig. 17.2). For paraffin-embedded sections of formalin-fixed tissue, the cresyl fast violet stain is reliable and relatively straightforward. As such it is by far the most commonly used Nissl preparation. Toluidine blue may also be used, whilst Einarson's gallocyanin method, being more suited to alcohol-fixed tissue, is largely unused (Kellett 1963).

Cresyl fast violet (Nissl) stain for paraffin sections	
Fixation	
Alcohol, Carnoy's or formalin.	
Sections	
Paraffin 7–10 μm or 25 μm (see Note b).	
Preparation of stain	
Cresyl fast violet	0.5 g
Distilled water	100 ml
Differentiation solution	
Glacial acetic acid	250 μl
Alcohol	100 ml

Method

1. Dewax sections and bring to water.
2. Cover with filtered cresyl fast violet; stain for 10–20 minutes.
3. Rinse briefly in distilled water.
4. Differentiate in 0.25% acetic alcohol until most of the stain has been removed (4–8 seconds).
5. Briefly pass through absolute alcohol into xylene and check microscopically.
6. Repeat steps 4 and 5 if necessary, giving less differentiation when repeating.
7. Rinse well in xylene and mount in Canada balsam or DPX.

Results

Nissl substance	purple-dark blue
Neurons	pale purple-blue
Cell nuclei	purple blue

Notes

a. If only Nissl substance is required to be demonstrated, the stain is acidified with 0.25% acetic acid.
b. Estimation of cortical neuronal density is made on 25 μm thick sections.
c. The cresyl violet method can be used as a counterstain when demonstrating myelin with the Kluver and Barrera method (see below).

Immunohistochemistry of neurons

The protein targets of antibodies used in immuno-histochemical preparations for the demonstration of neuronal elements can be classified into four main groups:

1. **Neuronal cytoskeletal proteins.** *Neurofilaments (NF)* are intermediate filaments specifically expressed by mature neurons. They are composed of protein subunits that are classified by molecular weight into NF-L, NF-M, and NF-H which may be variably phosphorylated (Gotow 2000). Antisera raised against different neurofilament proteins in different states of phosphorylation are available. NF-H, in particular, and NF-M, to a lesser extent, are normally unphosphorylated in the neuronal cell body, but become phosphorylated in the axons. Thus, antibodies to phosphorylated NF-H mark axons but not cell bodies in normal nervous system tissues. Antibodies to non-phosphorylated neurofilament will label neuronal somata (Trojanowski et al. 1986). *Microtubule-associated protein 2 (MAP-2)* is a protein involved with microtubule assembly and is expressed by neurons in dendrites and cell bodies (Maccioni & Cambiazo 1995; Shafit-Zagardo & Kalcheva 1998). It is therefore often used to as a marker of neuroepithelial differentiation (Wharton et al. 2002; Blumcke et al. 2004).

2. **Cytoplasmic proteins.** *PGP9.5* and *neuron-specific enolase (NSE)* are strongly expressed in neurons and can be reliably labeled by commercially available antisera. Unfortunately, they are not specific for neuronal cells, making interpretation tricky. They are best used in the context of a broad antibody panel (Ghobrial & Ross 1986; Wilson et al. 1988).

3. **Neuronal nuclear proteins.** *NeuN* is a neuron-specific DNA binding protein, which starts to be expressed around the time of initiation of terminal differentiation of the neuron (Mullen et al. 1992). Antibodies to NeuN therefore label neuronal nuclei, and neuronal components of other tumors (Edgar & Rosenblum 2008). However, in the context of neuro-oncology, it lacks specificity, being expressed to a variable degree in a diverse range of primary brain tumors. Therefore, NeuN is best used as part of a panel of antibodies in the investigation of clear cell primary brain tumors, but is of limited utility for other tumors (Preusser et al. 2006).

4. **Proteins associated with neurosecretory granules.** Antisera to these proteins can be useful to establish neuronal and neuroendocrine differentiation (Koperek et al. 2004; Takei et al. 2007). *Synaptophysin* is a membrane glycoprotein component of presynaptic neurosecretory vesicles. The cell body of normal neurons is usually unstained by synaptophysin (Fig. 17.3), resulting in early

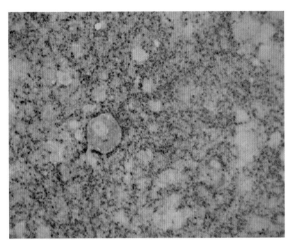

Figure 17.3 Large neuron from an area of cortical dysplasia stained with synaptophysin. Note intense staining within the neuropil and weak cytoplasmic staining.

claims that cell body labeling was a feature of neoplastic neuronal cells that differentiated them from native neurons (Miller et al. 1990). However, it is now evident that a population of normal neurons also show cell body labeling which detracts from the use of this feature as a diagnostic marker (Quinn 1998). Synaptophysin is a useful marker of neuroendocrine differentiation and so also stains cells in metastatic neuroendocrine tumors (Wiedenmann et al. 1987). *Chromogranin A* is a protein of the dense core matrix of neurosecretory granules, and antibodies to it can be used to identify cells containing dense core vesicles (Nolan et al. 1985). It is therefore used predominantly to elucidate neuroendocrine differentiation in tumors.

Techniques for staining axons and neuronal processes

The annals of neurohistology describe several methods to demonstrate various special structures of the neuron, including axons (viable and degenerate), dendrites, synapses, dendritic trees and peripheral nerve endings. Many of these were block impregnation and free-floating frozen section methods and are rarely performed in time-constrained modern diagnostic laboratories. Immunohistochemistry has largely replaced the old silver preparations for the demonstration of axons as it is reliable and produces adequate results for diagnostic neuropathology with ease. However, for formal quantitation of axons, many still find that Palmgren's method is superior to neurofilament immunohistochemistry (Chance et al. 1999). This technique has classically been used for staining axons of the peripheral nervous system. However, it is also an excellent preparation for staining central nervous system axons as well. Palmgren's method uses potassium nitrate to suppress staining of reticulin. It is considered that with the Palmgren method, cresyl violet preparations and immunohistochemistry for neurofilament and MAP-2, there is no longer requirement for older silver preparations such as that of Bielschowsky (Bielschowsky 1902) and Marsland (Marsland et al. 1954).

Silver techniques, such as the Palmgren method, require great care and attention to detail such as clean glassware and pure distilled water for a successful outcome. Stock solutions should be well maintained and not more than a few months old (in some cases less than a week).

Modified Palmgren's method for nerve fibers in paraffin-embedded material *(Palmgren 1948)*

Fixation
Formalin fixed tissue.

Sections
Paraffin sections 6–10 µm. Sections should be on coated slides.

Preparation of solutions
Acid formalin

Concentrated formaldehyde (40% w/v)	25 ml
Distilled water	75 ml
1% nitric acid	0.2 ml

Silver solution

30% silver nitrate	25 ml
20% potassium nitrate	25 ml
5% glycine	0.5 ml

Reducer

Pyrogallol	10 g
Distilled water	450 ml
Absolute ethanol	550 ml
1% nitric acid	2 ml

Fixing bath

5% sodium thiosulfate.

Method

1. Take sections to distilled water.
2. Treat sections with acid formalin for 5 minutes.
3. Wash in three changes of distilled water for 5 minutes.
4. Leave in filtered silver solution for 15 minutes at room temperature.
5. Without rinsing, drain the slide and flood the section with reducer that has been heated to 40–45°C. Rock the slide gently and add fresh reducer. Leave for 1 minutes. A beaker placed on a hot plate is useful for this stage.
6. Wash in three changes of distilled water. Examine microscopically and, if necessary, repeat from step 4, reducing the time in the silver solution and decreasing the temperature of the reducer to 30°C.
7. Wash in distilled water.
8. Fix in 5% sodium thiosulfate, 5 minutes.
9. Wash in tap water.
10. Dehydrate in alcohol. Clear and mount in DPX.

Result

Nerve fibers	brown or black

Notes

In the original method the silver solution contained 5% acetic acid rather than 5% glycine.

The only proviso when using glycine is that it must be made up fresh prior to use; as it is only stable for approximately one week. However the Palmgren silver, once made up, is stable for several weeks.

The silver incubation time may need to be increased for tissues which have had a short formalin fixation time, but as a rule of thumb you should see a slight yellow tinge to the tissues when the optimum time has been reached. The reducer keeps for several months.

The original method stated that it had to stand for 24 hours before use, but this is not the case. The reducer will darken with time, changing from pale yellow to dark amber. It is important that at the reduction step the slides are gently agitated to ensure an even reduction of the tissue; if the sections are not dark enough, they can be rinsed in distilled water and steps 4–6 repeated but with a shorter time in the silver solution.

The hotter the reducer, the faster the reduction will take place and it may well be uneven, leading to suboptimal preparations. Sections can be toned using gold chloride prior to fixing, which is an optional step.

The original method used an intensifying step prior to fixing: this employs aniline. Some have found this to be of little value. The method was originally designed for use with paraffin sections. However, it can be applied to cryostat sections which have been pretreated with 20% chloral hydrate overnight prior to carrying out the Palmgren method.

Examination of axons in peripheral nerve in diagnostic neuropathology now relies largely on toluidine blue-stained semi-thin resin-embedded tissue. Capricious techniques such as Eager's method for detecting degenerating axons are no longer in use (Eager et al. 1971).

The Golgi preparation and its variants are excellent for the visualization of the three-dimensional nature of the neuron and its dendritic processes. However, modern diagnostic neuropathology practice has no requirement for this. Golgi techniques are occasionally used in research (e.g. Garey 2010) although new antisera are increasingly allowing immunohistochemical indices of these aspects of cell morphology. It is suggested that the interested reader consider the Pugh and Rossi modification for use on paraffin-embedded tissue (Pugh & Rossi 1993) if a Golgi stain is to be attempted.

Myelin

Myelin forms an electrically insulating sheath around axons. It is approximately 80% lipid and 20% protein and is formed from sheet-like processes of glial cells that are concentrically wrapped multiple times around the axon. This greatly improves the speed and efficiency of impulse conduction along the axon. Myelin is formed by oligodendrocytes in the central nervous system and Schwann cells in the peripheral nervous system. A single oligodendrocyte may myelinate multiple axons in its vicinity, whereas a single Schwann cell may only myelinate a single segment of a single axon. Loss of myelin (as is seen in multiple sclerosis in the central nervous system or Guillain-Barré in the peripheral nervous system) can be severely debilitating.

Modern tinctorial stains for myelin are simple and reliable and can be performed on formalin-fixed paraffin-processed tissue. Many can be combined with a Nissl stain to demonstrate neuronal localization. Older methods may give more even and consistent staining, but are considerably more time consuming and have fallen from use (Weigert 1904; Loyez 1910; Weil 1928). Both luxol fast blue and solochrome cyanine preparations are now favored.

Luxol fast blue is a copper phthalocyanine dye which is employed in myelin staining of paraffin-processed tissue (Kluver & Barrera 1953). This can be combined with cresyl violet or hematoxylin to outline cellular architecture (Fig. 17.4) or with periodic acid-Schiff (PAS) to demonstrate myelin degradation products in demyelinating disease. It can be used on central nervous system tissue only.

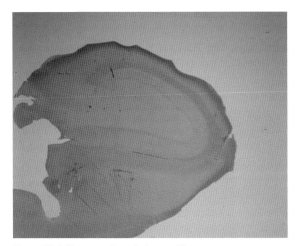

Figure 17.4 Macro section of a human hippocampus demonstrating geographical variation in myelin content. Luxol fast blue.

Luxol fast blue stain for myelin with cresyl violet counterstain (Kluver & Barrera 1953)

Fixation
Formalin.

Sections
Paraffin, 10–15 μm.

Preparation of solutions
Luxol fast blue

Luxol fast blue	1 g
Methanol (absolute)	1000 ml
10% acetic acid	5 ml

Mix reagents and filter.

Cresyl violet stock solution
Cresyl violet	0.5 g
Distilled water	100 ml

Acidified cresyl violet solution
Add 0.8 ml of 10% acetic acid to 100 ml of stock cresyl violet solution and filter before use.

Method
1. Take sections on slides to 95% alcohol (*not* water).
2. Stain in luxol fast blue solution, 2 hours at 60°C, or 37°C overnight.
3. Wash in 70% alcohol.
4. Wash in tap water.
5. Differentiate in 0.1% lithium carbonate solution until the gray and white matter are distinguished. This may be more easily controlled by using 0.05% lithium carbonate followed by 70–95% alcohol instead.
6. Wash in tap water.
7. Check differentiation under the microscope. Repeat step 5 if necessary.
8. Stain in cresyl violet solution, 10–20 minutes.
9. Drain sections and transfer to 70% alcohol. Avoid placing the section in water at this stage as the cresyl violet staining loses some of its intensity. Gently agitate the sections; the cresyl violet dye will flood out. The 70% alcohol differentiates the cresyl violet stain. Optimally, the cresyl violet should be removed, leaving the cell bodies and Nissl clearly visible. Do not over-differentiate; the 70% alcohol will take out the cresyl violet and to a certain extent the luxol fast blue. The cresyl violet counterstain will deepen the color of the luxol fast

blue stained myelin from turquoise to a deep blue.

10. Dehydrate, clear in xylene, and mount in DPX.

Result

Myelin	blue
Cells	violet-pink

Notes

a. If the section is over-differentiated with lithium carbonate/alcohol, the section can be restained with the luxol fast blue and then differentiated to obtain the optimum staining result. This may apply to tissues which have very low amounts of myelin (e.g. baby/neonatal brains). These tissues can be very challenging in achieving optimum staining. Unfortunately, once the cresyl violet counterstain has been applied the over-differentiation cannot be rectified.

b. Some histologists prefer to differentiate the cresyl violet using 0.25% acetic acid in 100% alcohol.

c. The use of thick sections is important for the visualization of myelin tracts.

d. Other counterstains may be used such as neutral red. This will result in the myelin appearing purple/blue due to a slightly different color balance, and is a matter of personal preference.

The solochrome cyanine stain is a simple and rapid technique for demonstration of myelin in both the central and peripheral nervous systems.

Page's solochrome cyanine technique for myelin in paraffin sections

Fixation
Formalin.

Sections
Paraffin, 6–10 μm. Cryostat section, 10 μm.

Preparation of solution

Solochrome cyanine RS	0.2 g
Distilled water	96 ml
10% iron alum	4 ml
Concentrated sulfuric acid	0.5 ml

Method

1. Take sections to water.
2. Stain for 10–20 minutes at room temperature.
3. Wash in running water.

4. Differentiate in 5% iron alum until all the nuclei are unstained. Wash frequently in distilled water, and examine microscopically.
5. Wash in running tap water.
6. Counterstain if desired.
7. Dehydrate, clear, and mount.

Result

Myelin sheaths	blue

Notes

a. The staining solution keeps well.

b. Neutral red, Neutral fast red, Piero-Ponceau S, or van Gieson can be used for counterstaining.

Immunohistochemistry for S-100 is useful in the diagnosis of tumors derived from Schwann cells both in the central nervous system and peripherally (Hirose et al. 1986; Winek et al. 1989). Many antisera are used as markers of myelination, the most useful being myelin basic protein and myelin associated glycoprotein (Itoyama et al. 1980a, 1980b; Ludwin & Sternberger 1984; Lindner et al. 2008). However, given the reliability and simplicity of the tinctorial stains, immunohistochemical myelin makers are largely unused in routine diagnostic neuropathology and remain the preserve of research laboratories.

Myelin loss may occur in a region of brain damaged by any of a number of processes such as trauma, neoplasia, multiple sclerosis or toxic insult. It may also occur secondary to the loss of axons emanating from a lesioned brain region. In modern practice, degeneration of myelinated tracts is most commonly demonstrated by showing loss of normal myelin staining by either luxol fast blue or solochrome cyanine preparations, or by showing a microglial reaction using CD68 immunohistochemistry (e.g., Ince et al. 2008). Historically, the Marchi technique (Swank & Davenport 1935) and neutral lipid stains have been used to detect early and late myelin degeneration products, respectively. However, the Marchi technique requires block staining or free-floating sections and lipid stains cannot be performed on paraffin-embedded material. Given these issues, the sensitivity of CD68 immunohistochemistry and the ease of the tinctorial preparations for normal myelin (see above), the Marchi and neutral lipid techniques have been rendered obsolete.

The neuroglia

The term neuroglia refers to the supporting cells of the central nervous system and comprises ependymal cells, astrocytes, oligodendrocytes, and microglia. As is becoming a recurrent theme, immunohistochemistry is increasingly replacing tinctorial stains for their identification.

Ependymal cells

Ependymal cells are epithelioid and line the ventricles of the brain and the central canal of the spinal cord. They are easily located with conventional stains such as H&E and immunohistochemistry for GFAP, vimentin and S-100. Immunohistochemistry for epithelial membrane antigen (Uematsu et al. 1989; Hasselblatt & Paulus 2003) labels both normal and neoplastic ependymal cells, whilst cytokeratin markers are negative.

Astrocytes

Astrocytes have multiple, fine processes and (in their reactive state) are 'star-shaped' (hence the name). On standard H&E sections, only the nucleus of resting astrocytes is distinct, as the cell body cannot be discerned from background neuropil. These nuclei are slightly larger with more open granular chromatin than that of the more compact oligodendrocyte. Modern neuropathology relies most heavily on GFAP (Fig. 17.5) immunohistochemistry for demonstration of astrocytes, although antibodies to S-100, αB-crystallin and glutamine synthetase may also be used. Metal-based and tinctorial methods such as Cajal's gold sublimate, PTAH (Chan & Lowe 2002) and Holzer (1921) are no longer in use as these are variously more expensive, more technically demanding or less specific than their immunohistochemical equivalents.

Figure 17.5 Reactive astrocytes in white matter, stained by anti-GFAP immunohistochemistry technique with hematoxylin nuclear counterstain. Fine GFAP-containing processes form a felt-like mat in which the stellate cell bodies are evident.

Astrocytes are principally classified into protoplasmic and fibrous forms. These are similar in function. However, whereas protoplasmic astrocytes have shorter, thicker, highly branched processes and are generally found in the gray matter, fibrous astrocytes have longer, thinner, less-branched processes and usually reside in white matter. Astrocytic reactions in the cerebellum are characterized by Bergmann or radial astroglia which have processes that run radially from the Purkinje cell layer of the cortex to the pial surface.

In response to injury of the brain parenchyma, astrocytes react by increasing in size with a more prominent, eosinophilic cytoplasm. The nucleus moves from a central to a more eccentric position within the cell cytoplasm and processes become more prominent. Astrocytic gliosis is a response to permanent injury, whereby astrocytes proliferate to fill tissue defects with a fibrous glial scar.

In neuro-oncology, astrocytic differentiation is best demonstrated by GFAP immunohistochemistry. GFAP immunoreactivity is also seen in other tumors including ependymoma, oligodendroglial tumors and choroid plexus tumors (Eng & Rubinstein 1978; Velasco et al. 1980; Eng 1983; Doglioni et al. 1987). Astrocytic tumors also label with vimentin and

S-100, but these are also seen in many other tumor types, rendering them of little use for differential diagnosis. Astrocytes occasionally show cross-reactivity as seen for the pan cytokeratin AE1/AE3 (Cosgrove et al. 1989). Therefore, it is expedient to use other cytokeratin markers such as CAM5.2 or MNF116 to exclude the diagnosis of epithelial cell tumors, such as metastatic adenocarcinoma.

The proliferation marker Ki-67 (MIB-1) is often used in the assessment of surgical neuropathology specimens as an aid to grading tumors and to help differentiate reactive from neoplastic astrocytic populations. The latter will tend to have a higher number of nuclei labeled with this marker.

An emerging and potentially more powerful tool for the diagnosis of diffuse oligodendroglial and astrocytic neoplasms is the use of antibodies to isocitrate dehydrogenase 1 (*IDH1*) carrying the R132H mutation. This is the most frequent mutation in diffuse gliomas (Hartmann et al. 2009). There is an emerging literature that appears to demonstrate that antisera to this mutant protein may be used to differentiate reactive gliosis from grade II and III astrocytomas (Camelo-Piragua et al. 2010; Capper et al. 2010) and oligodendrogliomas from lesions with similar morphologic appearances (Capper et al. 2011).

Oligodendrocytes

Oligodendrocytes are glial cells that form the myelin of the central nervous system and are present in both gray and white matter. As noted above, a single oligodendrocyte may myelinate axons from multiple neurons. In H&E and cresyl violet preparations, oligodendrocytes have small (7 μm) round to oval nuclei with compact chromatin. The cytoplasm is indistinct from the surrounding neuropil although oligodendroglial tumors may show artifactual perinuclear halos in paraffin sections. Silver preparations to demonstrate oligodendroglia (Penfield 1928; Stern 1932) are rarely used, now replaced by immunohistochemistry to myelin basic protein and myelin associated glycoprotein label oligodendrocyte processes (see above).

However, these epitopes are not expressed by oligodendroglial tumors (Nakagawa et al. 1986). Olig2 is a transcription factor that regulates oligodendroglial development and is expressed by the nuclei of oligodendrocytes and oligodendroglial tumors (Yokoo et al. 2004). Sadly, it is not specific for oligodendrogliomas as it labels other morphologically similar tumors (Preusser et al. 2007) and is also expressed by astrocytomas (Ligon et al. 2004). A reliable immunohistochemical marker to distinguish oligodendroglioma from astrocytomas has not yet been found. Finally, deletion of chromosomes 1p and 19q (most commonly investigated by fluorescence *in situ* hybridization) is a well-recognized molecular feature of oligodendrogliomas and appears to be associated with a better prognosis and response to treatment (Bourne & Schiff 2010).

Microglia

Unlike other glial cells, microglia are mesodermal in origin. They are believed to be derived from blood-derived monocytes that move into the brain during embryonic development (Kim & de Vellis 2005). Microglia serve as the resident innate immune system and, under certain pathological conditions, may develop into full-blown macrophages. They are involved in most, if not all, known forms of CNS pathology (Graeber & Streit 2010). Microglia are most commonly subclassified into resting, activated and 'amoeboid' forms. Resting microglia are classically ramified in morphology, whilst activated microglia are rod-shaped and amoeboid are (as the name suggests) amoeboid.

A number of established immunohistochemical markers for microglia are available, including CD68 (PGM1), human alveolar macrophage (HAM)-56, class II major histocompatibility complex (MHC; particularly in inflammatory states) and HLA-DR-II antibodies. Although these do not label other glial cells, they do label infiltrating macrophages from the circulation. Non-immunohistochemical preparations, such as that of Penfield (Penfield 1928) and Weil and Davenport (Stern 1932) are not specific, and they are no longer used.

Neurodegeneration

Neurodegenerative conditions are largely diseases of old age. As the population ages, these conditions place an increasing burden on health and social care systems. This, together with the escalation in research into neurodegeneration in recent years, has resulted in an increasing workload on neuropathology units.

Sadly, it is often the case that a definitive diagnosis of any neurodegenerative condition cannot be made without autopsy. In most studies, the accuracy of clinical diagnosis of the cause of a dementing illness is in the order of 75%. An autopsy does not benefit the deceased, but does have wider benefits, namely:

- Neuropathological autopsies can yield data and tissue to assist research.
- Neuropathological autopsies provide epidemiological data, allowing the prevalence of different neurodegenerative diseases to be monitored.
- Autopsy findings are often of considerable educational benefit for both senior and junior clinicians as well as pathologists.
- An increasing number of neurodegenerative conditions are familial, often with known causative mutations. Accurate neuropathological characterization can therefore guide genetic counseling.

The pathological characterization of neurodegenerative disease is a staged process. The first step is removal of the brain, sometimes with the spinal cord in addition. These are examined fresh and samples may be taken and snap-frozen for studies that require unfixed tissue. The brain is then fixed in formalin, ideally by suspending it by the basilar artery in a large volume of formalin for three or more weeks. Other methods, such as simply allowing the brain to rest on the bottom of the formalin container result in unacceptable distortion. Following formalin fixation, the brain is examined macroscopically both intact and after slicing (usually coronally). Appropriate blocks of tissue are taken, processed and paraffin embedded for microscopy.

In the majority of cases, neuropathological assessment of neurodegeneration tends to broadly focus on dementing illnesses and motor degeneration and there is considerable overlap between the two. Investigations of dementia tend to uncover one, or a combination of, three types of pathology, namely: Alzheimer's disease; vascular dementia (multi-infarct dementia); or dementia with Lewy bodies. A small number of dementia cases show frontotemporal lobar degeneration. The neurodegenerative diseases of the motor system that are diagnosed at autopsy tend to focus on motor neuron disease (also known as amyotrophic lateral sclerosis) and conditions that cause Parkinsonian clinical features. Other neurodegenerative diseases of the motor system (e.g., Huntington disease, spinocerebellar ataxia and Friedreich's ataxia) tend to be diagnosed by genetic tests.

The microscopic examination of the brain for neurodegeneration is often an iterative process, whereby an initial examination is performed using fairly standard tinctorial preparations (most favor H&E). After this, more specialist preparations (usually immunohistochemistry) are performed (Lowe 1998).

Many neurodegenerative diseases are characterized by accumulations (or inclusions) of protein, for the majority of which there are now commercially available antisera. These diseases are thus often classified by the particular protein that forms the pathological aggregates that characterize the disorders. These categories are: the tauopathies (e.g. Alzheimer's disease, Pick's disease, supranuclear palsy, corticobasal degeneration and argyrophilic grain disease), the synucleinopathies (Parkinson's disease, dementia with Lewy bodies and multiple system atrophy), prion disorders and TDP-43 proteinopathies (motor neuron disease, frontotemporal lobar degeneration with TDP-43). These inclusions are detailed in Table 17.1.

Ubiquitin is a small regulatory protein that binds misfolded or other aberrant proteins, and labels them for destruction by the proteasome. Many dementing illnesses are characterized by accumulations of ubiquitylated protein; the location and form of these accumulations can provide valuable

Table 17.1 Inclusion body immunostaining

Inclusion	Disease	Immunohistochemistry
Neurofibrillary tangle (Fig. 17.6a, b)	Alzheimer's disease	Tau protein, ubiquitin/p62
Lewy body (Fig. 17.7a)	Parkinson's disease	α-Synuclein, ubiquitin/p62
Cortical Lewy body (Fig. 17.7b)	Dementia with Lewy bodies	α-Synuclein, ubiquitin/p62
Motor neuron disease/FTLD inclusion (Fig. 17.8)	Motor neuron disease, some forms of FTLD	Ubiquitin/p62, TDP-43
Glial cytoplasmic inclusion	Multiple system atrophy	α-Synuclein, ubiquitin, p62
Glial cytoplasmic inclusion	Progressive supranuclear palsy Corticobasal degeneration	tau, ubiquitin/p62
Pick body	Pick's disease	Tau protein, ubiquitin/p62

diagnostic clues. Therefore, immunohistochemistry for ubiquitylated proteins is often a useful early step in neuropathological diagnosis. For this, we favor antibodies to p62. This protein binds ubiquitylated proteins and shuttles them to the proteasome (Wooten et al. 2006). Antibodies to p62 can be used to label pathological, ubiquitylated aggregates of tau, α-synuclein and TDP-43 (Kuusisto et al. 2008). Further, p62 immunohistochemistry has greater specificity for pathological aggregates than ubiquitin immunohistochemistry, leaving non-pathological features unlabeled.

As noted above, autopsies in neurodegeneration principally concern dementia and motor system degenerative diseases, many of which overlap. Of the dementing illnesses, the vast majority are diagnosed as Alzheimer's disease, vascular dementia, dementia with Lewy bodies and frontotemporal lobar degeneration. However, given the considerable public health concerns surrounding prion diseases, cases will also occasionally be assessed for consideration of this diagnosis.

Alzheimer's disease is characterized by ubiquitylated accumulations of tau and β-amyloid. Hyperphosphorylated tau forms flame-shaped neuronal intracytoplasmic inclusions known as neurofibrillary tangles and neuritic fibrillary deposits known as neuropil threads. β-Amyloid is formed from aggregates of peptides generated by the cleavage of amyloid precursor protein (a membrane-associated protein of unknown function) by β- and γ-secretases. Deposits of β-amyloid become surrounded by dilated and distorted neuronal processes to form senile plaques. Senile plaques and neurofibrillary tangles are the histological hallmarks of Alzheimer's disease (Figs 17.6 and 17.9).

Vascular dementia is an umbrella term for a variety of conditions characterized either by multiple large or small regions of infarction throughout the brain, or by smaller numbers of infarcts in functionally important structures such as the thalamus or hippocampus (Jellinger 2008). The picture is somewhat complicated by the fact that many cases with a heavy burden of vascular pathology will additionally have a coexistent burden of Alzheimer- or Lewy body-type pathology.

Dementia with Lewy bodies is characterized by neocortical and limbic neuronal cytoplasmic inclusions of α-synuclein – the Lewy bodies that give this condition the name. Lewy bodies were first described in Parkinson disease, where they are visible as round, intensely eosinophilic, hyaline intracytoplasmic neuronal inclusions in the substantia nigra and locus ceruleus of the midbrain and brainstem. They are composed of ubiquitylated α-synuclein and can therefore be detected by immunohistochemistry for

that in order to provide a full diagnostic service a laboratory should have access to optimized immunohistochemistry for hyperphosphorylated tau, β-amyloid, α-synuclein, p62 or ubiquitin (ideally the former), TDP-43, neurofilament and protease-resistant prion protein.

Stains for detection of the changes of Alzheimer's disease

As noted above, the two types of Alzheimer-type pathology are (1) features associated with hyperphosphorylated tau (principally neurofibrillary tangles and neuropil threads) and (2) features associated with β-amyloid (principally neuritic plaques and congophilic amyloid angiopathy). The tinctorial stains and immunohistochemical preparations used in the characterization of Alzheimer-type pathology reflect this dichotomy:

* Classically, Cross-modified Palmgren (Cross 1982) and the Gallyas technique (Gallyas 1971) have been used to demonstrate neurofibrillary tangles as well as the neuritic pathology associated with neuritic plaques. These have largely been replaced by immunohistochemistry for hyperphosphorylated tau (Fig. 17.6b).
* β-amyloid has historically been demonstrated by methenamine silver (which will also stain a minority of tangles; Fig. 17.9a) and thioflavine S. These have been replaced by immunohistochemistry after formic acid pretreatment (e.g. BA4; Fig. 17.9b).
* Some preparations can be used to detect both forms of pathology, although these tend to be less sensitive than those preparations that focus on one pathology. Thus, the modified Bielschowsky technique underestimates the β-amyloid pathology load (Lamy et al. 1989).

Guidelines for the dissection and staining of specimens in order to accurately characterize Alzheimer-type pathology have been laid down (Mirra et al. 1993; Alafuzoff et al. 2008; Alafuzoff et al. 2009).

Gallyas method for Tau pathology *(Gallyas 1971)*

This method gives excellent staining of neurofibrillary tangles, and the neuritic pathology surrounding plaques, although the amyloid component itself is unstained. It may also be used for a number of other neurodegenerative diseases (especially argyrophilic grain disease).

Fixation
Formalin-fixed tissues.

Sections
Paraffin-processed sections, 8 μm thick.

Solutions
1. 5% periodic acid
2. Alkaline silver iodide solution

Sodium hydroxide	40 g
Potassium iodide	100 g
Distilled water	500 ml
1% silver nitrate	35 ml

Dissolve the sodium hydroxide in water, then add the potassium iodide and wait until dissolved. Slowly add the silver nitrate and stir vigorously until clear. Then add distilled water to give a final volume of 1000 ml.

3. 0.5% acetic acid
4. Developer working solution
Add 3 volumes of stock solution II to 10 volumes of stock solution I. Stir and add 7 volumes of stock solution III. Stir and wait to clear.

Stock solution I
Sodium carbonate (anhydrous)	50 g
Distilled water	1000 ml

Stock solution II (dissolve consecutively)
Distilled water	1000 ml
Ammonium nitrate	2 g
Silver nitrate	2 g
Tungstosilicic acid	10 g

Stock solution III (dissolve consecutively)
Distilled water	1000 ml
Ammonium nitrate	2 g
Silver nitrate	2 g
Tungstosilicic acid	10 g
Formaldehyde (conc.)	7.3 ml

5. 0.1% gold chloride
6. 1% sodium thiosulfate ('hypo')
7. 0.1% nuclear fast red in 2.5% aqueous aluminum sulfate

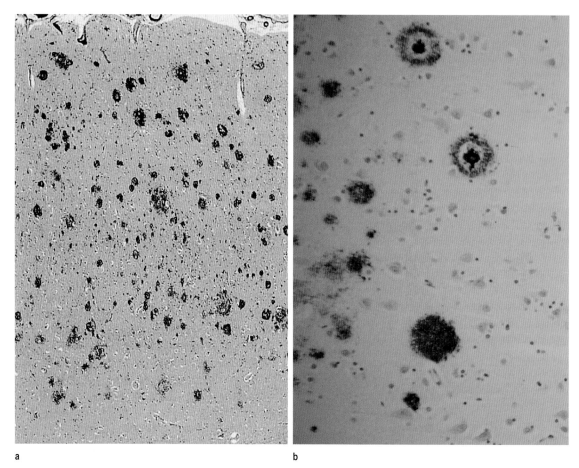

a   b

Figure 17.9 Methenamine silver (a) and immunohistochemistry for β-amyloid (b), showing senile plaques in cerebral cortex from cases of Alzheimer's disease.

Method

1. Take sections to distilled water.
2. Place in 5% periodic acid for 5 minutes.
3. Wash in distilled water for 5 minutes twice.
4. Place in alkaline silver iodide solution for 1 minute.
5. Wash in 0.5% acetic acid for 10 minutes.
6. Place in developer solution (prepare immediately before use) for 5–30 minutes.
7. Wash in 0.5% acetic acid for 3 minutes.
8. Wash in distilled water for 5 minutes.
9. Place in 0.1% gold chloride for 5 minutes.
10. Rinse in distilled water.
11. Place in 1% sodium thiosulfate solution for 5 minutes.
12. Wash in tap water.
13. Counterstain in 0.1% nuclear fast red for 2 minutes.
14. Wash in tap water.
15. Dehydrate, clear, and mount in DPX.

Results

Neurofibrillary tangles and plaque neurites	black
Nuclei	red

Methenamine silver method for senile plaques *(Yamaguchi et al. 1990)*

This preparation has largely been superseded by βA4 immunohistochemistry. It stains amyloid plaques well, but detects only a subset of neurofibrillary tangles.

Fixation

Formalin fixed.

Sections

Paraffin, 8 μm.

Solutions

Working solution

5% hexamine	50 ml
5% sodium tetraborate	2.5 ml
5% silver nitrate	2.5 ml

Add the reagents in the above order, i.e. silver nitrate last.

10% formalin in tap water

Method

1. Take sections to water.
2. Rinse in distilled water.
3. Place sections in working solution for 3–4 hours at 60°C.
4. Check microscopic appearance of plaques and tangles at regular intervals until stained black.
5. Rinse in distilled water.
6. Place sections in 10% formalin in tap water for 5 minutes.
7. Rinse in tap water.
8. Place sections in 5% sodium thiosulfate for 5 minutes.
9. Rinse in tap water.
10. Dehydrate, clear, and mount in DPX.

Results

Amyloid plaques	black
Some tangles (rare)	black
Background	yellow-brown

Modified Bielschowsky method for plaques and tangles *(Litchfield & Nagy 2001)*

This preparation is a reasonable compromise between plaque and tangle labeling. It can therefore be used for diagnostic purposes.

Fixation

Formalin fixed.

Sections

Paraffin sections, cut at 6–8 μm.

Solutions

20% silver nitrate solution

Silver nitrate	20 g
Distilled water	100 ml

Developer

Formalin	20 ml
Distilled water	100 ml
Concentrated nitric acid	1 drop
Citric acid	0.5 g

0.2% ammonia washing solution

Ammonia	0.2 ml
Distilled water	100 ml

'Hypo'

1% sodium thiosufate.

Method

1. Take sections to water.
2. Place slides in 20% silver nitrate for 20 minutes in a refrigerator (4°C).
3. Place slides in distilled water while performing step 4 below.
4. To the 20% silver nitrate (used in step 2) add ammonia, drop by drop, stirring vigorously until precipitate turns clear. Add two more drops of ammonia. Return slides to this solution for 15 minutes (4°C) in a fridge.
5. Place slides in 0.2% ammonia. This is a holding step whilst the working developer solution is made.
6. To 50 ml of the ammonical silver solution (from step 4), add 3 drops of the developer solution; place this in a clean Coplin jar. Drain the slides of the ammonia wash and place in the ammonical silver/developer solution. The development time will vary between 2 and 5 minutes approximately, depending on the ambient temperature. As the development proceeds the tissue will turn a golden brown. Check microscopically until the tangles and plaques are optimally demonstrated.
7. Wash in distilled water.
8. Fix sections in 'hypo' for 5 minutes
9. Wash in distilled water.
10. Dehydrate, clear, and mount in DPX.

Result

Tangles	black
Plaques	black
Background	brown

Notes

a. Some laboratories have found that variable ambient room temperature causes variability and inconsistency in staining. Performing the silver and ammonical silver stages at 4°C overcomes this problem. If this is not a concern for a particular laboratory, these steps can be performed at room temperature.

b. The original method used separate solutions of 20% silver at steps 1 and 4; however, with meticulous technique it is more cost-effective to use the same silver solution throughout.

Neuropathology laboratory specimen handling

Molecular neuroscience has flourished in recent years and neuropathology laboratories find that they are only one part of a larger team dedicated to the diagnosis and characterization of neurological disease. Thus, the neuropathology service remains central to the handling and storage of tissue as well as the procurement of that tissue (either by biopsy or autopsy) and must now do this in a manner that facilitates the work of other disciplines that use the tissue.

The principal histological specimens submitted to or taken by the neuropathology service are:

• Neurosurgical biopsies and excision specimens.
• Peripheral nerve biopsies.
• Muscle biopsies. See Appendix I and previous edition.
• Brain, spinal cord and other specimens taken at autopsy.

Brain and spinal cord biopsies and excision specimens

Given the declining autopsy rate that is seen internationally (Burton & Underwood 2007), surgical

samples of tissue from the CNS are coming (or have already come in many countries, including the UK) to represent the bulk of neuropathological practice.

The majority of these specimens are taken for the diagnosis and/or treatment of neoplasia. The tissue samples are often small and require very careful handling. Some centers prefer neurosurgical biopsies to be placed on a sterile polythene sheet which is folded over the specimen to reduce drying, contamination or loss. Other centers prefer samples to be placed directly into a clean pot. The biopsies should be transported rapidly to the neuropathology laboratory. If this is not possible, they may be placed in formalin fixative. Adequate formalin should be used (10 times the volume of tissue). On arrival at the laboratory, portions of tissue may be sampled for intraoperative diagnosis by smear, snap frozen for molecular analysis or intraoperative diagnosis of cryostat sections, or fixed in glutaraldehyde for electron microscopy. Following this, the remainder of the specimen is fixed in formalin.

Poorly handled tissue is a source of frustration for any neuropathology service. Anyone who has worked in such a laboratory will be well acquainted with the small tube into which a large tumor has been stuffed that requires a second 'neurosurgical' procedure to extract it, piecemeal, poorly fixed and terribly disrupted. The hopelessly desiccated fragment of tissue stuck to the bottom of a glass tube that has taken several hours to reach the laboratory is also well known. We could go on, but instead beg that histology staff strive to educate their neurosurgical and theater colleagues in the appropriate handling of tissue!

Intraoperative diagnosis from smear preparations and frozen sections

The histological and cytological detail that can be achieved from smear and frozen section preparations is substantially less than can be achieved from paraffin-based histology. Therefore, diagnoses made by these techniques can only ever be viewed as an approximation and subject to review following paraffin histology. As there is often only a small amount of tissue available, it is possible that performing an intraoperative diagnosis may compromise the ability to achieve a definitive diagnosis on paraffin-based histology as a feature that is crucial for diagnosis may be lost in the tissue used for smear or frozen section. It is therefore vital that prior to making smear or frozen section preparations from small biopsies the neuropathology staff are certain that this is necessary.

Representative, small pieces of tissue (approximately 1 mm in diameter) are dissected from the biopsy and placed at one end of a plain glass microscope slide. A second glass slide is used to crush the specimen and is then drawn across the slide to produce a uniform smear. Unlike blood film preparation, the two slides are held flat together during smearing, maintaining a gentle and even pressure. Alternatively, the tissue may be lightly touched to a single glass slide, allowing a few cells to adhere to the slide in order to minimize handling artifacts. Fresh postmortem tissue can be used to practice this method and gain familiarity with normal appearances. The slides are immediately fixed in acetic alcohol (Wolman's solution) and stained with H&E, aqueous toluidine blue or both. We find that the former gives better cytoplasmic definition and the latter more nuclear detail. This technique allows rapid sampling of several areas from a biopsy. All cell types in the CNS are readily identifiable by this method (Moss et al. 1997). Certain lesions may be too tough to smear, in which case a frozen section may be used.

Peripheral nerve biopsies

The situations in which peripheral nerve biopsy have been shown to provide clinically useful information include the management of infection, inflammatory and immune disorders (e.g., vasculitis and granulomatous diseases), amyloidosis and neoplasia (Dyck et al. 2005).

Peripheral nerve tissue is exceptionally delicate and prone to artifacts due to handling, and it is imperative that this is kept to a minimum. In this context it is worth recalling that myelin is a liquid,

such that pressure on the nerve at one point will result in pressure fluctuations that cause disruption at locations away from the site of compression. The fragility of nerve biopsies make it imperative that they should be performed only by specialist staff (usually a neurosurgeon or neurologist) who are trained and experienced in this procedure. The number of practitioners should be minimized so as to concentrate the expertise in these individuals. Useful technical guidelines for the taking, processing and interpretation of nerve biopsies have been published (Sommer et al. 2010).

Peripheral nerve biopsy should only be performed after consultation between the laboratory and clinical teams. A minimum of 20 mm, and preferably 30 mm, of nerve should be taken. Ideally, a member of the neuropathology technical staff should attend the biopsy room in order to receive the specimen as soon as possible. This should be placed gently on a piece of dry card, to which it will naturally adhere. The nerve should not be put in fixative, sutured, clamped, stapled, pinned or traumatized in any way.

On arrival at the laboratory, a fresh scalpel blade is used to divide the biopsy into at least three segments: one for paraffin-based histology, one for semi-thin preparations and electron microscopy and one for teased fiber preparations. Further portions may be taken for snap freezing. The 2 mm portions at the ends of the biopsy are usually damaged at surgical removal and are thus inappropriate for histology. They may, however, be frozen for molecular studies. Glutaraldehyde is the preferred fixative for processing to semi-thin sections and electron microscopy. Opinion is divided on the best fixative for paraffin-based nerve histology, although many prefer formalin (10% NBF).

Following glutaraldehyde fixation, the nerve may be cut into 1 mm pieces, osmicated and embedded (see also Chapters 22 and 8 on electron microscopy and plastic embedded sections, respectively). These blocks may be used for electron microscopy or the preparation of semi-thin (1–3 μm) sections. Semi-thin sections of transversely oriented tissue are cut and stained with toluidine blue or methylene blue-azure II-basic fuchsin.

For paraffin processing, fixed material is processed and cut at 6–8 μm. It is helpful to include a transverse and a longitudinal segment for examination. Different centers vary in the stains prepared as a matter of routine. However, these may include H&E, a trichrome stain to assess fibrosis, a myelin stain, an axon stain and an amyloid preparation such as Congo red. Many biopsies are performed for inflammatory disorders such as vasculitis. As these can be focal, patchy disorders, serial sections through the paraffin block should be performed. It may be necessary to augment this with immunohistochemistry.

Teased fiber preparations allow the examination of the pattern of myelin formation along individual axons (Asbury & Johnson 1978). This can give information on whether there have been past episodes of myelin loss with re-myelination, or whether there is myelin fragmentation due to axonal loss.

Methylene blue-azure II-basic fuchsin

This method is based on that of Humphrey and Pitman (1974).

Fixation
Glutaraldehyde.

Sections
Semi-thin resin sections.

Solutions

0.2 M sodium dihydrogen orthophosphate dihydrate

$NaH_2PO_4.2H_2O$	3.121 g
Distilled water	100 ml

0.2 M disodium hydrogen orthophosphate

Na_2HPO_4	2.839 g
Distilled water	100 ml

0.1 M phosphate buffer, pH 6.9

Methylene blue/azure A

Methylene blue	0.39 g
Azure A	0.06 g
Glycerol	30 ml
Methanol	30 ml
0.1 M phosphate buffer, pH 6.9	90 ml
Distilled water	150 ml

50% ethanol in deionized water

Basic fuchsin, stock solution

Basic fuchsin	0.5 g
50% ethanol	50 ml

Basic fuchsin, working solution

Basic fuchsin stock solution	1 ml
Deionized water	19 ml

Method
1. Filter methylene blue/azure A solution into Coplin jar.
2. Put into a water bath set at 65°C.
3. Stain sections in this solution for 30 minutes.
4. Rinse well in distilled, filtered water.
5. Do not allow sections to dry.
6. Filter basic fuchsin working solution onto slides and stain at room temperature for 4 minutes.
7. Rinse well in distilled water.
8. Drain, and allow to dry.
9. Mount in DPX.

Result

Myelin	blue
Other tissue elements	light blue
Collagen	pink/red
Elastin	red

Notes
a. If staining for leprosy bacilli in sections, stain in filtered working solution of basic fuchsin for a strict 2 minutes only. Follow this by washing well in distilled water.
b. Do not leave sections stained with methylene blue/azure A in distilled water before counterstaining as the blue will wash out and result will be too pale.

Preparation of teased nerve fibers (Asbury & Johnson 1978)

Nerve fibers can be processed to glycerine or unpolymerized Araldite for teasing. The latter method produces a firmer consistency to the individual fibers and is easier to work with. The stiffness of the fibers also relates to the amount of osmication and the concentration of the osmium used.

Tissue
Fresh nerve.

Fixation
Segment of nerve is fixed in 0.1 M phosphate-buffered 3.6% glutaraldehyde, for 4–16 hours.

Method

1. Wash twice in phosphate buffer, 15 minutes.
2. Under a stereomicroscope using two pairs of fine forceps, carefully remove the epineurium by only gripping and pulling the connective tissue. Separate the nerve into individual or small bundles of fascicles. This allows a uniform osmication, disregarding the variation in size of the specimen that one may have received.
3. Osmicate in 0.1 M phosphate-buffered 2% osmium tetroxide, 4 hours.
4. Wash twice in phosphate buffer, 15 minutes each.
5. Briefly rinse in distilled water and process through 50, 80, and 95% alcohol for 10 minutes each.
6. Dehydrate in two changes of 100% alcohol, 15 minutes each.
7. Process through two changes of propylene oxide, 15 minutes each.
8. Mix in equal parts of propylene oxide and Araldite CY212 resin for 1 hour.
9. Mix in unpolymerized Araldite CY212 resin overnight (the specimen can be kept in this resin at 4°C for up to 1 year).

Notes

a. Laboratories which do not have access to araldite processing can use a simplified method where, following fixation, the nerve biopsy is washed in distilled water (1 hour), osmicated (4 hours to overnight), washed in distilled water (1 hour), treated with 60% glycerol overnight, and then teased as described below.

b. Any remaining tissue from the protocol outlined in Note a can be subsequently paraffin processed and stained with H&E.

To tease fibers after preparation, place the processed nerve on a glass slide under a stereomicroscope in a pool of unpolymerized Araldite. Using fine forceps and sharp needles, remove the perineurium from a fascicle. Keep dividing the nerve bundles into halves until single or small bundles of two to three fibers (black) can be carefully teased out. When separating a smaller bundle from a larger one, it is helpful to hold onto the smaller one and pull the larger one slowly away. Slide the fiber across the slide in a trail of resin onto an adjacent slide. Care should be taken to insure that the fibers to be examined are aligned in parallel across the slide.

For diagnostic purposes, in order to avoid possible sampling errors, at least 100 fibers should be sampled (Dyck et al. 2005). However, in severely demyelinated cases, it may prove difficult to get enough black fibers. When enough fibers are obtained, use the fine forceps to pick up a small droplet of *partially polymerized* resin. Apply a thin line of the resin along one of the aligned ends of the parallel-arranged fibers (the resin should not touch the fibers at this stage). Trim a coverslip to size. Hold the coverslip at an angle to the surface of the slide and carefully touch the line of resin with the lower edge of the coverslip. Carefully lower the coverslip until it almost touches the slide, and let go. Lay the slide on a flat surface in a 37°C oven and let the resin slowly spread longitudinally along the fibers to fill the entire gap between the slide and the coverslip. Ring the coverslip with nail varnish. Any trapped bubbles should be left undisturbed. With practice, this mounting technique will allow the well-aligned, loosely attached fibers to remain undisturbed and without overlapping on the slide.

Muscle biopsies

The handling and preparation of muscle biopsies are covered in Appendix I and in previous editions.

Biopsy samples of skeletal muscle may be taken either using a biopsy needle or at open operation. The aim of histology is to provide an undistorted picture of muscle fiber architecture. A detailed evaluation of muscle disease relies heavily on enzyme histochemistry, which necessitates the use of cryostat sections of unfixed skeletal muscle (see Table 17.2).

The practice of performing immunohistochemisty for fast and slow myosins is beginning to replace ATPase enzyme histochemistry as a method for distinguishing fiber types. Major histocompatibility complex (MHC) class I proteins are overexpressed in some inflammatory myopathies, a feature that can be detected by immunohistochemistry (Dubowitz & Sewry 2007).

Table 17.2 Staining methods for muscle biopsies	
Method	**Demonstrates**
H&E	Morphology
Gomori trichrome	Inclusion bodies, connective tissue, ragged red fibers and tubular aggregates
PAS ± diastase	Glycogen
Oil red O	Lipids
ATPase, pH 9.4	Myosin loss and myofiber atrophy of Type 1 and 2 fibers
ATPase, pH 4.6	Type 2B myofibers
ATPase, pH 4.3	Type 2C myofibers
NADH-TR	Internal fiber architecture, mitochondria and tubular aggregates
Alkaline phosphatase	Regenerating myofibers, autoimmune connective tissue disorders
Acid phosphatase	Inflammatory cells; necrotic fibers; enhanced lysosomal enzyme activity
Non-specific esterase	Inflammatory cells, necrotic myofibers, enhanced lysosomal enzyme activity
Cytochrome c oxidase	Mitochondrial disorders
Succinic dehydrogenase	Mitochondrial disorders
Myoadenylate deaminase	Enzyme deficiency
Myophosphorylase	Type V glycogenosis (McArdle's disease)
Dystrophy-related immunohistochemical stains	Dystrophin 1, 2, and 3 (Figs 17.10a, b), sarcoglycans (α, β, γ, and δ), dysferlin, merosin, caveolin, emerin, calpain-3, spectrin

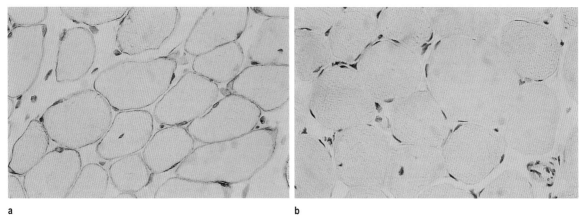

a   b

Figure 17.10 (a) In a normal muscle, dystrophin is localized beneath the cell membrane of muscle fibers. (b) In Duchenne muscular dystrophy, this staining pattern is absent.

A small portion of muscle may be fixed for electron microscopy if clinically indicated. The sample may be fixed lightly stretched, longitudinally in a special clip, or stretched out by pinning and fixed with a few drops of buffered glutaldehyde. After a few minutes, it will be stiffened and can be put into the main bulk of fixative. Staining of motor end-plates and axons may be performed on fresh tissues (Coers 1982). A detailed description of muscle histology and biopsy handling is given by Dubowitz and Sewry (2007).

Central nervous system tissues taken at autopsy

After removal and macroscopic examination in the autopsy room, the brain should be immersed in a 10-liter bucket of formalin. It should be suspended by the basilar artery from a piece of string tied to the two attachments of the bucket handle. This may be done by passing the string under the basilar artery, or by hooking the basilar artery to the string with a curtain hook or safety pin. The latter method is best avoided as the safety pin tends to rust. The brain should not be allowed to touch the bottom or sides of the bucket. The brain should then be left to fix for 3 or more weeks. The spinal cord may be suspended by the dura mater in a suitably long measuring cylinder with a weight attached to the dura mater at the lower end, to avoid artifactual contraction of the cord during fixation. While some laboratories prefer the minimization of tissue distortion that this method provides, others consider this is an unnecessarily complicated method and prefer to immerse the cord in the brain bucket beneath the fixing brain.

If molecular techniques are likely to be required, portions of brain and spinal cord may be snap-frozen in liquid nitrogen.

Whilst paraffin processing of neurosurgical material can be carried out using most routine overnight schedules, autopsy CNS material requires longer processing, depending upon block size. This can be anything from 48 hours to 5 days. Central nervous system tissue has a high lipid content due to the presence of myelin. This lipid makes it prone to processing artifact, largely due to poor dehydration. For this reason, some laboratories use isopropyl alcohol for the last two changes of alcohol to improve tissue dehydration during tissue processing.

Processing artifacts include:

- Sections blowing apart on the water bath.
- Tissue 'crazing' whereby sections start to disintegrate, resulting in 'crazy paving'-like cracking usually at the edge of the section.
- Sections lifting off the slide, especially in the context of immunohistochemistry on jumbo slides.
- Poor staining.

Most of these problems can be reduced by using a longer processing schedule and the use of coated/charged slides. Rushing fixation, processing or drying slides will lead to suboptimal preparations and frustration.

The prion diseases present special methodological problems for autopsy and subsequent tissue handling. The misfolded prion, being the transmissible element of these diseases, is a Group 3 Hazard and is extremely resistant to usual decontamination methods. Dissection of a brain where prion disease is a possibility should be done in an appropriate laboratory containment facility using disposable instruments and appropriate protective clothing. All contaminated tissues and fluids should be contained. Sampled tissues should be treated with formic acid prior to paraffin embedding (Brown et al. 1990). Work surfaces and instruments may be sterilized in 2M sodium hydroxide for 1 hour. Glassware can be cleaned in sodium hypochlorite (20,000 ppm). In cases of vCJD, prion protein (an infective hazard) also resides in lymphoid tissues such as tonsil, lymph node, spleen and bone marrow (Ironside et al. 2000). Detailed protocols for the handling of tissues that may be affected by prion disease have been published (Bell & Ironside 1993; World Health Organization 2004; Department of Health 2011).

Acknowledgments

Thanks to Sebastian Brandner for providing us with his protocol for methylene blue-azure II-basic fuschin staining and to Patrick Elliott of the Medical Illustration Department, Royal Hallamshire Hospital, Sheffield, for his illustration depicted in Figure 17.1.

References

Alafuzoff, I., Arzberger, T., Al-Sarraj, S., et al., 2008. Staging of neurofibrillary pathology in Alzheimer's disease: a study of the BrainNet Europe Consortium. Brain pathology 18 (4), 484–496.

Alafuzoff, I., Thal, D.R., Arzberger, T., et al., 2009. Assessment of beta-amyloid deposits in human brain: a study of the BrainNet Europe Consortium. Acta Neuropathologica 117 (3), 309–320.

Asbury, A.K., Johnson, P.C., 1978. Pathology of peripheral nerve. Saunders, Philadelphia.

Bell, J.E., Ironside, J.W., 1993. How to tackle a possible Creutzfeldt-Jakob disease necropsy. Journal of Clinical Pathology 46 (3), 193–197.

Bielschowsky, M., 1902. Die Silberimprägnation der Axenzylinder. Zentralblatt für Neurologie 21, 579.

Blumcke, I., Muller, S., Buslei, R., et al., 2004. Microtubule-associated protein-2 immunoreactivity: a useful tool in the differential diagnosis of low-grade neuroepithelial tumors. Acta Neuropathol 108 (2), 89–96.

Bourne, T.D., Schiff, D., 2010. Update on molecular findings, management and outcome in low-grade gliomas. Nat Rev Neurol 6 (12), 695–701.

Brown, P., Wolff, A., Gajdusek, D.C., 1990. A simple and effective method for inactivating virus infectivity in formalin-fixed tissue samples from patients with Creutzfeldt-Jakob disease. Neurology 40 (6), 887–890.

Burton, J.L., Underwood, J., 2007. Clinical, educational, and epidemiological value of autopsy. Lancet 369 (9571), 1471–1480.

Cairns, N.J., Bigio, E.H., Mackenzie, I.R., et al., 2007. Neuropathologic diagnostic and nosologic criteria for frontotemporal lobar degeneration: consensus of the Consortium for Frontotemporal Lobar Degeneration. Acta Neuropathol 114 (1), 5–22.

Camelo-Piragua, S., Jansen, M., Ganguly, A., et al., 2010. Mutant IDH1-specific immunohistochemistry distinguishes diffuse astrocytoma from astrocytosis. Acta Neuropathol 119 (4), 509–511.

Capper, D., Sahm, F., Hartmann, C., et al., 2010. Application of mutant IDH1 antibody to differentiate diffuse glioma from nonneoplastic central nervous system lesions and therapy-induced changes. Am J Surg Pathol 34 (8), 1199–1204.

Capper, D., Reuss, D., Schittenhelm, J., et al., 2011. Mutation-specific IDH1 antibody differentiates oligodendrogliomas and oligoastrocytomas from other brain tumors with oligodendroglioma-like morphology. Acta Neuropathol 121, 241–252.

Chan, K.K., Lowe, J., 2002. Techniques in neuropathology. In: Bancroft, J.D., Gamble, M., (Eds.), Theory and practice of histological techniques. Churchill Livingstone, Edinburgh, pp. 371–392.

Chance, S.A., Highley, J.R., Esiri, M.M., Crow, T.J., 1999. Fiber content of the fornix in schizophrenia: lack of evidence for a primary limbic encephalopathy. Am J Psychiatry 156 (11), 1720–1724.

Coers, C., 1982. Pathology of intramuscular nerves and nerve terminals. In: Mastaglia, F.L., Walton, J., (Eds.), Skeletal muscle pathology. Churchill Livingstone, Edinburgh, pp. 483–507.

Cosgrove, M., Fitzgibbons, P.L., Sherrod, A., et al., 1989. Intermediate filament expression in astrocytic neoplasms. Am J Surg Pathol 13 (2), 141–145.

Cross, R.B., 1982. Demonstration of neurofibrillary tangles in paraffin sections: a quick and simple method using a modification of Palmgren's method. Medical Laboratory Sciences 39 (1), 67–69.

Department of Health, 2011, 31/01/2011. Guidance from the ACDP TSE Working Group. Retrieved 29 March 2011 from http://www.dh.gov.uk/ab/ACDP/TSEguidance/index.htm.

Dickson, D.W., 1999. Tau and synuclein and their role in neuropathology. Brain Pathology 9 (4), 657–661.

Doglioni, C., Dell'Orto, P., Coggi, G., et al., 1987. Choroid plexus tumors. An immunocytochemical study with particular reference to the coexpression of intermediate filament proteins. Am J Pathol 127 (3), 519–529.

Dubowitz, V., Sewry, C.A., 2007. Muscle biopsy: a practical approach. Saunders Elsevier, Philadelphia.

Dyck, P.J., Dyck, P.J.B., Engelstad, J., 2005. Pathological alterations of nerves. In: Dyck, P.J.,

Thomas, P.K. (Eds.), Peripheral neuropathy. Elsevier Saunders, Philadelphia, pp. 733–829.

Eager, R.P., Chi, C.C., Wolf, G., 1971. Lateral hypothalamic projections to the hypothalamic ventromedial nucleus in the albino rat: demonstration by means of a simplified ammoniacal silver degeneration method. Brain Res 29 (1), 128–132.

Edgar, M.A., Rosenblum, M.K., 2008. The differential diagnosis of central nervous system tumors: a critical examination of some recent immunohistochemical applications. Arch Pathol Lab Med 132 (3), 500–509.

Eng, L.F., 1983. Immunocytochemistry of the glial fibrillary acidic protein. In: Zimmerman, H.M. (Ed.), Progress in neuropathology. Raven Press. New York, 5, pp. 19–39.

Eng, L.F., Rubinstein, L.J., 1978. Contribution of immunohistochemistry to diagnostic problems of human cerebral tumors. J Histochem Cytochem 26 (7), 513–522.

Gallyas, F., 1971. Silver staining of Alzheimer's neurofibrillary changes by means of physical development. Acta Morphologica Academiae Scientiarum Hungaricae 19 (1), 1–8.

Garey, L., 2010. When cortical development goes wrong: schizophrenia as a neurodevelopmental disease of microcircuits. J Anat 217 (4), 324–333.

Ghobrial, M., Ross, E.R., 1986. Immunocytochemistry of neuron-specific enolase: a re-evaluation. In: Zimmerman, H.M. (Ed.), Progress in neuropathology. Raven Press, New York, pp. 199–221.

Goebel, H.H., Wisniewski, K.E., 2004. Current state of clinical and morphological features in human NCL. Brain Pathol 14 (1), 61–69.

Goedert, M., 1999. Filamentous nerve cell inclusions in neurodegenerative diseases: tauopathies and alpha-synucleinopathies. Philosophical Transactions of the Royal Society of London. Series B, Biological Sciences 354 (1386), 1101–1118.

Gotow, T., 2000. Neurofilaments in health and disease. Med Electron Microsc 33 (4), 173–199.

Graeber, M.B., Streit, W.J., 2010. Microglia: biology and pathology. Acta Neuropathol 119 (1), 89–105.

Hartmann, C., Meyer, J., Balss, J., et al., 2009. Type and frequency of IDH1 and IDH2 mutations are related to astrocytic and oligodendroglial differentiation and age: a study of 1,010 diffuse gliomas. Acta Neuropathol 118 (4), 469–474.

Hasselblatt, M., Paulus, W., 2003. Sensitivity and specificity of epithelial membrane antigen staining patterns in ependymomas. Acta Neuropathol 106 (4), 385–388.

Hirose, T., Sano, T., Hizawa, K., 1986. Ultrastructural localization of S-100 protein in neurofibroma. Acta Neuropathol 69 (1–2), 103–110.

Holzer, W., 1921. Uber eine neue method der Gliafases Farbung. Zentralblatt für die gesamte. Neurologie und Psychiatrie 69, 354–360.

Humphrey, C.D., Pittman, F.E., 1974. A simple methylene blue-azure II-basic fuchsin stain for epoxy-embedded tissue sections. Stain Technology 49 (1), 9–14.

Ince, P.G., Clark, B., Holton, J., et al., 2008. Diseases of movement and system degenerations. In: Love, S., Louis, D.N., Ellison, D.W. (Eds.), Greenfield's neuropathology. Hodder Arnold, London, 1, pp. 889–1030.

Ironside, J.W., Head, M.W., Bell, J.E., et al., 2000. Laboratory diagnosis of variant Creutzfeldt-Jakob disease. Histopathology 37 (1), 1–9.

Itoyama, Y., Sternberger, N.H., Kies, M.W., et al., 1980a. Immunocytochemical method to identify myelin basic protein in oligodendroglia and myelin sheaths of the human nervous system. Ann Neurol 7 (2), 157–166.

Itoyama, Y., Sternberger, N.H., Webster, H.D., et al., 1980b. Immunocytochemical observations on the distribution of myelin-associated glycoprotein and myelin basic protein in multiple sclerosis lesions. Ann Neurol 7 (2), 167–177.

Jellinger, K.A., 2008. Morphologic diagnosis of 'vascular dementia' – a critical update. Journal of the Neurological Sciences 270 (1–2), 1–12.

Johnson, R.T., 2005. Prion diseases. Lancet Neurology 4 (10), 635–642.

Kellett, B.S., 1963. Gallocyanin-chrome alum: a routine stain for Nissl substance in paraffin sections. J Med Lab Technol 20, 196–198.

Kim, S.U., de Vellis, J., 2005. Microglia in health and disease. J Neurosci Res 81 (3), 302–313.

Kluver, H., Barrera, E., 1953. A method for the combined staining of cells and fibers in the nervous system. J Neuropathol Exp Neurol 12 (4), 400–403.

Koperek, O., Gelpi, E., Birner, P., et al., 2004. Value and limits of immunohistochemistry in differential diagnosis of clear cell primary brain tumors. Acta Neuropathol 108 (1), 24–30.

Kuusisto, E., Kauppinen, T., Alafuzoff, I., 2008. Use of p62/SQSTM1 antibodies for neuropathological diagnosis. Neuropathol Appl Neurobiol 34 (2), 169–180.

Lamy, C., Duyckaerts, C., Delaere, P., et al., 1989. Comparison of seven staining methods for senile plaques and neurofibrillary tangles in a prospective series of 15 elderly patients. Neuropathology and Applied Neurobiology 15 (6), 563–578.

Ligon, K.L., Alberta, J.A., Kho, A.T., et al., 2004. The oligodendroglial lineage marker OLIG2 is universally expressed in diffuse gliomas. J Neuropathol Exp Neurol 63 (5), 499–509.

Lindner, M., Heine, S., Haastert, K., et al., 2008. Sequential myelin protein expression during remyelination reveals fast and efficient repair after central nervous system demyelination. Neuropathology and Applied Neurobiology 34 (1), 105–114.

Litchfield, S., Nagy, Z., 2001. New temperature modification makes the Bielschowsky silver stain reproducible. Acta Neuropathologica 101 (1), 17–21.

Lowe, J., 1998. Establishing a pathological diagnosis in degenerative dementias. Brain Pathology 8 (2), 403–406.

Lowe, J., Mayer, R.J., Landon, M., 1993. Ubiquitin in neurodegenerative diseases. Brain Pathology 3 (1), 55–65.

Loyez, M., 1910. Coloration des fibers nerveuses par la méthode à l'hematoxyline au fer après inclusion à la celloidine. Compte Rendu des Séances de la Société de Biologie 69, 511.

Ludwin, S.K., Sternberger, N.H., 1984. An immunohistochemical study of myelin proteins during remyelination in the central nervous system. Acta Neuropathol 63 (3), 240–248.

Maccioni, R.B., Cambiazo, V., 1995. Role of microtubule-associated proteins in the control of microtubule assembly. Physiol Rev 75 (4), 835–864.

Mackenzie, I.R., Neumann, M., Bigio, E.H., et al., 2009. Nomenclature for neuropathologic subtypes of frontotemporal lobar degeneration: consensus recommendations. Acta Neuropathologica 117 (1), 15–18.

Mackenzie, I.R., Neumann, M., Bigio, E.H., et al., 2010. Nomenclature and nosology for neuropathologic subtypes of frontotemporal lobar degeneration: an update. Acta Neuropathologica 119 (1), 1–4.

Marsland, T.A., Glees, P., Erikson, L.B., 1954. Modification of the Glees silver impregnation for paraffin sections. J Neuropathol Exp Neurol 13 (4), 587–591.

Miller, D.C., Koslow, M., Budzilovich, G.N., Burstein, D.E., 1990. Synaptophysin: a sensitive and specific marker for ganglion cells in central nervous system neoplasms. Hum Pathol 21 (3), 271–276.

Mirra, S.S., Hart, M.N., Terry, R.D., 1993. Making the diagnosis of Alzheimer's disease. a primer for practicing pathologists. Archives of Pathology & Laboratory Medicine 117 (2), 132–144.

Moss, T.H., Nicoll, J.A.R., Ironside, J.W., 1997. Intra-operative diagnosis of CNS tumors. Arnold, London and New York.

Mullen, R.J., Buck, C.R., Smith, A.M., 1992. NeuN, a neuronal specific nuclear protein in vertebrates. Development 116 (1), 201–211.

Nakagawa, Y., Perentes, E., Rubinstein, L.J., 1986. Immunohistochemical characterization of oligodendrogliomas: an analysis of multiple markers. Acta Neuropathol 72 (1), 15–22.

Nolan, J.A., Trojanowski, J.Q., Hogue-Angeletti, R., 1985. Neurons and neuroendocrine cells contain chromogranin: detection of the molecule in normal bovine tissues by immunochemical and immunohistochemical methods. J Histochem Cytochem 33 (8), 791–798.

Palay, S.L., Palade, G.E., 1955. The fine structure of neurons. J Biophys Biochem Cytol 1 (1), 69–88.

Palmgren, A., 1948. A rapid method for selective silver staining of nerve fibers and nerve endings in mounted paraffin sections. Acta Zoologica 29, 377–392.

Penfield, W., 1928. A method of staining oligodendroglia and microglia (combined method). Am J Pathol 4 (2), 153–157.

Preusser, M., Laggner, U., Haberler, C., et al., 2006. Comparative analysis of NeuN immunoreactivity in primary brain tumors: conclusions for rational use in diagnostic histopathology. Histopathology 48 (4), 438–444.

Preusser, M., Budka, H., Rossler, K., Hainfellner, J.A., 2007. OLIG2 is a useful immunohistochemical marker in differential diagnosis of clear cell primary CNS neoplasms. Histopathology 50 (3), 365–370.

Pugh, B.C., Rossi, M.L., 1993. A paraffin wax technique of Golgi-Cox impregnated CNS that permits the joint application of other histological and immunocytochemical techniques. J Neural Transm Suppl 39, 97–105.

Quinn, B., 1998. Synaptophysin staining in normal brain: importance for diagnosis of ganglioglioma. Am J Surg Pathol 22 (5), 550–556.

Shafit-Zagardo, B., Kalcheva, N., 1998. Making sense of the multiple MAP-2 transcripts and their role in the neuron. Mol Neurobiol 16 (2), 149–162.

Sommer, C.L., Brandner, S., Dyck, P.J., et al., 2010. Peripheral Nerve Society Guideline on processing and evaluation of nerve biopsies. Journal of the Peripheral Nervous System: JPNS 15 (3), 164–175.

Stern, J.B., 1932. Neue Silberimprägnations Versuche zur Darstellung der Mikro- und Oligodendroglia (An Celloidin-serienschnitten anwendbare Methode). Zeitschrift für die gesamte Neurologie und Psychiatrie 138, 50.

Sulzer, D., Mosharov, E., Talloczy, Z., et al., 2008. Neuronal pigmented autophagic vacuoles: lipofuscin, neuromelanin, and ceroid as macroautophagic responses during aging and disease. J Neurochem 106 (1), 24–36.

Swank, R.L., Davenport, H.A., 1935. Chlorate-osmic formalin method for degenerating myelin. Stain Technology 10, 87–90.

Takei, H., Bhattacharjee, M.B., Rivera, A., et al., 2007. New immunohistochemical markers in the evaluation of central nervous system tumors: a review of 7 selected adult and pediatric brain tumors. Arch Pathol Lab Med 131 (2), 234–241.

Trojanowski, J.Q., Walkenstein, N., Lee, V.M., 1986. Expression of neurofilament subunits in neurons of the central and peripheral nervous system: an immunohistochemical study with monoclonal antibodies. J Neurosci 6 (3), 650–660.

Uematsu, Y., Rojas-Corona, R.R., Llena, J.F., Hirano, A., 1989. Distribution of epithelial membrane antigen in normal and neoplastic human ependyma. Acta Neuropathol 78 (3), 325–328.

Velasco, M.E., Dahl, D., Roessmann, U., Gambetti, P., 1980. Immunohistochemical localization of glial fibrillary acidic protein in human glial neoplasms. Cancer 45 (3), 484–494.

Weigert, C., 1904. Nervenfasern, Markscheide. Enzyklopädie der Mikroskopischen Technik. R. Krause. Berlin 3, 1622–1629.

Weil, A., 1928. A rapid method for staining myelin sheaths. Archives of Neurology and Psychiatry 20, 392.

Wharton, S.B., Chan, K.K., Whittle, I.R., 2002. Microtubule-associated protein 2 (MAP-2) is expressed in low and high grade diffuse astrocytomas. J Clin Neurosci 9 (2), 165–169.

Wiedenmann, B., Kuhn, C., Schwechheimer, K., et al., 1987. Synaptophysin identified in metastases of neuroendocrine tumors by immunocytochemistry and immunoblotting. Am J Clin Pathol 88 (5), 560–569.

Wilson, P.O., Barber, P.C., Hamid, Q.A., et al., 1988. The immunolocalization of protein gene product 9.5 using rabbit polyclonal and mouse monoclonal antibodies. Br J Exp Pathol 69 (1), 91–104.

Winek, R.R., Scheithauer, B.W., Wick, M.R., 1989. Meningioma, meningeal hemangiopericytoma (angioblastic meningioma), peripheral hemangiopericytoma, and acoustic schwannoma. A comparative immunohistochemical study. Am J Surg Pathol 13 (4), 251–261.

Wooten, M.W., Hu, X., Babu, J.R., et al., 2006. Signaling, polyubiquitination, trafficking, and inclusions: sequestosome 1/p62's role in neurodegenerative disease. J Biomed Biotechnol 2006 (3), 62079.

World Health Organization, 2004. Laboratory biosafety manual. World Health Organization, Geneva.

Yamaguchi, H., Haga, C., Hirai, S., et al., 1990. Distinctive, rapid, and easy labeling of diffuse plaques in the Alzheimer brains by a new methenamine silver stain. Acta Neuropathologica 79 (5), 569–572.

Yokoo, H., Nobusawa, S., Takebayashi, H., et al., 2004. Anti-human Olig2 antibody as a useful immunohistochemical marker of normal oligodendrocytes and gliomas. Am J Pathol 164 (5), 1717–1725.

Further reading

Dawson, T.P., Neal, J.W., et al., 2003. Neuropathology techniques. Arnold, London.

Dubowitz, V., Sewry, C.A., 2007. Muscle biopsy: a practical approach. Saunders Elsevier, Philadelphia.

Esiri, M.M., Perl, D.P., 2006. Oppenheimer's diagnostic neuropathology: a practical manual. Hodder Arnold, London.

Immunohistochemical techniques

Peter Jackson • David Blythe

Introduction

The introduction of prognostic and predictive markers in immunohistochemistry has made a tremendous beneficial impact on patient diagnosis and management. This has been made possible by the gradual development of immunohistochemical methodologies over the past 70 years which have allowed the identification of specific or highly selective cellular epitopes in formalin-fixed paraffin-processed tissues with an antibody and appropriate labeling system. The present trend in diagnostic laboratories is to try to avoid the use of frozen sections for immunohistochemical analysis as much as possible, and to perform immunohistochemical investigations on formalin-fixed paraffin-embedded tissue.

Many antibodies are now available to identify epitopes that survive the rigors of formalin fixation and processing to paraffin wax. In cases where morphology and clinical data alone do not allow a firm diagnosis, then immunohistochemistry is invaluable. The increasing use of prognostic and predictive markers permits the pathologist to make decisions that could profoundly affect patient management (Fig. 18.1).

In 1941 Albert H. Coons described a revolutionary new way of visualizing tissue constituents using an antibody labeled with a fluorescent dye. Visualization of the labeled complex was achieved by the use of a fluorescence microscope. The first fluorescent dye to be attached to an antibody was fluorescein isocyanate, but fluorescein isothiocyanate soon became the label of choice because the molecule was much easier to conjugate to the antibody and

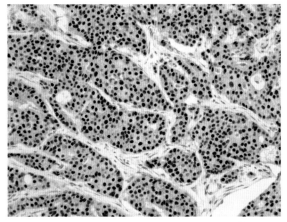

Figure 18.1 Formalin-fixed paraffin-embedded section of breast carcinoma showing strong expression of estrogen receptor. Pressure cooker antigen retrieval for 2 minutes using Vector antigen unmasking fluid.

the result was more stable (Riggs et al. 1958). Fluorescein compounds emit a bright green fluorescence when excited at a wavelength of 490 nm. The technique has enormously expanded and developed following the early work. New labels have been introduced, including red, yellow, and blue fluorochromes. This permits the simultaneous visualization of several separately labeled antibodies on a single preparation. Currently, fluorescein isothiocyanate and rhodamine are among the most popular fluorochromes. This methodology, whilst useful in some diagnostic areas, such as determining the nature of protein deposits in skin and renal diseases, and bacteria in infected material, has certain limitations. A fluorescence microscope is necessary to visualize the fluorochrome, and this has a tendency to fade. More importantly and probably the greatest disadvantage of immunofluorescence is that it is difficult to demonstrate the morphological detail of the labeled cell and the associated tissue components. The success of immunohistochemistry in some areas of pathology stimulated interest in the development of alternative antibody labeling techniques that would avoid the difficulties and limitations associated with immunofluorescence.

Many limitations were overcome with the introduction of enzymes as labels. Cells that have been labeled with an enzyme such as horseradish peroxidase, conjugated to an antibody, and visualized with an appropriate chromogen such as diaminobenzidine (DAB) (Nakane & Pierce 1966), can be counterstained with traditional nuclear stains such as hematoxylin. This permits the simultaneous evaluation of both specific immunohistochemistry and morphological detail. In 1970 Sternberger et al. described the peroxidase-anti-peroxidase (PAP) technique. In 1971, Engvall and Perlman reported the use of alkaline phosphatase labeling, and Cordell et al. (1984) described the alkaline phosphatase-anti-alkaline phosphatase (APAAP) technique. Heggeness and Ash (1977) proposed the use of avidin-biotin for immunofluorescence. This technique was modified by Guesden et al. (1979) and Hsu et al. (1981) who used a horseradish peroxidase label. Avidin-biotin labeling was superseded by streptavidin-biotin labeling, and was one of the more popular techniques used in diagnostic laboratories. However, labeled polymer detection systems are now the most popular choice for most diagnostic laboratories.

Over the last 30 years, many myths surrounding the preservation and presentation of antigens in formalin-fixed paraffin-embedded tissues have been dispelled. In the 1970s it was thought that routine paraffin processing destroyed many epitopes, and that certain antigens could never be demonstrated in paraffin sections. However it was found that many antigens are not lost, but are masked by the processes involved in formalin fixation and paraffin processing.

Certain epitopes, for example the proliferation antigen, Ki67 and T-cell antigens CD2, CD4, CD5 (Fig. 18.2), CD7 and CD8, can only be demonstrated

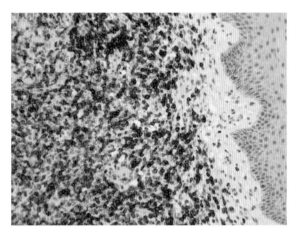

Figure 18.2 CD5 demonstration in a formalin-fixed paraffin-embedded section from a nasal biopsy showing extra nodal T-cell lymphoma.

in formalin-fixed, paraffin wax-processed tissue after heat pretreatment, and then only with certain monoclonal antibody clones. Antibodies such as those directed against the leukocyte common antigen (clones PD7/2B11) and the CD20 antigen (clone L26) produce enhanced staining after citrate buffer (pH 6.0) heating. Surprisingly, heat pretreatment allows for considerably greater dilution factors. The demonstration of antigens such as cyclin D1 (with clone DCS-6), on the other hand, is better in a high pH solution (Tris-EDTA, pH 10.0). However, the use of the cyclin D1 rabbit monoclonal antibody (clone SP4) produces very good results using citrate buffer, pH 6.0 (Fig. 18.3).

Immunohistochemistry theory

Definitions

Immunohistochemistry

This is a technique for identifying cellular or tissue constituents (antigens) by means of antigen-antibody interactions, the site of antibody binding being identified either by direct labeling of the antibody, or by use of a secondary labeling method.

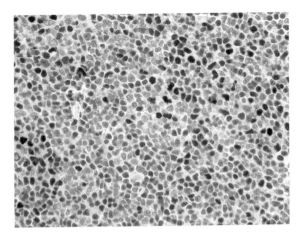

Figure 18.3 Formalin-fixed paraffin-embedded section of lymph node, showing cyclin D1 expression in a mantle cell lymphoma. Antigen retrieval with the pressure cooker and citrate buffer, pH 6.0, and Labvision rabbit monoclonal (clone SP4) primary antibody.

Antigens

An antigen is a molecule that induces the formation of an antibody and bears one or more antibody-binding sites. These are highly specific topographical regions composed of a small number of amino acids or monosaccharide units, being known as antigenic determinant groups or epitopes.

Antibody

Antibodies belong to the class of serum proteins known as immunoglobulins. The terms antibody and immunoglobulin are often used interchangeably. They are found in blood and tissue fluids, as well as many secretions. The basic unit of each antibody is a monomer. An antibody can be monomeric, dimeric, trimeric, tetrameric, or pentameric. The monomer is composed of two heavy and two light chains. If it is cleaved with enzymes such as papain and pepsin, two Fab (fragment binding antigen) fragments and an Fc (fragment crystallizable) fragment are produced. They are formed in the humoral immune system by plasma cells, the end cell of B-lymphocyte transformation after recognition of a foreign antigen. There are five types of antibody found in the blood of higher vertebrates: IgA, IgD, IgE, IgG, and IgM. IgG is the commonest and the most frequently used antibody for immunohistochemistry. The IgG molecule is composed of two pairs of light and heavy polypeptide chains linked by disulfide bonds to form a Y-shaped structure. The terminal regions of each arm vary in amino acid sequence and are known as 'variable domains'. This variability in amino acid content provides specificity for a particular epitope and enables the antibody to bind specifically to the antigen against which it was raised.

Antibody-antigen binding

The amino acid side-chains of the variable domain of an antibody form a cavity which is geometrically and chemically complementary to a single type of antigen epitope as described by Capra and Edmundson in 1977. The analogy of a lock (antibody) and key (antigen) has been used, and the precise fit required explains the high degree of antibody-antigen specificity seen. The associated antibody and antigen are held together by a combination of hydrogen bonds, electrostatic interactions, and van der Waals' forces.

Affinity

Affinity is the three-dimensional fit of the antibody to its specific antigen and is a measure of the binding strength between the antigenic epitope and its specific antibody-combining site.

Avidity

Avidity is a related property referring to the heterogeneity of the antiserum which will contain various antibodies reacting with different epitopes of the antigen molecule. A specific but multivalent antibody is less likely to be removed by the washing process than a monovalent antibody. Avidity therefore is the functional combining strength of an antibody with its antigen.

Antibody specificity

This refers to the characteristics of an antibody to bind selectively to a single epitope on an antigen.

Sensitivity

This refers to the relative amount of antigen that an immunohistochemical technique is able to detect. A technique with high sensitivity is able to detect smaller amounts of antigen than a technique with low sensitivity. If used to detect the same amount of antigen, the technique with high sensitivity would produce a larger signal than a method with low sensitivity.

Production of primary reagents

Polyclonal antibodies

Polyclonal antibodies are produced by immunizing an animal with a purified specific molecule (immunogen) bearing the antigen of interest. The animal will mount a humoral response to the immunogen and the antibodies so produced can be harvested by bleeding the animal to obtain immunoglobulin-rich serum. It is likely that the animal will produce numerous clones of activated plasma cells (polyclonal). Each clone will produce an antibody with a slightly different specificity to the variety of epitopes present on the immunogen. A polyclonal antiserum is therefore a mixture of antibodies to different epitopes on the immunogen. Some of these antibodies may cross-react with other molecules and will need to be removed by absorption with the appropriate antigen. The antiserum will probably contain antibodies to impurities in the immunogen. Antibodies raised against the contaminating immunogens are often of low titer and affinity, and can be diluted out to zero activity for immunolabeling. In consequence of the high possibility of a wide spectrum of naturally occurring antibodies being present in the host animal in response to previous antigen challenges, serum removed from the animal before injection of the immunogen is important as a negative or pre-immune control. For precise details of polyclonal antibody production see De Mey and Moeremans (1986).

Monoclonal antibodies

The development of the hybridoma technique by Kohler and Milstein in 1975 to produce monoclonal antibodies has revolutionized immunohistochemistry by increasing enormously the range, quality, and quantity of specific antisera. Detailed descriptions of the technique have been given by Gatter et al. (1984) and Ritter (1986).

The method combines the ability of a plasma cell or transformed B lymphocyte to produce a specific antibody with the *in vitro* immortality of a neoplastic myeloma cell line; a hybrid with both properties can be produced. With the technique of cloning, this cell can be grown and multiplied in cell culture or ascitic fluid, theoretically to unlimited numbers. By careful screening, hybrids producing the antibodies of interest, without cross-reactivity to other molecules, can be chosen for cloning. The original antigen need not be pure, for hybrids reacting to unwanted antigens or epitopes can be eliminated during screening. The result is a constant, reliable supply of one pure antibody with known specificity.

This approach to the production of monoclonals has dramatically increased the number of antibodies available for immunohistochemistry and has allowed for further evolution with the ability to identify more antigens in paraffin sections. Detailed comparisons of the values and limitations of polyclonal and monoclonal antibodies have been given by Warnke et al. (1983) and Gatter et al. (1984).

Lectins

Lectins are plant or animal proteins that can bind to tissue carbohydrates with a high degree of specificity according to the lectin and the carbohydrate group (Brooks et al. 1996). Since the carbohydrates may be characteristic of a particular tissue, lectin binding may have diagnostic significance (Damjanov 1987). They can be labeled in similar ways to antibodies, or identified by using lectin-specific antibodies as secondary reagents (Leatham 1986).

Labels

Enzyme labels

Enzymes are the most widely used labels in immunohistochemistry, and incubation with a chromogen using a standard histochemical method produces a stable, colored reaction end-product suitable for the light microscope. In addition, the variety of enzymes and chromogens available allow the user a choice of color for the reaction end-product.

Horseradish peroxidase is the most widely used enzyme, and in combination with the most favored chromogen, i.e. 3,3α-diaminobenzidene tetrahydrochloride (DAB), it yields a crisp, insoluble, stable, dark brown reaction end-product (Graham & Karnovsky 1966). Although DAB has been reported to be a potential carcinogen, the risk is now thought to be low (Weisburger et al. 1978).

Horseradish peroxidase is commonly used as an antibody label for several reasons:

- Its small size does not hinder the binding of antibodies to adjacent sites.
- The enzyme is easily obtainable in a highly purified form and therefore the chance of contamination is minimized.
- It is a stable enzyme and remains unchanged during manufacture, storage, and application.
- Endogenous activity is easily quenched.

Other chromogens are available, including: 3-amino-9-ethylcarbazole (Graham et al. 1965; Kaplow 1975), which gives a red final reaction product; 4-chloro-1-naphthol (Nakane 1968), producing a blue final reaction product; Hanker-Yates reagent (Hanker et al. 1977), producing a dark blue product; and α-naphthol pyronin (Taylor & Burns 1974), which produces a red-purple final reaction product.

Commercially available chromogens are available in kit form. For example Vector Laboratories produce a wide range of different colored chromogens such as Vector Red, Vector Blue, Vector VIP (purple) and BCIP/NBT(blue/violet) suitable as alternatives to DAB and more commonly for multi-labeling techniques.

It should be noted that some of these chromogens produce reaction products which are soluble in alcohol and xylene, and therefore the sections require aqueous mounting. Whilst neutral phosphate-buffered glycerin jelly is one of the more traditional aqueous media, other commercial products are now available that have improved preservation qualities and resolution compared with the traditional aqueous mountants. After drying in a hot oven, these mountants give a hard permanent covering of the section. For long-term storage it is advisable additionally to use a coverslip and resinous mountant on top of the hardened aqueous mountant. Commercially available permanent mounting media that are non-aqueous and both toluene- and xylene-free are also available (Vector Laboratories VectaMount TM) and they provide a permanent preparation for use with enzyme substrates such as Vector Red, Vector VIP and BCIP/NBT.

Endogenous peroxidase activity is present in a number of sites, particularly neutrophil polymorphs and other myeloid cells. Blocking procedures may be required, the hydrogen peroxide-methanol method (Streefkerk 1972) being the most popular. However, care should be taken with certain antigens – notably CD4, where too long an incubation in the blocking solution or too high a concentration of hydrogen peroxide can significantly diminish staining on formalin-fixed paraffin-embedded tissue. Performing the peroxidase block after the binding of the primary antibody to the tissue antigen is to be recommended for antibodies such as CD4.

Calf intestinal alkaline phosphatase is the most widely used alternative enzyme tracer to horseradish peroxidase, particularly since the development of the alkaline phosphatase-anti-alkaline phosphatase (APAAP) method in 1984 by Cordell et al. Fast red TR used with naphthol AS-MX phosphate sodium salt gives a bright red reaction end-product that is soluble in alcohol. New fuchsin has been reported as giving a permanent insoluble red product (Malik & Daymon 1982) when mounted in resinous mountant, but it is the experience of many workers in the field that the resistance of the reaction product to resinous mounting is inconsistent.

Endogenous alkaline phosphatase activity is usually blocked by the addition of levamisole to the substrate solution. Levamisole selectively inhibits certain types of alkaline phosphatase, but not intestinal or placental when used at a concentration of 1 mM. Twenty percent glacial acetic acid is a better blocker of endogenous alkaline phosphatase activity as it inhibits all types of alkaline phosphatase.

Some workers use glucose oxidase as a tracer and it can be developed to give a navy blue reaction (Suffin et al. 1979). This label lends itself to immunohistochemistry on animal tissue, as there is no endogenous enzyme activity in animals.

Bacterial-derived β-D-galactosidase has also been used as a tracer and can be developed using the indigogenic method to give a permanent turquoise-blue reaction end-product (Bondi et al. 1982). Endogenous enzyme activity is not a problem as the endogenous mammalian enzyme has a different optimum pH from the tracer enzyme.

As described, commercial companies have produced a range of different substrate kits, especially for peroxidase and alkaline phosphatase. Many of these not only produce reaction products that are resistant to organic solvents but also provide a range of contrasting colors for multi-labeling techniques.

Colloidal metal labels

When used alone, colloidal gold conjugates appear pink when viewed using the light microscope. A silver precipitation reaction can be used to amplify the visibility of the gold conjugates (Holgate et al. 1983a). In addition, both gold and silver-enhanced gold conjugates can be visually emphasized using polarized incident light (epi-illumination) microscopy (Ellis et al. 1988) (Fig. 18.4a, b).

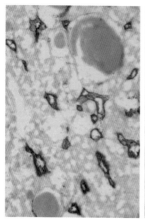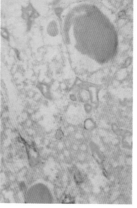

a   b
Figure 18.4 (a) Endothelial cells demonstrated by the immunogold silver staining method; (b) viewed by epi-polarized illumination.

Silver may also be used as a conjugate, and it gives a yellow color that is visible directly (Roth 1982). Other metals such as ferritin may be used, but they have not found wide usage among immunohistochemists using light microscope techniques. Colloidal gold has much wider usage with the electron microscope.

Fluorescent labels

These are discussed in detail in Chapter 19.

Radiolabels

The use of radioisotopes as tracers requires autoradiographic facilities, and developed from the need for quantitation in immunohistochemistry. Internally labeled antibodies are not widely available and labeling, at present, often limits the activity of the antibody. Techniques involving the use of radioisotopes as tracers have been discussed by Hunt et al. (1986).

Immunohistochemical methods

There are numerous immunohistochemical staining techniques that may be used to localize and demonstrate tissue antigens. The selection of a suitable technique should be based on parameters such as the type of specimen under investigation, the type of preparation under investigation (e.g., frozen sections, paraffin sections, resin sections or cytological preparations) and the degree of sensitivity required.

Traditional direct technique

The primary antibody is conjugated directly to the label. The conjugate may be either a fluorochrome (more commonly) or an enzyme (Fig. 18.5a). The labeled antibody reacts directly with the antigen in the histological or cytological preparation. The technique is quick and easy to use. However, it provides little signal amplification and lacks the sensitivity achieved by other techniques. Its use is mainly confined to the demonstration of immunoglobulin and complement in frozen sections of skin and renal

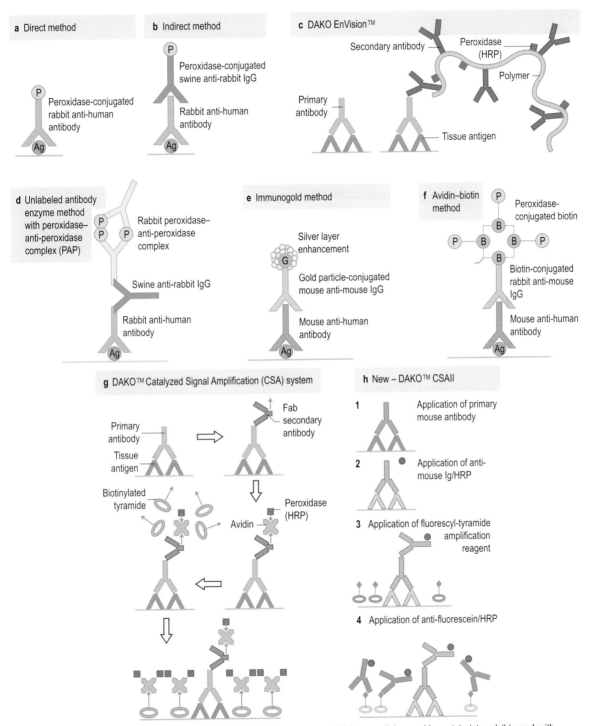

Figure 18.5 Schematic representation of immunohistochemical techniques. HRP, horseradish peroxidase. (c), (g) and (h) used with permission from Dakocytomation™ Systems.

biopsies. Low levels of antigen present in certain tumors may not be demonstrated by this technique and this could be crucial to an accurate and comprehensive diagnosis.

Two-step indirect technique

A labeled secondary antibody directed against the immunoglobulin of the animal species in which the primary antibody has been raised (Fig. 18.5b) visualizes an unlabeled primary antibody. Horseradish peroxidase labeling is most commonly used, together with an appropriate chromogen substrate. The method is more sensitive than the traditional direct technique because multiple secondary antibodies may react with different antigenic sites on the primary antibody, thereby increasing the signal amplification. The technique offers versatility in that the same labeled secondary antibody can be used with a variety of primary antibodies raised from the same animal species.

Polymer chain two-step indirect technique

This technology uses an unconjugated primary antibody, followed by a secondary antibody conjugated to an enzyme (horseradish peroxidase) labeled polymer (dextran) chain (Fig. 18.5c). This dextran chain has up to 70 enzyme molecules and 10 antibody molecules attached. Conjugation of both anti-mouse and anti-rabbit secondary antibodies enables the same reagent to be used for both monoclonal (rabbit and mouse) and polyclonal (rabbit) primary antibodies. The method is biotin free and therefore does not react with endogenous biotin. In addition to being quick, reliable, and easily reproducible, the technique offers great sensitivity. The technique is also useful for multi-color staining on single slide preparations. This technique is probably the most commonly used method in routine diagnostic use. There is a wide choice of commercially available polymer kits including EnVision™+ and FLEX+ from Dako, Novolink and Bond Polymer Refine from Leica, Immpress™ from Vector Laboratories, Excel + from Menarini and ultraVIEW from Ventana.

Unlabeled antibody-enzyme complex techniques (PAP and APAAP)

The original immunoenzyme bridge method using enzyme-specific antibody (Mason et al. 1969; Sternberger 1969) was rapidly superseded by an improved version using a soluble peroxidase-antiperoxidase complex (PAP) (Sternberger et al. 1970). These complexes are formed from three peroxidase molecules and two anti-peroxidase antibodies (Fig. 18.5d), and are used as a third layer in the staining method. They are bound to the unconjugated primary antibody, e.g. rabbit anti-human IgG, by a second layer of 'bridging' antibody that is usually a swine anti-rabbit applied in excess so that one of its two identical binding sites binds to the primary antibody and the other to the rabbit PAP complex.

Alkaline phosphatase antibodies raised in the mouse, by the same principle, can be used to form the alkaline phosphatase-anti-alkaline phosphatase complexes (APAAP). This method, first developed by Cordell et al. in 1984, lends itself to amplification by further application of the bridge and APAAP reagent. For unknown reasons, this form of amplification with the APAAP is not so successful with the PAP technique, and excessive background can sometimes be a serious drawback. These techniques have largely been replaced by streptavidin/biotin methods or polymer-based techniques.

Immunogold silver staining technique (IGSS)

The use of colloidal gold as a label for immunohistochemistry was introduced by Faulk and Taylor (1971). It can be used in both direct and indirect methods and has found wide usage in ultrastructural immunolocalization. It is not widely used in light microscope immunohistochemistry even after the advantages of silver development reported by Holgate et al. (1983a). In this method the gold particles are enhanced by the addition of metallic silver layers (Fig. 18.5e) to produce a metallic silver precipitate which overlays the colloidal gold marker and which can be seen with the light microscope. The technique uses silver lactate as the ion supplier and hydroquinone as the reducing agent in a protective colloid of gum arabic at pH 3.5. In some instances section pretreatment with Lugol's iodine and sodium after dewaxing and rehydration may be required to improve staining intensity. The method is generally accepted to be more sensitive than the PAP technique, but suffers from the formation of fine silver deposits in the background, especially in inexperienced hands. It can be confusing when trying to identify small amounts of antigen. Modifications to the original technique have been reviewed by De Mey et al. (1986).

(Strept) avidin-biotin techniques

Together with the indirect polymer-based techniques, the labeled streptavidin-biotin technique is the most widely used methodology in diagnostic immunohistochemistry. This is a three-step technique, which has an unconjugated primary antibody as the first layer, followed by a biotinylated secondary antibody (raised against the species of the primary animal). The third layer is either a complex of enzyme-labeled biotin and streptavidin, or enzyme-labeled streptavidin (Fig. 18.5f). The enzyme can be either horseradish peroxidase or alkaline phosphatase, used with a chromogen of choice.

These methods rely on the marked affinity of the basic glycoprotein avidin (MW 67 kDa) for the small (MW 244 Da) water-soluble vitamin biotin. However, avidin has two distinct disadvantages when used in immunohistochemistry. It has a high isoelectric point of approximately 10 and is therefore positively charged at neutral pH. As a result, it may bind non-specifically to certain negatively charged structures such as cell nuclei. Avidin, being a glycoprotein, also has a tendency to react with lectins via the carbohydrate moiety, again causing non-specific staining. These problems can be overcome by the substitution of streptavidin (MW 60 kDa) for avidin. Streptavidin has now largely replaced the use of avidin in immunohistochemical detection techniques.

Streptavidin can be isolated from the bacterium *Streptomyces avidini*, and like avidin it has four high-affinity binding sites for biotin. However, in practice due to the molecular arrangement of these binding sites, fewer than four biotin molecules actually bind.

Biotin (vitamin H) is easily conjugated to antibodies and enzyme markers. Up to 150 biotin molecules can be attached to one antibody molecule, often with the aid of spacer arms. By spacing the biotins, the large streptavidin has room to bind and maximize its strong affinity for biotin. The streptavidin-biotin technique can employ either enzyme label bound directly to the streptavidin (Guesden et al. 1979); alternatively, the enzymes are biotinylated and the biotinylated label, forming the streptavidin-biotin complex (Hsu et al. 1981), occupies 75% of the streptavidin-binding sites. Usually the latter is commercially supplied as two separate reagents, biotinylated label and streptavidin, and they are added together 30 minutes before use in order for the complex to form fully. Careful stoichiometric control ensures that some binding sites remain free to bind with the biotinylated secondary antibody. As a large number of biotins can be attached to a single antibody, then numerous labeled streptavidin molecules may be bound on top. This produces increased sensitivity compared to the previously described enzyme techniques and allows a higher dilution of the primary antibody. Tissues rich in endogenous biotin such as liver and kidney will require the use of an avidin/biotin block before applying the primary antibody.

Hapten labeling technique

Bridging techniques using haptens such as dinitrophenol and arsanilic acid have been advocated (Jasani et al. 1981, 1992). In this technique, the hapten is linked to the primary antibody and a complex is built up using an anti-hapten antibody and either hapten-labeled enzyme or hapten-labeled PAP complex.

Biotinylated tyramide signal amplification

Bobrow et al. first described the use of biotinylated tyramide to enhance signal amplification, in 1989. Subsequent work by Adams in 1992 and King et al. in 1997 enabled the development of a highly sensitive detection system. In conjunction with heat-induced epitope retrieval techniques, the use of biotinylated tyramide amplification enabled many antigens which had previously been unreactive in formalin-fixed paraffin-embedded tissue to be demonstrated. Antibodies could be used at far greater dilutions than in conventional techniques. The biotinylated tyramide amplification reagent was first available commercially from DuPont; this was subsequently followed by the CSA (Catalyzed Signal Amplification) kit from Dako.

The technique is based around the streptavidin-biotin technique. Application of the primary antibody is followed by subsequent incubations in biotinylated secondary antibody and then either horseradish peroxidase-labeled streptavidin or streptavidin-biotin-horseradish peroxidase complex. The critical stage is the subsequent treatment with the biotinylated tyramide amplification reagent. The bound peroxidase label in the presence of hydrogen peroxide catalyses the biotinyl tyramide to form free biotin radicals. These reactive biotin molecules bind covalently to proteins adjacent to the site of the reaction. Further incubation in either horseradish peroxidase-labeled streptavidin or streptavidin-biotin-horseradish peroxidase complex results in additional enzyme being deposited at the site of the reaction (Fig. 18.5g).

The technique does have certain disadvantages. Excessive background staining can be problematic, especially in tissues rich in endogenous biotin, although the use of a commercial avidin-biotin blocking kit reduces endogenous biotin demonstration. The incubation time in the biotinylated tyramide reagent is critical in preventing high background. Many users have experienced problems with consistency of results and reproducibility. Improved commercial reagents, in terms of antibodies and detection reagents, have now limited the impact and use of this technique. However, it still remains the method of choice for the demonstration of certain tissue antigens in formalin-fixed paraffin-embedded tissue and in formalin-fixed methyl methacrylate resin sections.

Biotin-free Catalyzed Signal Amplification (CSA II)

In an attempt to reduce the problems associated with endogenous biotin in conventional tyramide signal amplification, Dako produces a biotin-free system, available commercially as Catalyzed Signal Amplification system II (CSA II) for use with mouse monoclonal antibodies. Following incubation in primary antibody, a secondary anti-mouse immunoglobulin conjugated to horseradish peroxidase is bound to the primary antibody. The third layer involves peroxidase-catalyzed deposition of fluorescyl tyramide, which in turn is reacted with peroxidase conjugated anti-fluorescein, producing a greatly enhanced signal (Fig. 18.5h). This technique can be adapted easily to automated immunostaining protocols. Although a useful technique, in our hands the results fail to match the high sensitivity of conventional tyramide amplification.

Unmasking of antigen sites

A prerequisite for all routine histological and cytological investigations is to ensure preservation of tissue architecture and cell morphology by adequate and appropriate fixation (Chapter 4). The fixative of choice will depend on the individual laboratory; the most popular choice of fixatives for routine histology are formalin based, either as a 10% solution or with the addition of different chemical constituents. Prompt fixation of thin (3 mm) slices of tissue is essential to achieve consistent demonstration of tissue antigens. Delayed fixation or poor fixation may cause loss of antigenicity or diffusion of antigens into the surrounding tissue. Following fixation most material is routinely processed to paraffin wax to facilitate section cutting.

The concept that antigens can be masked by the chemical processes involved in formalin fixation and paraffin processing and that some form of unmasking of these antigens is required dates far back into the history of immunohistochemistry (Brandtzaeg 1983). The majority of antigen unmasking studies have been applied to formalin-fixed material. When formalin-based fixatives are used, intermolecular and intramolecular cross-linkages are formed with certain structural proteins. These are responsible for the masking of the tissue antigens. This adverse effect has been thought to be the result of the formation of methylene bridges between reactive sites on tissue proteins (Bell et al. 1987; Mason & O'Leary 1991). These reactive sites include primary amines, amide groups, thiols, alcoholic hydroxyl groups, and cyclic aromatic rings. The degree of masking of the antigenic sites depends upon the length of time in fixative, temperature, concentration of fixative, and availability of other nearby proteins able to undergo cross-linkage.

It must be remembered that tissue sections are unique to the laboratory of origin. Differences in the type and duration of fixation, together with variations in tissue processing schedules, reagents, and the manner by which sections are dried after microtomy, are important considerations. There are varying differences in the way these processes are performed by different laboratories. This lack of standardization of the basic processes of histology culminates in the production of a unique preparation. As a consequence, it is often found that one method of antigen unmasking may provide optimal results for one laboratory, but not for another. Therefore, each method of antigen unmasking should be carefully evaluated using the laboratory's own material. Indeed, digestion or heating times may need to be slightly modified to the times stated in antibody data sheets or published methodologies.

Most laboratories use automated immunohistochemical staining systems – some of which have the ability to perform on-board antigen retrieval, using either enzymes or more commonly heat. Most platforms offer the user the choice of two different antigen retrieval buffers (at different pH values) with variable heating times. Automated systems may also undertake the dewaxing, alcohol rinse and water wash steps prior to the antigen retrieval.

Manual methods for antigen unmasking include:

- Proteolytic enzyme digestion
- Microwave oven irradiation
- Combined microwave oven irradiation and proteolytic enzyme digestion
- Pressure cooker heating
- Decloaker heating
- Pressure cooker inside a microwave oven

- Autoclave heating
- Water bath heating
- Steamer heating

Before antigen unmasking pretreatments are employed, the sections are dewaxed, rinsed in alcohol, and washed in water.

Proteolytic enzyme digestion

Pretreating formalin-fixed routinely processed paraffin sections with proteolytic enzymes to unmask certain antigenic determinants was described by Huang et al. (1976), Curran and Gregory (1977), and Mepham et al. (1979). The most popular enzymes employed today are trypsin and protease, but other proteolytic enzymes such as chymotrypsin, pronase, proteinase K, and pepsin may also be used. The theory behind the unmasking properties of these proteolytic enzymes is not fully understood. Nevertheless, it is generally accepted that the digestion breaks down formalin cross-linking and hence the antigenic sites for a number of antibodies are uncovered.

For some antigens, proteolytic digestion can be detrimental to their demonstration, occasionally producing false-positive or false-negative results. Digestion times need to be tailored to individual antibodies and to fixation time. Under-digestion results in too little staining, because the antigens are not fully exposed. Over-digestion can produce false-positive staining, high background levels, and tissue damage. There can be a fine balance between under- and over-digestion when using proteolytic enzymes. Duration of enzyme digestion, enzyme concentration, use of a coenzyme, such as calcium chloride with trypsin, temperature, and pH must be optimized to produce consistent high-quality immunohistochemical staining. Different batches of enzyme may vary in quality and each new batch of enzyme should be tested prior to routine use. Enzymes produced specifically for immunohistochemical use are now widely available from commercial sources; these have been produced for use with automated immunostaining machines, are easy to use, and give good consistent results.

The use of heat-induced epitope retrieval techniques has largely replaced proteolytic digestion.

However, for the demonstration of immunoglobulins and complement in formalin-fixed paraffin-embedded renal biopsies and for a number of other individual antigens proteolytic digestion is still favored by many.

Heat-mediated antigen retrieval techniques

Heat-based antigen retrieval methods have brought a great improvement in the quality and reproducibility of immunohistochemistry. They have also widened its use as an important diagnostic tool in histopathology. The rationale behind the heat pretreatment methods is unclear and several different theories have been suggested. One of these is that heavy metal salts (as described by Shi et al. 1991) act as a protein precipitant, forming insoluble complexes with polypeptides, and that protein-precipitating fixatives display better preservation of antigens than do cross-linking aldehyde fixatives.

Another theory is that during formalin fixation intermolecular and methylene bridges and weak Schiff bases form intramolecular cross-linkages. These cross-linkages alter the protein conformation of the antigen, which may prevent it from being recognized by a specific antibody. It is postulated that heat-mediated antigen retrieval removes the weaker Schiff bases but does not affect the methylene bridges, so the resulting protein conformation is intermediate between fixed and unfixed.

Another possible theory was described by Morgan et al. (1997), who postulated that calcium coordination complexes formed during formalin fixation prevent antibodies from combining with epitopes on tissue-bound antigens. The underlying theory of calcium involvement is that hydroxymethyl groups and other unreacted oxygen-rich groups (e.g. carboxyl or phosphoryl groups) can interact with calcium ions to produce large coordinate complexes which can mask epitopic sites by steric hindrance. The high temperature weakens or breaks some of the calcium coordinate bonds, but the effect is reversible on cooling, because the calcium complex remains in its original position. The presence of a competing chelating agent at the particular temperature at which the coordinate bonds are

disrupted removes the calcium complexes. Evidence to support this theory comes from the chemical nature of some of the antigen retrieval reagents, such as citrate buffer and EDTA. In addition it has been shown that the inclusion of calcium ions with an unmasking reagent inhibits its effectiveness (Morgan et al. 1994).

Microwave antigen retrieval

Shi et al. (1991) first established the use of microwave heating for antigen retrieval. However, the use of heavy metal salts posed a significant risk to the health and safety of the users. Gerdes et al. (1992) used microwave antigen retrieval with a non-toxic citrate buffer at pH 6.0 and demonstrated the Ki67 antigen, which had previously thought to be lost during formalin fixation and paraffin processing. The results were equivalent to those seen in frozen sections. Cattoretti et al. (1993) established microwave oven heating as an alternative to proteolytic enzyme digestion. The method improved the demonstration of well-established antibodies such as CD45 and CD20 and enabled the demonstration of a wide range of new antibodies, such as CD8 and p53.

Numerous antigen retrieval solutions have been described; probably the most popular are 0.01 M citrate buffer at pH 6.0 and 0.1 mM EDTA at pH 8.0. Although an expanding range of commercially available antigen buffers at both high and low pH ranges is available, some are designed to improve the staining of specific antigens.

Most domestic microwave ovens are suitable for antigen retrieval and operate at 2.45 GHz, corresponding to a wavelength *in vacuo* of 12.2 cm (Fig. 18.6). Uneven heating and the production of hot spots have been reported by some workers using the microwave oven. However, by using a volume of buffer between 400 and 600 ml in a suitably sized microwave-resistant plastic container, the problems of uneven heating may be minimized. A batch of 25 slides in a plastic staining rack can be irradiated at one time and accurate, even antigen retrieval achieved. The actual heating time will depend on the following factors:

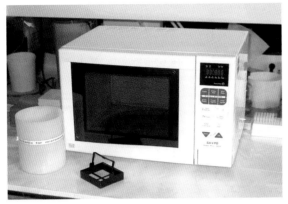

Figure 18.6 Domestic microwave oven.

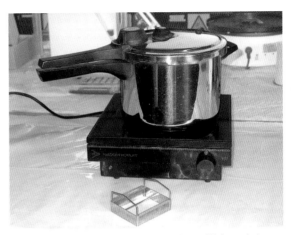

Figure 18.7 Stainless steel pressure cooker and halogen hot plate.

- Wattage of the oven. Most domestic ovens use a magnetron with an output between 750 and 1000 W. An important point to remember is that the output of the magnetron will decrease with age and frequency of use. The magnetron should be checked for efficiency annually.
- Choice of antigen retrieval buffer.
- Volume of buffer being used.
- Fixation of the tissues under investigation, in terms of fixative used and duration of fixation. This is an important factor, although not as critical as when using proteolytic enzyme digestion. Tissue fixed for extended periods of time will require extended irradiation times. Conversely, poorly fixed tissues may require a reduction in the heating time.
- Thickness of the tissue section: 3 μm sections require less antigen retrieval than 5 μm sections.
- Antigen to be demonstrated. Certain nuclear antigens may require increased heating times.

If extended heating times are used with a small volume of buffer, the buffer may need topping up with distilled or de-ionized water. This should be performed half-way through the total heating duration. At no stage should the sections be allowed to dry out during the antigen retrieval.

Pressure cooker antigen retrieval

Norton et al. (1994) suggested the use of the pressure cooker as an alternative to the microwave oven.

By using the pressure cooker, Norton et al. (1994) provided evidence that the batch variation and production of hot and cold spots in the microwave oven could be overcome. Pressure cooking is said to be more uniform than other heating methods. A pressure cooker at 15 psi (10.3 kPa) reaches a temperature of around 120°C at full pressure. It is this increased temperature that appears to be a major advantage when unmasking certain nuclear tissue antigens such as bcl-6, p53, p21, estrogen receptor, and progesterone receptor. The demonstration of these antigens can sometimes be weak when using microwave antigen retrieval.

It is preferable to use a stainless steel domestic pressure cooker, because aluminum pressure cookers are susceptible to corrosion from some of the antigen retrieval buffers (Fig. 18.7). The pressure cooker should have a capacity of 4–5 liters, thus allowing a large batch of slides to be treated at the same time. As with the microwave oven, the use of Superfrost Plus microscope slides or strong adhesives such as Vectabond or APES is required.

Steamer

Although quite a popular method in some parts of the world, steam heating appears to be less efficient than either microwave oven heating or pressure cooking (Pasha et al. 1995). Times in excess of 40 minutes are sometimes required, but the method does have the advantage in being less damaging to tissues than the other heating methods. Commercially available rice steamers are adequate for this purpose.

Water bath

Kawai et al. (1994) demonstrated that a water bath set at 90°C was adequate for antigen retrieval. However, by increasing the temperature to 95–98°C, antigen retrieval was improved and the incubation times could be decreased. The technique has the advantage of being gentler on the tissue sections because the temperature is set below boiling point. By using a lower temperature than other heating methods the antigen retrieval buffer does not evaporate and expensive commercial antigen retrieval solutions can be safely reused. The method has the disadvantage in that the antigen retrieval times are increased compared to other methods. This method is recommended with the Dako Hercept test for HER2 expression.

Autoclave

This method offers an alternative form of heat-mediated antigen retrieval, producing good results for nuclear antigens such as MIB1, p21, and p53.

Combined microwave antigen retrieval and trypsin digestion

This methodology is infrequently used today; brief proteolytic digestion can be carried out before or after microwave irradiation. Time trials need to be undertaken to ascertain the optimal pretreatment times; certainly, drastically reduced digestion times are required to prevent over-digestion of the tissue section.

Advantages of heat pretreatment

Some antigens previously thought lost in routinely processed paraffin-embedded sections are now recovered by heat pretreatment. Many antigens are retrieved by uniform heating times, regardless of length of fixation: e.g., up to several weeks in formal saline (Singh et al. 1993). The demonstration of heavy-chain immunoglobulins is more reliable and reproducible than when proteolytic digestion is employed. The dilution factors of some primary antibodies ascertained with traditional methods can be increased when using heat pretreatment.

Pitfalls of heat pretreatment

Care should be taken not to allow the sections to dry after heating, as this destroys antigenicity. The boiling of poorly fixed material also damages nuclear detail. Fibrous and fatty tissues tend to detach from the slide. This can sometimes be overcome by increasing the drying temperature to 56°C and using Superfrost Plus microscope slides. Alternatively, Vectabond or APES-coated slides can be dipped in 10% formal saline for 1–2 minutes and air dried before picking up the sections. This tends to improve the adhesion, probably by adding more aldehyde groups to the slide surface.

Not all antigens are retrieved by heat pretreatment, and the range of staining of some primary antibodies, for example PGP9.5, a neuroendocrine marker, is altered (Langlois et al. 1994).

Commercial antigen retrieval solutions

There are numerous commercial antigen retrieval solutions available. They can be either specialized high pH solutions (recommended for certain antibodies) or lower pH 6.0 for more general use. These solutions may be a mixture of different chemicals, such as citrate and EDTA. They offer advantages over the 'in house' retrieval solutions, in that they are ready to use, require no pH calibration, and are fully certified to comply with laboratory accreditation procedures. However, they can be expensive.

Most automated immunohistochemical staining systems employ commercial antigen retrieval buffers. As previously stated, these will be a high pH reagent and a lower more neutral pH.

There is an ever-growing range of antibodies available. Table 18.1 is intended as a guide only. Individual laboratories need to choose their preferred supplier and finalize the optimum dilutions

Table 18.1 Antibody clones/dilution chart

Antibody	Clone	Species	Supplier	Dilution
α1-Antichymotrypsin	–	Poly	Dako	1/100
α1-Antitrypsin	–	Poly	Dako	1/4000
α1-Fetoprotein	–	Poly	Dako	1/800
α1-Synuclein	KM51	M	Leica	1/50
Androgen receptor	AR441	M	Dako	1/50
Alzheimer precursor protein	22C11	M	Chemicon	1/2500
AUA	AUA-1	M	Skybio	1/100
ACTH	02A3	M	Dako	1/50
AE1	AE1	M	Biogenex	1/50
AE1 + AE3	AE1/3	M	Biogenex	1/100
Alk protein	ALK-1	M	Dako	1/50
Amyloid P component	–	Poly	Dako	1/2000
Bcl-2	124	M	Dako	1/100
Bcl-6	564	M	Leica	1/20
Ber EP4	Ber EP4	M	Dako	1/200
BOB-1	–	Poly	Santa Cruz	1/500
CA125	OV185H	M	Leica	1/100
Calcitonin	–	Poly	Dako	1/300
Caldesmon	h-CD	M	Dako	1/100
Calponin	CALP	M	Dako	1/100
CD1a	010	M	Immunotech	1/20
CD2	271	M	Leica	1/100
CD3	PS1	M	Leica	1/50
CD4	1F6	M	Leica	1/50
CD5	4C7	M	Leica	1/50
CD7	272	M	Leica	1/100
CD8	C8/144B	M	Dako	1/100
CD10	270	M	Leica	1/20
CD15	LeuM1	M	Becton Dickinson	1/50
CD20	L26	M	Dako	1/200
CD21	2G9	M	Leica	1/50
CD23	1B12	M	Leica	1/50
CD30	Ber-H2	M	Dako	1/50
CD31	JC70	M	Dako	1/50
CD34	Qbend 10	M	Dako	1/100
CD43	DF-T1	M	Dako	1/50

Table 18.1 *(continued)*

Antibody	Clone	Species	Supplier	Dilution
CD45	2B11 + PD7/26	M	Dako	1/200
CD45RA	4KB5	M	Dako	1/50
CD45RO	UCHL1	M	Dako	1/100
CD56	1B6	M	Leica	1/100
CD63	1/C3	M	Leica	1/50
CD68	PGM-1	M	Dako	1/200
CD71	309	M	Leica	1/10
CD75	LN-1	M	Leica	1/20
CD79a	JCB117	M	Dako	1/100
CD83	1H4b	M	Leica	1/50
CD99	12E7	M	Dako	1/50
CD117	–	Poly	Dako	1/200
CD138	MI 15	M	ABD Serotec	1/200
CEA	5A	M	Dako	1/600
c-erb B2	–	Poly	Dako	1/800
Chromogranin A	–	Poly	Dako	1/5000
CK7	OV-TL 12/30	M	Dako	1/100
CK14	LL002	M	Leica	1/50
CK20	Ks20.8	M	Dako	1/100
CK8/18	5D3	M	Leica	1/500
Cytokeratin	CAM5.2	M	Becton Dickinson	1/20
Cytokeratin	MNF116	M	Dako	1/100
Cytokeratin	LP34	M	Dako	1/10
Cyclin D1	SP4	M*	Labvision	1/20
Desmin	D33	M	Dako	1/200
Epithelial membrane antigen	E29	M	Dako	1/500
EGFR	113	M	Leica	1/100
Estrogen receptor	6F11	M	Leica	1/30
Factor VIII	–	Poly	Dako	1/2000
Fascin	5SK-2	M	Dako	1/500
FSH	C10	M	Dako	1/100
GFAP	–	Poly	Dako	1/300
Growth hormone	–	Poly	Dako	1/300
Glucagon	–	Poly	Dako	1/1500
Glycophorin C	Ret 40f	M	Dako	1/200
Granzyme B	Grb-7	M	Dako	1/25

Table 18.1 (continued)				
Antibody	**Clone**	**Species**	**Supplier**	**Dilution**
HLA-DR	TAL-1B5	M	Dako	1/100
H. pylori	–	Poly	Dako	1/200
IgA	–	Poly	Dako	1/800
IgD	–	Poly	Dako	1/200
IgG	–	Poly	Dako	1/1000
IgM	–	Poly	Dako	1/500
Kappa	–	Poly	Dako	1/2000
Lambda	–	Poly	Dako	1/2000
LMP-1	CS1-4	M	Dako	1/100
Lysozyme	–	Poly	Dako	1/1000
Mast cell tryptase	AA1	M	Dako	1/1000
Melanoma monoclonal	HMB45	M	Dako	1/50
Mesothelial cell	HBME-1	M	Dako	1/100
MIB1	Ki67	M	Dako	1/200
Myeloperoxidase	–	Poly	Dako	1/4000
MUM-1	Mum1p	M	Dako	1/50
MyoD1	5.8A	M	Dako	1/50
Myogenin	F5D	M	Dako	1/50
NFP	ZF11	M	Dako	1/250
OCT-2	–	Poly	Santa Cruz	1/500
PAX-5	24	M	Becton Dickinson	1/250
Progesterone receptor	PgR636	M	Dako	1/100
p21	SX118	M	Dako	1/15
p53	DO-7	M	Dako	1/40
PGP9.5	–	Poly	Dako	1/500
PLAP	–	Poly	Dako	1/100
PSAP	PASE/4LJ	M	Dako	1/1000
PSA	–	Poly	Dako	1/1000
PU-1	G148-74	M	Becton Dickinson	1/100
S100	–	Poly	Dako	1/250
Smooth muscle actin	1A4	M	Dako	1/150
Synaptophysin	Sy38	M	Dako	1/100
Tau	–	Poly	Dako	1/1500
Tdt	SEN28	M	Leica	1/100
TIA-1	2G9	M	Immunotech	1/100
TSH	0042	M	Dako	1/100

Table 18.1 (continued)				
Antibody	**Clone**	**Species**	**Supplier**	**Dilution**
TTF-1	8G7G3/1	M	Dako	1/50
Thyroglobulin	–	Poly	Dako	1/5000
Ubiquitin	–	Poly	Dako	1/1000
Vasointestinal polypeptide	–	Poly	Leica	1/200
Vimentin	V9	M	Dako	1/500
Zap-70	2F3.2	M	Upstate	1/100

M = monoclonal antibody, M* = rabbit monoclonal, Poly = polyclonal antibody.

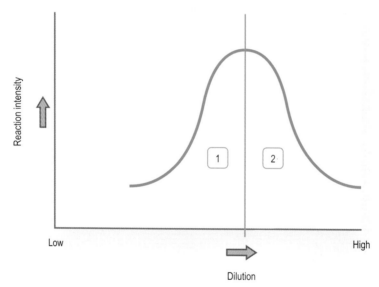

Figure 18.8 Antibody dilution curve.

based on their own sections and the techniques/automation appropriate to their laboratory.

Detection of low levels of antigen

Enhancement and amplification

The optimum dilution of primary antibody for diagnostic immunohistochemistry is defined as the concentration of the primary antibody which gives the optimal specific staining with the least amount of background staining. The optimal dilution will depend upon the type and duration of fixation. Serial dilutions of antibody will often give the distribution of reactivity shown in Figure 18.8.

Poor reaction in area 1 is due to steric hindrance of the labeling antibody accessing the primary antibody (the prozone effect). This is due to the primary antibody being used too concentrated.

Suboptimal reaction in area 2 is caused by inadequate presence of primary antibody: i.e. the primary antibody used is too diluted.

The optimum concentration of primary antibody is that measured below the apex of the peak and the use of several control sections with varying expression of antigen will aid the determination of a correct working dilution of primary antibody for that particular laboratory. Interlaboratory variations in the choice of fixative, duration of fixation, paraffin processing, section treatment, and the immunohistochemical detection system used make this dilution of primary antibody unique to the laboratory that produced the paraffin section and accounts for the great variation in the dilution of primary antibodies used from laboratory to laboratory.

The dilutions of primary antibodies and labeling systems for diagnostic immunohistochemistry should be ascertained on material where the antigen levels are adequate but not excessive. Occasionally situations arise where some tumors shed much of their antigen, e.g., prostatic tumors often express less prostate-specific antigen than normal prostatic glands. Enhancement and amplification by modification of demonstration techniques may be required to identify low levels of antigens. This can be achieved by the following methods:

1. Increasing the concentration of the primary antibody. Usually this can be accomplished with most monoclonals without increasing the background staining significantly, as this type of antibody, especially in the form of tissue culture supernatant, does not contain any non-specific contaminants. Polyclonal antibodies can give excessive background problems and it is advisable to use a casein blocking solution as described in the methods later in this chapter. Sometimes the addition of a small amount of detergent, e.g. 0.01% Tween, to the washes helps to reduce background staining. Further details on dealing with background appear later in the text.

2. Prolonging incubation with the primary antibody overnight, at 4–8°C or at ambient temperature, can enhance staining. Many immunohistochemists employ this methodology for their routine work because higher dilution of primary reagents is achieved, allowing costs to be reduced. Dilutions must not be excessive, otherwise low levels of

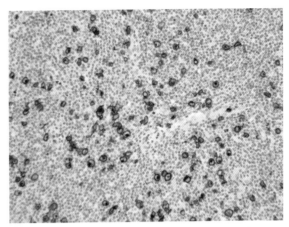

Figure 18.9 CD15 demonstration in a formalin-fixed paraffin-embedded section of Hodgkin's disease.

antigen will not be detected, resulting in false-negative staining.

3. Increasing the concentration of bridge reagent beyond the optimal dilution, or repeated application of the bridge reagent, marginally increases the sensitivity of the avidin-biotin systems. Furthermore, in the case of the CD15 primaries, which are IgM subclass antibodies, LeBrun et al. (1992) reported that an IgM link, as opposed to a broad-spectrum immunoglobulin bridge reagent, improves the rate of detecting CD15-positive Reed-Sternberg and Hodgkin cells (Fig. 18.9). Charalambous et al. not only confirmed this work in 1993, but they also indicated that when microwave antigen recovery was used in place of trypsin, further amplification was achieved.

4. Chemical enhancement of the reaction end-product of the peroxidase-diaminobenzidine method can be achieved by the addition of imidazole (Straus 1982), heavy metals such as copper or cobalt (Hsu & Soban 1982), osmication, or treatment with gold chloride. Colloidal gold labeling can be enhanced dramatically using silver salts with the IGSS technique (Holgate et al. 1983b).

5. Repeated applications of the bridge and label increase the sensitivity of the APAAP technique. Whilst the initial primary, bridge and label are incubated for 30 minutes each, the

repeated applications of bridge and label require only 10 minutes each. After two such repeats enhancement is usually sufficient for most antibodies.

6. Changing the chromogen substrate used. Some chromogen substrate solutions, especially for alkaline phosphatase, give a more intense reaction product than other reagents. For example nitro-blue tetrazolium is not only more intense than fast red but also can be left on overnight to give probably the most intense reaction of all chromogens available today. The only drawback is that the blue-black reaction product does not contrast well with hematoxylin counterstaining. Improved commercial formulae of traditional substrates are superior to 'in house' formulae.

7. Techniques for elevating the sensitivity of the extended polymer-labeled antibodies and other pre-diluted reagents are more restricted. The disadvantage of pre-diluted antibodies is that the dilutions selected are not necessarily suitable for the multitude of fixation and processing protocols employed. Hence, weak staining can only be overcome by increasing the incubation times, elevating the temperature to 37°C, or chemical enhancement of the diaminobenzidine reaction product, or other appropriate substrate.

8. Tyramide signal amplification. In 1989, Bobrow and fellow workers described a novel signal amplification method, catalyzed reporter deposition, and its application to immunoassays. In 1992 the same group proposed that this method would be suitable for immunohistochemistry. Erber et al. and King et al. in 1997 quite independently published data showing that this novel signal amplification system employed with avidin-biotin systems showed greater sensitivity than that provided by the more conventional avidin-biotin methods.

Multiple labeling techniques

The ability to label two or more different antigens in the same tissue section is playing a greater role

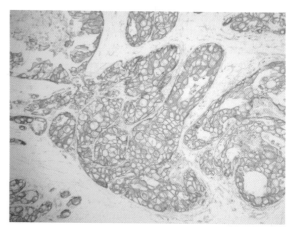

Figure 18.10 Double immunohistochemical staining of formalin-fixed paraffin-embedded section of breast carcinoma shows HER2 membrane staining with DAB as the chromogen and smooth muscle actin stained with Vector SG chromogen.

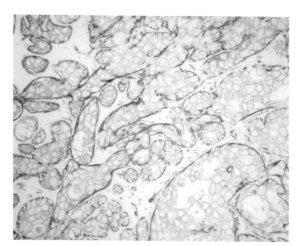

Figure 18.11 Double immunohistochemical staining shows the smooth muscle actin demonstrated with DAB and the HER2 with Vector SG.

in routine immunocytochemistry (Figs 18.10 and 18.11). The use of automated immunocytochemistry staining systems, a greater range of substrate chromogens and the use of commercially available double labeling kits has provided a much more robust method than was previously available. The user has the choice of using the same detection system with different substrates, or of using different detection systems for individual substrates.

The methodology involves sequential staining of each of the primary antibodies; practice will help the user determine the optimum order of labeling and the optimum substrates/chromogens to use. It is generally recognized that the primary antibody that gives the strongest final reaction product should be performed first (often with a DAB chromogen) followed by the weaker reaction. The choice of different enzyme-substrate combinations is important, as certain combinations work better and offer more contrast than others. The range of commercially available substrates from Vector Laboratories provides a wide choice. For example, when using alkaline phosphatase methods, the use of Vector Blue as the first substrate layer contrasts well when using Vector Red as the second substrate. For peroxidase methods the use of DAB as the first substrate contrasts well with Vector VIP as the second substrate.

Automation lends itself well to multiple labeling and this is facilitated by the availability of double labeling kits; e.g. Dako Envision™ DuoFLEX Doublestain system (HRP/AP) or the use of Leica Bond polymer Refine (DAB) with Bond Polymer Refine Red.

Immunohistochemistry in practice

Workload

As a result of heat antigen retrieval methods, there has been a continual increase in the numbers of antibodies effective on paraffin sections. Many of these antibodies can have a direct impact on diagnosis, prognosis, or treatment. As a consequence, the immunohistochemist is often overwhelmed with requests and either additional staff or automation are sought to cope with the increasing demand. If automation is selected, it does not mean that the immunohistochemist loses control of the activity. On the contrary, automation usually allows the immunohistochemist time to develop the service and improve the staining of some antigens. Increased workloads necessitate the use of automated immunostaining; this has brought about high productivity (with runs being performed overnight), quality assurance (logs of the staining runs readily

accessible) and reproducible high-quality immunostaining. Selection of a suitable autostainer should take into account factors such as:

- Capacity
- Flexibility
- Reliability
- Ease of use
- Cost per slide

It is highly recommended to trial the different autostainer options, and assess them with the laboratory's own material and their routine panels. Staining protocols are likely to need fine adjustment; automated immunostainers rarely give optimum demonstration at the first time of asking. Prioritization of the automated immunostainer criteria will differ between diagnostic and research facilities. The laboratory will need to decide between outright purchase, lease of the equipment or a reagent rental deal. Each method has its advantages and disadvantages. Purchase involves one payment but does not include maintenance (after the initial warranty) or replacement costs. Leasing of the equipment or a reagent rental deal will cover the maintenance costs and equipment is replaced as required. However, the cost of the latter two options is generally greater per slide.

Choice of technique

The choice of technique to suit the needs of particular types of work is governed by some important factors.

Frozen sections

Although the use of frozen sections for diagnostic purposes is decreasing, immunohistochemistry on frozen sections remains an important histological tool. Although frozen sections have certain inherent disadvantages compared to paraffin sections, including poor morphology, limited retrospective studies, and storage of material, the technique should be considered the gold standard when evaluating and assessing new antibodies. When evaluating a new antibody the results achieved on paraffin (or resin) sections can be compared to the results achieved on frozen sections.

The poor morphology often associated with frozen sections can be improved by ensuring the frozen sections are thoroughly dried both before and after the sections are fixed in acetone. The acetone not only assists with the preservation of the antigen and related morphology but also destroys most harmful infective agents.

Cytological preparations

The use of immunohistochemistry on cytological preparations is increasing. Acetone-fixed smears or cytospins are often preferred by the immunohisto-chemist, since acetone allows a wide range of primary antibodies to be employed without destroy-ing the target epitopes. Many cytology laboratories still insist on fixing cytological preparations in alcohol as opposed to acetone and consequently the number of antigens demonstrable may be limited, although perhaps the morphology is superior.

Formalin-fixed, routinely processed paraffin-wax sections

The aim of immunohistochemistry is to achieve reproducible and consistent demonstration of anti-gens with the minimum background staining whilst preserving the integrity of tissue architec-ture. Adequate and appropriate fixation is the cor-nerstone of all histological and immunohistochemical preparations. Good fixation is the delicate balance between under-fixation and over-fixation. Ideal fix-ation is the balance between good morphology and good antigenicity. The demonstration of many anti-gens depends heavily on the fixative employed and on the immunohistochemical method selected. Prompt fixation is essential to achieve consistent results. Poor fixation or delay in fixation causes loss of antigenicity or diffusion of antigens into the surrounding tissue. There is no one fixative that is ideal for the demonstration of all antigens, and certain antigens mandate the use of frozen sections – although the modern trend is to utilize fixed par-affin sections wherever possible. Most laboratories

use fixation based on formalin, such as unbuffered 10% formal saline or 10% neutral buffered forma-lin. Some groups prefer picric acid fixation (Bouin's) or mercuric fixation (formal mercury or B5). The choice of fixation among pathologists was initially based on morphological appearance and the clarity of established staining techniques using dyes which were the mainstay of diagnostic histopathology long before the advent of immunohistochemistry. As most pathology teaching and learning is based on these traditional techniques, with all the arti-facts they produce, immunohistochemistry has had to tailor itself to this type of material in order to become an effective diagnostic aid.

Blocking endogenous enzymes

If enzymes similar to those used as the antibody label are present in the tissue, they may react with the substrate used to localize the tracer and give rise to problems in interpretation. Inhibiting endoge-nous enzyme activity prior to staining can eliminate false-positive reactions produced in this way. Per-oxidase and substances giving a pseudo-peroxidase reaction are present in some normal and neoplastic tissues (e.g. leukocytes and erythrocytes) and various methods have been described for the destruction of their activity. The most frequently used method is preincubation of the sections in absolute methanol containing hydrogen peroxide (Streefkerk 1972). Incubation in absolute methanol containing 0.5% hydrogen peroxide for 10 minutes at room temperature has been reported to produce an almost complete abolition of endogenous peroxi-dase activity, without affecting the immunoreactiv-ity of antigens (Delellis et al. 1979). The mechanisms of inhibition and details of other methods have been reviewed by Straus (1976).

There are many types of alkaline phosphatase within the human body, and most endogenous alkaline phosphatase activity can be blocked using a 1 mM concentration of levamisole in the final incubating medium. The alkaline phosphatase used in the labeling system is usually intestinal in nature and remains unaffected by levamisole at the recommended concentration. Using 20%

acetic acid can block intestinal alkaline phosphatase. However, the acidic treatment may damage some antigens.

The other commonly used enzyme labels, glucose oxidase and bacterial β-D-galactosidase, do not present a problem. The former does not have active endogenous enzyme in mammalian tissue; the latter does, but the label and chromogen react at a different pH from the mammalian enzyme.

An alternative to chemical inhibition of endogenous enzyme activity has been described by Robinson and Dawson (1975), and is similar to multiple labeling. In this method, the endogenous peroxidases are first localized by using one chromogen and then, following immunohistochemical staining, the enzyme tracer is localized by an alternate chromogen which yields a reaction end-product in a contrasting color. Thus, endogenous activity and specific activity can be distinguished easily by their differently colored reaction end-products. A wide range of chromogenic substrates are now commercially available (Vector Laboratories), many of which produce colored end-products that are not removed or decolorized by the dehydrating and clearing agents commonly used in immunohistochemistry.

Blocking background staining

The major causes of background staining in immunohistochemistry are hydrophobic and ionic interactions and endogenous enzyme activity. Background staining may be specific (e.g., fibrinogen in blood vessels and immunoglobulins in serum-bearing tissues) or non-specific due to the apparent affinity of certain tissue components. Non-specific uptake of antigen, particularly the high affinity of collagen and reticulin for immunoglobulins, can cause high levels of background staining.

Hydrophobic interactions are the result of the cross-linking of amino acids, both within and between adjacent protein molecules. Proteins are rendered more hydrophobic by aldehyde fixation and the extent of hydrophobic cross-linking of tissue proteins is primarily a function of fixation.

Tissues that give background staining as a result of hydrophobic interactions include collagen and other connective tissues, epithelium, and adipocytes (Kraehenbuhl & Jamieson 1974). Hydrophobic bonding can be minimized by the addition of a blocking protein, by the addition of a detergent such as Triton X (Hartman 1973), or the addition of a high salt concentration, 2.5% NaCl, to the buffer (Grabe 1980). Some workers advocate the addition of the blocking serum to the diluted primary antibody (Delellis et al. 1979).

Non-specific staining is most commonly produced because the primary antibody is attracted non-immunologically to highly charged groups present on connective tissue elements. Positive staining is due not to localization of the antigen but to non-specific attachment of the primary antibody to connective tissues. Since the primary antibody is attached to connective tissue moieties, the subsequent labeling antibodies will be attracted not only to primary antibodies located on the specific antigen but also to the antibody bound to the connective tissue elements.

The most effective way of minimizing non-specific staining is to add an innocuous protein solution to the section before applying the primary antibody. The added protein should saturate and neutralize the charged sites, thus enabling the primary antibody to bind to the antigenic site only.

Traditionally, non-immune serum from the animal species in which the second (bridging) antibody was raised is used as a blocking serum. In practice any animal serum or protein (e.g. casein) can be used for this purpose as long as the protein used as a block cannot be recognized by any of the subsequent antibodies used in the technique.

In frozen sections and cytological preparations, tissue receptors for the Fc portion of antibodies may give rise to additional problems. Fc receptors are present on several cell types such as macrophages and monocytes, and are largely destroyed by formalin fixation and paraffin processing. If necessary Fab fragments of antibodies that lack the Fc portion should be used.

Several authors have also found that enzymatic digestion reduces non-specific background staining

(Huang et al. 1976; Curran & Gregory 1977; Denk et al. 1977).

Controls

Controls validate immunohistochemical results. It is essential that any method using immunohisto-chemistry principles include controls to test for the specificity of the antibodies involved. Polyclonal antibodies usually contain antibodies specific for several antigenic determinants on the antigen and, as many related molecules have components in common (e.g. gastrin and cholecystokinin), false-positive results can be obtained. Although monoclonal antibodies potentially eliminate this problem, epitope similarities are seen between some molecules and unwanted cross-reaction can occur.

The criteria for specificity have been outlined by Nairn (1976), and problems relating to specificity discussed by Petrusz et al. (1976, 1977). In general, for immunochemical staining to be specific it must be shown firstly that no staining occurs in the absence of the primary antiserum, and secondly that staining is inhibited by adsorption of the primary antibody with the relevant antigen prior to its use, but not by adsorption with other related or unrelated antigens. In practice, to evaluate the results of immunohistochemical staining, the following immunological and non-immunological specificity controls can be undertaken.

Negative control. This involves either the omission of the primary antibody from the staining schedule or the replacement of the specific primary antibody by an immunoglobulin which is directed against an unrelated antigen. This immunoglobulin must be of the same class, source, and species.

Positive control. As the absence of staining in a test section does not necessarily imply that the antigen is not present, the use of a section of known positivity is always advisable. Positive elements within test sections (e.g. normal reactive lymphocytes when staining with an antibody to the leukocyte common antigen to identify a suspected lymphoma) are the best form of positive control.

Absorption control. The ideal negative control is to demonstrate that immunoreactivity is abolished by pre-absorption of the specific primary antibody with the purified antigen. If staining does occur after absorption then the staining must be due to a contaminating antibody and not to the antigen-antibody interaction under investigation. This type of control is necessary in the characterization and evaluation of new antibodies. This may be regarded as the ultimate test for specificity (Fig. 18.12). It is rarely used in diagnostic work, as well-characterized commercial antibodies are available. For reasons of economy, absorption should be carried out at the highest possible dilution of the primary antibody compatible with consistent unequivocal staining, as the higher the concentration of antibody, the more antigen will be required for neutralization. The practicalities of this type of control have been described by Van Noorden et al. (1986).

An additional useful control is a blocking control in which the binding between the primary antibody and conjugated antibody in the traditional indirect method, or between the bridging antibody and the PAP in the unlabeled antibody method, is blocked. This is achieved by interposing between incubations of the two relevant antibodies incubation in unlabeled immunoglobulin of the type present in the labeled antibody.

When localizing immunoglobulin some workers consider it is advisable to include an anti-albumin 'control', as non-immunological cells in poorly fixed or postmortem tissue are known to passively take up immunoglobulin and other serum proteins. Anti-albumin-stained sections will help to identify these false-positive cells.

Finally, it can be beneficial to check the inhibition treatment for endogenous enzymes by staining a slide histochemically after the inhibition procedure. If residual activity is present, interpretation of the immunochemically stained slides may be aided by staining an untreated slide to reveal the sites of endogenous enzyme activity.

Practical aspects of immunohistochemical staining

The practical aspects of immunohistochemical staining are simple and straightforward, as the

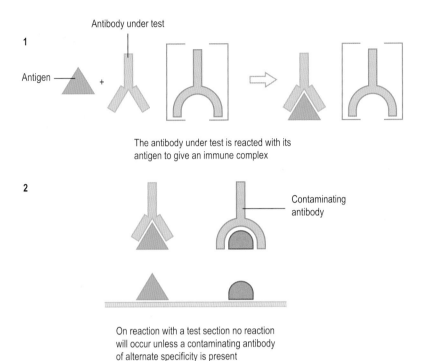

Figure 18.12 Absorption control.

techniques entail only sequential incubations in antibodies and labeling systems separated by washes in buffer. To obtain optimal staining and prevent the non-specific precipitation of antibody onto the sections, it is essential to ensure that each antibody is used at an appropriate dilution, does not evaporate off during incubation, and is completely removed, if unbound, before the next specific antibody or reagent is added.

Dilution of immune serum/antibodies

For optimal staining to occur it is necessary to use the primary specific antibody at the correct dilution (see Table 18.1). Incorrect dilutions can give rise to false-negative results, particularly in antigen-rich tissues (Bigbee et al. 1977).

When applying an untested antibody to a tissue section containing the relevant antigen, a broad dilution series should be used to insure that false-negative results do not occur. Selection of the cleanest dilution with intense signal, particularly on normal cells, is not always the optimal dilution for diagnostic material. Tumor cells can sometimes exhibit fewer antigens than the normal tissue background cells of origin. Dilutions that identify normal cells may be too dilute to demonstrate the tumor cells that originate from them. It is recommended that dilution factors are not set at the extreme end of the range and, where possible, it is useful to test out dilution factors on known neoplastic material when appropriate.

Theoretically, in multi-layer techniques each separate stage ought to be titrated against the other antibody stages and the optimal concentration selected for each antibody. In practice, most commercially supplied primary antibodies and labeling systems are provided with a recommended dilution range. It is usually only the primary antibody dilution that needs to be adjusted.

Washes

To prevent the formation of antigen-antibody complexes that will precipitate onto the sections and give rise to problems with interpretation and background staining, it is necessary to remove the unbound antibody before incubation in the next layer. This is achieved by washing the sections between antibody incubations in Tris-buffered saline (TBS). This solution may be made up in bulk for convenience.

For routine work, a few brief washes, with TBS, will usually suffice. In the past some workers recommended the addition of detergent, such as BRIJ 96 (Sigma), to the washing solutions (Heyderman & Monaghan 1979). Today the most popular surfactant is Tween 20, often used in concentrations of 0.01–0.05%.

Buffer solutions and heat-mediated antigen retrieval fluids

0.5 M Tris-buffered saline

Distilled water	10 liters
Sodium chloride	85 g
Tris (hydroxymethyl) aminomethane	60.5 g

Adjust pH to 7.6 with 50% hydrochloric acid.

Tris-buffered saline containing bovine serum albumin (BSA-TBS)

Tris (hydroxymethyl) aminomethane	12.14 g
Sodium chloride	45 g
Bovine serum albumin	5 g
Sodium azide	6.5 g
Distilled water	5 liters

Adjust final pH to 8.2 with 1 M hydrochloric acid.

Veronal acetate buffer

Sodium acetate trihydrate	0.972 g
Sodium barbitone	1.472 g
Distilled water	250 ml
0.1 M hydrochloric acid	2.5 ml

Heat-mediated antigen retrieval fluids

Citrate buffer

Citric acid (anhydrous)	21 g
Distilled water	10 liters

Adjust pH to 6.0 using 2 M sodium hydroxide.

Tris-EDTA

Tris	14.4 g
EDTA	1.44 g
1 M hydrochloric acid	1 ml
Tween 20	0.3 ml
Distilled water	600 ml

Add the Tris, EDTA, and acid to the distilled water and adjust pH to 10 with hydrochloric acid, then add the Tween.

Incubation methods

Manual

To prevent evaporation of antibodies, incubations must be carried out in a moist atmosphere. This is most easily obtained by placing the slides on Perspex strips which run the length of a lidded staining trough, in the bottom of which is a pool of water or a layer of moist tissue paper.

It is advisable to leave a small gap between adjacent slides so that cross-contamination of antibodies cannot occur. The use of moist incubation chambers means that it is not necessary to flood the slide with antiserum and, if the area around the section is dried thoroughly with a tissue before application of the antibodies and labeling systems, just a few drops of reagent should suffice. In addition, the use of a wax pen around the sections assists with retaining the reagents on the sections.

Semi-automated incubation methods

Shandon Sequenza coverplate system – when the coverplate and slide are charged with buffer during the assembly the surface tension created by the gap allows 80 µl of fluid to be held within the gap. This fluid is positively displaced by gravity flow following application of reagent into the upper chamber well, with 80 µl of the new reagent held between the gap during the incubation period. The system allows ease of washing between each of the incubation steps.

Automated incubation methods

Increased workloads necessitate the use of automated immunostaining. Automation ensures standardization of the technique and produces a high quality of immunostaining. Automated immunocytochemistry systems such as the Leica Bond III use a flat bed system with unique Covertile™ technology to facilitate uniform staining of the tissue. Reagent is gently applied at one end of the covertile and gently flows along under the covertile to fully cover the section and prevent drying out. The full immunocytochemical procedure including dewaxing and antigen retrieval is carried out using this automation. Automation such as the Dako Autostainer Link 48 also uses flatbed technology for the incubation and washing stages, with the antigen retrieval undertaken using the PT module Link prior to the slides being uploaded onto the machine. Automation such as the Ventana Benchmark Ultra use a kinetic mode system involving air-vortex mixers to mix the reagents, liquid coverslip to prevent drying out and thermoflex pad to provide precise heating across the whole slide. Dewaxing and antigen retrieval is carried out on-board. These are just three examples of automated immunocytochemistry staining systems; others exist and work very well.

Fixation and paraffin-wax block immunohistochemistry

Many publications have discussed the merits and drawbacks of particular fixatives for immunohistochemistry on diagnostic histopathological material, with some recommending specific fixatives for certain epitopes. Most diagnostic laboratories are faced with a request for certain antigens subsequent to the routine processing and hematoxylin and eosin stage. It is therefore important to establish a fixation and processing procedure that allows for good morphology and maximizes the ability of the immunohistochemist to identify the antigens that aid diagnosis. It should also, with prior arrangement with the surgeons and theater staff, be possible to receive fresh specimens soon after surgery in order that material can be selected for routine processing and frozen storage. The latter should be snap frozen using liquid nitrogen and stored at −80°C. If required, this material can be used for preparing imprints for fluorescence *in situ* hybridization (FISH) techniques or as a source of RNA and DNA for molecular biology techniques or for cutting frozen sections, for the demonstration of antigens not readily demonstrated in paraffin-wax sections.

Retrospective studies are often hampered by a lack of knowledge of the duration of fixation. Banks (1979) indicated that prolonged fixation reduces immunoreactivity. Acidic fixatives such as Bouin's

fluid can, over a 24-hour fixation period, reduce or destroy the immunoreactivity of some diagnostic antibodies, such as CD45RO (UCHL1). A similar picture is seen with mercury-containing fixatives. Formalin fixation can have a similar effect, but tends to occur over a period of weeks rather than days. Certain antibodies such as CD20 and CD45 are less affected by fixation times. According to Singh et al. (1993), microwave pretreatment enables the retrieval of antigens after formalin fixation of up to two years' duration. In general the use of heat-mediated antigen retrieval has enabled a greater consistency of immunohistochemical staining over a wide range of different fixatives and fixation times (Figs 18.13 and 18.14). Most individual laboratories will employ a single fixative used over a range of fixation times between 18 and 72 hours, for which a single standardized heat methodology can often be applied. For referral laboratories dealing with a wide range of material from different sources where the fixation regimes are unknown, more than one retrieval method may be necessary.

The advance in molecular technology has enabled the production of duplicate synthetic peptide sequences that survive routine processing techniques. One such peptide has been produced for the human CD3 antigen, fixed in a formalin fixative and subsequently used to raise a polyclonal antibody (Mason et al. 1989). This reagent has proved to

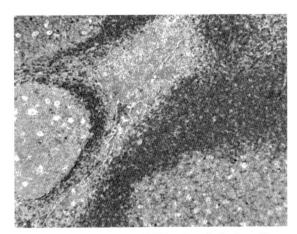

Figure 18.13 Demonstration of IgM in a formalin-fixed paraffin-embedded section of reactive tonsil, using a labeled streptavidin-biotin immunoperoxidase technique with DAB as the chromogen.

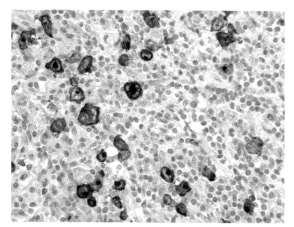

Figure 18.14 CD30 demonstration in a formalin-fixed paraffin-embedded section of Hodgkin's disease. Note the strong staining of both membrane and Golgi apparatus.

be successful in the detection of T cells and related lymphomas in routinely processed paraffin sections. With the aid of either proteolytic digestion or heat antigen retrieval, polyclonal anti-CD3 is an excellent example of how immunohistochemistry has adapted to the prevailing conditions in histopathology.

Other methods beyond routine techniques are occasionally needed, usually in research or specialist laboratories. One such example is the demonstration of hormones and neuropeptides that require special fixation (Van Noorden et al. 1986); for these hormones the use of freeze-dried material which is then vapor-fixed in *p*-benzoquinone or diethyl pyrocarbonate, and subsequently paraffin embedded, is recommended (Pearse & Polak 1975).

Method selection

The majority of immunohistochemists in the United Kingdom employ either a streptavidin-biotin system or a polymer chain two-step indirect method for routine work (data from the UK National External Quality Assessment Scheme for Immunocytochemistry). The peroxidase-diaminobenzidine reaction end-product, because of its resistance to processing to resinous mounting media and its long-term storage qualities, is also preferred. The storage qualities are particularly important when diagnoses are under review over prolonged periods of time.

Preparative techniques

Preparing paraffin wax sections for immunostaining

1. Cut 3–4 μm sections and place on clean electrostatically charged glass slides (we recommend Superfrost Plus slides). If using uncharged slides an adhesive should be used. Commercial products such as APES or Vectabond are successful in assisting with section adhesion.
2. Dry the sections overnight in a 37°C incubator. Alternatively the sections may be placed on a hot plate at 60°C for 15 minutes. Certain antigens, such as estrogen and progesterone receptors, show a reduction in staining when heated on a hot plate and therefore this is not recommended.
3. Where possible, sections should be cut fresh. Sections stored for several weeks prior to immunostaining may show reduced staining intensity. This is the case with estrogen and progesterone receptors.
4. Dewax sections in xylene and bring to absolute alcohol. Xylene substitutes such as Histoclear may be used. To ensure complete removal of wax the xylene/Histoclear may be warmed to 37°C in an incubator.
5. If required, remove fixation pigments.
6. Block endogenous peroxidase activity by incubating in 0.5% hydrogen peroxide in methanol for 10 minutes. This stage may be performed after the primary antibody has been bound onto the antigenic site. It is thought by many users that the methanol/hydrogen peroxide step may slightly alter some of the more labile antigenic epitopes, leading to weak demonstration. We have certainly found this to be the case with the demonstration of CD2 and CD4 in paraffin sections.
7. Rehydrate, wash well in running water.
8. Perform the required/preferred antigen retrieval techniques as detailed below.

Antigen retrieval techniques

Proteolytic enzyme methods

The digestion media outlined below must be freshly prepared as their activity decreases with time. Digestion methods with proteolytic enzymes are usually limited to sections taken from formalin-fixed, paraffin-embedded tissues, in order to enable those antigens that are blocked by the cross-linking of the formalin fixative to be uncovered for binding to the relevant antibody. However, not all antigens are blocked and therefore do not require this treatment.

Optimal times for digestion are dependent on fixation parameters. These vary according to specimen size, temperature of fixative, duration of fixation, and the rate of penetration of the fixative. With such variables a fixed digestion time does not always achieve optimal staining. Usually a uniform time, established on controls, is used in the initial stages. Antibodies such as those for pan-cytokeratin will react to a satisfactory standard even when the digestion time is suboptimal, but others such as immunoglobulin light chains require a more precise methodology.

The following methods should be used as a guideline only. We would recommend that individual laboratories determine individual digestion times on their own material.

Trypsin/chymotrypsin methodology

1. Incubate sections in pre-warmed distilled water at 37°C.
2. Prepare 0.1% trypsin in 0.1% calcium chloride in distilled water at 37°C. Adjust pH to 7.8 using 0.1 M sodium hydroxide solution.
3. Incubate the sections in the trypsin solution for 10 minutes at 37°C.
4. Wash sections in cold running tap water to prevent further digestion.
5. Proceed with the immunostaining method of choice.

   N.B. A successful alternative to trypsin is chymotrypsin (Sigma C-4129) (Miller et al. 1995).

Protease methodology

1. Incubate sections in pre-warmed distilled water at 37°C.
2. Prepare 0.1% protease (Sigma type XXIV, P-8038) in distilled water (at 37°C). Adjust pH to 7.8 using 1 M sodium hydroxide solution.
3. Incubate the sections in the protease solution for 6 minutes at 37°C.
4. Wash sections in cold running tap water to prevent further digestion.

5. Proceed with the immunostaining method of choice.

   Using 0.05% protease may be preferred. By using a less concentrated solution the possibility of over-digesting the tissue sections is decreased. Digestion times will require increasing but are not as critical as with the 0.1% protease solution.

Pepsin methodology

1. Incubate sections in pre-warmed distilled water at 37°C.
2. Prepare 0.4% pepsin solution in 0.01 M hydrochloric acid (pH 2.0) at 37°C.
3. Incubate the sections in the pepsin solution for 15–60 minutes at 37°C.
4. Wash sections in cold running tap water to prevent further digestion.
5. Proceed with the immunostaining method of choice.

   Certain antigens, e.g. basement membrane proteins, give improved staining if the digestion is performed by pepsin.

Heat-mediated antigen retrieval

There are now many heat retrieval methods employing different types of equipment and various retrieval solutions. The equipment includes microwave oven, pressure cooker, steamer, autoclave, water bath and the now widely used automated immunocytochemistry platforms with either on-board antigen retrieval technology or external antigen retrieval means. Among the various solutions, citrate buffer at pH 6.0, EDTA at pH 8.0, and Tris-EDTA (pH 9.9 or 10.0) are the most popular. However, with most laboratories using automated systems, appropriate commercial fluids – either a high pH option or a lower pH 6.0 option – are routinely employed.

In order to prevent section damage or detachment (due to the vigorous boiling of the antigen retrieval solution) the sections should be picked up on Superfrost Plus charged slides or on slides coated with a strong adhesive such as Vectabond (Vector Laboratories) or amino-propyltriethoxysilane (APES).

Microwave oven heating methodology (Fig. 18.6)

In 1994, Jessup reported that it is possible to achieve relatively even exposure of antigen across the tissue section by heating 10 slides in a plastic slide rack in a deep microwavable container (e.g. Addis 9400) holding 600 ml of fluid. This method has since been developed and a maximum of 25 sections can be heated per batch. With this type of tall narrow container, the height of the fluid above the slides is such that no topping up is needed, as there is no risk of the slides drying out over a 30-minute heating cycle. A loose lid is required to reduce the volume of fluid lost, but allows the steam to escape.

1. Using a plastic staining rack, place up to 25 sections in 600 ml of 0.01 M citrate buffer, pH 6.0.
2. Irradiate on high power (800 W) for 22 minutes.
3. Carefully remove the container from the microwave oven and flood with cold water.
4. Proceed with the immunostaining method of choice.

For suboptimally fixed material we recommend reducing the volume of buffer to 400 ml and the heating time to 15 minutes.

Pressure cooker antigen retrieval methodology

Use a 5-liter domestic stainless steel pressure cooker with an operating pressure of 103.4 kPa. To bring the pressure cooker to boil use either a halogen hot plate or domestic electric hot plate (Fig. 18.7). A maximum of three racks of 25 slides each can be pretreated at one time.

1. Add 1.5 liters of appropriate antigen retrieval buffer into the pressure cooker and bring to the boil (without securing the lid).
2. When the antigen retrieval buffer is boiling, carefully place the slide racks into the hot solution and seal the lid.
3. Allow the pressure cooker to reach full pressure 10.3 kPa (15 psi), incubate for 2 minutes (timing starts only when full pressure is reached).
4. Transfer the pressure cooker to a sink and run cold water over the lid until all of the pressure is released.
5. Flood the pressure cooker with cold water. Do not remove the slides until cool.
6. Proceed with the immunostaining method of choice.

Plastic pressure cookers are now available for heating in a microwave oven, but they have a lower operating pressure than the stainless steel versions and as a consequence the heating time at full pressure has to be significantly increased.

Steamer antigen retrieval methodology

This method uses a domestic rice steamer.

1. Place 1 liter of distilled water into the base of the steamer and insert a dry tray into the base.
2. Place steaming tray onto the dry tray.
3. Place the rice bowl into the steaming chamber.
4. Fill the incubation tray with 200 ml of appropriate antigen retrieval buffer and place in the chamber.
5. Place the lid onto the top of the steaming chamber.
6. Set the timer for 1 hour 15 minutes. The equilibration of the bath/rice chamber contents to 95°C is achieved after around 45 minutes.
7. Remove the lid and place the slides in the heated antigen retrieval buffer; replace the lid.
8. Incubate sections for 30 minutes.
9. Remove the antigen retrieval buffer from the chamber and allow the sections to cool for 15 minutes.
10. Wash sections in water.
11. Proceed with the immunostaining method of choice.

Water bath antigen retrieval methodology

This method uses a conventional laboratory water bath.

1. Place the appropriate antigen retrieval buffer in a plastic Coplin jar.
2. Place the Coplin jar into the water bath and heat to 95–98°C (do not allow to boil).
3. Place slides into the preheated buffer and incubate for 30 minutes.
4. Remove the container from the water bath and allow cooling for 15 minutes at room temperature.
5. Wash sections in water.
6. Proceed with the immunostaining method of choice.

Examples of immunostaining protocols for routine diagnostic antigens

Testing all the clones available for a particular epitope would be too costly. Most manufacturers and suppliers provide a data sheet with each of their antibodies, which will give recommendations as to their use. If a more independent guide is sought then the *Manual of Diagnostic Antibodies for Immunohistology* by Leong et al. (1999) is recommended.

The following information is based on the experiences of the University College London Immunohistochemistry Laboratory, the Hematological Malignancy Diagnostic Service, and the Department of Histopathology and Molecular Pathology at the Leeds Teaching Hospitals NHS Trust.

Immunohistochemistry for immunoglobulin light chains in formalin-fixed paraffin-wax sections

This is one of the most difficult of all techniques to perform. The retention of the immunoglobulin in the appropriate cells with good fixation is a prerequisite of producing good light chain demonstration. Furthermore, light chain restriction is an important criterion when identifying B-cell lymphoma and this restriction is one of few markers of malignancy available to immunohistochemists today. Prompt fixation in either a buffered or unbuffered 10% formalin solution is essential. Lymph nodes and other dense lymphoid tissue should be sliced as soon as possible in order to facilitate the penetration of the fixative. Ideally, fixation of 18–72 hours is acceptable, but once fixation time is extended to several weeks, demonstration of light chain immunoglobulin becomes increasingly difficult.

Accuracy of staining has been verified by comparing immunohistochemical results on sections with flow cytometric analysis of fresh lymphoid tissue. Flow cytometric analysis requires fresh (not previously frozen) tissue to be perfused with an isotonic solution and any red cell contamination to be lysed with ammonium chloride. The lymphocytes are labeled with a fluorescently conjugated primary antibody, washed with an isotonic solution, and analyzed on a flow cytometer. Flow cytometric analysis is the optimum method for immunophenotyping lymphomas on fresh tissue; however, many laboratories do not have the resources to undertake this and many lymphomas present as formalin-fixed paraffin-embedded blocks.

Sections of reactive tonsil provide the ideal control material for light chain demonstration. Tonsil sections should show marked demonstration of the mantle zone and follicle center B cells together with intense plasma cell staining (Fig. 18.15). The T-cell zone should have little staining. Background immunoglobulin, caused essentially by non-specific uptake, is seen on follicular dendritic cells, some connective tissue and epithelia.

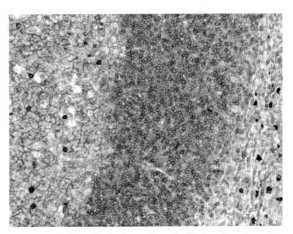

Figure 18.15 Formalin-fixed paraffin-embedded section of reactive tonsil demonstrating kappa light chain immunoglobulins. Strong staining of plasma cells, follicular dendritic cells, and mantle zone B cells are clearly visible. Antigen retrieval using the microwave oven and citrate buffer, pH 6.0.

If there is any doubt, it is important to establish on the test material that small round B cells (see Appendix VII) are present, with a series of B markers. This will usually assist with identifying B cells at different maturation stages. Once achieved, immunoglobulin staining can be compared with the control section. If there are only a few plasma cells and little else staining then it is almost certain that the antigen retrieval has been underachieved. Increasing the antigen retrieval times on duplicate sections will increase the reactivity, and perinuclear space and surface staining of the light chains on the B cells will indicate optimal retrieval. In addition, intense cytoplasmic staining of immunoglobulin in plasma cells should be seen. Excessive antigen retrieval, by heat or by proteolytic digestion, will cause staining of large amounts of reticulin and could remove some of the cells and protein structures from the slide.

Reliable light chain demonstration on paraffin sections can be achieved using either two-step indirect polymer-labeled methods with diaminobenzidine as the preferred chromogen (or by polymerase chain-based techniques). If manual antigen retrieval is used we would recommend antigen retrieval using microwave oven heating with citrate buffer. However, optimum results are seen using automated immunocytochemistry platforms.

The choice of antigen retrieval will depend upon the individual laboratory and their fixation and processing regimes. Polyclonal primary antibodies are recommended.

Immunohistochemistry for the assessment of HER2 expression

The assessment of HER2 in human tumor cells has recently become important since the amplified gene is predictive of response to the novel humanized HER2 antibody Herceptin®/trastuzumab. Historically the major factors directing the appropriate treatment for breast cancer have been those regarding prognosis, such as indicators of how long the average patient is likely to survive. As a result, the relative aggressiveness of a tumor has been gauged and the appropriate treatment regime has been planned. Recently the concept of predictive factors has risen to the fore. Unlike prognostic factors, which are concerned with the likelihood of a particular outcome, the predictive factors are concerned with identifying features of a tumor that will direct specific targeted therapies or a more probable outcome with combinations of chemotherapeutic agents.

HER2 is a member of the epidermal growth factor receptor (EGFR) family of molecules and is encoded for by the HER2 proto-oncogene on the long arm of chromosome 17. HER2 is overexpressed in 10–20% of primary breast cancers. Overexpression indicates poor prognosis. Breast cancers showing over-expression are candidates for treatment with trastuzumab (Herceptin). Studies show that trastuzumab can reduce the risk of occurrence by one-half and mortality by one-third in early-stage breast cancer patients.

Formalin-fixed paraffin sections immunostained to demonstrate HER2 are examined microscopically and scored. Only invasive breast cancer cells should be scored. Non-invasive tumors (ductal carcinoma *in situ*) are not assessed. It is recommended that formalin-fixed paraffin sections should be antigen retrieved using the water bath antigen retrieval method and citrate buffer, pH 6.0, as antigen retrieval solution, to ensure optimal immunostaining.

When assessing HER2 staining, the following scoring system is used:

0 No staining at all or very slight partial membrane staining in less than 10% of tumor cells.

1+ Faint barely perceptible membrane staining in more than 10% of tumor cells. Cells stained in only part of the membrane.

2+ Weak to moderate complete membrane staining observed in more than 10% of tumor cells.

3+ Strong complete membrane staining in more than 30% of tumor cells. See Figure 18.16.

Application of fluorescence *in situ* hybridization (FISH) for HER2 assessment (Fig. 18.17)

- The centromeric region of chromosome 17 is marked with a green fluorescent signal and the HER2 gene with a red signal.

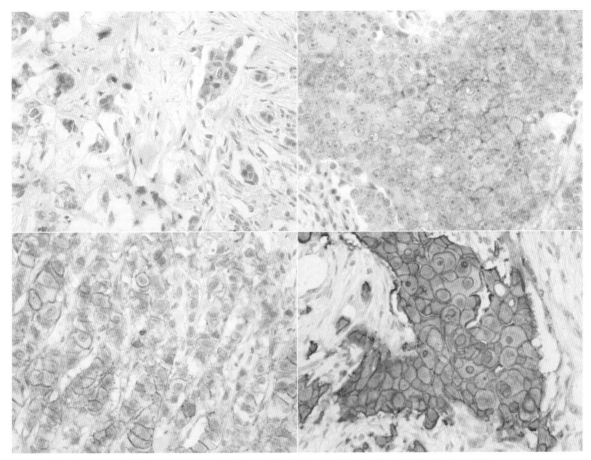

Figure 18.16 Breast tumor HER2 assessment graded 0 (top left), 1+ (top right), 2+ (bottom left), 3+ (bottom right).

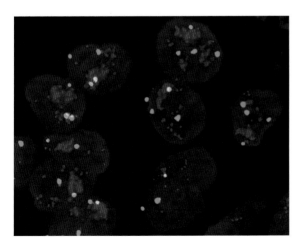

Figure 18.17 FISH HER2 demonstration, showing amplification of the HER2 gene (red fluorescence).

- Assess 20–60 cells: count the number of red:green signals in each cell.
- The overall gene-to-chromosome ratio is calculated.
- A tumor is designated *positive* if gene-to-chromosome ratio is >2.2 and *negative* if <1.8. For gene counts which fall in between 1.8 and 2.2 we class as *equivocal* then assess more cells and make a call in conjunction with the IHC.

Application of chromogenic *in situ* hybridization (CISH) as an alternative to FISH (Figs 18.18 and 18.19)

- Similar technique to FISH but allows the chromogenic visualization of the HER2 gene

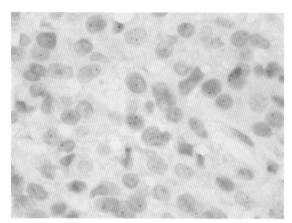

Figure 18.18 CISH HER2 demonstration, showing single signal count.

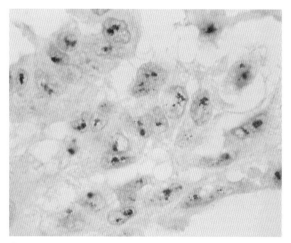

Figure 18.19 CISH HER2 demonstration showing signal clusters.

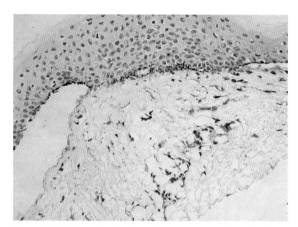

Figure 18.20 Formalin-fixed paraffin wax-processed section of skin with a bullous pemphigoid blister, immunostained for IgG using protease digestion and an indirect technique. The bullous lesion and basement membrane clearly show IgG deposition.

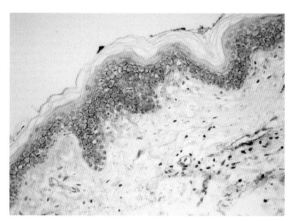

Figure 18.21 IgG demonstration in a bullous pemphigus formalin-fixed paraffin-embedded section of skin.

and/or chromosome 17 on either the same or separate slides.

- Often reported as either a direct count if signal quality allows or may be reported as signal clusters.

Immunohistochemistry on renal and skin biopsies

Direct immunofluorescence tests performed on skin biopsy and renal biopsy specimens to demonstrate specific patterns of immunoglobulin and complement deposition have clarified the diagnostic entities within the group of vesiculobullous diseases and glomerular nephritis. In glomerulonephritis there is usually immunoglobulin and complement deposition in relation to the glomerular basement membrane. In skin the bullous lesions are thought to be caused by an autoimmune response producing large amounts of antibody that is deposited either on the epidermal basement membrane or intercellularly in the epidermis. The pemphigus group of diseases is characterized by antibodies, usually IgG, directed against the intercellular substance of squamous epithelium. The pemphigoid group of bullous diseases is characterized by antibody, usually IgG, directed against the basement membrane zone (Figs 18.20 and 18.21).

McIver and Mepham reported in 1982 that immunoperoxidase was their established method for demonstrating immunocomplexes in renal biopsies. Also in the same year Turbitt et al. described an immunoperoxidase method to demonstrate autoantibodies in the bullous lesions of pemphigoid and pemphigus.

Today, even with the disadvantage of having to split the biopsy for frozen and paraffin processing (and for electron microscopy for renals), the method of choice for many, certainly in the UK, is still frozen section immunofluorescence coupled with paraffin section morphology. While the frozen fluorescence technique requires a high degree of skill, there is no doubt that the paraffin-wax method provides a difficult technical challenge. Furthermore, such is the capriciousness of this method that maintaining the standards of an established immunoperoxidase technique for these purposes requires a dedicated and highly skilled immunohistochemist. There are some important reasons why opinion is divided as to the preferred technique.

Wax-embedded paraffin sections of renal biopsies

In most cases renal disease affects the glomeruli. Hence this is an important technique, especially when glomeruli are absent in the portion selected for fluorescence and electron microscopy, but are found in the paraffin-processed sample. It is essential that proteolytic digestion is employed, and an indirect peroxidase labeling system is recommended as this avoids endogenous biotin staining. Relatively inexpensive polyclonal antibodies, used at extremely high dilutions, can be effectively employed in this technique (Figs 18.22 and 18.23).

Protocol outline

1. Fix for 3–24 hours in a formalin fixative, e.g. 10% formal saline, 10% neutral buffered formalin.
2. Proteolytic digestion is necessary and is best achieved by using 0.1% protease type XXIV (Sigma) for 45 minutes.
3. Non-immune serum is essential, especially when polyclonal antibodies are employed.

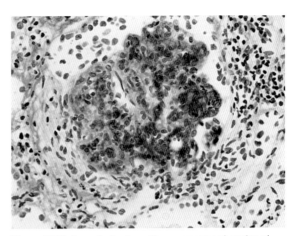

Figure 18.22 Formalin-fixed paraffin wax-processed section of renal biopsy with IgA nephropathy, immunostained for IgA using protease digestion and labeled with an indirect immunoperoxidase staining method. IgA is clearly demonstrated.

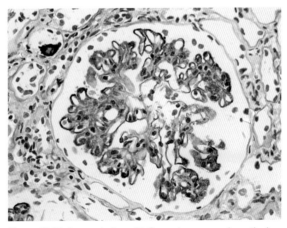

Figure 18.23 Demonstration of IgG membranous nephropathy in a formalin-fixed paraffin-embedded renal biopsy.

4. Polyclonal antibodies, as described in Table 18.2, are used at high dilutions for 60 minutes followed by swine anti-rabbit peroxidase-labeled secondary antibody for 25 minutes. A high-quality DAB is employed as the chromogen.

An alternative protocol was published by Boyd SM and Ronan JE (*Dakofacts* Vol. 8. No. 1) that uses trypsin digestion with EnVision reagents.

Table 18.2 Immunocomplexes in renal biopsies

Antibody	Species	Supplier	Dilution	Pretreatment
IgA	Rabbit	Dako	1/20,000	Protease
IgM	Rabbit	Dako	1/500	Protease
IgG	Rabbit	Dako	1/20,000	Protease
C3c	Rabbit	Dako	1/800	Protease
C1q	Rabbit	Dako	1/400	Protease
Fibrinogen	Rabbit	Dako	1/30,000	Protease
Kappa	Rabbit	Dako	1/20,000	Protease

Table 18.3 Immunocomplexes in skin biopsies

Antibody	Species	Supplier	Dilution	Pretreatment
IgA	Rabbit	Dako	1/25,000	Protease
IgG	Rabbit	Dako	1/25,000	Protease
IgM	Rabbit	Dako	1/20,000	Protease
C1q	Rabbit	Dako	1/10,000	Protease
C3c	Rabbit	Dako	1/20,000	Protease
Fibrinogen	Rabbit	Dako	1/30,000	Protease
Lambda	Rabbit	Dako	1/20,000	Protease

Immunoperoxidase staining method for formalin-fixed paraffin wax-embedded skin biopsies

Reports suggest (W. Merchant, personal communication) that this technique can be effective on paraffin sections. However, it must be considered one of the most capricious methods employed by immunohistochemists today. Direct immunofluorescence on frozen sections is generally preferred as its relatively low level of sensitivity, compared with avidin-biotin peroxidase, reduces the labeling of non-specifically bound immunoglobulins and complement in the various tissue elements. The following immunoperoxidase protocol (Saeerda Kauser, Zeshaan Ejaz, personal communications) has, at the time of writing, proved to be successful in a number of cases, but is not always reliable.

Protocol outline

1. Fix for 3–24 hours in formalin, e.g. 10% formal saline, 10% neutral buffered formalin, and routinely process to paraffin wax.

2. Cut sections at 3–4 μm onto Superfrost Plus slides and dry overnight at 37°C.

3. Treat sections with 0.1% protease XXIV (Sigma) in Tris-buffered saline, pH 7.6, for 10 minutes.

4. Minimize non-specific binding by treating sections with 10% casein solution (Vector Laboratories) for 10 minutes.

5. Incubate sections in primary antibody at the dilutions shown in Table 18.3 for 30 minutes.

6. Treat sections with Dako EnVision reagent for 30 minutes.

7. Visualize with DAB for 5 minutes.

8. Besides using positive controls for each particular antibody, it is essential that normal skin should always be employed to monitor the background levels.

This highly sensitive method ensures good labeling of dilute primary antibody binding to the target. The background levels of normal non-specifically bound immunoglobulins and complement are subdued. This latter point is achieved because the high dilutions of primary antibody, coupled with the short incubation times and Tween TBS washes, insure weak labeling of the less-concentrated non-specific uptake staining that so often causes considerable interpretation difficulties. In Figure 18.20 the basement membrane is quite clearly positive for IgG.

Frozen-section immunofluorescence

Advantages of this method are:

- It usually involves a simple, rapid, and sensitive direct technique.
- It is easily reproduced.
- Histopathologists, experienced with fluorescent antibody techniques in renal and skin biopsies, find little difficulty with interpretation.

Disadvantages:

- The production of good-quality frozen sections from small biopsies sometimes requires a high degree of skill.
- A fluorescence microscope is required.
- Immunofluorescent labeling has poor storage qualities, and can often fade within days of the sections being immunostained.
- The morphology of the tissue is not easily seen, and hence a substantial part of the biopsy is processed to paraffin wax.

Paraffin-wax section immunoperoxidase

Advantages of this method are:

- All or a substantial part of the biopsy (except for renals where a small portion is processed

for electron microscopy) is formalin fixed and paraffin processed.

- Immunolocalization and morphology are clearly seen in the same section.
- Peroxidase has good long-term storage qualities, especially if diaminobenzidine chromogen is employed.
- An expensive fluorescence microscope is not required.
- Processing, section cutting and storage of blocks are compatible with a routine diagnostic service.

Disadvantages:

- A more time-consuming, sensitive technique, employing proteolytic enzyme antigen retrieval, is required.
- Proteolytic digestion must be tailored to fixation time.
- The technique requires a high degree of skill to insure a reliable level of reproducibility.
- To the experienced histopathologist interpretation offers little difficulty. However, for those with experience of only frozen-section immunofluorescence, paraffin-wax immunoperoxidase interpretation is more difficult.

Immunohistochemistry on frozen section and non-gynecological cytology smears

Frozen sections

1. Cut 6 μm frozen sections and place on Superfrost Plus microscope slides or adhesive-coated slides.
2. Air dry the sections at room temperature overnight (in urgent cases dry for a minimum of 1–2 hours).
3. Fix sections in absolute acetone at room temperature for 20 minutes. Allow sections to air dry. If required the sections may be stored at this stage at −20°C or lower. Prior to storage, the slides should be wrapped in foil and then placed in the freezer with a desiccant. When

required, the sections should be allowed to return to room temperature before unwrapping.

4. Rehydrate in TBS, apply optimally diluted primary antibody. Antibodies should be diluted in TBS; avoid the use of commercial antibody diluents or the use of detergents such as Triton or Tween. Chromatolysis and loss of nuclear membranes on frozen sections is compounded by the action of detergents.

5. For frozen sections an endogenous peroxidase-blocking step is not included, as this can be damaging to the antigens to be demonstrated. The use of a negative control for the identification of endogenous peroxidase activity is preferable. If the endogenous peroxidase activity is excessive, then an alternative enzyme tracer, such as alkaline phosphatase, should be considered.

Cytology preparations

Smears, imprints, cytospins, etc., should be air dried for 1–3 hours and then fixed or stored as outlined for frozen sections.

Immunohistochemical staining techniques

Avidin-biotin techniques

In these techniques either peroxidase or alkaline phosphatase may be used as the enzyme label.

Labeled streptavidin/streptavidin-biotin complex technique for monoclonal antibodies

1. Rinse sections in TBS, then incubate in 10% casein solution for 10 minutes.
2. Drain off excess casein.
3. Incubate in optimally diluted primary antibody for 60 minutes.
4. Wash slides in TBS.
5. Incubate in optimally diluted biotinylated secondary antibody for 30 minutes.
6. Wash slides in TBS.
7. Incubate in optimally prepared labeled streptavidin or streptavidin-biotin complex for 30 minutes. When using a streptavidin-biotin complex the reagents should be mixed 30 minutes before use in order for the complex to form.

8. Wash slides in TBS.
9. Incubate in DAB substrate solution.
   Wash in running water, counterstain in hematoxylin, dehydrate, clear, and mount.

Modifications required for rabbit primary antibody

Step 5. Replace with biotinylated swine anti-rabbit secondary. Many of the commercial streptavidin-biotin kits are supplied with a multi-species secondary link which can be used for both mouse and rabbit primary antibodies.

N.B. When using a goat primary antibody an appropriate biotinylated secondary antibody raised against the goat species must be used.

Polymer techniques

Dako EnVision detection technique

1. Rinse sections in TBS, then incubate in 10% casein solution for 10 minutes.
2. Drain off excess casein.
3. Apply optimally diluted primary monoclonal antibody for 60 minutes.
4. Wash slides in TBS.
5. Incubate with EnVision polymer reagent for 30 minutes.
6. Wash slides in TBS.
7. Incubate in freshly prepared DAB solution for 10 minutes.
8. Rinse in TBS and transfer to running water.
9. Counterstain in hematoxylin, dehydrate, clear, and mount.

Novolink polymer detection technique

1. Following antigen retrieval, rinse sections in TBS.
2. Drain off excess TBS and block endogenous peroxidase activity using peroxidase block, for 5 minutes.
3. Wash in TBS for 5 minutes.
4. Incubate with protein block for 5 minutes.
5. Wash in TBS.
6. Apply optimally diluted primary antibody for 60 minutes.
7. Wash slides in TBS.

8. Incubate with post primary block for 30 minutes.
9. Wash slides in TBS.
10. Incubate with Novolink polymer for 30 minutes.
11. Wash slides in TBS.
12. Incubate in freshly prepared DAB solution for 10 minutes.
13. Rinse in TBS and transfer to running water.
14. Counterstain in hematoxylin, dehydrate, clear, and mount.

Tyramide signal amplification techniques

Tyramide signal amplification of the labeled streptavidin-biotin method

1. Rinse sections in TBS, then incubate in 10% casein solution for 10 minutes.
2. Drain off excess casein.
3. Incubate in optimally diluted primary antibody for 60 minutes.
4. Wash slides in TBS.
5. Incubate in biotinylated secondary antibody for 20 minutes.
6. Wash slides in TBS.
7. Incubate in labeled streptavidin (or streptavidin-biotin complex) for 20 minutes.
8. Wash slides in TBS.
9. Incubate slides in biotinylated tyramide reagent for 5 minutes.
10. Wash in TBS.
11. Re-incubate sections in labeled streptavidin (or streptavidin-biotin complex) for 20 minutes.
12. Wash slides in TBS.
13. Incubate in DAB substrate solution.
14. Wash in running water, counterstain in hematoxylin, dehydrate, clear, and mount.

   N.B. The incubation in biotinylated tyramide should be strictly adhered to otherwise unacceptably high levels of background staining can be encountered.

Dako CSAII detection method

1. Rinse sections in TBS, then incubate in 10% casein solution for 10 minutes.
2. Drain off excess casein.
3. Incubate in optimally diluted primary antibody for 15–60 minutes.

4. Wash slides in TBS.
5. Apply anti-mouse immunoglobulins-HRP reagent for 15 minutes.
6. Wash slides in TBS.
7. Incubate in amplification reagent for 15 minutes. *N.B.* This incubation should be undertaken in the dark.
8. Wash slides in TBS.
9. Apply anti-fluorescein-HRP for 15 minutes.
10. Wash slides in TBS.
11. Incubate in DAB substrate solution.
12. Wash in running water, counterstain in hematoxylin, dehydrate, clear, and mount.

Alkaline phosphatase techniques

Alkaline phosphatase-anti-alkaline phosphatase (APAAP) for monoclonal antibodies

1. Rinse sections in TBS.
2. Drain off excess TBS and incubate in 10% casein for 10 minutes.
3. Incubate in primary antibody at optimal dilution for 30–40 minutes.
4. Wash in TBS.
5. Incubate in optimally diluted unconjugated rabbit anti-mouse bridge antibody for 30 minutes.
6. Wash in TBS.
7. Incubate in alkaline phosphatase-anti-alkaline phosphatase complex at the optimal dilution for 30 minutes.
8. Wash in TBS.
9. Incubate in substrate medium of choice: for example, fast red solution.
10. Wash in running tap water.
11. Counterstain and mount as desired.

Notes

a. The reaction end-product may be enhanced by repeating steps 5–8 once or twice with a reduction of the incubation times to 10 minutes.

b. As the alkaline phosphatase label is usually intestinal, it is resistant to blocking with levamisole at the concentrations described and hence it is included in the substrate mixture. Levamisole blocks most other types of alkaline phosphatase.

Immunogold techniques

These techniques lend themselves to electron micros-copy more than to the light microscope. The labeling intensity of gold alone, even using 20 nm colloidal gold, is usually not sufficiently intense to be of value for light microscopy. However, the work of Holgate et al. (1983a, 1983b) showed that silver enhancement increased the sensitivity of the method considerably. The Lugol's iodine and thiosulfate step appears to be essential for this technique to work on routinely processed paraffin sections. This method uses bovine serum albumin in Tris-buffered saline (BSA-TBS).

Indirect immunogold technique for monoclonal antibodies

Method

1. Take sections to distilled water.
2. Treat sections with Lugol's iodine for 5 minutes, clear with 2.5% sodium thiosulfate, and then wash well in running tap water.
3. Take sections to BSA–TBS (0.1% bovine serum albumin in TBS, pH 8.2), drain and wipe off excess around section.
4. Incubate in 1/20 normal goat serum (NGS) in BSA-TBS for 10 minutes.
5. Drain, wipe off excess serum.
6. Incubate in primary antibody optimally diluted in BSA-TBS for 30–60 minutes.
7. Gently wash in TBS.
8. Incubate in gold-conjugated secondary antibody at optimal dilution in BSA-TBS for 60 minutes.
9. Repeat step 7.
10. Wash in 0.1 M phosphatase buffered saline (PBS), pH 7.6, for three 2-minute changes.
11. Post-fix with 2% glutaraldehyde in PBS for 10–15 minutes.
12. Wash well in several changes of distilled water and enhance staining with silver. (See silver enhancement procedure below.)
13. Counterstain, dehydrate, clear, and mount.

Silver enhancement

The intensity of the gold label may be enhanced by incubation of the sections in a silver solution.

Solutions

a. Citrate buffer stock solution

Trisodium citrate	23.5 g
Citric acid	25.5 g
Distilled water	100 ml

b. Silver solution

Silver lactate	110 mg
Distilled water	15 ml
Prepare fresh.	

c. Hydroquinone solution

Hydroquinone	950 mg
Distilled water	15 ml
Prepare fresh.	

d. Gum acacia

50% gum acacia solution	7 ml

e. Silver enhancement solution

Silver lactate solution	15 ml
Hydroquinone solution	15 ml
Molar citrate buffer	10 ml
Distilled water	60 ml
50% gum acacia solution	7 ml

Method

1. Rinse the sections in 0.2 M citrate buffer for 2 minutes.
2. Incubate the sections in freshly prepared silver enhancement solution at room temperature, protected from the light. Development will take place in approximately 5 minutes.
3. Wash well in distilled water.
4. Wash in 2% sodium thiosulfate, 1 minute.
5. Wash well in running water.
6. Counterstain if desired.
7. Dehydrate, clear, and mount.

Visualization substrates for alkaline phosphatase methods

The methods for the visualization of alkaline phos-phatase activity are based on the coupling of substi-tuted naphthol to a suitable azo dye. The most commonly used dyes are fast red TR and hexazo-tized new fuchsin. Nitro-blue tetrazolium methods are also gaining popularity, as they seem to be most sensitive. The following is recommended for histo-logical preparations.

Fast red TR solution

Naphthol-AS-MX phosphate, free acid	4.0 mg
N,N-dimethyl formamide	0.2 ml
1 M Tris-HCl buffer, pH 8.2	9.8 ml
Levamisole	2.4 mg
Fast red TR salt	10 mg

Dissolve the naphthol-AS-MX phosphate in *N,N*-dimethyl formamide in a glass vial and then add the Tris buffer. Add and dissolve the levamisole and fast red TR salt and immediately filter onto the sections. Incubate the sections for 10–20 minutes and, as the bright red reaction product is soluble in alcohol, mount in an aqueous medium. A blue reaction product can be obtained by using 4 mg fast blue BB instead of fast red TR salt in the above recipe. Counterstaining with hematoxylin would not be appropriate with blue salt.

Alternative fast red substrate solution recommended for cytological preparations

This solution described by Ponder and Wilkinson (1981) would appear to be more effective against endogenous alkaline phosphatase in pleural aspirates than the previous solution (Happerfield, personal communication).

Solution

Naphthol AS-BI phosphoric acid sodium salt	5.0 mg
N,N-dimethyl formamide	0.2 ml
Veronal acetate buffer, pH 9.2	9.8 ml
Levamisole	2.5 mg
Fast red TR salt	5.0 mg

This solution is prepared by dissolving the naphthol AS-BI in *N,N*-dimethyl formamide in a glass vial. Add the buffer, levamisole, and mix. Immediately before staining, dissolve the fast red salt in the substrate solution and filter before use.

Hexazotized new fuchsin (Malik & Daymon 1982)

Naphthol-AS-BI phosphate	5.0 mg
N,N-dimethyl formamide	60 µl
1 M Tris-HCl buffer, pH 8.7	10 ml
1 M levamisole	10 µl
4% sodium nitrite (freshly prepared)	50 µl
5% new fuchsin in 2 M HCl	20 µl

Add the new fuchsin to the sodium nitrite, mix for 30–60 seconds and then add the Tris buffer and levamisole. Immediately before staining, add the naphthol AS-BI phosphate, dissolved in the *N,N*-dimethyl formamide, and filter directly onto the sections. Incubate for 20 minutes. The reaction end-product is bright red, but whilst this is considered to be resistant to dehydration, clearing in xylene, and mounting in resinous mounting media, it is not always consistent. Therefore, it is advisable to water-mount. A modified new fuchsin method proposed by Stein et al. in 1985 is more complex than the first, but many users agree that the final reaction product is much more intense.

Modified new fuchsin method

Solution 1

1 M 2-amino-2-methyl-1,3-propanediol	18 ml
1 M Tris-HCl buffer, pH 9.7	50 ml
Sodium chloride	600 mg
Levamisole	28 mg

Solution 2

Naphthol AS-BI phosphate	35 mg
N,N-dimethyl formamide	0.42 ml

Dissolve the naphthol AS-BI phosphate in *N,N*-dimethyl formamide.

Solution 3

New fuchsin (5 g in 100 ml 2 N HCl)	0.14 ml
Sodium nitrite (freshly prepared, 40 mg in 1 ml distilled water)	0.35 ml

Mix the new fuchsin with the freshly prepared sodium nitrite and incubate this mixture for 60 seconds at room temperature whilst agitating.

Mix solutions 1 and 2 and then add solution 3. Adjust the pH to 8.7 by adding HCl. Mix well, filter through ordinary filter paper directly onto slides, and incubate for 20 minutes.

Nitro-blue tetrazolium method for alkaline phosphatase (McGadey 1970)

Buffer solution

0.2 M Tris-HCl, pH 9.5, containing 10 mM $MgCl_2$

Solution A

5 mg 5-bromo-4-chloro-3-indolyl phosphate (BCIP) is dissolved in 0.1 ml dimethyl formamide (DMF) and then in 1.0 ml of the above buffer.

Solution B

5 mg nitro-blue tetrazolium is dissolved in 0.1 ml DMF.

Solutions A and B are added, with continuous stirring, to 30 ml of the above buffer and filtered. Once filtered, incubate immediately for 20 minutes. The intense blue-black reaction product at the site of alkaline phosphatase activity is soluble in alcohol and xylene: hence aqueous mounting is recommended.

More detailed descriptions of these and various other methods are available in many books published on immunohistochemical methodology (Bullock & Petrusz 1982, 1983, 1985; Polak & Van Noorden 1986; Jasani & Schmid 1993; Kirkham & Hall 1995). Data sheets and instructions with the wide range of commercially available substrates/chromogens are included with the products.

References

Adams, J.C., 1992. Biotin amplification of horseradish peroxidase in histochemical stains. Journal of Histochemistry and Cytochemistry 40, 1457–1463.

Banks, P.M., 1979. Diagnostic applications of an immunoperoxidase method in hematopathology. Journal of Histochemistry and Cytochemistry 27, 1192.

Bell, P.B., Rundquist, I., Svenson, I., Collins, U.P., 1987. Formaldehyde sensitivity of a GFAP epitope removed by extraction of the cytoskeleton with high salt. Journal of Histochemistry and Cytochemistry 35, 1375–1380.

Bigbee, J.W., Kosek, J.C., Eng, L.E., 1977. The effects of primary antiserum dilution on staining of 'antigen-rich' tissue with the peroxidase anti-peroxidase technique. Journal of Histochemistry and Cytochemistry 25 (6), 443–447.

Bobrow, M.N., Harris, T.D., Shaughnessy, K.J., Litt, G.J., 1989. Catalysed reporter deposition, a novel method of signal amplification in a variety of formats. Journal of Immunological Methods 125, 279–285.

Bobrow, M.N., Litt, G.J., Shaughnessy, K.J., et al., 1992. The use of catalyzed reporter deposition as a means of signal amplification in a variety of formats. Journal of Immunological Methods 150 (1–2), 145–149.

Bondi, A., Chieregatti, G., Eusebi, V., et al., 1982. The use of β-galactosidase as a tracer in immunohistochemistry. Histochemistry 76 (2), 153–158.

Brandtzaeg, P., 1983. Tissue preparation methods for immunocytochemistry. In: Bullock, G.R., Petrusz, P. (Eds.), Techniques in immunocytochemistry. Vol. 1, Academic Press, New York, pp. 1–75.

Brooks, S.A., Leathem, A.J.C., Schumacher, U., 1996. Lectin histochemistry. Microscopy handbook 36. Bios Scientific Publishers, Oxford.

Bullock, G.R., Petrusz, P. (Eds.), 1982. Techniques in immuno-cytochemistry, Vol. 1. Academic Press, New York.

Bullock, G.R., Petrusz, P. (Eds.), 1983. Techniques in immuno-cytochemistry, Vol. 2. Academic Press, New York.

Bullock, G.R., Petrusz, P. (Eds.), 1985. Techniques in immuno-cytochemistry, Vol. 3. Academic Press, New York.

Capra, J.D., Edmundson, A.B., 1977. The antibody combining site. Scientific American 236 (1), 50–59.

Cattoretti, G., Pileri, S., Parravicini, C., 1993. Antigen unmasking on formalin-fixed paraffin embedded tissue sections. Journal of Pathology 171 (2), 83–98.

Charalambous, C., Singh, N., Isaacson, P.G., 1993. Immunohistochemical analysis of Hodgkin's disease using microwave heating. Journal of Clinical Pathology 46 (12), 1085–1088.

Coons, A.H., Creech, H.J., Jones, R.N., 1941. Immunological properties of an antibody containing a fluorescent group. Proceedings of the Society of Experimental Biology and Medicine 47, 200–202.

Cordell, J.L., Falini, B., Erber, W., et al., 1984. Immunoenzymatic labelling of monoclonal antibodies using immune complexes of alkaline phosphatase and monoclonal anti-alkaline phosphatase (APAAP complexes). Journal of Histochemistry and Cytochemistry 32 (2), 219–229.

Curran, R.C., Gregory, J., 1977. The unmasking of antigens in paraffin sections of tissue by trypsin. Experientia 33 (10), 1400.

Damjanov, I., 1987. Biology of disease, lectin cytochemistry and histochemistry. Laboratory Investigations 57, 5–20.

Delellis, R.A., Sternberger, L.A., Mann, R.B., et al., 1979. Immunoperoxidase techniques in diagnostic pathology. American Journal of Clinical Pathology 71 (5), 483.

De Mey, J., Moeremans, M., 1986. Raising and testing polyclonal antibodies for immunocytochemistry. In: Polack, J.M., Van Noorden, S. (Eds.), Immunocytochemistry: modern methods and applications. Wright, Bristol, pp. 3–12.

De Mey, J., Hacker, G.W., Dewaele, M., Springall, D.R., 1986. Gold probes in light microscope. In: Polak, J.M., Van Noorden, S. (Eds.), Immunocytochemistry: modern methods and applications, second ed. Wright, Bristol, pp. 71–88.

Denk, H., Syre, G., Weirich, E., 1977. Immunomorphologic methods in routine pathology. Application of immunofluorescence and the unlabeled antibody-enzyme (peroxidase-antiperoxidase) technique to formalin fixed paraffin embedded kidney biopsies. Beiträge zur Pathologie 160 (2), 187–194.

Ellis, I.O., Bell, J., Bancroft, J.D., 1988. An investigation of optimal gold particle size for immunohistological immunogold and immunogold-silver staining. Journal of Histochemistry and Cytochemistry 36 (1), 121–122.

Engvall, E., Perlman, P., 1971. Enzyme-linked immunosorbent assay (ELISA). Qualitative assay of immunoglobulin G. Immunochemistry 8 (9), 871–874.

Erber, W.N., Willis, J.I., Hoffman, G.J., 1997. An enhanced immunocytochemical method for staining bone marrow trephine sections. J Clin Pathol 50 (5), 389–393.

Faulk, W.P., Taylor, G.M., 1971. An immunocolloid method for the electron microscope. Immunochemistry 8 (11), 1081–1083.

Gatter, K.C., Falini, B., Mason, D.Y., 1984. The use of monoclonal antibodies in histopathological diagnosis. In: Antony, P.P., MacSween, R.N.M. (Eds.), Recent advances in histopathology, Vol. 12. Churchill Livingstone, Edinburgh, pp. 35–67.

Gerdes, J., Becher, M.H.G., Key, G., Cattoretti, G., 1992. Immunohistological detection of tumor growth fraction (Ki67) in formalin fixed and routinely processed tissues. Journal of Pathology 168, 85–87.

Graham, R.C., Karnovsky, M.J., 1966. The early stages of absorption of injected horseradish peroxidase in the proximal tubules of mouse kidney: ultrastructural cytochemistry by a new technique. Journal of Histochemistry and Cytochemistry 4, 291.

Graham, R.C. Jr, Ladholm, U., Karnovsky, M.J., 1965. Cytochemical demonstration of peroxidase activity by 3-amino-9-ethylcarbazole. Journal of Histochemistry and Cytochemistry 13, 150–152.

Grabe, D., 1980. Immunoreactivities of gastrin (G) cells II. Non-specific binding of immunoglobulins to G-cells by ionic interactions. Histochemistry 65 (3), 223–237.

Guesden, J.L., Terynck, T., Avrameas, S., 1979. The use of avidin-biotin interaction in immunoenzymatic techniques. Journal of Histochemistry and Cytochemistry 8, 1131–1139.

Hanker, J.S., Yates, P.E., Metx, C.B., Rustini, A., 1977. A new specific, sensitive and non-carcinogenic reagent for the demonstration of horseradish peroxidase procedures. Journal of Histochemistry 9, 789–792.

Hartman, B.K., 1973. Immunofluorescence of dopamine B hydroxylase. Application of improved methodology to the localization of the peripheral and central noradrenergic nervous system. Journal of Histochemistry and Cytochemistry 21, 312–332.

Heggeness, M.H., Ash, J.F., 1977. Use of the avidin-biotin complex for the localization of actin and myosin with fluorescence microscopy. Journal of Cell Biology 73, 783.

Heyderman, E., Monaghan, P., 1979. Immunoperoxidase reactions in resin embedded sections. Investigative Cell Pathology 2, 119–122.

Holgate, C., Jackson, P., Cowen, P., Bird, C., 1983a. Immunogold-silver staining: new method of immunostaining with enhanced sensitivity. Journal of Histochemistry and Cytochemistry 31, 938–944.

Holgate, C., Jackson, P., Lauder, I., et al., 1983b. Surface membrane staining of immunoglobulins in paraffin sections of non-Hodgkin's lymphomas using immunogold-silver staining techniques. Journal of Clinical Pathology 36, 742–746.

Hsu, S.M., Soban, E., 1982. Colour modification of diaminobenzidine (DAB) precipitation by metallic ions and its application to double immunohistochemistry. Journal of Histochemistry and Cytochemistry 30, 1079–1082.

Hsu, S.M., Raine, L., Fanger, H., 1981. Use of avidin-biotin-peroxidase complex (ABC) in immunoperoxidase techniques: a comparison between ABC and unlabeled antibody (PAP) procedures. Journal of Histochemistry and Cytochemistry 29, 577–580.

Huang, S., Minassian, H., More, J.D., 1976. Application of immunofluorescent staining in paraffin sections improved by trypsin digestion. Laboratory Investigation 35, 383–391.

Hunt, S.P., Allanson, J., Mantyh, P.W., 1986. Radioimmunochemistry. In: Polak, J.M., Van Noorden, S. (Eds.), Immunocytochemistry. Modern methods and applications, second ed. Wright, Bristol, pp. 99–114.

Jasani, B., Schmid, K.W., 1993. Immunocytochemistry in diagnostic pathology. Churchill Livingstone, Edinburgh.

Jasani, B., Wynford-Thomas, D., Williams, E.D., 1981. Use of monoclonal anti-hapten antibodies for immunolocalisation of tissue antigens. Journal of Clinical Pathology 34, 1000–1002.

Jasani, B., Thomas, N.D., Navabi, H., et al., 1992. Dinitrophenol (DNP) hapten sandwich staining (DHSS) procedure. A 10 year review of its principle reagents and applications. Journal of Immunological Methods 150, 193–198.

Jessup, E., 1994. Antigen retrieval techniques for the demonstration of immunoglobulin light chains in formalin-fixed paraffin embedded sections. UK NEQAS Newsletter 4, 12–16.

Kaplow, L.S., 1975. Substitute for benzidine in myeloperoxidase stains. American Journal of Clinical Pathology 63, 451.

Kawai, K., Scrizawa, A., Hamana, T., Tsutsumi, Y., 1994. Heat induced antigen retrieval of proliferating cell nuclear antigen and p53 protein in formalin fixed paraffin embedded sections. Pathology International 44, 759–764.

King, G., Payne, S., Walker, F., Murray, G.I., 1997. A highly sensitive detection method for immunohistochemistry using biotinylated tyramine. Journal of Pathology 183 (2), 237–241.

Kirkham, N., Hall, P. (Eds.), 1995. Progress in pathology. Churchill Livingstone, Edinburgh.

Kohler, G., Milstein, C., 1975. Continuous cultures of fused cells producing antibody of pre-defined specificity. Nature 256, 495–497.

Kraehenbuhl, J.P., Jamieson, J.D., 1974. Localisation of intracellular antigens by immunoelectron microscopy. International Review of Experimental Pathology 12, 1–53.

Langlois, N.E.I., King, G., Herriot, R., Thompson, W.D., 1994. Non enzymatic retrieval of antigen permits staining of follicle centre cells by the rabbit polyclonal antibody to protein gene product 9.5. Journal of Pathology 173, 249–253.

Leatham, A., 1986. Lectin histochemistry. In: Polak, J.M., Van Noorden, S. (Eds.), Immunocytochemistry: modern methods and applications, second ed. Wright, Bristol, pp. 167–187.

LeBrun, D.P., Kamel, O.W., Dorfman, R.F., Warnke, R.A., 1992. Enhanced staining for Leu M1 (CD15) in Hodgkin's disease using a secondary antibody specific for immunoglobulin M. American Journal of Clinical Pathology 97, 135–138.

Leong, A.S.-Y., Cooper, K., Leong, F.J.W.-M., 1999. Manual of diagnostic antibodies for immunohistology. Greenwich Medical Media, London.

McGadey, J., 1970. A tetrazolium method for non-specific alkaline phosphatases. Histochemie 23, 180–184.

McIver, A.G., Mepham, B.L., 1982. Immunoperoxidase techniques in human renal biopsy. Histopathology 6, 249–267.

Malik, N.J., Daymon, M.E., 1982. Improved double immuno-enzymatic labelling using alkaline phosphatase and horseradish peroxidase. Journal of Clinical Pathology 35, 1092–1094.

Mason, J.T., O'Leary, T.J., 1991. Effects of formaldehyde fixation on protein secondary structure: a calorimetric and infrared spectroscopic investigation. Journal of Histochemistry and Cytochemistry 39 (2), 225–229.

Mason, T.E., Pfifer, R.F., Spicer, S.S., et al., 1969. An immuno-globulin enzyme bridge method for localising tissue antigens. Journal of Histochemistry and Cytochemistry 17, 563.

Mason, D.Y., Cordell, J., Brown, M., et al., 1989. Detection of cells in paraffin wax embedded tissue using antibodies against a peptide sequence from the CD3 antigen. Journal of Clinical Pathology 42, 1194–1200.

Mepham, B.L., Frater, W., Mitchell, B.S., 1979. The use of proteolytic enzymes to improve immunoglobulin staining by the P.A.P. Technique. Histochemical Journal 11, 345.

Miller, K., Auld, J., Jessup, E., et al., 1995. Antigen unmasking in formalin-fixed routinely processed paraffin wax-embedded sections by pressure cooking: a comparison with microwave oven heating and traditional methods. Advances in Anatomical Pathology 2, 60–64.

Morgan, J.M., Navabi, H., Schmidt, K.W., Jasani, B., 1994. Possible role of tissue bound calcium ions in citrate-mediated high temperature antigen retrieval. Journal of Pathology 174, 301–307.

Morgan, J.M., Navabi, H., Jasani, B., 1997. Role of calcium chelation in high-temperature antigen

retrieval at different pH values. Journal of Pathology 182 (2), 233–237.

Nairn, R.C., 1976. Fluorescent protein tracing, fourth ed. Churchill Livingstone, Edinburgh.

Nakane, P.K., 1968. Simultaneous localisation of multiple tissue antigens using the peroxidase-labelled antibody method: a study on pituitary glands of the rat. Journal of Histochemistry and Cytochemistry 16, 557–560.

Nakane, P.K., Pierce, G.B., 1966. Enzyme-labeled antibodies: preparation and localisation of antigens. Journal of Histochemistry and Cytochemistry 14, 929–931.

Norton, A.J., Jordon, S., Yeomans, P., 1994. Brief high temperature heat denaturation (pressure cooking): a simple and effective method of antigen retrieval for routinely processed tissues. Journal of Pathology 173, 371–379.

Pasha, T., Montone, K.T., Tomaszeweski, J.E., 1995. Nuclear antigen retrieval utilizing steam heat (abstract). Laboratory Investigation 72, 167A.

Pearse, A.G.E., Polak, J.M., 1975. Bifunctional reagents as vapour and liquid phase fixatives for immunochemistry. Histochemical Journal 7, 179–186.

Petrusz, P., Sar, M., Ordonneau, P., Dimeo, P., 1976. Specificity in immunochemical staining. Journal of Histochemistry and Cytochemistry 24, 1110.

Petrusz, P., Sar, M., Ordronneau, P., Dimeo, P., 1977. Reply to letter of Swaab et al.: 'Can specificity ever be proved in immunocytochemical staining'. Journal of Histochemistry and Cytochemistry 25, 390.

Polak, J.M., Van Noorden, S. (Eds.), 1986. Immunochemistry. Practical applications in pathology and biology, second ed. Wright, Bristol.

Ponder, B.A., Wilkinson, M.M., 1981. Inhibition of endogenous tissue alkaline phosphatase with the use of alkaline phosphatase conjugates in immunohistochemistry. Journal of Histochemistry and Cytochemistry 29 (8), 981–984.

Riggs, J.L., Seiwald, J.R., Burkhalter, J.H., et al., 1958. Isothiocyanate compounds as fluorescent labeling agents for immune serum. American Journal of Pathology 34, 1081–1097.

Ritter, M.A., 1986. Raising and testing monoclonal antibodies for immunocytochemistry. In: Polak, J.M., Van Noorden, S. (Eds.), Immunocytochemistry: modern methods and applications. Wright, Bristol.

Robinson, G., Dawson, I.M.P., 1975. Immunochemical studies of the endocrine cells of the gastrointestinal tract: 1. The use and value of peroxidase conjugated antibody techniques for the localisation of gastrin-containing cells in the human pyloric antrum. Histochemical Journal 7, 321–333.

Roth, J., 1982. Applications of immunocolloids in light microscopy. Preparation of protein A-silver and protein A-gold complexes and their application for the localization of single and multiple antigens in paraffin sections. Journal of Histochemistry and Cytochemistry 30, 691–696.

Shi, S.R., Key, M.E., Kalra, K.L., 1991. Antigen retrieval in formalin-fixed paraffin-embedded tissues: an enhancement method for immunohistochemical staining based on microwave oven heating of sections. Journal of Histochemistry and Cytochemistry 39, 741–748.

Singh, N., Wotherspoon, A.C., Miller, K.D., Isaacson, P.G., 1993. The effect of formalin fixation time on the immuno-cytochemical detection of antigen using the microwave. Journal of Pathology (Suppl), 382A.

Stein, H., Gatter, K., Asbahr, H., Mason, D.Y., 1985. Use of freeze-dried paraffin embedded sections for immuno-histologic staining with monoclonal antibodies. Laboratory Investigation 52, 676–683.

Sternberger, L.A., 1969. Some new developments in immuno-cytochemistry. Mikroskopie 25, 346–361.

Sternberger, L.A., Hardy, P.H., Cuculis, J.J., Meyer, H.G., 1970. The unlabelled antibody enzyme method of immunohistochemistry: preparation and properties of soluble antigen-antibody complex (horseradish peroxidase-antiperoxidase) and its use in identification of spirochaetes.

Journal of Histochemistry and Cytochemistry 18, 315.

Straus, W., 1976. Use of peroxidase inhibitors for immunoperoxidase procedures. In: Feldmann, G. (Ed.), First International Symposium on Immunoenzymatic Techniques. North Holland, Amsterdam.

Straus, W., 1982. Imidazole increases the sensitivity of the cytochemical reaction for peroxidase with diaminobenzidine at a neutral pH. Journal of Histochemistry and Cytochemistry 30, 491–493.

Streefkerk, J.G., 1972. Inhibition of erythrocyte pseudo-peroxidase activity by treatment with hydrogen peroxide following methanol. Journal of Histochemistry and Cytochemistry 20, 829.

Suffin, S.C., Muck, K.B., Young, J.C., et al., 1979. Improvement of the glucose oxidase immunoenzyme technique. American Journal of Clinical Pathology 71, 492–496.

Taylor, C.R., Burns, J., 1974. The demonstration of plasma cells and other immunoglobulin-containing cells in formalin-fixed, paraffin-embedded tissues using peroxidase-labelled antibody. Journal of Clinical Pathology 27, 14–20.

Van Noorden, S., Stuar, M.C., Cheung, A., et al., 1986. Localization of pituitary hormones by multiple immuno-enzyme staining procedures using monoclonal and polyclonal antibodies. Journal of Histochemistry and Cytochemistry 34, 287.

Warnke, R.A., Gatter, K.C., Mason, D.Y., 1983. Monoclonal antibodies as diagnostic reagents. Recent Advances in Clinical Immunology 3, 163.

Weisburger, E.K., Russfield, A.B., Homburger, F., et al., 1978. Testing of twenty-one environmental aromatic amines or derivatives for long-term toxicity or carcinogenicity. Journal of Environmental Pathology and Toxicity 2, 325–356.

Recommended further reading

Immunoenzyme Multiple Staining Methods, Royal Microscopical Society, Microscopy Handbook Series 45 by C.M.van der Loos.

Immunofluorescent techniques

19

Graeme Wild

Introduction

Immunofluorescence is a laboratory technique whereby antigens are detected by specific antibodies that are conjugated directly to a readily identifiable fluorescent label. It was first described in 1941 by Coons, Creech and Jones to identify pneumococcal antigens in tissues. The method has been refined, and has become well established in the identification and localization of antigen deposits and cells within tissue sections. The fluorochrome conjugated to the antibody absorbs ultraviolet or visible light of a particular wavelength to reach an unstable excited state as its electrons gain energy. The fluorochrome subsequently emits light of a different, usually longer, wavelength to that of the excitation light as the electrons return to their ground state. Molecules that are commonly used in immunohistological tissue examination are fluorescein isothiocyanate (FITC), which absorbs at 494 nm and emits green light at 518 nm, or tetramethyl rhodamine isothiocyanate, which has an excitation wavelength of 550 nm and emits red light at 580 nm (Allan 2000).

The original work of Coons and colleagues used a method called direct immunofluorescence, where the specific primary antibody is conjugated directly with the fluorochrome and viewed under a fluorescent microscope. Indirect immunofluorescence was introduced by Weller and Coons in 1954. It is distinct from the direct method in that the specific primary antibody is unlabeled and is detected in a second stage by the use of a fluorochrome-labeled anti-species specific immunoglobulin antiserum.

Immunofluorescent methods can be used to detect antigens such as double-stranded DNA antibodies as well as cell surface receptors on lymphocytes, to name but two examples. The advantage of tissue immunofluorescence methods over other immunological methods, such as enzyme-linked immunosorbent assay (ELISA), is the ability to not only identify the presence of antigen but also identify the deposition site within the tissue section.

Success in immunofluorescent staining techniques is dependent upon many factors, including:

- Preservation of substrate antigens and quality of tissue sections
- Affinity and specificity of antibodies and conjugates
- The detection method
- The microscope
- Quality control of staining procedures

Preservation of substrate antigens

Tissue antigens demonstrable by immunofluorescent techniques include viruses, protozoa, bacteria, enzymes, hormones, plasma proteins, cells and cell constituents. The antigen must remain sufficiently insoluble *in situ*, but should not so denatured that it loses reactivity with its specific antibody. A variety of methods are available to preserve different antigens. The use of air-dried unfixed cryostat sections of skin or renal biopsies allows the detection of chemically sensitive or otherwise labile antigens present in the tissue. In practice, unfixed cryostat sections or cell preparations are used whenever possible unless the antigen under investigation is known to be soluble, in which case suitable fixation such as cold 10% neutral buffered formalin can be used. Ethanol and acetone are other alternatives but it should be noted that tissue morphology is suboptimal with these methods.

Biopsy tissue should be transported to the laboratory in Michel transport medium at pH 7.0 (Michel et al. 1972) and processed for freezing as soon as possible by washing in wash solution. The tissue can remain in Michel medium for several days, but extended time in the transport medium can increase autofluorescence and background staining (Carson 1997). The Michel medium should be kept in capped containers and the pH checked at regular intervals as it can absorb CO_2 and become acidic – resulting in variable staining and causing other tissue artifacts.

For best quality, frozen tissue sections should be cut from unfixed tissue that has been snap frozen. Slow freezing can cause ice crystal formation, which can distort tissue morphology and antigen structure and so should be avoided. Renal and skin biopsies can be mounted in OCT compound on a chuck and frozen in a cryostat at a temperature of –25°C. The tissue can be wrapped in aluminum foil and stored at –20°C if there is to be a delay in cutting the sections. Frozen sections 5 µm thick are cut on a microtome in the cryostat and mounted on clean slides followed by air-drying. The use of positively charged slides may help in the adherence of the section to the slide and prevent the section floating free or becoming fragmented during the washing stages.

Method for preparing frozen tissue sections

1. The biopsy should be carefully removed from the Michel transport medium with forceps and placed in biopsy wash solution for a minimum of 30 minutes. The Michel medium reversibly denatures proteins within the tissue and the washing step restores the proteins to their former state.

2. Remove the tissue from the wash solution and place onto a glass slide to remove excess wash solution.

3. A small amount of OCT compound is placed on a metal chuck that has been cooled to –25°C. The biopsy tissue is then placed in the OCT and orientated so that it is on a level plane. The OCT turns from transparent to a dense white as it freezes. Before the OCT freezes on its upper surface more is added to form a mound over the top of the tissue. This ensures that the biopsy is completely covered and has some protection from dehydration.

4. The chuck with frozen OCT and biopsy tissue should be left at –25°C for at least 30 minutes before cutting. The chuck can be wrapped in aluminum foil and stored at –20°C if sectioning is to be delayed.

5. The covering OCT is removed by sectioning at 15 µm until the tissue is exposed.

6. The tissue should be cut in 5 µm sections and attached to clean microscope slides that are at ambient temperature. One or two sections are attached to each slide, depending on laboratory protocols.

7. For renal biopsies the sections are checked at regular intervals for the presence of glomeruli by staining with toluidine blue and viewed under a light microscope. Skin biopsy sections should be checked for the presence of an epidermal layer.

8. Sections should be allowed to air dry for a minimum of 30 minutes.

9. The slides are wrapped in aluminum foil and stored at –20°C until ready for staining.

Primary antibodies and conjugates

Most of the reagents used in immunofluorescence staining procedures are available from commercial sources. However, it is useful to be familiar with the methods of production and characterization of these materials in order to compare similar products from different suppliers and also for troubleshooting procedures.

A preparation of highly purified or recombinant antigen is an absolute requirement for the production of monospecific antiserum having a high affinity and avidity. Antibody specificity can be determined by reacting it against the purified antigen used to immunize the animal. It can also be tested against the unpurified source of the protein such as whole human serum: for example, if the antibody is against a specific human serum protein. This checking for monospecificity can be achieved by gel diffusion, immunoelectrophoresis or passive hemagglutination, and should result in the production of one precipitin line in both the purified antigen and the unpurified source. Antibody concentrations of relatively high titer are required for conjugation with fluorochromes.

Serum proteins have differing capacities to combine or conjugate with fluorochromes. In particular, immunoglobulins have less affinity for FITC than other more 'negatively charged' proteins such as albumin and β-proteins. These latter molecules when conjugated can also combine with tissue components via electrostatic forces and thus give high levels of non-specific staining. Thus, purified immunoglobulin free from other serum proteins is a prerequisite for conjugation. Immunoglobulin molecules are composed of heavy and light chains. The heavy chains identify the isotype of the antibody and the light chains are common to all immunoglobulin types. Consequently, an antibody raised to a particular immunoglobulin type may also cross-react with all other immunoglobulin types due to the presence of antibodies to the light chains. These contaminating light chain antibodies should be removed by absorption against free light chains and leave only antibody reacting against the heavy chain component; i.e., γ, α or μ chain specific.

Conjugates may be prepared from:

1. Immunoglobulin-rich fractions of serum prepared by salting-out procedures
2. Chromatographically prepared fractions, usually on diethyl aminoethane (DEAE)

ion exchange columns, consisting mainly of IgG
3. Pure IgG fractions obtained by immunoabsorption on affinity chromatography columns
4. F(Ab)2 fractions of IgG obtained by proteolytic cleavage of purified IgG (from step 3 above).

The four methods are progressive in terms of the purity of their antibody preparation, and each can be used with success in different situations. For most routine applications, reagents prepared using purification methods 1 or 2 are adequate, particularly when they can be used at high dilution. Reagents prepared with method 2 are useful when background staining is a problem. Conjugates made from F(Ab)2 fragments are used when the binding of the conjugated antibody to Fc receptors is to be avoided. They may also be useful in double staining techniques where cross-reactions between antibodies produced in different species are a problem.

The absorption and emission characteristics of several commonly used fluorochromes are summarized in Table 19.1 (Allan 2000). FITC is the most widely used fluorochrome in immunofluorescent microscopy. It has a wide absorption spectrum that covers the ultraviolet to blue light range and has a characteristic apple-green emission. An advantage of FITC is that the apple-green fluorescence is rarely seen as autofluorescence in mammalian tissues. Rhodamine absorbs maximally in green light and has an orange-red emission light and can be used in a two color technique where two different antigens can be identified on the same section by antibodies conjugated with FITC or rhodamine.

The conjugation of fluorochrome with antibody can be a complex reaction and is dependent on the

Table 19.1 Spectral characteristics of commonly used fluorochromes

Fluorochrome	Absorption maximum (nm)	Emission maximum (nm)	Observed color
Fluorescein (FITC)	494	518	green
Rhodamine (TRITC)	550	580	red
Texas Red™	595	615	red
R-Phycoerythrin (PE)	565	575	orange/red

Allan, V.J., 2000. Protein localization by fluorescence microscopy. Oxford University Press, Oxford.

type of fluorochrome. FITC and rhodamine can be linked covalently to free terminal amino and carboxyl groups, free amino groups on lysine side chains and free carboxyl groups in aspartic and glutamic acid residues. The reactions occur at pH 9.5 and the degree of conjugation is both time and temperature dependent. The ideal fluorochrome to antibody ratio is between 2 and 4.

Over-conjugation of the antibody will give high background staining as the molecules have a net negative charge and will bind to tissue non-specifically. This can also result in poor reactivity of the antibody due to interference with antigen binding sites. Under-conjugation gives a preparation that will produce unsatisfactory low-level fluorescence.

Free chromophore in the conjugate preparation must be removed to prevent non-specific staining. The free chromophore can be removed by dialysis against 0.15 M sodium chloride at 4°C. The presence or absence of fluorescence in the dialysate can be seen under UV examination. An alternative is to use gel filtration column chromatography using Sephadex G50. A method for testing commercial conjugate preparations for free dye is described by Johnson and Holborrow (1986).

It is good laboratory practice to evaluate the sensitivity and specificity of all antiserum and conjugates used in immunofluorescence. In assessing the sensitivity of the reagents, a checkerboard test will indicate the optimal working dilution for a particular antibody or conjugate. For indirect immunofluorescence, serial dilutions of the antiserum or conjugate are tested against serial dilutions of the unlabeled primary antibody and the tissue sections assessed for the least amount of background fluorescence which still allows identification of the target antigen. The conjugate working dilution in direct immunofluorescence can be determined by examining serial dilutions of the conjugate on a tissue section containing known protein deposits (e.g., renal sections from an IgA nephropathy or skin sections from known pemphigus or pemphigoid patients).

Specificity checking of a working strength conjugate on a tissue section with known deposits shows whether or not it will cross-react with other antigens. Anti-IgG γ-chain-specific conjugate for example should not react with other classes of immunoglobulin such as IgA, IgM or kappa/lambda (κ/λ) light chains.

Some anti-animal immunoglobulin specific conjugates used in indirect immunofluorescence may cross-react with human immunoglobulins, and in such cases it is essential that the cross-reacting antibodies are removed by absorption with human immunoglobulin. Cross-reactivity can be assessed by incubating the conjugated antibody directly on a tissue section containing human immunoglobulin and examining the slide for fluorescence.

Staining procedure

Staining of renal and skin biopsies can involve both direct and indirect procedures, depending on the availability of suitable monospecific conjugated antiserum directed against human proteins. If such reagents are not available or the antigen is present in small amounts and greater sensitivity is needed, then an indirect staining or sandwich technique is required where unlabeled primary antibody is incubated with the tissue and then a conjugated antibody directed against the animal species of the primary anti-body is used to detect binding: e.g., FITC rabbit anti-goat IgG as secondary antibody for the primary IgG goat anti-human C4d. Avidin and biotinylated reagents can also be used in indirect immunofluorescence.

Antibodies present in serum that are directed against tissue antigens such as anti-nuclear or anti-mitochondrial antibody can be identified with indirect immunofluorescence using mouse or rat tissue as the substrate. In this case the autoantibody in the serum acts as the unlabeled primary antibody and is detected using a goat anti-human IgG conjugate. Using indirect immunofluorescence in this way permits the screening of many different serum samples for various antibodies with only a single conjugated secondary antibody being required.

Typically, skin biopsy samples are examined for deposits of IgG, IgA, IgM, kappa (κ), lambda (λ), complement C3 and complement C1q. Renal biopsy samples are stained for IgG, IgA, IgM, κ, λ, C3, C1q, C4d and amyloid P. Additionally, renal transplant biopsies are examined for lymphocyte infiltration using CD3, CD4, CD8 and CD19.

Biopsy staining procedure *(for both direct and indirect immunofluorescence)*

1. Circle the biopsy section on the slide with an isolator hydrophobic marker pen to prevent mixing of adjacent antiserum and label the slide with the antibody specificity.
2. Wash the slide in phosphate buffered saline (PBS) for 5 minutes.
3. Remove slides from the wash tank and remove residual PBS by tapping the edge of the slide against a pad of tissue paper. The slide should be wiped around the isolator ring if required but care should be taken not to wipe the section off the slide. The section should not be allowed to dry out.
4. Flood the section with working-strength antibody or conjugated antibody and incubate for 30 minutes.
5. Wash the slides in PBS for 10 minutes.
6. Remove slides from the wash tank and remove residual PBS by tapping the edge of the slide against a pad of tissue paper. The slide should be wiped around the isolator ring if required, but care should be taken not to wipe the section off the slide. The section should not be allowed to dry out. If the sections have been stained with conjugated antiserum (i.e., direct immunofluorescence) then proceed to step 10 or step 7 if incubated with unconjugated antiserum (i.e., indirect immunofluorescence).
7. Wash the slides in PBS for 10 minutes.
8. Flood the section with the second stage conjugated antibody and incubate for 30 minutes.
9. Wash the slides in PBS for 10 minutes.
10. Mount all slides in buffered glycerol using coverslips.
11. Store the slides at 4°C until review.

Microscopy

The fluorescent microscope should deliver light of a specific wavelength to cause excitation of the fluorochrome, and then collect the emitted light for viewing through the eyepiece. This is achieved by applying excitation energy at the maximum absorption wavelength of the fluorochrome so that the maximum amount of light is emitted. The light source and filter arrangement of the microscope are important factors in achieving satisfactory results.

As the energy output of a fluorochrome is relatively low, a light source capable of delivering sufficient excitation wavelength photons to produce visible fluorescence is essential. Many fluorescent microscopes use mercury vapor or xenon as a light source and these are contained in quartz capsules under pressure. The light output for both of these bulbs diminishes over time due to blackening of the quartz capsule and a change in the spectral emission profile. High-pressure capsules are explosive and this risk increases the longer the bulb is in use and so to avoid this occurring and the added danger of mercury contamination it should be changed every 200–300 hours. If a mercury light source is used, it should be regularly checked for uniform fluorescence across a field and the bulb reaaligned if this is not satisfactory.

More recently the light-emitting diode (LED) has been introduced as a light source for immunofluorescence microscopy. These have several advantages over mercury bulbs in that they do not produce large quantities of heat, have a lifetime of 8000–10,000 hours, present no explosion risk and do not have warm-up or cool-down times. LED light sources are capable of producing high-intensity monochromatic light and do not require bulb realignment.

Excitation and emission filters act complementary to each other and have transmission ranges that are appropriate for the fluorochrome being used. Colored glass filters were originally used but these have been superseded by broad- or narrow-band interference filters. Unlike glass filters, the interference filters have a high transmission and a near vertical cut-off. The excitation filter allows light corresponding to the excitation wavelength of the fluorochrome to be directed on to the tissue section and all other wavelengths removed. Microscopes with a monochromatic LED source do not require excitation filters. Barrier filters are selected to absorb reflected excitation light and prevent it reaching the eyepieces but allow transmission of the emitted light from the fluorochrome.

Most fluorescent microscopes use a system of epi-illumination rather than transmitted light dark-ground illumination. In epi-illumination systems the excitation light is directed through the objective lens and onto the section. Fluorescent light passes from the sample through the same objective lens and is viewed through the eyepiece. A dichroic mirror between the objective and eyepiece allows selective reflection of the excitation light onto the section and then selective transmission of the fluorescent light wavelength only. The dichroic mirror only allows excitation light to pass one way and so prevents reflection of this wavelength from the tissue sample back to the eyepiece. Because the objective lens also acts as a condenser, the area viewed is equal to the area illuminated and so increasing the objective magnification will give a brighter image and more fluorescence intensity. Epi-illumination has several advantages over transmitted light illumination in that the light path passes through fewer glass surfaces and so less light is lost, oil immersion of the objective lens is not required, and the use of excitation and barrier filters with a dichroic mirror allows rapid changeover – if a two-color fluorescence technique is being used.

A drawback of immunofluorescence microscopy is that fluorescence from the chromophore fades with time, especially if it is exposed to excitation light for extended periods. The slides cannot therefore be used to provide a permanent record of the staining results and so photo documentation of the tissue sections is necessary. Good photographic images can be obtained where the sections show unequivocal staining against a darker background. Anti-fade reagents in the mounting medium reduce the rate of fluorescence fade and so can give shorter exposure time, which is especially useful if multiple exposures of a particular area of tissue are required. The camera system attached to the fluorescent microscope should ideally allow all the available light to enter the camera and not employ beam splitters for simultaneous observation and photography with the subsequent reduction in available light.

Quality control

Quality control is an essential component of good laboratory practice and is necessary to ensure consistency and reliability of the results generated. Evaluating the sensitivity and specificity of all antiserum and conjugates used by the laboratory has been discussed above. Every batch of immunofluorescence slides prepared should include slides with known antigen deposits as quality control slides. Microscopic examination of these slides should include an evaluation of the fluorescence intensity and amount of background staining compared to previous results as well as the identification and location of the deposits and the integrity of the tissue. The batch should be rejected if the quality control slide results are aberrant. Negative slides can also be included to indicate non-specific binding.

High background, or false-positive, staining may occur because of inadequate washing of the slides following antibody or conjugate incubation. It may also occur if the sections have been allowed to dry out during processing. High background staining may also be due to a high fluorochrome to protein ratio, from free chromophore in the conjugate or over-incubation of the tissue with reagent.

Diagnostic histopathology

Many tissue immunofluorescence techniques have been replaced by the use of flow cytometry and tissue immunoperoxidase staining. Immunofluorescence used in conjunction with light and electron microscopy provides a powerful tool in the diagnosis of renal disease and some skin diseases.

Renal disease

The immunofluorescence examination of frozen sections of renal tissue obtained by percutaneous needle biopsy or wedge biopsy allows the detection and distribution of antigens to be observed within the kidney. Different glomerular diseases show different and often specific patterns of distribution. Some of these patterns are illustrated in Figures 19.1–19.5 and

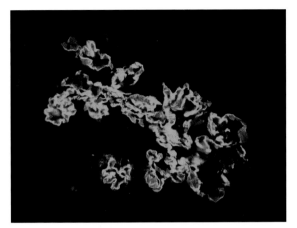

Figure 19.1 Renal biopsy, demonstrating glomerular basement membrane staining pattern, as seen in Goodpasture's syndrome.

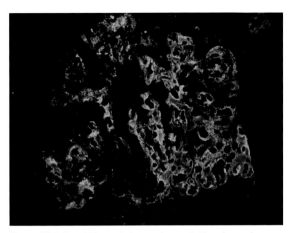

Figure 19.4 Renal biopsy in lupus, demonstrating glomerular staining for IgG.

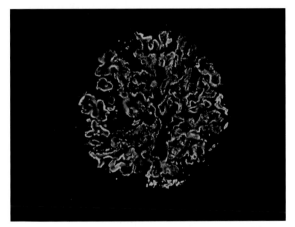

Figure 19.2 Renal biopsy, demonstrating membranous staining pattern with antibody to C3.

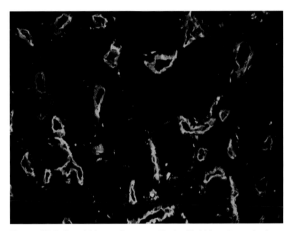

Figure 19.5 Renal biopsy from a patient with kidney transplant rejection, demonstrating staining of peritubular capillaries for C4d.

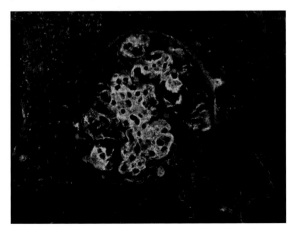

Figure 19.3 Renal biopsy in lupus, demonstrating glomerular staining for C1q.

are discussed in detail in Jennette et al. (1998), Walker (2009), Satoskar et al. (2007) and Crosson (2007). Most of these investigations use direct immunofluorescence with FITC-labeled primary antibodies. Other antigens such as C4d deposition in transplant kidneys with suspected antibody-mediated rejection (Collins 1999) require an indirect method.

Any fluorescent staining on the slide should be reported as antigen type (IgG, C3, κ, λ, CD3, etc.), intensity (+, ++, +++), location (mesangial, peripheral, basement membrane, etc.), pattern (linear, granular), and extent (focal, diffuse, global, segmental).

Table 19.2 Immunofluorescent patterns in selected skin diseases

Skin disease	Substances present	Location of deposits
Pemphigus	IgG, C3	Intercellular epidermis
Pemphigoid	C3, IgG	Basement membrane zone (linear pattern)
Bullous systemic lupus erythematosus	IgG, C3 (±IgM, IgA) (granular)	Basement membrane zone
Dermatitis herpetiformis	IgA and C3 (granular)	Dermal papillae of perilesional skin (granular pattern)

Farmer, E.R., Hood, A.F., 2000. Pathology of the skin, second ed. McGraw-Hill, New York.

Skin disease

Certain skin diseases have characteristic patterns of immunoglobulin deposition, usually in the upper dermis or at the dermo-epidermal junction. Immunofluorescent investigation is particularly useful in the diagnosis of bullous disorders, systemic lupus erythematosus and vasculitides. Some of the more common examples are summarized in Table 19.2 and discussed in more detail in Farmer and Hood (2000).

References

Allan, V.J., 2000. Protein localization by fluorescence microscopy. Oxford University Press, Oxford.

Carson, F.L., 1997. Histotechnology: a self-instructional text, second ed. ASCP Press, Chicago.

Collins, A.B., Schneeberger, E.E., Pascual, M.A., et al., 1999. Complement activation in acute humoral renal allograft rejection: diagnostic significance of C4d deposits in peritubular capillaries. Journal of the American Society of Nephrology 10, 2208–2214.

Coons, A.H., Creech, H.J., Jones, R.N., 1941. Immunological properties of an antibody containing a fluorescent group. Proceedings of the Society for Experimental Biology and Medicine 47, 200–202.

Crosson, J.T., 2007. Transplant rejection under the microscope. Transplant Proceedings 39 (3), 662–666.

Farmer, E.R., Hood, A.F., 2000. Pathology of the skin, second ed. McGraw-Hill, New York.

Jennette, J.C., Olson, J.L., Schwartz, M.M., Silva, F.G., 1998. Heptinstall's pathology of the kidney, fifth ed. Lippincott-Raven, Philadelphia.

Johnson, G.D., Holborow, E.J., 1986. Preparation and use of fluorochrome conjugates. In: Weir, D.M., Herzenberg, L.A. (Eds.), Immunochemistry. Handbook of experimental immunology. Blackwell, Oxford.

Michel, B., Milner, Y., David, K., 1972. Preservation of tissue-fixed immunoglobulins in skin biopsies of patients with lupus erythematosus and bullous disease – preliminary report. Journal of Investigative Dermatology 59, 449–452.

Satoskar, A.A., Burdge, K., Cowden, D.J., et al., 2007. Typing of amyloidosis in renal biopsies: diagnostic pitfalls. Archives of Pathology and Laboratory Medicine 131 (6), 917–922.

Walker, P.D., 2009. The renal biopsy. Archives of Pathology and Laboratory Medicine 133, 181–188.

Weller, T.H., Coons, A.H., 1954. Fluorescent antibody studies with agents of varicella and herpes zoster propagated in vitro. Proceedings of the Society for Experimental Biology and Medicine 86, 789–794.

Immunohistochemistry quality control

20

Tracy Sanderson • Gregory Zardin

Introduction

Since its introduction into routine histopathology in the 1980s, immunohistochemistry has become established as an integral part of the diagnostic process. The use of immunohistochemical staining has developed within the diagnostic arena of an increasing range of infectious, neoplastic and reactive disease processes. Immunohistochemistry is now also able to provide prognostic or predictive information such as the likely response to specific treatments. Examples of such 'pharmaco-diagnostic' markers include estrogen (ER) and progesterone (PR) receptors and HER2/neu overexpression as well as CD117 (c-Kit) and CD20.

Reflecting the increasing diagnostic and prognostic role played by immunohistochemistry, the markers are known to generate results which may directly impact upon the patient care pathway. Consequently, it is vital that these investigative procedures are properly controlled by monitoring quality, both internally and externally.

External quality monitoring of clinical laboratories is achieved by participation in an external quality assurance scheme, such as UKNEQAS and NordiQC. Whilst in some countries participation in such schemes is a mandatory requirement in order to gain laboratory accreditation, the function of these schemes is primarily to monitor and improve the performance of the participating laboratory over a range of immunohistochemical tests.

It is important to ensure the correct internal quality control measures are in place. Immunohistochemisty is a complicated process and it is essential that the biomedical scientist has a sound understanding of all the requirements and procedures involved.

There should be staff experienced in identifying and resolving associated diagnostic procedural problems in order to be able to provide effective and efficient quality control within the laboratory. In addition to technical understanding, the laboratory scientist should also have knowledge of the expected staining patterns for the antibodies in both pathological and non-pathological tissues. Good communication between the biomedical scientist and the pathologist must be maintained, particularly during the introduction and validation of new antibodies and procurement of positive control material.

Detailed documentation and an audit trail throughout the process are necessary for potential backtracking and troubleshooting. Such audit trail details can include antigen retrieval methods, antibody dilution data, control tissue samples, temperatures and incubation times. The advent of automated platforms for immunohistochemistry has improved this aspect of quality control, but vigilance is still required. These automated platforms generally use standardized protocols for antigen retrieval and staining procedures, which makes overall control of the process easier. The generation and storage of automated run logs by these platforms make full reagent traceability possible. The logs can also be interrogated in the event of abnormal staining to identify errors such as missed steps due to low reagent levels.

Factors affecting stain quality

Tissue factors

Fixation

Tissue fixation has a significant influence on immunohistochemistry as most antigens are altered during this process (Williams et al. 1997). The purpose of fixation is to preserve tissue and prevent further degradation by the action of tissue enzymes or micro-organisms. As discussed in an earlier chapter, good fixation requires tissue to have adequate time in the fixative to allow the solution to penetrate, retaining uniform cellular detail throughout the tissue. However, in the routine laboratory this ideal may be compromised as it is difficult to define a standard tissue size, fixation time, and fixative for each specimen type. Tissues need to be adequately, but not over-fixed, so that antigenicity is preserved without excessive alteration. Prolonged fixation can result in the irretrievable loss of many antigens, particularly membrane-associated antigens such as CD20 and immunoglobulin (Ig) light chains (Miller et al. 1995; Ashton-Key et al. 1996). Lack of adequate fixation, or delay in fixation, may also be equally detrimental to labile antigens (Donhuijsen et al. 1990; von Wasielewski et al. 1998; GEFPICS-FNCLCC 1999).

Any fixative used must be compatible with immunohistochemical staining methods and formalin is still the most universal of fixatives. Formulations differ between laboratories and include 10% neutral buffered formalin (NBF), 10% formalin in tap water, 10% formal saline, and 10% NBF with saline (Angel et al. 1989; Williams 1993; Williams et al. 1997). Even though it may be the pathologist's choice, it can create a challenge for demonstrating certain antigens. Dabbs (2006) characterizes formalin as:

a satisfactory fixative for both morphology and immunohistochemistry provided that a simple and effective antigen retrieval technique is available to recover those antigens that are diminished or modified.

Williams et al. (1997) investigated the effect of fixation on immunostaining to establish whether a specific preparation schedule would allow for the optimal demonstration of all antigens. Of the fixatives tested, 10% formal saline, 10% NBF (except for CD45RO), and 10% zinc formalin (except for CD3) gave the most consistent results overall and showed excellent antigen preservation. More recently, alcohol-based fixatives have been considered as an alternative to formalin (van Essen et al. 2010) and produced satisfactory immunohistochemistry

staining. Other fixatives which may still be used in some laboratories include Bouin's, B5 (mercury), zinc formalin, 10% formal-acetic and Carson's, which also have an influence on the reproducibility of staining, each presenting a change in pH, length of required exposure and different artifacts.

Fixatives dictate many factors for immunohistochemical staining, such as dilution, antibody incubation time, retrieval method (if applicable), type of retrieval solution, and special pretreatments (e.g. pigment removal). Depending upon the type of fixative used, the protocols may require slight modifications. With the advent of heat-induced epitope retrieval (HIER) (Shi et al. 1991) many of the problems associated with fixation have been reduced and, in conjunction with automated techniques, good-quality staining is achievable on most tissue sections.

Processing

As with fixation, all tissue must be appropriately processed to produce successful immunohistochemical staining. Tissue that is inadequately processed will potentially produce poor-quality sections, with poor adhesion to the slides – especially fatty tissue such as breast and skin. Modern tissue processors all have the option to include vacuum and temperature variation at each step, allowing for greater optimization of the procedure. However, high temperatures can be detrimental to antigens that are heat labile. It is recommended that paraffin with a low-temperature melting point be used for this reason.

Regarding paraffin processing of tissues for immunohistochemistry, as with fixation, there is no standard protocol for the optimal demonstration of all antigens, as concluded by Williams et al. (1997). In a study of laboratories in the UK, Williams (1993) found nearly as many different schedules as the number of laboratories participating in the survey. Of the nine tissue-processing factors investigated, only two had any significant effect on immunoreactivity. Increasing the temperature of processing from ambient to 45°C, as well as longer processing times for dehydration and wax infiltration, were both found to improve immunostaining. Other factors including type of processor, type and quality of reagents, time in clearing agent, use of vacuum, most of which had been suggested as possible causes of poor processing (Horikawa et al. 1976; Trevisan et al. 1982; Anderson 1988; Slater 1988), were found to have no effect on subsequent immunohistochemistry.

Microwave processing is now being introduced into some laboratories to speed the processing time and reduce turnaround time for diagnostic specimens, and has been used successfully in conjunction with routine antibody staining. Acceptable staining was achieved when compared to tissues processed in a conventional processor (Emerson et al. 2006). As with all processing, if the tissue is not completely fixed then artifacts will be introduced.

One important point is that any control tissues used in the laboratory should be processed using the same protocols established for patient samples.

Reversal of fixation/epitope retrieval

The quality and reproducibility of immunohistochemical staining relies upon the reversal of fixation, which results in the targeted epitope being exposed, allowing for the antigen binding site to be available. The revolution of reversing the hydrogen cross-bonds formed by formalin was introduced by Shi et al. (1991). There are now numerous methods for epitope retrieval including protein digestion techniques or, more commonly, heating the slides in a buffered solution. Cattoretti et al. (1993) introduced the solution most commonly used in standardized retrieval methods. They used a citrate buffer at pH 6.0, which is inexpensive, stores easily, and is readily available commercially or easily prepared in the laboratory. Other buffers used include EDTA-based solutions at a higher pH range, which produce more intense staining of some antibodies. These methods have allowed for the successful demonstration of a much greater range of antigens in tumors, including proliferation markers and oncogene expression. The use of automated immunostainers has brought greater standardization of retrieval methods, as these use standard retrieval solutions with defined reproducible protocols. Non-automated laboratories may have a number of variables that require internal standardization in the antigen retrieval technique including the choice of heating method (e.g. pressure cooker, microwave, etc.), retrieval solution, pH, temperature, volume of the fluid, and the temperature and exposure time while heating and cooling slides.

Equipment commonly used to perform epitope retrieval includes the modified pressure cooker, initially reported by Norton et al. (1994), microwaves, waterbath or a pretreatment module. Some automated platforms have on-board retrieval where individual slide bays can be heated with the appropriate solution on the slide.

Other factors required for successful retrieval include the proper drying and complete removal of water from slides. In addition to avoiding wrinkles or tears in the tissue, these factors will all assist the adhesion of tissue to the slide. With respect to enzymatic proteolytic 'epitope retrieval', such as trypsin digestion prior to immunostaining, the choice of enzyme usually dictates the temperature and pH of the solution, as different enzymes have different preferential pH and temperatures. For example, the optimal values for a mammalian-derived trypsin are pH 7.8 at 37°C, with 0.1% calcium chloride included as an activator (Huang et al. 1976). The concentration of enzyme required is dependent on the proteolytic qualities of the product being used. A typical concentration used for many commercial trypsins employed in immunohistochemistry protocols is 0.1%. The concentration, pH, and temperature are then usually held constant, while the time of digestion is varied. The time required for optimal digestion will vary, depending on the antigen under investigation, the quality (proteolytic capabilities) of the trypsin and the length of formalin fixation. For antigens that are only present in small amounts, e.g. immunoglobulin light chains on the surface of B cells, the time for optimal digestion may vary from case to case, depending on how long each case has been fixed in formalin.

Reagent factors

Production of high-quality staining is dependent upon the correct storage, handling and application of the reagents used. Once a protocol has been developed, it is important to ensure the reproducibility of the stain. To achieve this, the storage conditions and expiration dates of in-house and commercial reagents must be monitored as the preparation and use of each reagent must be consistent. Details of the storage and preparation of all reagents used in each staining run must be documented as part of the audit trail to allow back-tracking and troubleshooting.

Reagent monitoring is one area in which the use of an automated staining system with bar-code reagent labeling can be of assistance both in alerting the operator to reagents which have reached their expiry date and in the automated creation of audit trails and quality control documentation.

Buffers and diluents

The buffer and diluent used for wash steps and antibody dilution will affect the results of immunostaining. The pH of these reagents needs to be monitored and must be checked and documented prior to use. If it falls outside of the range proscribed by the established protocol, corrections must be made or the reagent discarded.

Many antibody diluents contain additives such as sodium azide to stabilize and maintain the protein. Although this extends the shelf life of the antibody, the additives may interfere with, or inhibit, staining if present at excessive levels.

Antibodies

The storage temperature of an antibody is critical to its stability. Commercially available antibodies should be accompanied by a specification sheet, containing storage and handling instructions.

Concentrated antibodies tend to have a longer shelf life than pre-diluted 'ready to use' antibody preparations. Concentrated antibodies can be mixed with glycerine to prevent ice crystal formation, aliquoted into cryovials, then 'snap' frozen and stored in a −80°C freezer. This greatly extends their shelf life; compliance with the expiry date printed on the antibody packaging is important. The storage temperature for antibodies and reagents should also be monitored closely, as any fluctuation in temperature may cause increased deterioration of reagents. Frost-free −20°C freezers should hence be avoided for the storage of antibodies due to damage caused by the freeze-thaw cycles that these types of freezer perform.

Procedural factors

The automation of immunostaining is perhaps the easiest way of improving the reproducibility and consistency of the staining. Although the use of automation is increasing, many laboratories still perform at least some immunohistochemical staining manually. Other laboratories perform semi-automated staining (for example manual epitope retrieval). The production of good manual procedures is important for these stains and also for use in case of failure of automated staining machinery. These procedures must be clear, easy to follow and sufficiently detailed to ensure a minimum of inter-operative variation. Adherence to these protocols and the reduction of human error is the goal in order to ensure consistent stain quality.

Block and slide storage conditions

Processed blocks should be kept in a cool dry place. Resealing paraffin blocks following cutting can help protect the tissue from everyday elements such as air drying, excessive moisture or physical damage. The use of fresh cut controls for each run would be ideal but this is not always feasible in a busy laboratory. Repeated sectioning of a control tissue block can also result in loss of usable tissue, although some laboratories now have a control on the same slide as the test section.

Pre-cutting control slides is more time efficient and serial sections result in minimal tissue loss. The correct storage of pre-cut slides is important and frequently overlooked as a potential source of error in staining. Some studies have found deterioration of antigens in stored sections (Raymond & Leong 1990; Bromley et al. 1994; Prioleau & Schnitt 1995). Others have found no deterioration of some markers investigated, including estrogen receptor (ER), CD3, CD20, CD45RO, vimentin, and Ig light chains, in sections stored for up to four months at room temperature (Williams et al. 1997; Eisen & Goldstein 1999).

The viability of the antigen and speed of antigen deterioration in cut tissue sections is highly dependent upon the antigen under consideration and the temperature used for section adhesion. For example, whilst antigens such as CD30 and PSA seem relatively robust, CD117 (C-kit) deteriorates quickly and should be cut fresh.

The temperature at which the slides are dried can also affect the immunoreactivity of the antigens. It is advisable to dry all slides for immunohistochemical staining at 37°C. Urgent cases can generally be dried at 60°C for up to 4 hours. The exception to this is HER2, where it is recommended that sections should not be dried at 60°C for more than 1 hour.

An appropriate number of control slides and blocks should be kept with these factors in mind. This stock level will vary depending on the workload in each individual laboratory.

Monitoring stain quality

Whenever a new batch of reagent is used, its details and the efficacy must be recorded, checked and compared with the previous batch. Reagents from different batches should never be mixed. Any enzymes used must be validated prior to use, due to a high degree of inter-lot variation. It should be noted that poor storage or shipping conditions can result in a reduction in enzyme activity. Antibody validation documentation should be available and is best kept in combination with the antibody specification sheet. This may be in either paper or electronic form. Detection system reagent validation is best performed by using a panel of several different antibodies. This should include different antigen retrieval methods and cover a variety of different staining patterns (nuclear, cytoplasmic, and membrane staining). A clean (i.e. non-reacting) negative control is just as important as the intensity of positive staining patterns, and such controls must be carefully checked.

Validation of antibodies

It is important that all antibodies used in diagnostic testing are fully validated in the laboratory and detailed records are kept of the validation process. This should include demonstration of the reactivity of the antibody, validation of the procedure and quality checking of positive and negative controls used with that antibody. Before introducing a new antibody into the laboratory repertoire it is important to research details of the clone required. Most commercial antibodies have data sheets available on-line which should include a number of facts for consideration. These should indicate the host in which the antibody was raised (e.g. rabbit, mouse, or goat), location of the target antigen, concentration of the antibody, recommended application (e.g. frozen tissue, formalin-fixed paraffin-embedded tissue), recommended positive and negative control tissue sources, classification (e.g. analyte-specific reagent, research use only, or *in vitro* diagnostic) and reference materials for the application of the antibody. The specification sheet also typically includes suggested staining protocols.

Most antibodies used in diagnostic pathology laboratories are classified as 'research use only' or 'analyte-specific reagent'. This means that it is the responsibility of the diagnostic laboratory to validate and document the sensitivity and specificity of the antibody. This process can be simplified if an appropriate antibody classified for '*in vitro* diagnostic' (IVD) use can be sourced. The vendor has assumed responsibility for the validation and application of these antibodies.

The suggested protocol should serve as a baseline whilst working up the antibody and each laboratory should optimize the stain. If no protocol is suggested by the manufacturer, journal articles can be a good source of baseline protocols.

Selection of the most appropriate epitope retrieval method is important to ensure the maximum sensitivity of the stain. Antibodies are pH sensitive and it has been shown that staining intensity is better when the epitope retrieval step is performed at a pH specific to each antibody. It has also been shown that an antibody may not be specific or work as well if a proper pH is not maintained during the retrieval step. Selection of the detection complex used may also be influenced by the primary antibody. Some antibodies have been found to work better with an alkaline phosphatase detection system than with a horseradish peroxidase system and vice versa. Antibodies commonly used in pigmented tissues such as melanoma markers may benefit from a red (or other) chromogen end-point, as the endogenous pigment can disguise the more commonly used brown DAB chromogen.

Staining protocol development generally consists of trial and error, making sequential alterations in order to achieve optimal signal-to-noise ratio. In real terms this means strong, crisp target antigen staining with little or no background staining. If the staining is too strong, then further dilution of the primary antibody may improve staining specificity. If target antigen staining fades and the background remains, then the addition of a blocking step, change of epitope retrieval or changing the detection system used (e.g. to a polymer-based system) may improve the result. Changing the antibody diluent may help to increase the antibody's reactivity, while at the same time lowering background staining. Weak staining may be improved with an increase of the antibody concentration (e.g. from 1:50 to 1:25).

Negative staining can be more difficult to resolve and may be the result of multiple factors. It is advisable to rule out human or mechanical error by repeating the staining before making further modifications. If the stain remains negative, change one variable at a time and document each reagent, step and reaction time. Negative staining may be resolved by increasing the antibody concentration, changing the epitope retrieval method, changing the solution pH, changing the antibody diluent to one of a different pH, changing the base composition or using an amplification step as part of the detection system. It is also important to ensure that the tissue stained should exhibit positive staining and the slides are freshly cut.

The duration of formalin fixation to which the tissue has been exposed may affect the reversal of protein cross-linking. Over-fixation of tissue may require more aggressive epitope retrieval methods to achieve satisfactory retrieval. This must be considered if the control or test tissue available for protocol development and validation has been stored in formalin for an extended period of time.

The final stain protocol must be confirmed on both positive and negative tissue controls prior to implementation. False-positive staining of negative control tissue suggests that the concentration of the antibody is too high.

Once an antibody dilution and staining method has been established and validated, each step of the procedure must be clearly documented and maintained in written or electronic form. This should include the antibody lot, expiration date, dilution, details of blocking steps performed (serum, avidin-biotin, and hydrogen peroxide), secondary and label (detection), chromogen tested, and the duration of each step.

Control slides

Control slides can include both reagent substitution and internal or external tissue controls. A positive control for each antibody should be used with every staining run. It is important to obtain a reliable, known, positive control tissue for use with each antibody offered by the laboratory. Control tissue selection should be supported by publications and the selection process should be documented. Many commercial antibody specification sheets make recommendations regarding controls, and most cite references which are of use when selecting control tissue.

The acquisition of appropriate control tissue requires knowledge of the desired tissue type (e.g. kidney, liver, etc.) and whether the target antigen is expressed in normal or tumor tissue. It is helpful if the person validating a control has knowledge of the prospective control tissue's diagnosis in the case of tumor controls to assist in the evaluation of expected staining patterns. In order to be comparable to the test section it is important that the fixation and processing of control tissue should be the same as the patient tissue being tested. Ideally, target antigens in positive controls should be distributed across the

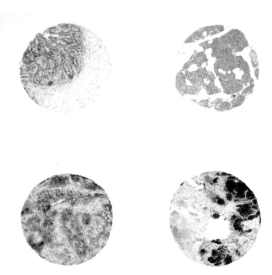

Figure 20.2 High-power image of a multi-tissue control stained with an antibody to polyclonal CEA, demonstrating both normal tissue and tumor staining, in addition to a negative normal tissue core.

Figure 20.1 Low-power image of a multi-tissue control stained with an antibody to polyclonal carcinoembryonic antigen (CEA). Using carefully chosen 'donor' tissues, both positive and negative tissue controls can be demonstrated on the same slide.

entire sample and, if possible, should be present at a range of densities in order to monitor the sensitivity as well as specificity of the stain.

Whilst a separate positive control should be included for each antibody, a single tissue type is often suitable for use as an external control for several different antibodies. For example, a section of appendix can be used for testing antibodies to low molecular weight cytokeratins, EMA, vimentin, desmin, SMA, CEA, S-100, NSE, CD45, CD20, CD3, CD4, CD8, CD79a, bcl-2, Ki-67, etc. (Balaton 1999). One way of creating a control block containing multiple positive and negative tissues suitable for a wide range of antibodies is to use a tissue micro-array (Figs 20.1 and 20.2). A composite block, containing representative punches from multiple tissue types in a single block, can be used for the majority of stains offered by a laboratory. With careful tissue selection the block should not have to contain an overlarge number of punches in order to achieve this goal. A drawback of this approach is that, whilst it simplifies daily quality control, it requires a large amount of available control material, particularly in larger laboratories offering a wide range of antibodies.

Internal and external positive controls

Many tissues contain native components that serve as internal positive controls for immunohistochemical staining: e.g. the crypts of normal colon stain with polyclonal CEA (Fig. 20.3). These internal controls are in many ways better than external tissue controls, since they demonstrate that the test tissue was appropriately fixed and processed. Although external positive tissue controls do not show this, they are required for some tests where there is no

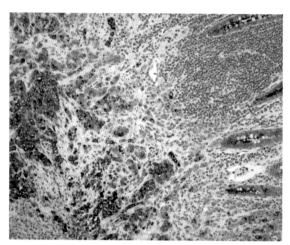

Figure 20.3 Section of colon, demonstrating staining of normal crypts for polyclonal CEA, serving as an internal positive control.

internal positive control in the tissue under investigation, such as those performed for infectious agents. External controls are also needed whilst working up an antibody for inclusion into the laboratory repertoire, and are also of use in assisting the day-to-day monitoring of the stain where it is preferable to use the same tissue with a known pattern of staining. If an internal control is not present, and/or if there is doubt over the retention of antigenicity in the test tissue, then this can be checked by staining with vimentin. However, since vimentin is a relatively robust antigen it is possible that its viability could be maintained whilst more labile antibodies such as CD3 may be lost.

Daily slide review

All slides should be reviewed and quality assessed prior to being sent out of the laboratory. This can be performed by an appropriately trained laboratory scientist or a pathologist. The reviewer should be able to distinguish acceptable signal-to-noise ratio and recognize interpretable results. At a minimum, the positive control slides should be screened for expected results.

Without stained controls the results of many immunohistochemical assays cannot be validated. The controls should also demonstrate the sensitivity

(i.e., tissue with low expression of the target antigen stains positive) and specificity (i.e., negative controls are not stained and background staining is absent) of the stain. Controls indicate whether the staining protocols have been followed correctly, whether day-to-day and worker-to-worker variations have impacted upon stain quality, and whether the reagents used continue to be in good working order.

External quality assurance

Whilst daily internal monitoring of stain quality through the use of control slides is vital, it is also important to ensure inter-laboratory consistency of quality and results. This is best achieved through participation in an external quality assurance scheme such as UKNEQAS or NordiQC. These schemes are arranged into different modules, each covering common stains performed in different areas of pathology. Examples of modules are breast pathology (HER2, ER, PR, etc.), neuropathology (NFP, GH, TSH, etc.) and general pathology (desmin, CD3, Ki67, etc.). Participants choose which modules they wish to participate in, and are sent slides to stain with relevant selected antibodies. The stained slides are returned to the scheme organizer often accompanied by one of the laboratories in-house control slides used for the requested antibody. Submitted slides are assessed and scored independently by the scheme organizer and participating laboratory, who will then receive both individual feedback on the slides submitted and general feedback on results from all participants. The methods used to produce the highest scoring slides are taken as 'best practice' and made available for all laboratories to consider. Any laboratory producing consistently poor results will be offered advice by the scheme organizers to help improve future results.

Through participation in such schemes the laboratory can assure service users that the results they produce are not only consistent but also that they are in concordance with the national consensus. This is particularly important for laboratories using prognostic and predictive markers which may impact on patient care (Rhodes et al. 2001; Ibrahim et al. 2008; Bartlett et al. 2009). In many countries participation in such schemes is a prerequisite for the accreditation of the laboratory.

Troubleshooting

Troubleshooting problems in immunohistochemistry can be difficult due to the complexity of the technique and the number of variables involved. However, good documentation of the processes involved can help with backtracking to potential sources of error. The use of bar codes on slides and reagents on automated staining systems has helped to reduce some of the common human errors, but machines are not entirely reliable and have their own associated problems. One of the advantages of an automated system is the ability to see on screen records of staining logs and reagent preparation details, which can help to identify problems promptly.

A key element to producing good-quality immunohistochemical staining is in the preparation of the slides. Poorly fixed or processed tissue tends to be more difficult to section, being prone to detachment from the slide, especially given the harsh nature of some pretreatment protocols. Furthermore, poor section quality can lead to problems with interpretation if visualization of the staining is occluded or the tissue morphology is damaged. This includes section thickness, damage (such as holes or scores) and excessive heat exposure (causing dry sections). An experienced laboratory scientist with a good understanding of all the processes and techniques involved should be able to identify and resolve all of the problems that may arise.

The most common problems that are likely to occur are either false-negative or false-positive staining, and the potential sources of error for these are discussed below.

False-negative staining

The absence of staining of an antigen that should be present in the tissue can present in various patterns. The easiest to identify is when the positive control slide and the patient (test) slide are completely negative. After checking that the correct positive control section has been used, the source of the problem needs to be identified and rectified, before the stain is repeated.

In the second type of false-negative staining the positive control slide is negative, but the patient slide shows positive staining in either the area of interest, or in some internal component that acts as a positive control. If this internal control stains according to the expected pattern it may not be necessary to repeat the stain as long as the failure of the control is documented. The cause of the failure of staining in the positive control still needs to be determined to ensure it is still viable to be used in future staining runs.

The third pattern of false-negative staining occurs when the positive control slide stains appropriately, but the patient slide is completely negative. This is more difficult to detect because at first glance it may appear that the patient test is just negative. In this instance it is important to check for any internal positive control components within the tissue, and if these are also negative the stain should be repeated. If the negatively stained section was part of a panel of antibody tests, then it may help with the assessment if the negative result is appropriate when compared to the other test results. A number of factors can cause false-negative staining.

Process failure

This can be caused by human or mechanical error if there is automation of the process. Human errors usually occur because the standard procedure has not been followed, but commonly such errors involve missing a step, or performing steps out of sequence, incorrect reagent preparation, or reagent incubation time not being delivered. Shortening steps may not allow for chemical or immunological reactions to complete.

Process automation has cut out some potential errors by bar-coding slides and reagent bottles. However, it is still possible for slides to be incorrectly labeled, or for reagents to be wrongly prepared unless they are commercial, ready-to-use reagents. Another potential problem is reagents

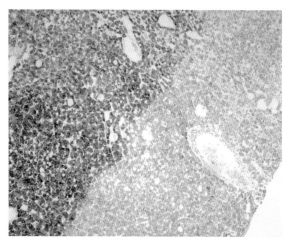

Figure 20.4 Adenocarcinoma stained on a horizontal immunostainer with an antibody to cytokeratin 7, demonstrating incomplete coverage of the tissue section by staining reagent.

being skipped if the instrument runs out of wash buffer, thereby compromising staining. Incorrect programming of an instrument can occur, but should be picked up before a staining run is started. A common artifact that can be seen is uneven staining of the section caused by incomplete coverage by one or more of the reagents (Fig. 20.4).

Instrumentation failure can also occur through pump failure, clogged or damaged probes, or because electrical components wear out. The computer can have software glitches or experience external network problems if interfaced with a laboratory or hospital system. Equipment should be well maintained and regular maintenance is helpful to keep instruments in good working order.

Positive control selection

Positive control material should have previously been tested for validation before use. If the positive control slide is negative and the patient slide positive, there are three main problems that could have occurred. Firstly, the wrong control could have been used, which may happen when inexperienced staff members are working in the laboratory. It can help to clearly label pre-cut control sections with the antibody or antibody group they can be used for, such as cytokeratins, or to have a list of antibodies and

the appropriate control section required. The second problem might be that the area of interest in the control slide might have been cut through. This can be prevented by testing the first and last slide of each batch of sections, in order to validate that the control is still demonstrating appropriate staining. Thirdly, some antigens are more labile, and their antigenicity deteriorates with time in cut sections, resulting in weak or negative staining. If this is suspected, a fresh section should be cut and stained to make sure the block still contains viable control tissue. Once any of these antigens have been identified or there are antibodies that are used infrequently, it is advisable for the laboratory to only keep a small stock of pre-cut sections, or to cut them freshly as required in order to prevent further occurrence.

Incomplete deparaffinization

Failure to remove paraffin wax from the slide may interfere with the ability of the antibody to penetrate the tissue and thus may inhibit antibody binding. Reagents used for de-waxing and dehydration should be changed regularly, and paraffin wax with a high plastic content may require longer times in xylene with agitation to assist with complete removal. Some pretreatment solutions de-wax and pretreat in one step. It is important to monitor the use and temperature of the reagents and follow the manufacturer's recommendations for use to ensure that they continue to perform at an optimal level. Changing or rotating solutions regularly is recommended to ensure that deterioration of these reagents does not introduce unnecessarily weak or false-negative staining, which is often overlooked as a potential problem.

Epitope retrieval

It is essential that the correct epitope retrieval protocol has been performed on the sections, as not all retrieval solutions work for all antibodies used in the laboratory. For example, the antibody BerEP4 will generally not work if pretreated in high pH EDTA-based retrieval solutions. The retrieval protocol should have already been defined as part of the optimization of a new antibody and should be strictly adhered to; otherwise, it will most likely result in false-negative staining. Therefore, slides should be clearly labeled and sorted for the specific retrieval procedure required. This is generally less of an issue on automated platforms as the retrieval step is part of the set staining protocol. The retrieval will either be carried out on the machine, or a slide label will have been attached to the slide with the appropriate protocol details printed on it, making it easier to indentify the correct pretreatment.

When HIER protocols are performed, it is advisable to monitor the temperature of the solution to check that it has reached the correct setting, and that it has been maintained for the required length of time. Failure so to do may result in substandard reversal of fixation and possible negative staining. Many of the automated systems are able to monitor and log retrieval temperatures electronically and can be easily viewed on screen.

If enzyme digestion is employed as the retrieval method, care should be taken to ensure that the correct time and temperature protocol is used depending on the digestion agent and the antibody in question. Over-digestion of the tissue can result in loss of morphology of the tissue, at which point the antigen may have been destroyed, resulting in negative staining.

Temperature

Chemical reaction rates are affected by temperature, so it is important to monitor all aspects of the procedure where heating or cooling is required, either during pretreatment or staining. Some automated stainers use heat during various steps to speed up chemical reactions and these can develop faults. However, regular maintenance and monitoring should help to prevent these occurrences. Antibodies are proteins, and as such their structure can be modified by heat, which may decrease the sensitivity of antibody binding during the staining process. It is also important not to overlook the general room temperature of the laboratory where immunohistochemical staining takes place. With numerous fridges and staining machines working, the core temperature of the room can rise by several

degrees if there is no air-conditioning system in place. Some staining machine manufacturers have recommendations about minimum and maximum advised working temperatures.

Antibody preparation

All commercially available antibodies should be labeled with an expiry date and come with a datasheet detailing the correct storage requirements of the antibody. Most concentrated and pre-diluted antibodies are recommended to be stored at 2–8°C. Those that are less stable may need to be aliquoted and frozen at −20°C. Antibodies stored at 2–8°C will still decline over a period of time, as oxidation occurs on exposure to air and at some point will decline rapidly and produce a false-negative result. This deterioration may be picked up by close monitoring of the positive control section if the expected level of staining starts to decrease.

Human error in the preparation of an antibody dilution may occur. Pipettes should be regularly maintained and calibrated at least annually. Staff should be trained in the correct mechanical use of the pipette, as well as choosing the appropriate size of pipette for a particular volume range. Antibody dilutions should be documented to include the date that the antibody dilution is made in order to identify when a possible preparation error may have occurred.

Chromogen incompatibility

Various detection systems are available for visualization of the antibody, and it is important to understand the compatibility of chromogen and enzyme label. The standard combination is horseradish peroxidase (HRP) enzyme used with diaminobenzidine (DAB) chromogen, but other chromogens such as amino ethyl carbazole (AEC) work with HRP as well. Fast red chromogen and BCIP/NBT react only with an alkaline phosphatase enzyme. Reading the manufacturer's recommendations for preparation and shelf life of a prepared chromogen is important. These problems should not occur on automated platforms, as the detection reagents are generally supplied as a ready-to-use kit with bar-coded bottles that cannot be confused. When using alkaline phosphatase-based detection, care should also be taken from counterstaining to mounting as some enzyme labels are alcohol soluble and cannot be dehydrated.

False-positive staining

False-positive staining is often easier to troubleshoot than false-negative staining, although it is potentially much more serious. If the false-positive staining is interpreted by the pathologist as real (i.e. positive) staining, then the patient may be incorrectly or unnecessarily treated. An experienced laboratory scientist should be able to identify possible false-positive staining, and should then either repeat the test or bring it to the attention of the pathologist to discuss any action required. When false-positive staining is observed in a patient slide only, it may be due to different fixation or processing of the patient tissue. In these instances it may be helpful to run a negative patient slide alongside the repeat test to check for non-specific false-positive staining. As with false-negative staining, there are a number of factors which can cause the problem.

Poor quality of fixation

With greater emphasis on meeting targeted diagnostic turnaround times, the laboratory can be put under pressure to process samples through as quickly as possible. However, this can greatly impact the quality of tissue processing. When fixation and processing times are too short, tissue may not be adequately dehydrated. The result is that the tissue may be partially unprocessed, or that the center of the tissue will be alcohol fixed during processing. In this case the immunohistochemical staining pattern of the patient test tissue can be quite variable, compared to that of the control section on which the dilution and method have been developed (Fig. 20.5).

Technical preparation

As mentioned previously, it is important to start with good-quality sections for immunohistochemical

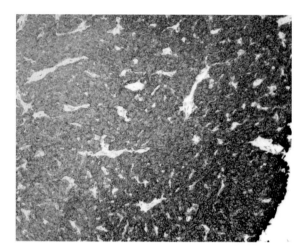

Figure 20.5 Section of poorly fixed thymus stained with an antibody to AE1/AE3 cytokeratin cocktail, demonstrating a gradient of staining from the formalin-fixed outer edge to the alcohol-fixed center.

staining, as this is a common cause of false-positive staining. Poorly fixed and/or processed tissue is more difficult to cut and has a greater tendency to detach from the slide. Therefore, all sections should be picked up onto positively charged slides to assist with tissue adhesion and to prevent detachment during potentially harsh pretreatments. They should all be cut at the same thickness and need to be as flat and wrinkle free as possible. The waterbath used for floating out the sections should be wiped after every case to prevent floaters and squamous cells being transferred to the next section (see Fig. 20.6).

Poor section quality can result in streaks, overall blushing across the tissue, or patches of non-specific positive staining. Calcified tissue can cause scores or holes which may affect staining, but any decalcification treatment must be kept to a minimum as the acidic reagents can be deleterious to the end result. Wrinkles, tears, and folds create areas in which the reagents are not properly rinsed away and remain trapped underneath or on top of the tissue (Figs 20.7–20.9), so that by the time the chromagen is applied those areas are intensified and may make it impossible to interpret the staining.

Once cut, the sections need to be dried on properly before staining to help with adhesion. Oven-drying must be monitored and maintained at a constant temperature, as tissue exposed to high temperatures for long periods of time may demonstrate edge arti-fact (Fig. 20.10). If sections are not going to be stained immediately, they should be dried at 37°C and then stored at room temperature once dried on.

Epitope retrieval

As discussed earlier, the use of retrieval solutions must be monitored to ensure the correct protocol is performed each time. Variations of pH or temper-ature of the solution will interfere with staining results. One possible effect of incorrect retrieval is non-specific staining due to the amplification of endogenous biotin in the tissue (O'Leary 2001), which is observed with avidin-biotin detection systems. Some antibodies do not require any pre-treatment, and exposure to a retrieval solution or step may create non-specific nuclear staining (Fig. 20.11).

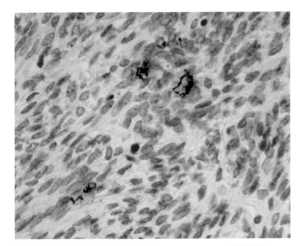

Figure 20.6 Section of lymph node stained with an AE1/AE3 cytokeratin antibody cocktail, demonstrating squamous cell contaminants that result from the technician placing ungloved fingers into the water bath, also known as floaters.

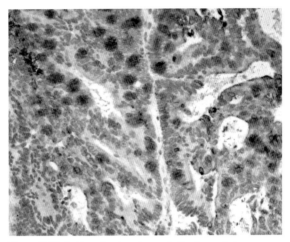

Figure 20.8 Section of colon, demonstrating trapped chromogen due to poor tissue adhesion to the slide.

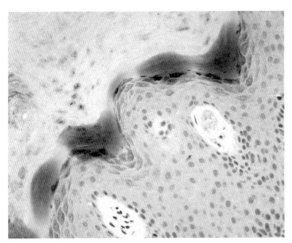

Figure 20.7 Section of skin intended as a negative control, demonstrating trapped chromogen under the keratin layer due to tissue lifting.

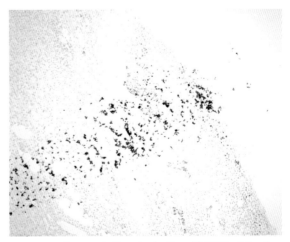

Figure 20.9 Section of skin stained with an AE1/AE3 cytokeratin antibody cocktail, demonstrating chromogen streaking across the section due to poor rinsing. Staining is present across an area expected to be negative.

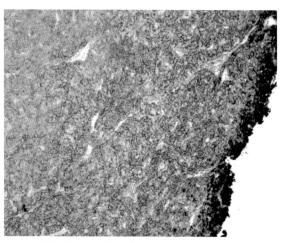

Figure 20.10 Tissue section, demonstrating edge artifact due to excessive drying.

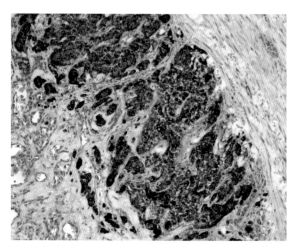

Figure 20.12 Over-digested carcinoma stained with an AE1/AE3 cytokeratin antibody cocktail. Excessive staining creates difficulty in identifying true positive staining.

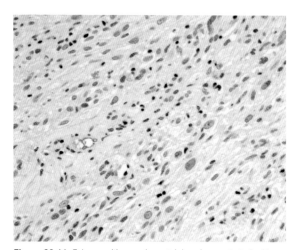

Figure 20.11 False-positive nuclear staining demonstrated with an antibody to polyclonal myosin due to unnecessary heat-induced epitope retrieval.

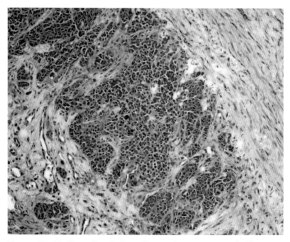

Figure 20.13 Over-digested carcinoma (same case as in Fig. 20.12) intended as a negative reagent control slide, confirming that much of the staining observed in the patient AE1/AE3 section is non-specific staining.

Care should be taken not to over-digest the tissue when using proteolytic enzymes. This can be caused by extending the time beyond that determined to be the optimal digestion time within the individual laboratory, or by performing the digestion step at a warmer temperature than has been determined in the laboratory's validation process. Excessive heat will typically increase the rate of digestion. If the section is not sufficiently rinsed following the digestion step and the enzyme is not removed completely, it will continue to digest the tissue. All of these factors lead to over-digestion of proteins, which may then diffuse into or deposit onto the tissue, leading to diffuse non-specific staining. The occurrence of over-digestion should be apparent by the subsequent damage to tissue morphology (Figs 20.12 and 20.13).

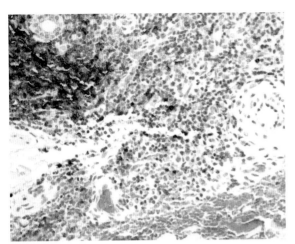

Figure 20.14 Lymphoid tissue stained with an antibody to CD3, demonstrating non-specific staining of red blood cells (intrinsic peroxidase activity) due to inadequate quenching with hydrogen peroxide solution.

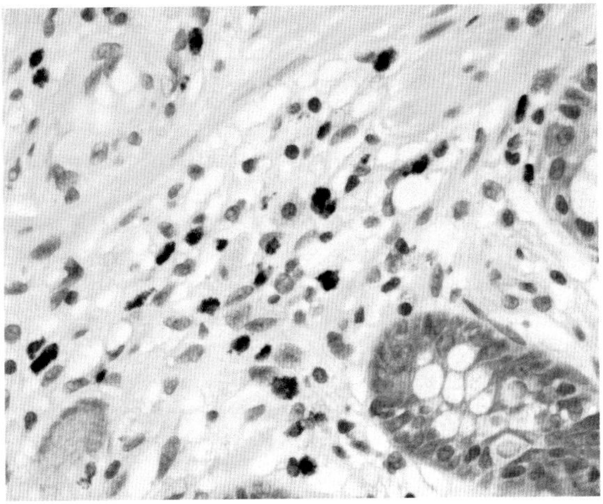

Figure 20.15 Section of colon intended as negative reagent control, demonstrating mast cell staining due to inadequate quenching of endogenous peroxidase activity within mast cells.

Tissue drying (wetting agents)

Once the tissue has been de-waxed for staining the sections should be kept moist and fully covered by each reagent. The amount of visible artifact will depend on whether just the edges or the entire section has dried out, in which case the whole section will demonstrate non-specific staining. Wetting agents such as detergents may be added to the rinse buffer, in order to keep the tissue from drying out between and during the staining steps. Detergents also assist with rinsing off unbound antibodies and other reagents, keeping the staining clean. Too much of these reagents can interfere with the staining as well, so controlling the concentration in the rinsing buffer is recommended.

Intrinsic tissue factors

There are two main intrinsic tissue factors that need to be considered as possible causes of non-specific staining.

Endogenous peroxidase is commonly found in red blood cells and other tissue components (Fig. 20.14) and this can react with DAB in horseradish peroxidase detection systems if not treated. This can be blocked by treatment with a 3% hydrogen peroxide solution applied prior to staining to quench the peroxidase activity.

Hydrogen peroxide should be stored in dark bottles and the blocking solution should be freshly prepared before use. Staining may be observed in mast cells in a negative tissue control when inadequate quenching occurs (Fig. 20.15).

Biotin is a vitamin found in high concentration in a number of tissues, including the liver, kidney and brain. This can lead to non-specific staining when using an avidin-biotin detection system, but can be reduced by the addition of a blocking step. To achieve this, avidin is applied first for 15 minutes, rinsed with buffer, and then biotin is applied for 15 minutes, followed by another rinse in buffer. Protein block or the application of the primary follows the avidin-biotin blocking step. Non-specific biotin will be easiest to identify in the negative control slide (Figs 20.16 and 20. 17).

Antibody concentration

All antibodies, whether concentrated or pre-diluted, should have their working dilution validated prior to implementation into the laboratory. Commercially prepared diluents are readily available and generally provide greater stability of diluted

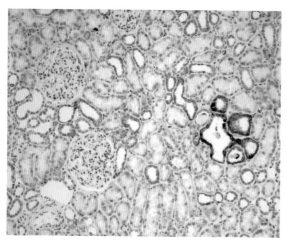

Figure 20.16 Section of kidney intended as a negative reagent control using an avidin-biotin detection system, demonstrating non-specific biotin in some tubules.

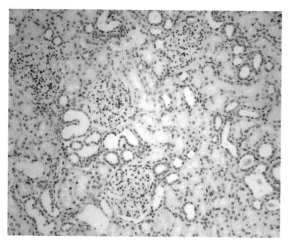

Figure 20.17 Section of kidney (same case as in Fig. 20.16) properly blocked with avidin-biotin, demonstrating the expected absence of staining (negative reagent control).

1:4, 1:8, and so on), starting from the neat concentration, using both positive and negative control tissues. If non-specific staining is observed, the dilution should be taken out further until a good signal-to-noise ratio is achieved.

Polyclonal antibodies are more sensitive than specific. Using monoclonal antibodies reduces non-specific staining, due to their specificity and affinity for one epitope.

Detection system

The choice of detection system used can impact on the quality of staining, but may be affected by other factors such as cost, or reagent rental agreements associated with the type of automated platform being used. In recent years the most commonly used system has been avidin/biotin or streptavidin/biotin, but (as mentioned above) these systems can cause problems, specifically when staining tissue types that contain intrinsic biotin. These are now being replaced by the introduction of polymer or synthetic-based systems that have allowed for the elimination of biotin-induced non-specific staining. Another advantage of the polymer-based systems is that they can shorten staining times by eliminating the need for multiple blocking steps. However, polymer-based systems are not a cure-all for every antibody as some polymeric complexes are large and can have difficulty reaching some epitopes, depending on their location. With the variety of detection systems now available, the laboratory has the opportunity to continually evaluate and improve the quality of the staining produced, provided it can be achieved within the financial constraints of the department.

Chromogen

In general, chromagen solutions should be freshly prepared just before use and according to the manufacturer's instructions, if using a kit. Commercially available products provided for use on automated stainers may be stable for extended periods of time, once mixed in accordance with the manufacturers' instructions. Alkaline phosphatase chromogens are sensitive to light and heat, making them

antibodies. The pH of the diluent is important to maintain the antibody in its proper structure as any deterioration can create non-specific staining and reduce the overall quality of the staining.

The concentration of a pre-diluted ready-to-use antibody has been determined by the manufacturer and may not have been tested with different detection systems. These antibodies should be validated before use by performing serial dilutions (e.g. 1:2,

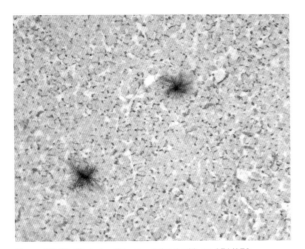

Figure 20.18 Merkel cell tumor stained with an AE1/AE3 cytokeratin antibody cocktail using alkaline phosphatase detection with red chromogen, demonstrating crystals on the surface. Crystal deposits could have been avoided by filtering the chromogen.

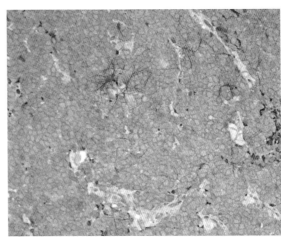

Figure 20.19 Merkel cell tumor stained with an antibody to neuron-specific enolase using alkaline phosphatase detection with red chromogen, demonstrating 'spider web-like' precipitate across the section.

susceptible to lysis/loss after preparation. Peroxidase chromogens can also break down, but not as quickly. Once chromogen activity is depleted, it will either create a blush across the tissue or deposit debris. Chromogen precipitate and streaking can be reduced with adequate mixing, rinsing, and filtering of the chromogen prior to application (Figs 20.18 and 20.19).

Extended time in primary, secondary, or chromogen and inadequate rinsing with buffer between steps may also cause non-specific staining.

Species cross-reactivity

While many commercial kits are available that are ready to use, it is important that the user should understand the formulation of the kit. Those kits that use 'universal' secondary reagents are directed at many primary antibody targets. This information is especially important if staining animal tissue; for example, goat anti-mouse IgG in the kit can cross-react with mouse tissue, creating a non-specific background stain. Mouse tissue typically will demonstrate blood vessel staining due to such cross-reactivity. This staining mimics endothelial cell positive staining. To avoid such non-specific

staining, primary antibodies raised in a different species, and secondary reagents not directed against mouse IgG, should be used. If a primary antibody is to be used that originated in the same species being stained, special blocking steps can be introduced to minimize non-specific binding. Kits containing such blocking reagents are commercially available.

Automation error

The use of automated platforms has assisted in improving staining quality and consistency but is not foolproof and can create unique artifacts of its own. Depending on the type of instrument used insufficient rinsing can be a problem – which may be amplified during the chromogen application. Horizontal staining instruments require very careful leveling on installation, to prevent reagents slipping off the slide and causing incomplete coverage of the sections. A faulty probe can result in empty or partial draws of reagents, with the result that it may then dispense air bubbles onto the slide (Fig. 20.20). In instruments that blow over the top of the tissue to mix reagents, the probe height must be set correctly or it can create a bull's eye pattern (Figs 20.21 and 20.22).

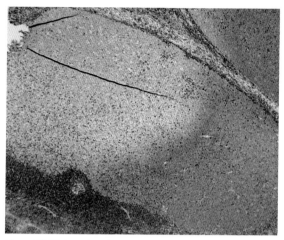

Figure 20.20 Lymph node stained with an antibody to Bcl-2, demonstrating poor tissue coverage due to air bubbles, and non-specific staining due to poor rinsing.

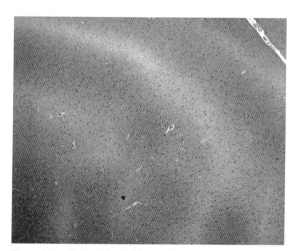

Figure 20.21 Brain stained with an antibody to polyclonal ubiquitin using alkaline phosphatase detection with red chromogen. Bull's eye pattern created on a horizontal stainer with the blowing head too close to tissue.

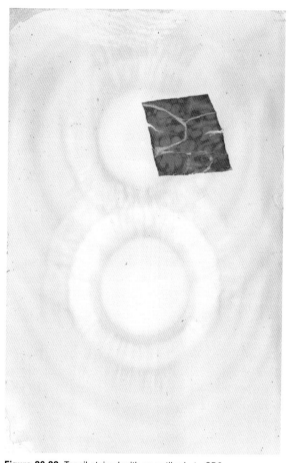

Figure 20.22 Tonsil stained with an antibody to CD3, demonstrating bull's eye artifact on the slide, visible to the naked eye, created by the autostainer's blowing head being too close to the slide.

References

Anderson, G., 1988. Enclosed tissue processors. IMLS Gazette 32, 141–142.

Angel, C.A., Heyderman, E., Lauder, I., 1989. Use of immunochemistry in Britain: EQA forum antibody usage questionnaire. Journal of Clinical Pathology 42, 1012–1017.

Ashton-Key, M., Jessup, E., Isaacson, P.G., 1996. Immunoglobulin light chain staining in paraffin-embedded tissue using a heat mediated epitope retrieval method. Histopathology 29, 525–531.

Bartlett, J.M., Ibrahim, M., Jasani, B., et al., 2009. External quality assurance of HER2 FISH and ISH testing: three years of the UK National External

Quality Assurance Scheme. Am J Clin Pathol 131, 106–111.

Bromley, C.M., Palecheck, P.L., Benda, J.A., 1994. Preservation of estrogen receptor in paraffin sections. Journal of Histotechnology 17, 115–118.

Cattoretti, G., Pileri, S., Parravicini, C., et al., 1993. Antigen unmasking of formalin-fixed, paraffin-embedded tissue sections. Journal of Pathology l71, 83–98.

Dabbs, D.J., 2006. Diagnostic immunohistochemistry, second ed. Churchill Livingstone, New York.

Donhuijsen, K., Schmidt, U., Hirche, H., et al., 1990. Changes in mitotic rate and cell cycle fractions caused by delayed fixation. Human Pathology 21, 709–714.

Eisen R.N., Goldstein N., 1999. Observations on antigen preservation in unstained sections. In: Proceedings of the National Society for Histotechnology, 25th Symposium, 1–11.

Emerson, L.L., Tripp, S.R., Baird, B.C., et al., 2006. A comparison of immunohistochemical stain quality in conventional and rapid microwave processed tissues. American Journal of Clinical Pathology 125, 176–183.

GEFPICS-FNCLCC, 1999. Recommendations pour l'evaluation immunohistochimique. Annals of Pathology 19, 336–343.

Horikawa, M., Chisaka, N., Yokoyama, S., Onoe, T., 1976. Effect of stirring during fixation upon immunofluorescence. Results with distribution of albumin-producing cells in liver. Journal of Histochemistry and Cytochemistry 24, 926–932.

Huang, S.N., Minassian, H., More, J.D., 1976. Application of immunofluorescent staining on paraffin sections improved by trypsin digestion. Laboratory Investigation 35, 383–390.

Ibrahim, M., Miller, K., 2008. HER-2 testing: the value of national audit, external quality assessment (UK NEQAS) and laboratory accreditation (CPA-UK-Ltd). Histopathology 53 (s1), 41.

Miller, K.D., Singh, N., Wotherspoon, A.C., 1995. Current trends in immunocytochemistry. Progress in Pathology 1, 99–119.

Norton, A.J., Jordon, S., Yeomans, P., 1994. Brief high temperature heat denaturation (pressure cooking): a simple and effective method of antigen retrieval for routinely processed tissues. Journal of Pathology 173, 371–379.

O'Leary, T.J., 2001. Standardization in immunohisto-chemistry. Applied Immunohistochemistry and Molecular Morphology 9, 3–8.

Prioleau, J., Schnitt, S.J., 1995. p53 antigen loss in stored paraffin slides. New England Journal of Medicine 332, 1521–1522.

Raymond, W.A., Leong, A.S., 1990. Oestrogen receptor staining of paraffin-embedded breast carcinomas following short fixation in formalin: a comparison with cytosolic and frozen section receptor analyses. Journal of Pathology 160, 295–303.

Rhodes, A., Jasani, B., Balaton, A.J., et al., 2001. Study of interlaboratory reliability and reproducibility of estrogen and progesterone receptor assays in Europe. Documentation of poor reliability and identification of insufficient microwave antigen retrieval time as a major contributory element of unreliable assays. Am J Clin Pathol 115, 44–58.

Shi, S.-R., Key, M.E., Kalra, K.L., 1991. Antigen retrieval in formalin-fixed, paraffin-embedded tissues: an enhancement method for immunohistochemical staining based on microwave oven heating of tissue sections. Journal of Histochemistry and Cytochemistry 39, 741–748.

Slater, D.N., Cobb, N., 1988. Enclosed tissue processors. IMLS Gazette 32, 543–544.

Trevisan, A., Gudat, F., Busachi, C., et al., 1982. An improved method for HBcAg demonstration in paraffin-embedded liver tissue. Liver 2, 331–339.

van Essen, H.F., Verdaasdonk, M.A.M., Elshof, S.M., et al., 2010. Alcohol based tissue fixation as an alternative for formaldehyde: influence on immunohistochemistry. J Clin Pathol; 63, 1090–1094.

Von Wasielewski, R., Mengel, M., Nolte, M., 1998. Influence of fixation, antibody clones, and signal amplification on steroid receptor analysis. Breast Journal 4, 33–40.

Williams, J.H., 1993. Tissue processing and immunocytochemistry. UK NEQAS Immunocytochemistry News 2, 2–3.

Williams, J.H., Mepham, B.L., Wright, D.H., 1997. Tissue preparation for immunocytochemistry. Journal of Clinical Pathology 50, 422–428.

Molecular pathology 21

Diane L. Sterchi • Caroline Astbury

Introduction

Molecular pathology seeks to apply gene expression against morphology and use gene expression analysis to validate large numbers of targets. A glossary of common definitions and terminology can be found at the end of this chapter.

Molecular pathology techniques have been used in the clinical laboratory to aid in the diagnosis and monitoring of treatment regimens of many infectious diseases such as HIV, hepatitis B, and tuberculosis (Netterwald 2006). These tests are usually performed on serological or other body fluids, such as sputum and seminal fluid. Currently the most well-known and most advertised molecular testing is for human papillomavirus (HPV) and human epidermal growth factor receptor 2 (HER2).

Clinical and research laboratories may use additional molecular pathology techniques, such as blotting methods which are used to study extracted ribonucleic acid (RNA) and deoxyribonucleic acid (DNA). Blotting methods consist of extracting DNA and/or RNA from homogenized tissues and then analyzing them using dot, Southern and Northern blotting filter hybridization methods (Sambrook et al. 1989). Blotting techniques such as these are powerful tools for the qualitative analysis of extracted nucleic acid from fresh or frozen cells and frozen tissues.

The polymerase chain reaction (PCR) is included in molecular pathology methods. PCR is a common method of creating copies of specific fragments of DNA. It rapidly amplifies a single DNA molecule into many billions of copies. In one application of the technology, small samples of DNA, such as those found in a strand of hair at a crime scene, can produce sufficient material to carry out forensic tests. PCR may also be used in addition to *in situ* hybridization (ISH) to study a specific genome of a tissue (Innis et al. 1990).

All of this leads to the role the histology laboratory plays in molecular pathology. In the histology laboratory the main method used in molecular pathology is ISH. John et al. (1969) and Gall and Pardue (1969) described the technique of ISH almost simultaneously.

ISH is a method of localizing and detecting specific mRNA sequences in preserved tissue sections or cell preparations by hybridizing the complementary strand of a nucleotide probe to the sequence of interest.

The method consists of denaturing (breaking apart) DNA and RNA strands using heat. A probe (a labeled complementary single strand) is incorporated with the DNA/RNA strands of interest. The strands will anneal with complementary nucleotides bonding back together with their homologous partners when cooled (Fig. 21.1). Some will anneal with the original complementary strands, but some will also anneal or hybridize with the probe. As probes increase in length, they become more specific. The chances of a probe finding a homologous sequence other than the target sequence decreases as the number of nucleotides in the probe increases. A longer probe can hybridize less specifically than shorter probes. Optimal probe size for ISH is small fragments of about 200–300 nucleotides. However, probes may be as small as 20–40 base pairs (bp) or as large as 1000 bp.

The detection of specific nucleic acid sequences (RNA, viral DNA or chromosomal DNA) in cells,

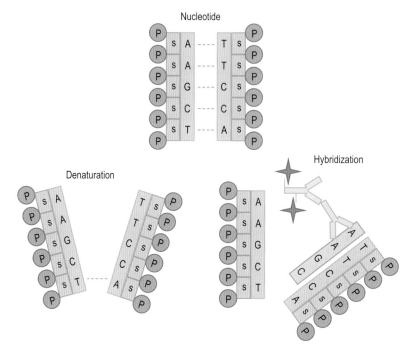

Figure 21.1 The genetic information for humans is encoded in billions of nucleotides (the building blocks of the DNA code) arranged in a double-helix molecule. Nucleotides consist of a base, a sugar (S), and a phosphate (P). The DNA code is written in an alphabet that uses four letters to represent each of the bases: (A) = adenine, (T) = thymine, (C) = cytosine, (G) = guanine. These bases will form pairs. (A) will only pair with (T). (G) will only pair with (C). Therefore, double-stranded DNA consists of two strands of homologous nucleotides. The genetic code in DNA is in triplets such as ATG. The base sequence of that triplet in the partner strand is therefore TAC.

tissues or whole organisms by ISH has numerous applications in biology, clinical and anatomical pathology, as well as in research.

ISH methods may employ radiolabeled probes that are visualized on a photographic film or photographic emulsion. However, most of these probes do not work well on routinely fixed, processed tissues and require the use of frozen sections. They may need 20–50 days of exposure before the results are visible. The development of non-radiolabeled probes that perform well on routine surgical and autopsy specimens has extended the field of anatomic pathology.

Detection of mRNA by using ISH is particularly useful if the protein product is quickly degraded or rapidly transported out of the target cell.

In ISH detection, immunohistochemistry (IHC)-like methods may be incorporated to detect the labeled (biotin, digoxigenin (DIG)) probe. So, the question arises, why not just do IHC? After all IHC is well-established, reliable, and less time consuming than ISH. IHC has been employed in the clinical and research arenas for several decades and has become a routine procedure in the histology laboratory. Furthermore, IHC has provided diagnostic procedures and a close look at the proteins within and on the cell membranes. The advantages of ISH over IHC include:

- High degree of specificity.
- DNA and mRNA are not as sensitive to formalin fixatives.
- Probe-target hybrid is stronger than antibody-antigen complex.
- Provides an alternative means of detection when reliable antibodies are not available.
- Provides a diagnosis at the molecular level.

It is important to understand the 'how and why' of the different stages in the ISH process in order for the testing to result in a functional outcome. This revised chapter continues to focus on the 'how and why' of ISH, and includes a review of automated ISH versus the manual processes (Sterchi 2008). It also includes a revised comprehensive review of fluorescence *in situ* hybridization (FISH) staining procedures and analysis.

Applications

There are many modifications of ISH methods that relate to application needs. Although the demonstration of DNA and RNA sequences by ISH is a valuable research tool, according to Warford and Lauder (1991) and Mitchell et al. (1992), it is also used diagnostically in:

- detection of abnormal genes
- identification of viral infection
- tumor phenotyping

ISH comes in many forms and methods, and over the past 10 to 20 years the methodology has expanded significantly. At one time only FISH was the 'standard' method for ISH. Now there are methods that allow visualization of the stain using a bright field microscope, reducing the need for a fluorescence microscope. However, FISH still has an advantage over chromogenic methods for labeling specific nucleic acid sequences in cells and tissues. It is a 'direct' technique, so it is faster and in some cases it does not require IHC-like detection. These probes employ fluorescent (fluorescein) tags that glow under ultraviolet light to detect the hybridization. FISH allows the use of multiple probes on the same tissue that may spatially or spectrally overlap. The literature suggests that it is possible to distinguish at least four or five different fluorescent signals in a single sample (Haugland & Spence 2005), whereas chromagens are often limited to one or two color options per slide. FISH, also known as molecular cytogenetics, has enabled a huge advance in the diagnostic and prognostic capability of the clinical cytogenetic laboratory. FISH can also vividly paint chromosomes or portions of chromosomes with fluorescent molecules (thus, the term 'chromosome painting').

ISH can provide cytological information on the location and alteration of genomic sequences in chromosomes. Traditionally, the technique has been applied to metaphase chromosome spreads (Davis et al. 1984; Lux et al. 1990), but it has been shown to be applicable to interphase nuclei (Hopman et al. 1988; Poddighe et al. 1992). Routine paraffin wax preparations of tissues can be used and 'interphase cytogenetics', as the method is termed, can provide direct information on chromosomal abnormalities in unselected tumor cell populations.

Viral identification can be undertaken using a variety of methods, of which only immuno-histochemistry and ISH provide simultaneous morphological information. The sensitivity of immunohistochemistry for the visualization of viral antigens, and ISH for the demonstration of cytomegalovirus, correlate well (Van den Berg et al. 1989). Most viral ISH methods use probes for DNA. Others, such as in the demonstration of the Epstein-Barr virus (Fig. 21.2), the detection of a virally encoded RNA transcript, provide results that are more sensitive than the use of antibodies and may even approach that of the PCR (Pringle et al. 1992).

The light chain portion kappa and lambda mRNA may be detected in normal and neoplastic B cells in human lymphoid tissue. Restriction of either kappa or lambda mRNA denotes monoclonality of lymphoid neoplasms and is useful in distinguishing between neoplastic and reactive lymphoid proliferations. Due to the destruction of RNAases by formalin fixation, kappa and lambda sequences are conserved in routine surgical tissues. (See Data Sheet Kappa and Lambda Probe ISH Kit, Novacastra.) (Fig. 21.3.)

Chromogenic *in situ* hybridization (CISH) is a method 'that enables the detection of gene expression in the nucleus using a conventional histochemical reaction' (White 2005); it is used for the detection of abnormal genes and to identify a gene therapy treatment direction. CISH can be used as an alternative in screening archived breast cancer tissue samples for HER2/neu (type 1 growth factor receptor gene) (Madrid & Lo 2004). Automated CISH techniques were used for detecting light chain expression in paraffin sections on plasma cell dyscrasias and B-cell non-Hodgkin lymphomas

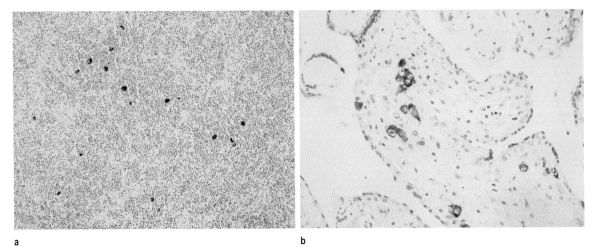

Figure 21.2 Example of automatic chromogenic *in situ* hybridization (CISH) staining. (a) Epstein-Barr virus-encoded RNA (EBER) and (b) cytomegalovirus (CMV). (Photographs courtesy of Leica Microsystems, Inc.)

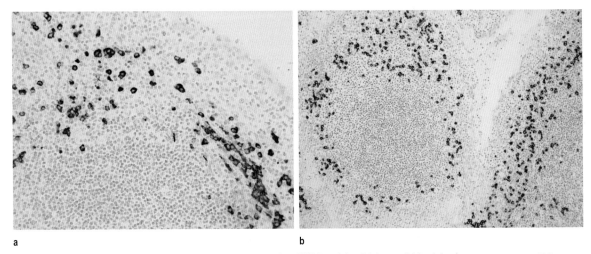

Figure 21.3 Example of automatic chromogenic *in situ* hybridization (CISH) staining (a) kappa (b) lambda. (Photographs courtesy of Leica Microsystems, Inc.)

'appeared superior to IHC' in that the ISH resulted with no background staining (Beck et al. 2003).

Silver precipitation *in situ* hybridization (SISH) is an emerging ISH method that works well with formalin fixed paraffin embedded (FFPE) tissues. It is also similar to FISH performance in detecting the location of genomic targets using probes. The major advantage of CISH and SISH is the possibility of long term storage of the stained slides. The chromagens or silver signals do not quench over time, unlike FISH signals (Fig. 21.4).

In situ zymography (ISZ) is a method that uses specific protease substrates to detect and localize protease activities in tissue sections. In the regulation of biological processes, proteases modulate several cellular functions. Several molecular techniques identify and characterize proteases in cells and tissue, such as a Northern blot and reverse transcription-polymerase chain reaction (RT-PCR) but ISZ works as well. One of its drawbacks is that unfixed fresh frozen tissues must be used. In contrast, its advantages are that it costs less than

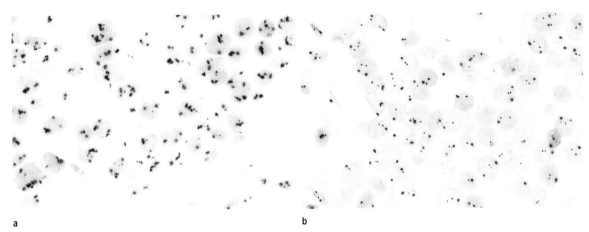

a   b

Figure 21.4 Example of automatic silver (silver deposition technology) *in situ* hybridization (SISH) staining. (a) HER2 and Chr17. (b) HER2 and Chr17. (Photographs courtesy of Ventana Medical Systems, Inc.)

conventional ISH methods, there are two approaches (one uses a photographic emulsion, the other uses a fluorescent-labeled substrate) and it is applicable to almost any protease (Yan & Blomme 2003).

Immunolabeling electron microscopy (IEM) in combination with ISH has been used in detecting severe acute respiratory syndrome (SARS). Viral immunogold labeling and ultrastructural ISH were used to analyze the morphogenesis of this recently emergent virus. A negative-sense riboprobe was used for the ultrastructural ISH (Goldsmith et al. 2004).

Polymerase chain reaction-ISH (PISH) is another form of ISH. Viral RNA is detected by RT-PCR, using formalin-fixed paraffin-embedded tissue (FFPE). PISH results have been compared to IHC on staining for Newcastle disease in veterinary medicine. Newcastle disease is an avian viral infection that has a potential for rapid spread and may cause serious economic impact and international trade restrictions in the poultry industry (Wakamatsu et al. 2005). PISH is also used in the detection of human papillomavirus in uterine cervical neoplasia (Xiao et al. 2001).

The identification of mRNA sequences by *in situ* hybridization may be the technique of choice for the rapid and sensitive identification of viral infection. Another advantage of *in situ* hybridization for viral detection is that some viral coat antigens are not expressed at certain stages of the viral replication cycle, thus negating the use of immunohistochemical methods.

ISH methods have been developed over the years so that most FFPE tissues, including decalcified tissues, can be used (Janneke et al. 1999).

Another area in which *in situ* hybridization and immunochemistry can be viewed as complementary techniques is in the phenotyping of tumors. Many monoclonal and polyclonal antibodies are available for phenotyping and these may be employed in sensitive and rapid techniques. When problems arise in the interpretation of immunohistochemical results, mRNA phenotyping by *in situ* hybridization can be helpful (Pringle et al. 1990, 1993; Kendall et al. 1991; Ruprai et al. 1991).

Common reagents

Listed here are names of reagents that are used in ISH techniques. The formulae for preparing these reagents are located in Appendix VIII. The majority of these reagents can be purchased pre-mixed or in a kit for easy mixing. Keep in mind that different reagents may be suggested with some ISH methods and automatic IHC equipment often provide pre-package reagents as ready to use (RTU) with their equipment. Purchasing the reagents pre-mixed or in kits is convenient and safer, and it provides some reassurance that they are mixed according to manufacturer's specifications and guaranteed by the vendor. This may cut down the possibility of human error.

1. Diethylpyrocarbonate (DEPC) treated water
2. 2% aminoalkylsilane (positively charged slides)
   These slides may be purchased pre-coated
   Make sure they are RNA/DNA free
3. Proteinase K
   Aliquot and freeze below −20°C
4. Hyaluronidase
5. 0.1 M triethanolamine (TEA), freshly made
6. 1 M Tris (this is to make buffers that vary in pH: buffer #1, pH 7.5; buffer #2, pH 9.5)
7. 1 M magnesium chloride
8. 5 M sodium chloride
9. Maleic acid buffer a washing buffer
10. 20× Saline sodium citrate (SSC) buffer (this is also used to make 2× SCC and 1× SCC buffers)
11. Denhart's solution
    (may cause increase in background)
12. Prehybridization solution
13. Hybridization solution
14. Detection method reagents:
    a. Streptavidin-alkaline phosphatase
    b. Anti-digoxigenin
    c. Horseradish peroxidase (HRP)
15. Colorimetric detection reagents:
    a. 5-bromo-4-chloro-3-indolyl phosphate (BCIP) nitro-blue tetrazolium salt (NBT)
    b. 3-amino-9-ethylcarbazole (AEC)
    c. Diaminobenzidine (DAB)

Probes and their choice

Probe choice is based on the type of sequence you are trying to detect. The technologist needs to optimize the conditions used as much as possible. The strength of the bonds between the probe and the target plays an important role. The strength decreases in the order RNA-RNA to DNA-RNA. Various hybridization conditions such as concentration of formamide, salt concentration, hybridization temperature, and pH influence this stability.

A probe is a labeled fragment of DNA or RNA used to find its complementary sequence or locate a particular clone. The choice of probes will depend on availability, sensitivity, and resolution required. The sensitivity of the probe will also depend on the degree of substitution and the size of the labeled fragments. Degree of substitution refers to the original nucleotide substituted by the labeled analogues. The sensitivity of detection correlates with the amount of label substituted. In general, probes with 25–32% substitution yield the highest sensitivity. There are several different types of probe. Each has unique characteristics that must be considered for each application.

Probes for DNA:

• Double-stranded DNA
• Single-stranded DNA
• Oligodeoxyribonucleotides

Probe for RNA:

• Single-stranded complementary RNA, a riboprobe

Probe type and means of synthesis

There are essentially four types of probe that can be used in performing *in situ* hybridization. Oligonucleotide probes are usually 20–50 bases in length. They are produced synthetically by an automated chemical synthesis employing a specific DNA nucleotide sequence (of your choice). These probes are resistant to RNases and are small, thus allowing easy penetration into the cells or tissue of interest. However, the small size has a disadvantage in that it covers fewer targets. The label should be positioned at the 3′ or the 5′ end. To increase sensitivity one can use a mixture of oligonucleotides that are complementary to different regions of the target molecule. Oligonucleotide protocols can be standardized for many different probes regardless of the target genes being sought. Another advantage of oligonucleotide probes is that they are single stranded, therefore excluding the possibility of renaturation.

Single-stranded DNA probes cover a much larger size range (200–500 bp) than oligonucleotide probes. They can be prepared by a primer extension on single-stranded templates by RT-PCR of RNA, or by an amplified primer extension of a PCR-generated fragment in the presence of a single antisense primer, or by the chemical synthesis of oligonucleotides. PCR-based methods are much easier and probes can be synthesized from small amounts of starting material. Moreover, PCR allows great flexibility in the choice of probe sequences by the use of appropriate primers.

Double-stranded DNA probes can be prepared by nick-translation, random primer, or PCR in the presence of a labeled nucleotide, and denatured prior to hybridization in order for one strand to hybridize with the mRNA of interest. They can also be produced by the inclusion of the sequence of interest in bacteria, which is replicated, lysed, and then the DNA is extracted and purified. The sequence of interest is removed with restriction enzymes. Random priming and PCR give the highest specific activities. These probes are less sensitive than single-stranded probes, since the two strands have a tendency to rehybridize to each other, thus reducing the concentration of probe available for hybridization to the target. Nevertheless, the sensitivity obtained with double-stranded probes is sufficient for many purposes, although they are not widely used today.

RNA probes (cRNA probes or riboprobes) are thermostable and are resistant to digestion by RNases. These probes are single stranded and are the most widely used in ISH. RNA probes are generated by *in vitro* transcription from a linearized template using a promoter for RNA polymerase that must be available on the vector DNA containing the template (SP6, T7, or T3). RNA polymerase is used to synthesize RNA complementary to the DNA substrate. Most commonly, the probe sequence is cloned into a plasmid vector so that it is flanked by two different RNA polymerase initiation sites enabling either sense-strand (control) or antisense (probe) RNA to be synthesized. The plasmid is linearized with a restriction enzyme so that plasmid sequences are not transcribed, since these may cause high backgrounds. Single-stranded probes provide advantages over double-stranded probes such as:

- The probe does not self-anneal in solution, so the probe is not exhausted.
- Large probe chains are not formed in solution; thus, probe penetration is not affected.

If high sensitivity is required, single-stranded probes should be used (Table 21.1).

Probe preparation and labeling

To visualize where the probe has bound within your tissue section or within your cells, you must attach a detectable label to your probe before hybridization. Two major choices must be made for the preparation of a probe:

- What type of nucleic acid is to be used (DNA or RNA, single or double stranded)?
- What type of label is to be incorporated into the probe?

A vital consideration is the length of the probe, and the means by which this is controlled depends on the type and the method of synthesis. There are two methods of probe labeling. They are:

- Direct: the reporter molecules (enzyme, radioisotope or fluorescent marker) are directly attached to the DNA or RNA.
- Indirect: a hapten (biotin, digoxigenin, or fluorescein) is attached to the probe and detected by a labeled binding protein (typically an antibody).

Methods for incorporating labels into DNA are nick translation and random primer methods.

Oligonucleotide probe labeling

5'-end labeling

The 5' end of DNA or RNA undergoes direct phosphorylation of the free 5'-terminal OH groups. The free 5'-OH substrates can be labeled using T4 polynucleotide kinase. This method is usually used

Table 21.1 Probe types

Probe	Labeling	Advantages	Disadvantages
dsDNA	Random primers	Easy to use Subcloning unnecessary Choice of labeling methods High specific activity Possibility of signal amplification (networking) Readily available	Re-annealing during hybridization (decreased probe availability) Probe denaturation required, increasing probe length and decreasing tissue penetration Hybrids less stable than RNA probes
ssDNA	Primer extension	No probe denaturation needed No re-annealing during hybridization (single strand) More sensitive Stable	Technically complex Subcloning required Hybrids less stable than RNA probes Template binding
ssRNA	DNA polymerase transcription	High specific activity No probe denaturation needed No re-annealing Unhybridized probe enzymatically destroyed, sparing hybrid	Subcloning needed Less tissue penetration RNase labile May have higher levels of non-specific binding to tissue components, thus increasing the chance of higher background and lower penetration of the probe into the tissue
Oligo	5′ end 3′ end 3′ tailing	No cloning or molecular biology expertise required Stable Good tissue penetration (small size) Constructed according to recipe from amino acid data No self-hybridization Limited labeling methods Short oligonucleotide sequences can be directly manufactured Can use multiple probes, no competition between probes	Limited labeling methods Lower specific activity, so less sensitive Dependent on published sequences Less stable hybrids

for radiolabeling. Non-radiolabels use a covalent linker.

3′-end labeling

Terminal dexoxynucleotidyl transferase (TdT) is used to add a labeled residue to the 3′ end of a synthetic oligonucleotide that is approximately 14–100 nucleotides in length. These probes provide excellent specificity but only moderate sensitivity. See the oligonucleotide 3′-end labeling procedure on page 555 of sixth edition.

3′ tailing

A tail containing labeled nucleotides is added to the free 3′ end of double- or single-stranded DNA using TdT. These probes are more sensitive than the 3′-end labeled versions, but can produce more non-specific background. Oligonucleotide tailing kits are commercially available.

It should be noted that the use of commercially available labeling kits can greatly assist in making methods simpler to undertake while providing results of an assured standard.

Purification of labeled probes

There are several methods that can be used to test the purification. If the probe is homemade or purchased it must be tested for its sensitivity to the selected target. Here is a list of methods that can be used, but it is advisable to follow the manufacturers' recommendation on their use:

- Sephadex G-50 column
- Sephadex G-50 chromatography
- Selective precipitation

Estimating the labeling efficiency and testing the probe

It is always good practice to estimate the yield of labeled nucleic acids. This confirms a successful labeling reaction before performing the staining.

Before using a labeled probe, it is useful to prepare and demonstrate test strips to gauge the degree of label incorporation. This may be done by using the normal detection procedure for the ISH method on dots of labeled nucleic acid sequence and a labeled control applied at matching descending concentrations on a positively charged nylon membrane. Some technicians will prepare several test strips from one labeled sequence to compare the sensitivity of different detection systems. The nylon membrane is subjected to an immunological detection which can be either a colorimetric or chemiluminescent method depending on the protocol used. Direct comparison of the signal intensities of sample and control allows estimation of labeling yield. Kits for this technique are commercially available in which the labeled control already exists on a test strip. A much quicker method for estimating the yield of labeled nucleic

acids is to use a bioanalyzer, since this can give quantitative results in as little as 30 minutes.

A method for estimating labeling efficiency of the nucleic acid using a dilution series followed by a spot test is described below.

Preparation of the dilution series

1. Dilute the labeling probe using dilution buffer to a starting concentration of 2.5 pmol/μl.
2. Make a dilution series of purified probe in Eppendorf tubes to give nucleic acid concentrations of 300 pg/μl, 100 pg/μl, 30 pg/μl, 10 pg/μl, 3 pg/μl, and one tube containing diluent only. Ensure that all tube volumes are equal. Repeat the same dilution series with your control or used pre-labeled (with control) test strips.
3. Apply 1 μl drops from each tube onto the nylon membrane (Roche). The control dilutions should be lined up with the test sample dilution concentration. For an example of placing spots, see Figure 21.5.
4. Label the position of each application with a pencil on the side of the strip (not on the strip).
5. Fix the nucleic acid to the membrane by either baking the membrane for 30 minutes at 120°C or using a UV light.
6. Wash the membrane briefly in washing buffer.
7. Immerse in blocking solution for 10 minutes.
8. Incubate with reagents used in ISH detection technique.

Note: Dilute reagents in blocking solution and use this solution for washing.

9. Detect enzyme using the same solutions and procedure as for ISH method.
10. Rinse in double-distilled water and blot dry.

Commercially made probes

Custom designed, pre-made cloned DNA and oligonucleotide sequences and labeling kits are commercially available. Their use can make methods simpler

Probe concentrations in pg/μl

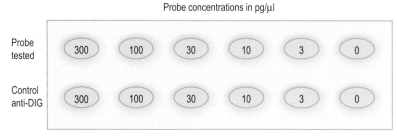

Control concentrations in pg/μl

Figure 21.5 Diagram of 'dot test' for estimating the labeling efficiency and testing the probe.

to undertake while providing results of an assured standard. Depending on the type of laboratory you have and how many ISH requests you receive, pre-mixed reagents and pre-labeled probes can be cost-effective. The kits, reagents, or ordering the labeled probes can cut down on precious technologist time, and they come with instructions – a benefit for the novice technologist. However, this does not mean that the theory behind ISH can be ignored. The technologist must understand ISH to order labeled probes and the ISH kits.

Probe concentration

For DNA probes the concentration of the probe will be ~0.5–2 μg/ml. Oligonucleotide probes can be used with, or without, acetylation. Probes without acetylation pretreatment of the sample will have a concentration of ~50–200 ng/ml and may provide more intense results with minimal background. For probes with acetylation pretreatment, a higher concentration of oligonucleotide probe may be used without incurring non-specific background staining.

Length of probe

As mentioned previously, one must consider the length of the probe. Longer probes give weaker signals and they penetrate less effectively into the cross-linked (fixed) tissue. The extent of weaker signals and penetration depends also on the nature of the tissue, the choice of fixative and whether a pretreatment has been carried out.

The length of probe can be controlled in either the synthesis reaction or the subsequent partial cleavage. In nick-translated probes, the DNA length is determined by the amount of DNase in the reaction, whereas in random priming the length is determined by concentration of the primer. Long RNA probes may show poor tissue penetration, whereas chemical shortening (hydrolysis) enhances tissue penetration, and may also increases the likelihood of non-selective binding to other non-targeted gene sequences.

Once a probe is prepared, its size should be checked. If the probe is too small, it may yield low signals with high background. It is necessary to know whether a reduction in probe size (length) will improve both the signal for the tissue and the preparation method used.

Detection

The choice of detection system will be principally determined by the probe label used and secondly by the ISH procedure type. One must consider the sensitivity and resolution required.

Colorimetric detection substrate systems include horseradish peroxidase with either 3-amino-9-ethylcarbazole (AEC) or 3,3′-diaminobenzidine tetra-hydrochloride (DAB) substrates. AEC forms a red-brown product which is alcohol soluble; therefore aqueous mounting media are required. Methyl green/blue has been the most often used counter-stain in earlier publications but is losing popularity. DAB forms a permanent, insoluble, brown product that is compatible with solvent-based mounting media. Alkaline phosphatase systems can use 5-bromo-4-chloro-3-indolyl phosphate/nitro-blue tetrazolium (BCIP/NBT) or fast red. BCIP/NBT forms a purple/blue alcohol-insoluble stain. Eosin is a compatible counterstain if a nuclear target is expected, or nuclear fast red if the target is cytoplasmic. Fast red forms an intense red product which is alcohol soluble and an aqueous mounting media is required. Methyl green or blue is compatible if a nuclear target is expected, or light hematoxylin if the target is cytoplasmic.

Detection methods can be either direct or indirect. Incorporation of a stable hapten to a probe is the cornerstone of non-radiographic detection. Hybridized probes can be detected by enzymatic reactions that produce a colored precipitate at the site of hybridization. The most commonly used enzymes for this application are alkaline phosphatase (AP) and horseradish peroxidase (HRP). Although these enzymes can be conjugated directly to nucleic acid probes, such enzyme-coupled probes are often inappropriate for ISH to tissue preparations because probe penetration is hampered by the presence of the conjugated enzyme. Therefore, indirect methods are preferred (Knoll & Lichter 1995).

Biotin, fluorochromes (fluorescein), and digoxigenin (DIG) are the most common labels used. Probes that are labeled with these reporter molecules are usually detected by an AP or HRP conjugate to avidin (for biotin) or antibodies (for DIG). Fluorescein and DIG have an advantage over biotin in that they produce lower levels of background signals in tissues that contain high amounts of endogenous biotin.

Direct detection of a fluorescent label is often employed for the demonstration of multiple chromosome targets (Nederlof et al. 1989), but when single target sequences are to be identified, indirect methods may be used.

To reduce non-specific staining (particularly of collagen) by indirect detection reagents it is advisable to pre-incubate preparations in a Tris (Triton X-100 or Tween) buffer solution containing bovine serum albumin. It may also prove beneficial to use this solution as the diluent for the primary detection reagent. However, at this step it is more important to use a Fab fragment of an antibody as this may reduce background staining.

Indirect detection procedures offer increased sensitivity. The selection of the enzyme and substrate (De Jong et al. 1985) should be included in weighing the benefits of different detection systems. A substrate system that employs conjugated antibodies such as anti-DIG or anti-FITC that are conjugated with AP together with the application of a colorimetric BCIP/NBT that can be cycled to produce an insoluble blue/black precipitate over a period of 24 hours is recommended. Another substrate system one could use for a more intense fluorescent signal is a fluorescent 2-hydroxy-3-naphthoic acid-2'-phenylanilide phosphate (HNPP) with fast red TR.

The main advantages of this procedure are low levels of non-specific staining, simplicity, and the use of an enzyme substrate system that can produce an insoluble blue/black precipitate.

Many commercially available probes for ISH are labeled with biotin. When used in combination with streptavidin detection systems, high sensitivity can be achieved. A disadvantage of this combination is having a widespread endogenous tissue distribution. Substantial quantities of endogenous biotin are, for example, present in the liver and kidney (Wood & Warnke 1981), as well as in other tissues, such as pituitary, submandibular gland, thyroid, and parathyroid. Furthermore, proliferating cells may often produce enough biotin to make the discrimination between true and false-positive results difficult. However, methods of blocking endogenous biotin have greatly improved and work well to prevent false positives.

Digoxigenin (Herrington et al. 1989) in combination with a Fab fragment-enzyme conjugate detection system currently provides results of equal or superior sensitivity to biotin, with extremely low non-specific background staining. Another label that may be used in conjunction with a single-step detection method is fluorescein. Using this label it is possible to undertake rapid ISH methods in which target sequences of moderate to high copy number can be demonstrated in a working day.

Sample preparation

Fixation

Fixation is an initial step in specimen preparation or can be an intermediate step in a protocol, as in methods using cryostat sections. The duration, type, and temperature of fixation may also differ according to preparation. Together, these factors will have an effect, not only on the preservation of the tissue but also on the retention of nucleic acid and the resistance of DNA and RNA to nuclease digestion. The choice of fixative will have an influence on the conservation of nucleic acids and their availability for hybridization. Specimens that are immersion-fixed prior to paraffin embedding appear to be unaffected by 'normal' contamination levels of nucleases, thus indicating that only the hybridization solutions need to be scrupulously free of the enzymes.

The functional groups involved in base pairing are protected in the double-helix structure of duplex DNA. RNA is fairly unreactive to cross-linking agents.

Methanol/acetic acid fixation is recommended for metaphase chromosome spreads. Cryostat sections may be fixed with 4% formaldehyde (~30 minutes), Bouin's fixative, or paraformaldehyde vapor fixation. This fixation also helps to secure the tissue to the slide.

Proteins surround DNA and RNA target sequences and the extensive cross-linking of these proteins may mask the target nucleic acid. Therefore, 'permeabilization' procedures may be required.

After the tissue is removed from the patient or animal, it must be fixed to prevent autolysis, inhibit bacterial/fungal growth, and make it resistant to damage from subsequent processing. There are two main groups of fixatives, coagulant and non-coagulant, classified by their reaction with soluble proteins. Ethanol and mercuric chloride are coagulant fixatives. They are not the preferred fixative for use with ISH, since ethanol dehydrates, coagulates,

and precipitates cellular proteins, nucleic acids, and carbohydrates. Covalent bonding does not occur with ethanol fixatives and the tissue components, so mRNA is not anchored within the tissue and is likely to be lost during post-fixation processing procedures. For ISH, non-coagulant, cross-linking aldehydes (formaldehyde, paraformaldehyde, and glutaraldehyde) are recommended.

Tissues fixed for ISH should retain mRNA within the tissue but not raise background. Both background and signal are generally higher on perfused-fixed paraffin tissue sections than on frozen sections. The signal-to-noise (S/N) ratio on perfused-fixed tissue sections is better.

Most commonly, tissue specimens are routinely fixed in 10% buffered formalin, processed overnight in an automatic tissue processor, and embedded in paraffin wax. Fixation time of 8–12 hours is optimal. Keep in mind that the longer the fixation, the more rigorous the enzyme digestion is required to optimize the signal. Alcohol-fixed tissues should be post-fixed with an aldehyde fixative to prevent the diffusion of mRNA (if you are looking at RNA).

Slide/section preparation

Sections are cut at 4–6 μm on an alcohol-cleaned microtome using positively charged or hand-coated slides. Sections are drained well and then air-dried at room temperature. After deparaffinization, slides are placed in an alcohol-cleaned staining container of DEPC water. The staining container is then placed in the heated water bath at 23–37°C and held until the start of ISH. Gloves must be worn to prevent contamination, and all utensils, such as brushes and forceps, should be cleaned with alcohol and kept within the cleaned area designated for ISH.

Proteolytic digestion

The use of formaldehyde-based fixatives prior to paraffin embedding of specimens will mask nucleic acid sequences. Digestion is a important step when performing ISH. Digestion improves probe penetration by increasing cell permeability with minimal tissue degradation. Although the nucleic acid is not directly affected by proteolytic digestion, it is important to control this step carefully. Under-digestion will result in insufficient exposure of the nucleic acid, while over-digestion can sufficiently weaken the protein structure surrounding the sequence, bringing about its loss into subsequent solutions. mRNA sequences tend to be loosely associated with proteins, while DNA targets are intimately associated with histone and other nuclear proteins. Due to these differences, the concentration of proteolytic enzyme required to unmask mRNA will be less than that necessary to expose DNA.

The selection of the proteolytic enzyme is important. This should be of molecular biology grade to ensure the absence of nuclease activity. Proteinase K and pepsin are two enzymes commonly used for digestion. Proteinase K has an advantage over other proteolytic enzymes because during incubation it digests any nucleases that might be present. However, higher concentrations of the enzyme may be required, depending on the tissue fixation time.

Nuclease digestion is used as a negative control. Treatment of same tissue/patient tissue sections with RNase A will demonstrate that ISH signals are due to RNA hybridization.

Proteoglycan digestion is required for bone and cartilage. Kidney and brain may also need proteoglycan digestion, if the signal is weak. Post-fixation in 4% paraformaldehyde is necessary after digestion to prevent tissue loss. In addition, post-fixation after digestion (for all digestions) prevents leaching and will inhibit RNase activity.

When ISH methods are used to demonstrate mRNA sequences, non-specific attachment of digoxigenin and fluorescein-labeled oligonucleotides to epithelial tissues can create non-specific results. To minimize this interaction, preparations can be acetylated after proteolytic digestion and before post-fixation. Acetylation decreases non-specific binding of the probe to the tissue. Positive charges on the tissue are neutralized by reducing electrostatic binding of the probe.

Prehybridization is intended to reduce non-specific binding. Sites in the tissue become saturated with the components of the prehybridization solution preventing non-specific binding. The purpose of the prehybridization solution is to equilibrate the specimen with the hybridization solution prior to the addition of the probe, and to allow anionic macromolecules to block sites of potential non-specific probe interaction. The prehybridization solution contains all the ingredients of the hybridization mixture except the probe. Non-complementary sequences such as bovine serum albumin (BSA at 1 mg/ml), Denhardt solution (Ficoll, BSA, and polyvinylpyrrolidone all at 0.02%), and tRNA are used to reduce non-specific binding. Most data indicate that blocking is required, but a separate prehybridization step may not be necessary. In some cases, adequate blocking may be accomplished during the hybridization step. Electrostatic binding of probes to the tissue and slides can be neutralized by treatment in TEA buffer containing 0.1 M triethanolamine.

Hybridization

Hybridization occurs after denaturization, during cooling, in the presence of a complementary probe, and permits hydrogen bonding of the two strands of nucleic acids. The probe must form stable hydrogen bonds with the target with minimal hybridization with non-target sequences. The probe and target sequences must be single stranded. Simultaneously heating the probe and target to high temperatures may increase the consistency and sensitivity of detection. This can only be met if care is taken to precisely control this step of the ISH procedure. Control is achieved through balancing the various components of the hybridization solution and hybridizing at an optimal temperature for the correct length of time.

If a DNA probe is employed or a DNA target demonstrated, then it is essential that these are rendered single stranded. This is achieved by using dry heat with the hybridization solution placed over the specimen, which is then covered with a coverslip, plastic sheet, or cap. The denaturation will differ according to the percentage of guanine-cytosine base pairs within the target sequence of interest. When there is a high percentage of guanine-cytosine base pairs present, the third hydrogen bond associated with the base pair will occur at a higher melting temperature (T_m) than in the sequences in which adenosine and thymidine pairing predominates. Overheating to temperatures greater than 100°C at this stage may compromise specimen preservation.

At the molecular level, hybridization involves an initial nucleation reaction between a few bases, followed by hydrogen bonding of the remaining sequences. The control of temperature during hybridization is crucial, as variations will influence the specificity (stringency) of annealing. RNA and DNA hybrids are formed optimally at about 25°C, below their T_m, but when lower temperatures are used some partial homologous annealing may occur. Although this situation should be avoided, it can be usefully employed to screen for sequences with partial homology (e.g. human papillomavirus subtypes). By incorporating formamide, a helix-destabilizing reagent, the annealing may be maintained using lower temperatures (e.g. at 37°C, at which the tissue preservation is not affected).

Stringency can also be altered by adjusting the availability of monovalent cations in the hybridization solution. These cations are usually supplied by sodium chloride and they regulate the degree of natural electrostatic repulsion between the probe and target sequences. When used at high concentration their effect is to produce conditions of low stringency, while at low concentrations only sequences with complete homology can hybridize.

Anionic macromolecules are often included in the hybridization solution to reduce non-specific interactions of the probe. Sonicated and denatured salmon sperm DNA can shield non-homologous nucleic acid sequences from the probe and reduce the opportunity for cellular electrostatic interactions. Dextran sulfate will also reduce the possibility of cellular electrostatic interactions and locally concentrate the probe, enhancing the rate of hybridization. Particular attention should be taken to ensure that hybridization solutions are prepared using reagents free from nuclease contamination.

The rate of annealing will be influenced by time and temperature as well as by the composition of the hybridization solution as discussed above. Due to steric constraints, ISH proceeds at a slower rate than in blotting methods. However, high probe concentrations can be used to compensate for this factor. Hybridization times of 1–2 hours for biotinylated and fluorescein-labeled probes are often effective. However, with digoxigenin-labeled probes, overnight hybridization may be required to provide high sensitivity.

Post-hybridization washes are used to adjust the stringency of hybridization. The sections must be rinsed with solutions that contain high concentrations of salt to remove the unbound probe. Subsequent washing with solutions containing decreasing salt concentrations and increasing temperature reduces mismatching of base pairs. Longer probes and those with higher G + C content are more stable. Increases in temperature and formamide concentration are the destabilizing factors. By reducing the concentration of formamide in the hybridization solution, while maintaining a constant temperature, the annealing conditions will become less stringent, thereby increasing the sensitivity of mRNA detection when using fluorescein-labeled oligonucleotide probes.

Controls

It is essential to include controls to verify ISH results. A positive and no-hybridization control should always be included when undertaking an ISH procedure. The positive control should contain the target sequence being demonstrated and be prepared the same as the test samples. It should receive the same solutions and go through the same procedural steps as the test samples. This will provide a gauge for the overall performance of the technique. If the same positive control is used from run to run, it will help validate the ISH staining reproducibility.

Other controls may be incorporated to test the results' validity. The number and type of controls to be incorporated into the technique is determined at the discretion of the laboratory's personnel and standard operating procedures. As mentioned under the digestion section earlier in this chapter, nuclease digestion can be used as a negative control.

Equipment and reagent preparation

DNA and RNA can be degraded by nuclease activity. Indeed, high concentrations of DNase and RNase are useful in confirming the nucleic acid type specificity of hybridization. However, at much lower concentrations, nucleases present on the skin may contaminate solutions used in hybridization methods sufficiently to degrade the quality of naked DNA and RNA. For this reason, in addition to the wearing of gloves, elaborate precautions are often taken to ensure the absence of nucleases from solutions used in hybridization techniques.

Treatment of solutions and glassware to destroy nuclease activity

DNase is destroyed by autoclaving. RNase is resistant to heat inactivation and therefore other procedures should be used as described below.

Preparation of DEPC-treated water

Add diethylpyrocarbonate (DEPC) (Sigma D5758) to pure water to a final concentration of 0.1%. This should be done in a fume hood. Shake well to dissolve and allow it to stand overnight. Autoclave the solution and container the following day.

Preparation of DEPC-treated solutions

Prepare solutions, then add DEPC to 0.1%. Shake and leave overnight, then autoclave.

Note

Adding full-strength DEPC directly to a buffer may alter the buffering properties. Solutions that require a buffer of that type should be made up in RNase-free glassware using pre-mixed autoclaved DEPC-treated water.

Preparation of glassware

Treat glassware at 200°C overnight or, if delicate:

1. Wash in a mild/low suds soap or RNase Away solution.
2. Rinse in double-distilled nuclease-free water until detergent is removed.
3. Soak in 3% aqueous hydrogen peroxide, 10 minutes.
4. Rinse in DEPC-treated water.
5. Dry and protect from dust.

Most laboratories purchase DEPC-treated water and use sterile plastic disposable containers in place of the glassware. The information in this chapter is for those laboratories that prefer to prepare their own DEPC water and use glass bottles for buffer storage.

Universal ISH method (no frills or specialized equipment)

Day 1

1. Deparaffinize slides completely. Three changes of xylene and/or substitute for 4–8 minutes each.

Note

Incomplete deparaffinization may cause a weak reaction.

2. Dehydrate through two changes 100% (ethanol) EtOH, 1 change 95% EtOH for 3 minutes each. Rinse in DEPC-treated water or use slides already in warmed DEPC-treated water. Rinse in warmed (23–37°C) Tris/saline buffer #1, pH 7.5, and drain.
3. De-proteinize sections in freshly prepared proteinase K solution at 23–37°C, in a moist chamber for 15 minutes.
4. Rinse in Tris/saline buffer #1 at room temperature for 5 minutes. If necessary, digest proteoglycans and/or acetylation before going to next step.
5. Dehydrate slides through one change of 95% EtOH and two changes 100% EtOH for 2 minutes each. Air-dry for 5 minutes. This step is omitted if prehybridizing (next step).
6. Apply the prehybridization solution by putting 1–2 drops (60–100 µl) on the sections. Incubate in a moist chamber at room temperature for 1 hour. Blot off all excess prehybridization solution before adding the probe.

7. Apply hybridization fluid (probe) and cover with a heat-resistant film (microwave wrap, coverslips, or chambers). The probe is tailed with either biotin-dUTP or digoxigenin-dUTP.

8. Initiate hybridization by denaturing slides for 5–10 minutes at 92–100°C (try not to exceed 100°C). Use a preheated 'metal' tray to set slides on for optimal denaturization. Cool slides to 37–42°C and incubate in humidity chamber for 18–24 hours. Agitation may enhance reaction. Since this method is not using a commercial kit, the staining continues on day 2.

Day 2

9. Rinse slides twice in 2× SSC and twice in 1× SSC for 5 minutes each at 37°C.

10. Apply a 5% blocking solution at 37°C for 10 minutes.

11. Rinse in buffer #1 for 2 minutes, followed by a 10-minute rinse in buffer #2.

12. Add 1–2 drops of detection reagent to each slide (streptavidin-AP or anti-digoxigenin-AP). Incubate in a humidity chamber for 20–30 minutes at 37°C. During the incubation period, prepare the substrate and warm to 37°C.

13. Rinse slides in three changes of 1× SSC for 5 minutes each.

14. Incubate in substrate for 30–60 minutes at 37°C.

15. Stop reaction by washing in buffer at 37°C for 2 minutes. Rinse in two changes of distilled water (DW) for 2 minutes each.

16. Rinse in two changes of DW for 2 minutes each.

17. Counterstain; this is dependent on the chromogen selected. For BCIP/NBT use nuclear fast red, eosin, or methyl green. For DAB use hematoxylin or methyl green. Go on to step 18 if using BCIP/NBT or DAB. For AEC use methyl green and coverslip out of distilled water using an aqueous mounting medium. Do not go through alcohols or clearing.

18. Dehydrate in increasing concentrations of alcohol.

19. Clear using xylene and coverslip in permanent mounting resin (Doran & Sterchi 2000).

Automation

There are several versions of automation for comparing with the universal manual ISH method.

Automation types can be placed in the following categories:

1. Fully automated: this is where the cut section/slide comes out of the oven and straight into the stainer. The slide is deparaffinized, digested, prehybridized, hybridized, and detected all in one piece of equipment. This type of equipment can be expensive, but is necessary for large volumes of ISH.

2. Mainly automated:
   a. Requires that the histologist must remove the paraffin before placing it on the stainer.
   b. As above, but the digestion must also be performed before placing the slide on the stainer.

All these options are time-efficient and cost-effective, since they use less reagents than manual staining. Often the hybridization time is less than 2 hours.

3. Semi-automated: usually the manual paraffin removal, digestion, prehybridization and hybridization are performed either manually or using a hybridizer or a thermocyler before finishing the detection part of the staining. Commercial stand-alone hybridizers perform prehybridization and hybridization automatically. Some do not require removal of the slides for the washes and the temperatures and times are programmed into the equipment. The fully programmable ones for prehybridizing, hybridizing and washes are great for laboratories that have IHC stainers only.

Any equipment that will cut down on the hands-on time and provide more consistent and reliable results is advantageous.

Troubleshooting

Tissue sections fall off

- adhesive absent/insufficient poly-L-lysine or amino-alkylsilane (AS) on slide
- insufficient adhesion time/temperature

Table 21.2 Suggested digestion times adjusted to fixation time		
Fixation time (hours)	Enzyme	Digestion time (minutes)
4	Pepsin, trypsin, or proteinase K	10
15	Pepsin, trypsin, or proteinase K	90
24	Pepsin, trypsin, or proteinase K	120

- over-digestion (too long/too concentrated)
- overzealous coverslip removal (use pliable wrap, AS slips, or well covers)
- denaturation too long or temperature too high (93–98°C is ideal)
- excessive slide agitation

Weak staining (tissue preparation)

- slides incompletely deparaffinized (add an additional xylene/substitute step to insure that all the paraffin has been removed)
- slides not dehydrated or drained prior to addition of probe (water in tissue will dilute probe)
- over-fixation (increase digestion time)
- insufficient digestion (increase time, concentration, or type of digesting reagent) (see Table 21.2)

Weak staining (hybridization/detection)

- probe insufficiently biotinylated
- probe concentration too dilute (hybridize longer)
- probe or target DNA insufficiently denatured (increase time of denaturation, check the temperature of the hot start)
- incomplete hybridization (prehybridize, increase hybridization time, lower temperature if too high, or check stringency)

- buffer wrong pH (should be alkaline, pH 9.5)
- reagents too cold (warm reagents to 23°C)

High background

- skipped blocking step
- probe too concentrated
- slides dried out during incubations
- washes omitted or shortened
- detergent wash buffer not used after label incubation
- incubated substrate too long

'Negative' positive control

- wrong probe
- reagents bad (improper storage)
- digestion absent (enzymes are unstable)
- denaturation absent (increase temperature)
- omitted step in protocol
- mixed detection reagents improperly

Inconsistent staining (stringency conditions)

Stringency conditions occur if a related but non-homologous probe binds to the target:

- non-homologous sequences hybridize/some mismatch (low stringency – high salt concentration, low temperature, low formamide concentration)
- complete binding only if homologous (high stringency – low salt concentration, high temperature, high formamide concentration)

Digestion

If there is absent or a weak signal, digestion needs to be increased by 10 minutes.

A quick test for sufficient digestion is to place the slide under the microscope; using a 40× objective one cell is observed. When 20 dots can be counted in the nucleus, digestion is complete.

Oligonucleotide 3′-end labeling with DIG-ddUTP

Terminal transferase is used to add a single modified dideoxyuridine triphosphate (DIG-ddUTP, biotin-ddUTP, or fluorescein-ddUTP) to the 3′ ends of an oligonucleotide. In this method, DIG-ddUTP will be used. The method described here is from Roche Applied Science Laboratory; it has been modified from the Boehringer Mannheim procedure. The reagents in this procedure may be purchased in a kit (Roche).

Contents of labeling reagents: the amounts to prepare listed here are the amounts supplied in the kit. The kit will accommodate 25 labeling reactions. If you require other amounts, just adjust your volume calculations for less or more.

1. Reaction buffer, pH 6.6 (this is a 5× concentrated solution)

1 M potassium cacodylate

0.125 M Tris-HCl

1.25 mg/ml bovine serum albumin

Prepare 50–100 µl

2. CoCl₂ solution

25 mM cobalt chloride

Prepare 50–100 µl

3. DIG-ddUTP solution

1 mM digoxigenin-11-ddUTP in double distilled water

Prepare 25 µl

4a. Terminal transferase 1 (newer method)

25 µl terminal transferase, in the following:

60 mM potassium phosphate (pH 7.2 at 4°C)

150 mM potassium chloride

1 mM 2-mercaptoethanol

0.5% Triton X-100

50% glycerol

Prepare a solution with a concentration of 400 units/µl

4b. Terminal transferase 2 (older method)

1 µl (50 units) terminal transferase, in the following:

200 mM potassium cacodylate

200 mM potassium chloride

1 mM EDTA

0.2 mg/ml bovine serum albumin

50% glycerol

Add enough double-distilled water to make a final volume of 20 µl

5. 0.2 M EDTA (pH 8.0) made in double distilled water

Procedure

1. Dissolve 100 pmol of the purified oligonucleotide in 10 µl of sterile double distilled water.
2. Add the following to a sterile microcentrifuge tube on ice:

    4 µl of 5′ concentrated reaction buffer

    4 µl of 25 mM cobalt chloride (CoCl₂)

    1 µl DIG-ddUTP solution. For this labeling we will use DIG-ddUTP.

    1 µl of terminal transferase (400 units/µl)
3. Mix and centrifuge briefly.
4. Incubate at 37°C for 15 minutes, then place on ice.
5. Stop the reaction by adding 2 µl of 0.2 M EDTA (pH 8.0)

Genetic testing: fluorescence *in situ* hybridization (FISH)

The current methods for genetic testing of hereditary and oncological human disease are vast and continuously evolving, as faster, more reliable, and cheaper techniques are developed. One such method of genetic testing is a specialized form of ISH: fluorescence *in situ* hybridization (FISH), also known as molecular cytogenetics. FISH utilization has enabled a huge advance in the diagnostic and prognostic capability of clinical and research laboratories for both constitutional and acquired disorders. We now concentrate on this one technique of genetic testing.

Methodology

The basic steps in a FISH procedure include the fixation of the DNA, as either metaphase chromosomes or interphase nuclei, on a slide; the DNA is then denatured *in situ*, so that it becomes single stranded. This target DNA is then hybridized to specific DNA probe sequences, which are labeled with fluorochromes to allow for their detection. The labeled probe is added in excess, so probe binding to target DNA occurs. Fluorescence microscopy then allows the visualization of the probe on the target material; analysis of the probe signals includes observation of gain of signals, loss of signals, positioning of signals, or fusion of signals.

Probes

Most probes used in the clinical laboratory in the United States are commercially available and tend to fall into three categories:

1. Repetitive sequences (such as the centromeres or alpha-satellite regions of chromosomes).
2. Whole chromosome sequences (including the short arm, centromere, and long arm of the chromosome).
3. Unique sequences (ranging in size from < 1 kb to >1 Mb of DNA).

With the availability of data from the Human Genome Project (www.genome.ucsc.edu), virtually any sequence of DNA may be used as a FISH probe for the study of specific regions of the chromosome. Several laboratories utilize the Human Genome Project to create 'homebrew' probes, such as bacterial artificial chromosomes.

Labeling

Commercially available probes are usually directly labeled, such that the fluorochrome is directly attached to the probe nucleotides. This technique involves no other detection of the probe before analysis. Probes may also be indirectly labeled, via incorporation of a hapten (such as biotin or digoxigenin) into the DNA via nick translation, for example. The probes are then detected using a fluorescently labeled antibody (such as strepavidin and anti-digoxigenin). Currently, directly labeled probes may be labeled in green (such as SpectrumGreen™ or fluorescein), red (SpectrumOrange™ or Texas Red), blue (SpectrumAqua™), or gold (SpectrumGold™). The ability of a fused green and red FISH signal to be seen as yellow under a fluorescent microscope is

helpful in several hematological FISH studies, as detailed below.

Tissue types

FISH can be applied to a variety of clinical specimens, providing there is DNA in the sample. Cultured cells, such as amniocytes, chorionic villi, lymphocytes, bone marrow aspirates, or from solid tumors, will generally yield metaphase spreads. Metaphase spreads are used routinely in the clinical cytogenetics laboratory and are stained with a variety of special stains to allow interpretation of chromosomal regions and rearrangements; these spreads may also be used for FISH analysis. Analysis of FISH on metaphase spreads allows the exact position of the target signals to be determined, as well as whether they are in their normal location or not. One major advantage of FISH is that it does not require cultured cells or metaphase spreads, and can therefore be applied to interphase or non-dividing cells, including uncultured amniocytes (used for rapid prenatal diagnosis), peripheral blood smears (used in immediate newborn blood analysis), or bone marrow aspirate smears. In addition, FISH may be performed on paraffin block sections, disaggregated cells from paraffin blocks, touch preparations from lymph nodes or solid tumors. Therefore, FISH may be used when metaphase chromosomes are unavailable, such as from archival material or when using samples of poor quality.

Clinical applications of FISH

In the clinical laboratory, FISH is used for both congenital and acquired chromosomal analyses. Standard banding techniques (G-banding) allow for the detection of chromosomal rearrangements of approximately 3–5 Mb. FISH is a necessary adjunct in delineating rearrangements, such as subtle deletions or duplications, which are beyond the level of resolution of standard G-banding. FISH is also used to identify the many recurring translocations observed in oncology specimens, both at the initial diagnosis stage and as a monitor of residual disease.

Prenatal chromosome studies

One of the major advantages of FISH is the ability to detect numerical abnormalities (aneuploidy) in uncultured cells from amniotic fluid or chorionic villi. The turnaround time is generally 24 to 48 hours. In high-risk pregnancies, including those associated with advanced maternal age (older than 35 years), abnormal ultrasound findings, or abnormal maternal screening results, FISH is used as an adjunct to standard cytogenetic analysis to provide aneuploidy screening for chromosomes 13, 18, 21, as well as the X and Y chromosomes. Aneuploidy of these chromosomes accounts for the most common abnormalities detected prenatally (Fig. 21.6). FISH technology on prenatal samples has been found to be effective, sensitive, and specific (Tepperberg et al. 2001).

Microdeletion and microduplication syndromes

Microdeletion or contiguous gene syndromes are caused by a deletion of genetic material, which results in the loss of several genes from one chromosomal region. Generally, these deletions are <2 Mb in size. There are several, clinically recognized, microdeletion syndromes (Table 21.3), for which commercial FISH probes are available (Fig. 21.7). Microduplication syndromes are caused by a gain of genetic material, often in the same regions of the chromosome in which microdeletions are observed. The same FISH probes used for microdeletion analyses may be used for microduplication analyses; the major difference is that interphase nuclei must be scored as well as metaphase cells.

Acquired abnormalities

FISH probes have been developed for the majority of recurrent chromosomal aberrations found in hematological malignancies (Table 21.4). One of the commercial suppliers of hematological FISH probes is Abbott Molecular Inc., an Abbott Laboratories Company (Des Plaines, IL). Their hematological FISH probes are currently divided into four types:

1. Dual-color/single-fusion probes
With the dual-color, single-fusion probes, the DNA probe hybridization targets are located on one side of each of the two genetic breakpoints in the specific translocation (for example, chromosomes 9 and 22 in the case of the Philadelphia chromosome associated with chronic myelogenous leukemia or acute lymphoblastic leukemia).

2. Extra-signal probes
The extra-signal (ES) probes are designed to reduce the frequency of normal cells with an abnormal FISH signal pattern due to random co-localization of probe signals in the nucleus. In this type of probe set, one larger probe (labeled in one color) spans one breakpoint in the specific translocation, while the other probe (labeled in another color) flanks the breakpoint of the other gene involved in the translocation.

3. Dual-color/break-apart probes
Dual-color, break-apart probes are used when a specific gene may have several different chromosomal partners, for example the MLL gene, rearrangements of which are seen in both acute myelogenous leukemia and acute lymphocytic leukemia. These dual-color, break-apart probes are designed so that

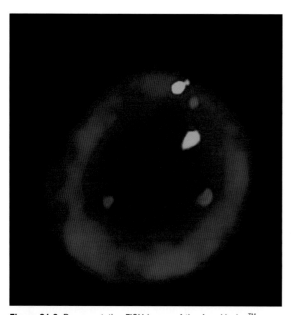

Figure 21.6 Representative FISH image of the AneuVysion™ (Abbott Molecular Inc., Des Plaines, IL) probe set with probes for chromosome 13 (labeled in SpectrumGreen™) and chromosome 21 (SpectrumOrange™) on an interphase cell from an uncultured amniocyte sample. Three red signals are seen for chromosome 21, indicating that this fetus has Down's syndrome.

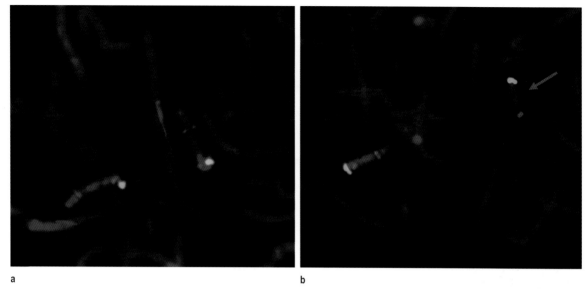

a   b

Figure 21.7 Fluorescent *in situ* hybridization (FISH) images of the SNRPN probe set used in the diagnosis of Prader-Willi and Angelman syndromes, with SNRPN at 15q11.2 and PML at 15q22 labeled in SpectrumOrange™, and D15Z1 at 15p11.2 labeled in SpectrumGreen™. The D15Z1 and the PML probes are used as internal controls in this probe set. (a) A partial metaphase spread from a peripheral blood specimen. This is the normal signal pattern, with two green signals and four red signals, indicating there is no deletion of any of these probes. (b) A partial metaphase spread from a peripheral blood specimen, showing a deletion of one SNRPN locus at 15q11.2 (red arrow), indicating that this patient has the clinical diagnosis of either Prader-Willi syndrome or Angelman syndrome.

Table 21.3 Common constitutional microdeletion syndromes

Syndrome	Chromosomal region	Critical gene(s)
1p36 deletion syndrome	1p36.3	Unknown
Angelman	15q11.2	UBE3A
Kallmann	Xp22.31	KAL1
Miller-Dieker	17p13.3	LIS1
Prader-Willi	15q11.2	SNRPN
Smith-Magenis	17p11.2	RAI1
Sotos	5q35	NSD1
Steroid sulfatase deficiency	Xp22.31	STS
Velocardiofacial/DiGeorge	22q11.2	TUPLE1 (HIRA)
Williams	7q11.2	ELN

the DNA sequence on either side of the breakpoint in a specific gene is labeled in two colors; when the gene is disrupted due to a translocation, the probe is seen as two separate colors (red and green), rather than as one fused signal pattern (yellow).

4. Dual-color/dual-fusion probes (Fig. 21.8) This probe set is designed to reduce the number of normal nuclei showing an abnormal signal pattern due to random co-localization; large probes (in different colors) span both breakpoints involved in the

Table 21.4 Common commercially available FISH probes for hematological diseases

Chromosomal aberration	Gene(s)	Associated disease[a]
t(1;19)(q23;p13.3)	PBX1/TCF3	ALL
t(2;5)(p23;q25)	ALK	NHL
3q27	BCL6	CLL, NHL
del(4)(q12q12)	FIP1L1-PDGFRA	HES
t(4;14)(p16;q32.3)	FGFR3/IgH	MM
Trisomy 4	4cen[b]	ALL
-5/del(5q)	EGR1	AML, MDS
6q23	MYB	CLL
-7/del(7q)	D7S486[c]	AML, MDS
t(8;14)(q24;q32)	MYC/IgH	ALL, NHL, MM
t(8;21)(q22;q22)	ETO/AML1	AML
Trisomy 8	8cen[b]	AML,CML,MDS, NHL
9p21 rearrangements	P16 (CDKN2A)	ALL
t(9;22)(q34;q11.2)	ABL1/BCR	CML, ALL, AML
Trisomy 10	10cen[b]	ALL
del(11)(q22.3)	ATM	CLL
t(11;14)(q13;q32)	CCND1/IgH	NHL, MM
t(11;18)(q21;q21.1)	API2/MALT1	NHL
11q23 rearrangements	MLL	ALL, AML
t(12;21)(p13;q22)	TEL/AML1	ALL
12p13 rearrangements	ETV6	ALL, AML
Trisomy 12	12cen[b]	CLL
del(13)(q14.2)	RB1	MDS/MPD
del(13)(q14.3)	D13S319[c]	CLL, NHL, MM
t(14;16)(q32;q23)	IgH/MAF	MM
t(14;18)(q32;q21)	IgH/BCL2	NHL
t(14;18)(q32;q21.1)	IgH/MALT1	NHL
14q11 rearrangements	TCRαδ	ALL
14q32 rearrangements	IgH	NHL, MM
t(15;17)(q22;q21.1)	PML/RARA	APL
inv(16)(p13q22) or t(16;16)(p13;q22)	CBFβ	AML
del(17)(p13.1)	TP53	CLL, MM, NHL
Trisomy 17	17cen[b]	ALL
del(20)(q11q13)	D20S108[c]	MDS

[a]Abbreviations: ALL = acute lymphocytic leukemia; AML = acute myelogenous leukemia; APL = acute promyelogenous leukemia; CLL = chronic lymphocytic leukemia; CML = chronic myelogenous leukemia; HES = hypereosinophilic syndrome; MDS/MPD = myelodysplastic syndrome/myeloproliferative disorder; MM = multiple myeloma (plasma cell myeloma); NHL = non-Hodgkin's lymphoma (including follicular lymphoma, Burkitt's lymphoma, anaplastic large cell lymphoma, diffuse large cell lymphoma, mantle cell lymphoma and mucosa-associated lymphoid tissue (MALT) lymphoma).

[b]cen = centromere of chromosome (not a gene).

[c]An STS (sequence-tagged site) marker (not a gene).

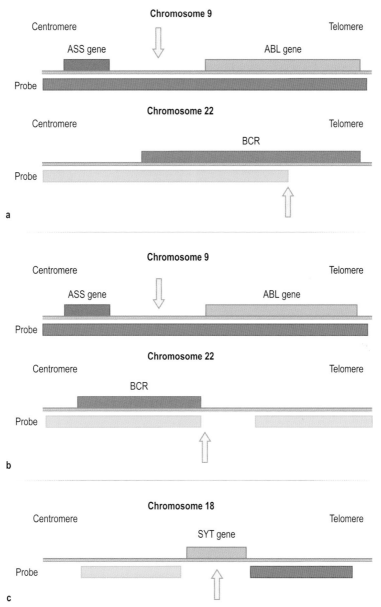

Figure 21.8 (a) Diagram illustrating the design of a dual-color, extra-signal probe set. This probe set is used to identify the Philadelphia chromosome, which results from the translocation between chromosomes 9 (labeled with SpectrumOrange™) and 22 (SpectrumGreen™) in chronic myelogenous leukemia (CML) and some cases of acute lymphocytic leukemia (ALL). The arrows indicate the breakpoints on the chromosomes. The extra signal is due to the presence of the ASS gene, also labeled in SpectrumOrange™, which remains on the derivative chromosome 9, following the translocation. (b) Diagram illustrating the design of the dual-color, dual-fusion signal probe set. This probe set is also used to identify the translocation between chromosomes 9 and 22 seen in CML and some cases of ALL. The arrows indicate the breakpoints on the chromosomes. The two fusion signals arise due to the fusion of part of the red signal on chromosome 9 with part of the green signal on chromosome 22, and vice versa. (c) Diagram illustrating the design of a dual-color, break-apart probe. This probe is used to identify translocations involving the SYT gene on chromosome 18 seen a majority of synovial sarcomas. The probe is labeled in both SpectrumGreen™ and SpectrumOrange™, forming a yellow or fused signal in a normal cell; a translocation in an abnormal cell will disrupt this fused yellow signal, creating a separate red and green signal. (Diagrams adapted from product information with permission from Abbott Molecular Inc.)

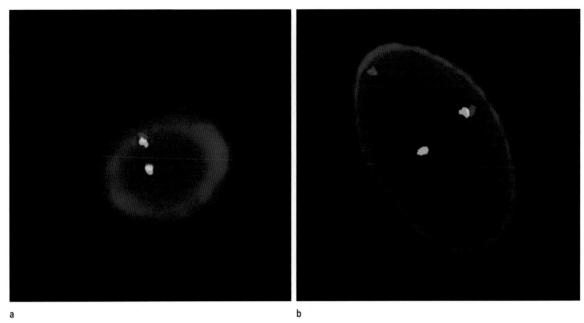

a   b

Figure 21.9 Representative FISH images of the SYT dual-color, break-apart probe on interphase cells from a bone marrow sample. The SYT gene is located on chromosome 18 and translocations involving this region are seen in the majority of synovial sarcoma patients. (a) Two yellow or fused signals (both SpectrumOrange™ and SpectrumGreen™ present) are seen, which is the normal signal pattern. (b) One fused yellow signal is seen, representing the normal chromosome 18, as well as a separate red and green signal, indicating that a translocation has occurred. The SYT gene is translocated to the X chromosome and forms an abnormal fusion protein with either the SSX1 or SSX2 gene. This analysis was performed in an interphase cell and, therefore, the specific translocation partner of the SYT gene cannot be determined.

rearrangement. In a truly abnormal cell, two fusion signals are generally seen, representing the specific chromosomal translocation, as well as a red and a green signal, representing the normal and uninvolved chromosomes.

Solid tumors

Solid tumors are often difficult to grow in culture, and metaphase spreads can be hard to obtain and/or analyze. FISH is useful in detecting specific rearrangements in interphase cells of solid tumors that have diagnostic and prognostic implications. Some soft tissue masses, such as synovial sarcoma, may be difficult to diagnose by morphology alone. A break-apart, dual-color FISH probe has been designed which is telomeric and centromeric to the SYT gene. In a normal cell, two yellow or fused signals are

seen, while in an abnormal cell, one yellow, one red, and one green signal are seen, representing the disruption and translocation of the SYT gene (Fig. 21.9). Such translocations bring the SYT gene on chromosome 18 into contact with either the SSX1 or SSX2 gene on the X chromosome (Geurts van Kessel et al. 1997). Chromosomal rearrangements involving the DDIT3 (formerly CHOP) gene on chromosome 12 are common in myxoid/round cell liposarcomas (Aman et al. 1992). This FISH probe, also a break-apart probe, will detect a translocation involving the DDIT3 gene, but not the specific chromosomal translocation partner. Another break-apart probe involves the FOXO1 (formerly FKHR) gene on chromosome 13, which, when fused with the PAX3 gene on chromosome 2 or the PAX7 gene on chromosome 1, is associated with alveolar rhabdomyosarcoma (Mehra et al. 2008).

Neuroblastoma

Amplification and overexpression of the MYCN oncogene on chromosome 2 is seen in childhood neuroblastoma and is associated with rapid tumor progression and a poor prognosis (Ambros et al. 2009). The MYCN FISH probe is used to detect extra copies or amplification of the gene. Analysis is usually performed on interphase cells, from bone marrow biopsies, fresh or snap-frozen tumor, or paraffin-embedded tumor samples. MYCN amplification is considered to be present when there is more than a 4-fold increase in the MYCN signal number compared to the reference probe signal (generally the centromere of chromosome 2); for example, if there are two signals seen for the centromere of chromosome 2, there must be at least 9 signals present for the MYCN probe for the result to be deemed amplified. Amplification may be seen as either double minutes (dmin) or homogeneously staining regions (hsr) (Storlazzi et al. 2010).

Breast cancer

Breast cancer is the second most common cause of cancer death among women in the United States (American Cancer Society, 2010). A great deal of money and research has been targeted toward the improvement of early detection and effective therapies. This area of genetic testing has arisen because of the advances made in the field of pharmacogenomics, in which therapeutic drug development is dependent upon genetic variations in an individual. One of the major advantages of FISH is the ability to study paraffin-embedded tissue, permitting the analysis of both fresh and archival samples. This has been extremely helpful in the analysis of breast cancer tissue specimens. The HER2 (ERBB2) gene on chromosome 17 has been shown to be overexpressed or amplified in approximately 25% of breast cancers (Kallioniemi et al. 1992). Amplification of the HER2 gene and/or overexpression of its protein product is associated with poor prognosis, an increased risk of recurrence, and a shortened survival time (Press et al. 1997). There are two types of test commonly used to determine HER2 status: immunohistochemistry, which measures the level of expression of the gene; and FISH, which measures the number of copies of the gene. Assessment of HER2 status (Pegram and Slamon, 2000) is useful for determining chemotherapy responsiveness and selection for targeted monoclonal antibody therapy (Herceptin® (trastuzumab), Genentech, Inc., South San Francisco, CA). FISH (for example, the Path-Vysion™ DNA probe kit from Abbott Molecular Inc.) has been approved by the United States Food and Drug Administration (FDA) as the most sensitive and specific methodology for HER2 detection. The highest Herceptin® response is seen in FISH-positive breast cancer patients. Therefore, knowledge of the status of HER2 amplification is vital to treatment strategies for some breast cancer patients.

The PathVysion™ FISH procedure for the detection of HER2 amplification involves in brief, 4 μm sections of paraffin-embedded breast cancer tumor samples being prepared. The tumor areas are scored by a pathologist, and FISH analysis with a probe set consisting of the HER2 gene in combination with the alpha-satellite probe for the centromere of chromosome 17 is performed. The number of HER2 and chromosome 17 signals is scored, the ratio of the two is determined, and a ratio of greater than 2.2 is taken to indicate amplification of the HER2 gene (Fig. 21.10). These results are then interpreted in conjunction with clinical and pathological findings to determine the best treatment option for patients with stage II, node-positive breast cancer.

Bladder cancer

Bladder cancers are among the most frequent of adult cancers, expected to account for approximately 14,680 deaths (men and women) in the USA in 2010 (American Cancer Society, 2010). Chromosomal aberrations, such as aneuploidy for chromosomes 3, 7, 9, and 17, have been found to be associated with histological progression in bladder cancer (Nemoto et al. 1995). An FDA-approved FISH test has been developed by Abbott Molecular Inc., the UroVysion™ assay, results from which should be used in conjunction with current standard diagnostic procedures for bladder cancer. The assay consists of a panel of probes for the centromeric regions of

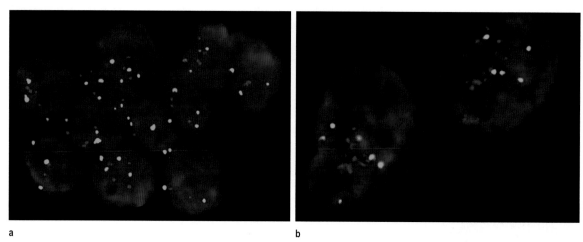

a   b

Figure 21.10 Representative FISH images of the PathVysion™ (Abbott Molecular Inc., Des Plaines, IL) probe set with probes for the centromere of chromosome 17 (labeled in SpectrumGreen™) and the HER2 probe (labeled in SpectrumOrange™) on a paraffin-embedded sample of two patients with breast cancer. (a) The signal ratio of the two probes was determined to be 1.13 in this sample and, therefore, no amplification of the HER2 gene was seen. (b) The signal ratio of the two probes was determined to be 5.48 in this sample and, therefore, amplification of the HER2 gene was determined to have occurred.

chromosomes 3, 7, and 17, as well as a probe for a region on the short arm of chromosome 9 (9p21). Gain of chromosomes 3, 7, and 17, and/or homozygous loss of chromosome 9p21 are both associated with recurrence of bladder cancer (Fig. 21.11); the UroVysion™ assay may also be used as an aid for the initial diagnosis of bladder cancer in patients with hematuria. This FISH assay is performed on voided urine and is capable of detecting approximately 95% of recurrent transitional cell carcinomas (Wolff 2007).

General FISH procedure

Sample requirements

1. Fixed metaphase or interphase chromosomes on a microscope slide or coverslip are required. One should not bake the slides (as is performed for slides that will be G-banded for routine chromosome analysis). Aging of slides is essential to obtaining good FISH signals, as it hardens the DNA, removes water, and may increase signal intensity. If slides are made and used in a FISH analysis the same day, then artificial aging must be performed, by placing slides for a minimum of 2 hours in a 37°C oven. Alternatively, if the slides have been stored at room temperature for less than 3 weeks, then the slides may be aged in 2x SSC at 73°C for 2 minutes or at 37°C for 60 minutes (followed by dehydration in an ethanol series).

2. For analysis with metaphase FISH probes, at least 15 metaphases per 22 × 22 mm area are required for a complete analysis.

Solutions

20× SSC

Sodium chloride	175.32 g
Sodium citrate	88.20 g
Double distilled (dd) H_2O	800 ml

pH to 7.0 with 1 M HCl. Bring to 1 liter with ddH₂O. Filter through a 0.4 µm filtration unit. Store at room temperature. Expiration: 6 months.

2× SSC

20× SSC	50 ml
ddH₂O	450 ml

Store at room temperature. Expiration: 6 months.

Ethanol series

	70%	80%	95%	100%
Ethanol (ml)	350	400	475	500
ddH₂O (ml)	150	100	25	0

Store at room temperature.

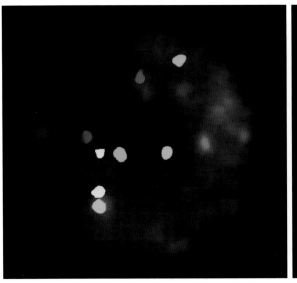
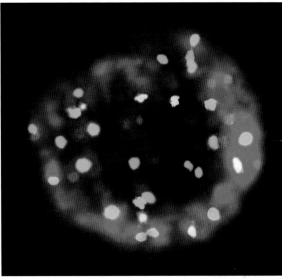

a   b

Figure 21.11 Representative FISH images of the UroVysion™ (Abbott Molecular Inc., Des Plaines, IL) probe set with probes for the centromeres of chromosome 3 (labeled in SpectrumRed™), chromosome 7 (SpectrumGreen™), and chromosome 17 (SpectrumAqua™). The chromosome 9p21 probe is labeled in SpectrumGold™. (a) Two signals with each of the probes can be seen in this cell from a urine sample of a patient previously diagnosed with bladder cancer; this is the normal signal pattern. (b) This FISH image is from an abnormal cell found in a urine sample of a patient previously diagnosed with bladder cancer. The extra copies of chromosomes 3, 7, and 17 indicate aneuploidy of these chromosomes and perhaps a recurrence of the bladder cancer.

Denaturation solution (70% formamide/ 2× SSC)

Formamide	35 ml
20× SSC	5 ml
ddH₂O	10 ml

Bring pH to 7.0 with 1 M HCl. Store at 4°C. Expiration: 1 week.

Post-wash solution (2× SSC/0.1% Nonidet P-40 (NP-40))

20× SSC	100 ml
ddH₂O	899 ml
NP-40	1 ml

Bring pH to 7.0 ± 0.2 with 1 M NaOH. Mix well. Store at room temperature. Discard used solution at the end of each day. Expiration: 6 months.

Post-wash solution (0.4× SSC/0.3% NP-40)

20× SSC	20 ml
ddH₂O	977 ml
NP-40	3 ml

Bring pH to 7.5 ± 0.2 with 1 M NaOH. Mix well. Store at room temperature. Discard used solution at the end of each day. Expiration: 6 months.

DNA counterstain

Propidium iodide and DAPI (4′,6-diamidino-2-phenylindole) are fluorescent dyes used to counterstain DNA. Propidium iodide dyes the chromosomes red/orange, while DAPI stains chromosomes blue. Different concentrations of DAPI are available. Abbott Molecular Inc. provides both DAPI I and DAPI II. DAPI I is recommended when a more intense counterstain is required. It provides a distinct banding pattern. DAPI II provides a weaker counterstain, which is useful when viewing smaller probes (unique sequences and centromeric regions).

FISH set-up

This set-up procedure is the basic procedure for use with either commercially available probes or home brew probes. The denaturation times and temperatures may need to be adjusted depending on the specific probe used (whole chromosome paint versus centromere-specific probes, for example) and the tissue type (peripheral blood specimen slide versus amniocyte coverslip). Different commercially available probes are provided either pre-denatured and in solution with the appropriate hybridization buffer, or require to be prepared with the appropriate hybridization buffer and distilled water (step 5) before denaturation. The two alternatives to denaturation of the slides/coverslips and probes are listed in step 7 (denaturation solution) and step 12 (all-in-one co-denaturation and hybridization system). The stringency of the post-wash solutions is important to remove non-specifically bound probe. The stringency of the post-wash solutions may be altered by changing the salt concentration, the temperature, or the time in each solution. Some specimen types require pretreatment before denaturation, which removes cytoplasmic proteins of the cell membrane, allowing greater accessibility of the DNA. Pretreatment is generally performed using fresh pepsin in an acid solution.

Day one

1. Place denaturation solution in water bath at 73°C (if following step 7).
2. Examine slide or coverslip to determine optimal target area.
3. Treat slide(s) in 2× SSC at 37°C for at least 30 minutes.
4. Dehydrate the slide(s) in a cold ethanol series (70%, 85%, and 100%) for 2 minutes each. Allow slides to dry. Store slide(s) in covered slide box until ready to denature.
5. Pre-warm probe to room temperature for about 5 minutes. If probe does not need to be denatured, aliquot 10 μl for each 22 × 22 mm target area; if probe needs to be denatured, aliquot 7 μl hybridization buffer, 2 μl ddH₂O, and 1 μl probe into a microcentrifuge tube. Keep probe in darkness as much as possible. Return probe to freezer as soon as possible.
6. Vortex probe briefly and centrifuge for 2–3 seconds.
7. Denature the slide(s) for exactly 2 minutes in the pre-warmed denaturant at 73°C.

Note

A maximum of three slides should be denatured at one time to maintain the correct denaturation temperature. In addition, denaturation temperatures and times may vary depending on tissue type and type of probe.

8. Dehydrate the slide(s) in a cold ethanol series (70%, 80%, and 100%) for 2 minutes each.
9. Wipe the back of the slide(s) and place on a 37°C slide warmer to dry completely. Leave slide(s) on slide warmer until ready to apply probe mixture.
10. Denature aliquoted probe mix for 5 minutes in a 73°C water bath. Vortex probe briefly and centrifuge for 2–3 seconds.
11. Apply 10 μl probe mix to target area and cover with a 22 × 22 mm glass coverslip. Seal with rubber cement.
12. If not denaturing probes and slides separately, probes and slides can be co-denatured on, for example, the ThermoBrite™ Denaturation and Hybridization system from Abbott Molecular Inc. for 2 minutes at 73°C.
13. Following either form of denaturation: incubate slide(s) at 37°C overnight in a humidified chamber (place moist sponge or paper towels in an airtight, opaque container).

Note

Slide(s) may be left in the ThermoBrite™ instrument for hybridization at 37°C for 4–16 hours. A minimum of 4 hours of hybridization is recommended for any probe.

Day two

14. Warm glass Coplin of 0.4× SSC/0.3% NP-40 to 73 ± 1°C. Do not wash more than three slides at a time, to ensure the correct wash temperature is maintained.
15. Remove coverslip and rubber cement from hybridized slide(s). Keep slides covered as much as possible and away from the light.
16. Wash slide(s) in 0.4× SSC/0.3% NP-40 at 72°C for 2 minutes. Agitate slide(s) for 1–3 seconds.
17. Wash slide(s) in 2× SSC/0.1% NP-40 at room temperature for 1 minute. Agitate slide(s) for 1–3 seconds.
18. Allow the slide(s) to dry while protected from the light.
19. Apply 2 μl of DAPI I or DAPI II to slide(s) and cover with appropriately sized glass coverslip.

Note: DAPI is a carcinogen

For batching FISH samples, or running a FISH procedure with many steps and solution changes, automated FISH processing may be advantageous. One such pre-programmed automated system is supplied by Abbott Molecular Inc., the VP 2000™ Processor, which may be used for a variety of functions, such as deparaffinization and pretreatment of FISH samples, histology/cytology staining, special stains of chromosomes, and routine slide washing.

Specific FISH procedure: HER2 FISH (PathVysion™)

Sample requirements

Formalin-fixed, paraffin-embedded breast cancer tissue specimens should be cut into approximately 4 μm sections. Slides are then floated in a protein-free water bath at 40°C. Each section is mounted on the positive side of an organosilane-coated slide in order to minimize the loss of tissue during processing. The slides are air dried. A hematoxylin and eosin (H&E) slide, scored by a pathologist, should accompany each specimen, with the areas of tumor to be scored clearly delineated. Control slides (one negative and one positive slide) must be run at the same time as the clinical, patient slides in each specimen processing run, to ensure accuracy of signal analysis and to monitor assay performance. If the FISH assay on the control slides does not work, then the patient analysis cannot be reported. In addition, control slides must be run with each new lot of the PathVysion™ probe kit. A more detailed reference of the procedure may be obtained from the PathVysion™ HER2 DNA Probe Kit product data sheet (Abbott Molecular Inc.).

Solutions needed for the VP 2000™ Processor

70%, 85%, 95% ethanol

Posthybridization wash buffer. Note: only one wash buffer used in this procedure.

2x SSC/0.3% NP-40

Protease I reagent

25 mg pepsin/lyophilized per 50 ml 0.01 M HCl. Make fresh.

Pretreatment reagent (1 M sodium thiocyanate)

Keep covered at ambient temperature. Expiration: 6 months.

0.2 M HCl

Keep covered at ambient temperature. Expiration: 6 months.

10% buffered formalin

PathVysion™ HER2 DNA probe kit *(Abbott Molecular Inc.)*

DAPI I

Day one

Bake slide(s) overnight at 56°C (hot plate or oven).

Day two

Slide pretreatment (as run on the VP 2000™ Processor)

1. Deparaffinization in Hemo-De (non-toxic solvent similar to xylene) for 5 minutes at ambient temperature.
2. Repeat twice.
3. 95% ethanol for 1 minute at ambient temperature.
4. Repeat.
5. 0.2 M HCl for 20 minutes at ambient temperature.
6. Rinse in water for 3 minutes at ambient temperature.
7. Pretreatment reagent for 30 minutes at 80°C.
8. Rinse in water for 3 minutes at ambient temperature.
9. Protease treatment for 10 minutes at 37°C.
10. Rinse in water for 3 minutes at ambient temperature.
11. Fixation in 10% buffered formalin for 10 minutes at ambient temperature.
12. Rinse in water for 3 minutes at ambient temperature.
13. Dehydrate for 1 minute each in ethanol series (70%, 85%, and 95% ethanol).
14. Air dry on drying station for 3 minutes at 25°C.
15. Proceed to FISH procedure.

Notes

1. Before each run on the VP 2000™ Processor, each basin should be filled with 470 ml of the appropriate reagent. After approximately 15 runs, all solutions should be discarded and the basins refilled with fresh reagents.
2. The fixative step 11 helps to reduce tissue loss during denaturation.

FISH procedure

See general FISH procedure described previously. It is recommended that denaturation solution (step 7) is used to denature the slide(s). Denature slide(s) at 72 ± 1°C for 5 minutes.

Day three

1. Wash slide(s) in 2× SSC/0.3% NP-40 at 73 ± 1°C for 2 minutes.
2. Air dry slides in the dark.
3. Apply 20 µl DAPI I counterstain and cover with a glass coverslip.

Signal analysis

Using a 40× objective, scan several areas of tumor cells within the area corresponding to the H&E area, as designated by the pathologist. Select an area of good nuclei distribution. Using a 100× objective, begin analysis in the upper left quadrant of the selected area and, scanning from left to right, count the number of signals within the nuclear boundary of each evaluable interphase cell. Do not score nuclei with no signals or signals of only one color.

1. Thirty interphase cells are analyzed by one technologist and the results are confirmed by a second technologist. Note: A minimum of 20 interphase cells must be analyzed.
2. Results are recorded as the number of signals for the HER2 probe and the number of signals for the CEP (chromosome enumeration probe) 17 probe (the centromere of chromosome 17).
3. The ratio of the average copy number of HER2 to CEP 17 signals is calculated.
4. If the ratio of HER2 to CEP 17 signals is borderline (between 1.8 and 2.2), then a second technologist will count an additional 30 interphase cells and a new ratio is calculated.
5. A schematic drawing of the section of the tissue analyzed should be made to indicate the area analyzed by each technologist.

Interpretation of results

1. The ratio of the average copy number of HER2 to CEP 17 signals is calculated. If the number is less than 1.8, then the results are reported as not amplified.
2. If the ratio is ≥2.2, the results are reported as amplified.
3. If the ratio is between 1.8 and 2.2, the results are reported as equivocal.

Troubleshooting

One of the most common problems encountered with paraffin-embedded FISH analysis is under- or over-digestion of the tissue sample. If the tissue looks under-digested (too much cytoplasm, weak or no signals), then the incubation time in the pretreatment solution should be increased to 15–60 minutes. Over-digested tissue appears faded, with a loss of cell borders. A repeat sample must be run, with a decrease in the pretreatment time to 15–25 minutes and a decrease in the protease solution to 5–7 minutes. In addition, the denaturation time and temperature may be adjusted to increase the accessibility of the sample DNA to the probe. Formalin fixation, tissue size, and sample quality may all also affect the FISH results.

General scoring analysis criteria for FISH

The scoring analysis criteria described here are based on the minimum requirements of the College of American Pathologists (CAP) guidelines, as well as recommendations by the American College of Medical Genetics (ACMG).

Metaphase scoring criteria

General information

1. Only complete metaphases (i.e. with 46 chromosomes) should be scored. An exception may be made when the number of complete metaphases is low and all the chromosomes of interest are present in one field of view.
2. Analysis of 10 metaphase cells on all clinical samples is required for a complete study. If necessary, additional metaphase cells may be analyzed.
3. Record coordinates and results of at least two representative metaphase spreads analyzed on analysis sheet. At least two images should be captured if the analysis is abnormal; at least one image should be captured if the analysis is normal.

Table 21.5 Troubleshooting FISH

Problem	Possible cause	Possible solution
Slide background	Inadequate post-hybridization wash	Ensure correct wash solution and temperature. Re-wash slide
	Inadequate cleaning of glass slides	Clean slides in ethanol and wipe dry with lint-free paper
Weak or no signal	Specimen inadequately denatured	Ensure correct denaturation solution and temperature. Increase denaturation time
	Specimen slides not aged	Age slides for 24 hours at ambient temperature before use
	Probe not added	Allow probe to thaw completely before use. Vortex probe. Pipette slowly
	Probe inadequately denatured	Ensure correct temperature of water bath
	Counterstain is too bright	Remove coverslip. Re-wash in 2x SSC/ 0.1% NP-40 at ambient temperature. Dehydrate slides; reapply counterstain
	Probes improperly stored	Store probes at −20°C (in dark)
Distorted chromosome morphology	Specimen over-denatured	Ensure correct denaturation solution and temperature. Repeat on new specimen with reduced time of denaturation

4. In cases suspected of mosaicism (more than one cell line present), additional metaphase cells should be counted.

Interphase scoring criteria

General information

1. At least 200 individual interphase cells should be analyzed. Only cells that are in a monolayer with discrete borders are countable. Overlapping cells should not be counted. Not all cells are appropriate for analysis and may be skipped.
2. Signals should be discrete (not diffuse). Signals should be counted as two signals if they are greater than one signal-width apart. Signals that are closer than one signal-width apart should be counted as one signal.
3. Signals should be counted as yellow (fusion of orange and green) if they are on top of each other. A green signal and an orange signal with

discrete borders are considered separate (i.e. not a fusion (yellow) signal).

Troubleshooting FISH

There are various problems that may be encountered when setting up a FISH experiment, ranging from over-denaturation of the DNA, to weak or no FISH signals. Table 21.5 highlights some of the more common problems and their solutions; however, the list is by no means exhaustive. Commercially available probes are supplied with package inserts which generally cover a wide array of possible problems with FISH set-up and analysis.

Validation of FISH probes in the clinical laboratory

The majority of probes and materials used for clinical FISH studies in the United States are considered to be analyte-specific reagents (ASRs). They are exempt from the Food and Drug Administration (FDA) regulations (probes that are FDA-approved include PathVysion™ and UroVysion™). Therefore, these probes must be independently validated by each clinical laboratory. The College of American Pathologists (CAP) and the Standards and Guidelines for Clinical Genetics Laboratories issued by the ACMG state that each probe must be validated for sensitivity (the expected signal pattern is observed) and specificity (the probe is localized to the correct chromosome and chromosomal region). If the probe is to be used on interphase cells, a reportable reference range for that probe must be established. Reportable reference ranges are generally established from a database of cytogenetically characterized cases, so that the percentage of cells exhibiting an 'abnormal' signal pattern by random chance can be determined. Thus, a normal cut-off for each probe can be established. Biannual or continual evaluation of the performance characteristics of each probe in clinical use is also required by CAP.

FISH nomenclature

The ISCN 2009, an International System for Human Cytogenetic Nomenclature, addresses FISH nomenclature. The appropriate FISH nomenclature should accompany each FISH report on a patient, indicating whether the FISH test was performed on metaphase (ish) or interphase (nuc ish) cells, the probe name, the number of signals observed, and for metaphase analyses, the chromosomal location. For example, a result indicating a deletion of the SNRPN gene (see Fig. 21.6) is written as: ish del(15)(q11.2q11.2) (SNPRN-), indicating that one chromosome 15 did not have the SNRPN signal, confirming a diagnosis of either Angelman or Prader-Willi syndrome. A normal HER2 result would be written as: nuc ish(D17Z1,HER2)x2[X], with [X] representing the number of interphase cells analyzed; the result indicates that two signals for both the centromere of chromosome 17 and the HER2 gene were seen, and there was no amplification of the HER2 gene. An abnormal HER2 result may be written as: nuc ish(D17Z1x2),amp(HER2)[20/30], indicating that

there were two signals seen for the control probe and amplification was observed for the HER2 probe in 20 out of 30 of the interphase cells counted.

Summary

This section describes only one specialized area of genetic testing: the use of FISH in clinical laboratories. Advances in genetic testing seem to occur on an almost daily basis, including new FISH probes, pharmacogenetics, targeted therapies, and Next Gen sequencing, including exome sequencing. The increasing usage of other technologies such as microarrays (SNP, oligonucleotide, or expression arrays) in clinical laboratories will certainly reduce the utilization of FISH in the future, but it will still remain a valid and user-friendly way of answering many diagnostic and prognostic questions.

Glossary and definitions of the terminology used in this chapter and in ISH techniques

Amplification

Production of additional copies of a gene sequences. This multiplication of the sequence makes it easier to identify.

Anneal

To join two strands of complementary nucleic acids.

Antisense RNA

An RNA which is complementary to mRNA.

Base

A building block of the nucleotide. Four different bases for DNA: (A) – adenine, (T) – thymine, (C) – cytosine, (G) – guanine. In RNA, the thymine is replaced by (U) – uracil.

Base pair (bp)

Two bases which are complementary to each other and joined by hydrogen bonds.

cDNA

A complementary sequence of DNA that has been synthesized from an initial template of RNA by the enzyme reverse transcriptase.

Codon

A set of three consecutive nucleotides in DNA or mRNA that directs the incorporation of an amino acid during protein synthesis or signals the start or stop of translation. Multiple codons will code for the same amino acid.

Complementary sequence

Nucleic acid sequence of bases that can form a double-stranded structure by matching base pairs. For example, the complementary sequence to C-A-T-G (where each letter stands for one of the bases in DNA) is G-T-A-C.

Denature

To dissociate a double-stranded region of nucleic acid into the homologous single strands by breaking the hydrogen bonds. This is usually achieved by heating.

DNA

Deoxyribonucleic acid is the genetic material in chromosomes.

DNA polymerase

An enzyme that synthesizes new DNA using a parental DNA strand as the template.

Downstream

A region extending from the 3' end of the gene.

Endonuclease

Any enzyme that starts to degrade DNA or RNA within the nucleic acid sequence. These enzymes are used as molecular scalpels to cut DNA or RNA at precise points.

Gene

A DNA segment that codes for a polypeptide.

Gene cloning

The selection, application, and production of an individual nucleotide sequence.

Gene library

A collection of nucleotide sequences that have been artificially inserted into microorganisms or viruses and propagated.

Genome

The total amount of DNA present in a cell.

Hybridization

The action whereby two complementary single-stranded pieces of nucleic acids are joined to form a double-stranded segment.

In situ

In the normal location. An *in situ* tumor is one that is confined to its site of origin and has not invaded neighboring tissue or gone elsewhere in the body.

In situ hybridization

A technique that identifies and quantifies nucleic acid sequences within cells.

Kilobase

A measure of length of nucleic acids. One kilobase (kb) equals 1000 nucleotides of single-stranded nucleic acid; kbp refers to kilobase pairs of double-stranded DNA.

Melting temperature

The temperature at which the hydrogen bonds between complementary nucleotides will break, causing the dissociation of double-stranded nucleic acid. It is dependent on the $G + C$ content of the DNA.

Missense mutation

A single base substitution in DNA that changes a codon for one amino acid into a codon for a different amino acid.

mRNA

Messenger RNA carries the message of the DNA to the cytoplasm of the cell where protein is made. Single-stranded RNA synthesized from a DNA template during transcription binds to ribosomes and directs protein synthesis.

Mutation

A change in the sequence of nucleotides in DNA.

Nucleotide

The unit of DNA or RNA that consists of a phosphate group, a sugar and a base.

Oligonucleotide

A short piece of nucleic acid that can be used as a hybridization probe.

Probe

A single-stranded piece of labeled DNA or RNA that will bind to a complementary sequence (target).

Random priming

A method for labeling double-stranded DNA to produce a probe.

Recombinant DNA

The production of a single piece of DNA from two different sources.

Replication

The process by which an exact copy of parental DNA or RNA is made with the parental molecule serving as a template.

Reverse transcriptase

An enzyme that will synthesize a complementary sequence of DNA from an RNA template.

RNA

Ribonucleic acid. A nucleic acid that plays an important role in protein synthesis and other cell activities.

RNA polymerase

An enzyme that catalyzes the synthesis of RNA from a DNA template, using nucleotide triphosphates as substrates.

RNases

Ubiquitous RNA degrading enzymes.

rRNA

Ribosomal RNA is a component of ribosomes and functions as a non-specific site for making polypeptides.

Sense strand

The DNA strand that RNA polymerase copies to produce mRNA, rRNA, or tRNA.

Stringency

Conditions employed in hybridization reactions used to control the specificity of probe binding. The highest stringency conditions ensure the probe will bind only to completely complementary sequences. Lower stringency conditions will allow binding to sequences with some mismatching.

Template

A strand of DNA or RNA that specifies the base sequence of a newly synthesized complementary strand of DNA or RNA.

Transcription

The process by which a DNA sequence is copied into a complementary RNA sequence.

tRNA

Transfer RNA is a short-chain type of RNA present in cells that transfers specific amino acids in the formation of proteins.

Acknowledgments

The author would like to acknowledge Maureen Doran for her technical sharing with this edition. Special thanks also go to the companies, Leica and Ventana who provided the photographs of automated ISH.

References

Aman, P., Ron, D., Mandahl, N., et al., 1992. Rearrangement of the transcription factor gene CHOP in myxoid liposarcomas with t(12;16) (q13;p11). Genes, Chromosomes and Cancer 5 (4), 278–285.

Ambros, P.F., Ambros, I.M., Brodeur, G.M., et al., 2009. International consensus for neuroblastoma molecular diagnostics: report from the International Neuroblastoma Risk Group (INRG) Biology Committee. British Journal of Cancer 100, 1471–1482.

Beck, R.C., Tubbs, R.R., Hussein, M., et al., 2003. Automatic colorimetric *in situ* hybridization (CISH) detection of immunoglobulin (Ig) light chain mRNA expression in plasma cell dyscrasias and non-Hodgkin lymphoma. Diagn Mol Pathol 12, 14–20.

Davis, M., Malcolm, S., Rabbitts, T.H., 1984. Chromosome translocation can occur on either side of the c-myc oncogene in Burkitt lymphoma cells. Nature 308, 286–288.

De Jong, A.S.H., Van Kessel-Van Vark, M., Raap, A.K., 1985. Sensitivity of various visualization methods for peroxidase and alkaline phosphatase activity in immunoenzyme histochemistry. Histochemical Journal 17, 1119–1130.

Doran, M., Sterchi, D.L., 2000. Let's do *in situ* (workshop no. 67). National Society for Histotechnology, Milwaukee, WI.

Gall, J.G., Pardue, M.L., 1969. Formation and detection of RNA-DNA hybrid molecules in cytological preparations. Proceedings of the National Academy of Sciences USA 63, 378–383.

Geurts van Kessel, A., dos Santos, N.R., Simons, A., et al., 1997. Molecular cytogenetics of bone and soft tissue tumors. Cancer Genetics and Cytogenetics 95 (1), 67–73.

Goldsmith, C.S., Tatti, K.M., Ksiazek, T.G., et al., 2004. Ultrastructural characterization of SARS coronavirus. Emerging Infectious Diseases 10 (2), 320–326.

Haugland, R.P., Spence, M.T.Z. (Eds.), 2005. The handbook: a guide to fluorescent probes and labeling technologies, tenth ed. Invitrogen, Paisley.

Herrington, C.S., Burns, J., Graham, A.K., et al., 1989. Interphase cytogenetics using biotin and digoxigenin labeled probes II: simultaneous differential detection of human and papilloma virus nucleic acids in individual nuclei. Journal of Clinical Pathology 41, 601–606.

Innis, M.A., Gelfand, D.H., Sminsky, J.J., et al. (Eds.), 1990. PCR protocols: a guide to methods and applications. Academic Press, New York.

Janneke, C., Alers, P.-J.K., Kees, J., et al., 1999. Effect of bone decalcification procedures on DNA *in situ* hybridization and comparative genomic hybridization: EDTA is highly preferable to a routinely used acid decalcifier. Journal of Histochemistry and Cytochemistry 47 (5), 703–709.

John, H.A., Birnstiel, M.L., Jones, K.W., 1969. RNA-DNA hybrids at the cytological level. Nature 223, 582–587.

Hopman, A.H., Ramaekers, F.C., Raap, A.K., et al., 1988. *In situ* hybridization as a tool to study numerical chromosome aberrations in solid bladder tumors. Histochemistry 89, 307–316.

Kallioniemi, O.P., Kallioniemi, A., Kurisu, W., et al., 1992. *ERBB2* amplification in breast cancer analyzed by fluorescence *in situ* hybridization. Proceedings of the National Academy of Sciences USA 89 (12), 5321–5325.

Kendall, C.H., Roberts, P.A., Pringle, J.H., et al., 1991. The expression of parathyroid hormone messenger RNA in normal and abnormal parathyroid tissue. Journal of Pathology 165, 111–118.

Knoll, J.H.M., Lichter, P., 1995. Current protocols in molecular biology. In situ hybridization and detection using nonisotopic probes. Wiley, New York.

Lux, S.E., Tse, W.T., Menninger, J.C., et al., 1990. Hereditary spherocytosis associated with deletion of human erythrocyte ankyrin gene on chromosome 8. Nature 345, 736–739.

Madrid, M.A., Lo, R.W., 2004. Chromogenic in situ hybridization (CISH): a novel alternative in screening archival breat cancer tissue samples for HER-2/neu. Breast Cancer Research 6 (5), R593–R600.

Mehra, S., de la Roza, G., Tull, J., et al., 2008. Detection of FOXO1 (FKHR) gene break-apart by fluorescence in situ hybridization in formalin-fixed, paraffin-embedded alveolar rhabdomyosarcomas and its clinicopathologic correlation. Diagnostic Molecular Pathology: the American Journal of Surgical Pathology Part B 17 (1), 14–20.

Mitchell, B.S., Dhami, D., Schumacher, U., 1992. In situ hybridization: a review of methodologies and applications in the biomedical sciences. Medical Laboratory Sciences 49, 107–118.

Nederlof, P.M., Robinson, D., Abuknesha, R., et al., 1989. Three-color fluorescence in situ hybridization for the simultaneous detection of multiple nucleic acid sequences. Cytometry 10, 20–27.

Nemoto, R., Nakamura, I., Uchida, K., et al., 1995. Numerical chromosome aberrations in bladder cancer detected by in situ hybridization. British Journal of Urology 75 (4), 470–476.

Netterwald, J., 2006. Molecular testing? Emerging technologies show promise for helping to prevent spread of the epidemic disease. Advance for Medical Laboratory Professionals April, 17–18.

Pegram, M., Slamon, D., 2000. Biological rationale for HER-2/neu (c-erbB2) as a target for monoclonal antibody therapy. Seminars in Oncology 27 (5), 13–19.

Poddighe, P.J., Ramaekers, F.C.S., Hopman, A.H.N., 1992. Interphase cytogenetics of tumors. Journal of Pathology 166, 215–224.

Press, M.F., Bernstein, L., Thomas, P.A., et al., 1997. HER-2/neu gene amplification characterized by fluorescence in situ hybridization: poor prognosis in node-negative breast carcinomas. Journal of Clinical Oncology 15 (8), 2894–2904.

Pringle, J.H., Ruprai, A.K., Primrose, L., et al., 1990. In situ hybridization of immunoglobulin light chain mRNA in paraffin sections using biotinylated or hapten-labeled oligonucleotide probes. Journal of Pathology 162, 197–207.

Pringle, J.H., Barker, S., et al., 1992. Demonstration of Epstein-Barr virus in tissue sections by in situ hybridization for viral RNA. Journal of Pathology 167 (Suppl), 133A.

Pringle, J.H., Baker, J., Colloby, P.S., et al., 1993. The detection of cell proliferation in normal and malignant formalin-fixed paraffin-embedded tissue sections using in situ hybridization for histone mRNA. Journal of Pathology 169 (Suppl), 144A.

Ruprai, A.K., Pringle, J.H., Angel, C.A., et al., 1991. Localization of immunoglobulin light chain mRNA expression in Hodgkin's disease by in situ hybridization. Journal of Pathology 164, 37–40.

Sambrook, J., Fritsch, E.F., Maniatis, T., 1989. Molecular cloning – a laboratory manual, second ed. Cold Spring Harbor Laboratory Press, Cold Spring Harbor.

Sterchi D., 2008. Molecular pathology – in situ hybridization. In: Bancroft, J.D., Gamble, M. (Eds.), Theory and practice of histological techniques, sixth ed. Churchill Livingstone Elsevier, London.

Storlazzi, C.T., Lonoce, A., Guastadisegni, M.C., et al., 2010. Gene amplification as double minutes or homogeneously staining regions in solid tumors: origin and structure. Genome Research 20 (9), 1198–1206.

Tepperberg, J., Pettenati, M.J., Rao, P.N., et al., 2001. Prenatal diagnosis using interphase fluorescence *in situ* hybridization (FISH): 2-year multi-center retrospective study and review of the literature. Prenatal Diagnosis 21 (4), 293–301.

Van den Berg, F., Schipper, M., Jiwa, M., et al., 1989. Implausibility of an aetiological association between cytomegalovirus and Kaposi's sarcoma shown by four techniques. Journal of Clinical Pathology 42, 128–131.

Wakamatsu, N., King, D.J., Seal, B.S., et al., 2005. Detection of Newcastle disease virus RNA by reverse transcription polymerase chain reaction using formalin-fixed, paraffin-embedded tissue and comparison with immunohistochemistry and *in situ* hybridization. [abstract] American Association of Veterinary Laboratory Diagnosticians 48, 166.

Warford, A., Lauder, I., 1991. *In situ* hybridization in perspective. Journal of Clinical Pathology 44, 177–181.

White, J., 2005. An introduction to chromogenic *in situ* hybridization. Journal of Histotechnology 28, 229–234.

Wolff, D.J., 2007. The genetics of bladder cancer: a cytogeneticist's perspective. Cytogenetic and Genome Research 118, 177–181.

Wood, G.S., Warnke, R., 1981. Suppression of endogenous avidin binding activity in tissues and its relevance to biotin-avidin detection systems. Journal of Histochemistry and Cytochemistry 29, 1196–1204.

Xiao, Y., Sato, S., Oguchi, T., et al., 2001. High sensitivity of PCR *in situ* hybridization for the detection of human papillomavirus infection in uterine cervical neoplasias. Gynecologic Oncology 82 (2), 350–354.

Yan, S.J., Blomme, E.A.G., 2003. *In situ* zymography: a molecular pathology technique to localize endogenous protease activity in tissue sections. Veterinary Pathology 40, 227–236.

Websites

American Cancer Society. Cancer Facts and Figures 2010. Online. Available: http://www.cancer.org/research/cancerfactsfigures/index.

American College of Medical Genetics. Standard and Guidelines for Clinical Genetic Laboratories. Online. Available: http://www.acmg.net.

College of American Pathologists Laboratory Accreditation Checklists. Online. Available: http://www.cap.org/apps/docs/laboratoryaccreditation/checklists/checklistftp.html.

UCSC Genome Bioinformatics. Online. Available: http://genome.ucsc.edu.

Further reading

Darby, I.A. (Ed.), 2000. *In situ* hybridization protocols, second ed. Humana Press, Totowa, NJ.

Shaffer, L.G., Slovak, M.L., Campbell, L.J. (Eds.), 2009. ISCN 2009: an international system for human cytogenetic nomenclature. S. Karger, Basel.

Wilkinson, D.G. (Ed.), 1999. *In situ* hybridization: a practical approach, second ed. Oxford University Press, New York.

Transmission electron microscopy 22

Anthony E. Woods • John W. Stirling

The fundamental advantage of transmission electron microscopy (TEM) over conventional light microscopy is that the electron microscope has a resolution approximately 1000 times better than the light microscope. With this greater resolving power the transmission electron microscope is able to reveal the substructure or ultrastructure of individual cells. The physical basis of this benefit lies in the formula:

$$R = \frac{0.61\lambda}{NA}$$

where R, the resolution, represents the capacity of the optical system to produce separate images of objects very close together, λ is the wavelength of the incident illumination, and NA is the numerical aperture of the lens.

Critically, for any given lens, resolution is directly related to the wavelength of the source radiation. For example, the limit of resolution of a bright-field microscope using glass lenses and white light is around 200 nm, whereas a fluorescence microscope operating with shorter wavelength ultraviolet light is capable of resolving objects around 100 nm apart.

By comparison, using electromagnetic lenses and a beam of electrons accelerated to a potential of 100 kV, an electron microscope is theoretically capable of resolving approximately 0.001 nm. Although flaws in lens design restrict this potential, contemporary transmission electron microscopes are capable of resolving structures of 0.2 nm or less.

Tissue preparation for transmission electron microscopy

The basic preparation methods for routine TEM are provided in this chapter. More detailed discussions

of these, plus alternative and specialized procedures, can be found elsewhere (Glauert 1972; Robards & Wilson 1993; Allen & Lawrence 1994; Glauert & Lewis 1998; Hayat 2000). A flow chart summarizing the steps required for preparing the basic range of diagnostic TEM specimens is given in Figure 22.1.

The fundamental principle underlying TEM is that electrons pass through the section to give an image of the specimen. However, the electron beam is only capable of penetrating around 100 nm, so, to obtain a high-quality image and optimize the resolution of the instrument, it is necessary to section the tissue to a thickness of around 80 nm.

Sectioning at this level requires tissues to be embedded in extremely rigid material. Clearly the wax embedding media used in light microscopy are not suitable. In routine TEM synthetic embedding resins are used which are capable of withstanding the vacuum in the electron microscope column and the heat generated as the electrons pass through the section. Although hydrophilic media are available, in most circumstances, hydrophobic epoxy resins are preferred.

Specimen handling

In order to preserve the ultrastructure of the cell it is crucial that samples are fixed as soon as possible after the biopsy is taken. The most sensitive cellular indicators of autolytic/degenerative change are the mitochondria and endoplasmic reticulum, both of which may show signs of swelling (a reflection of osmotic imbalance) only a few minutes after the cells are separated from a blood supply.

The standard approach is to immerse the specimen in fixative (preferably pre-cooled to 4°C)

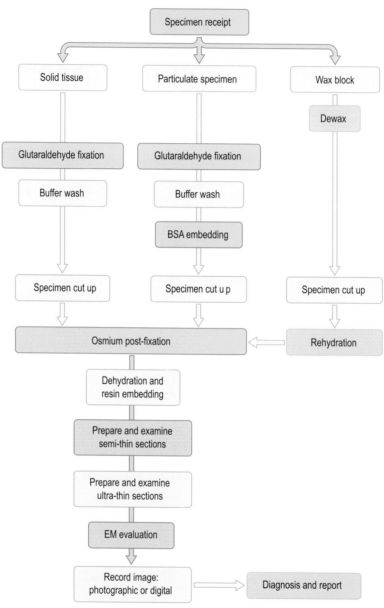

Figure 22.1 Flow chart illustrating the major steps in the preparation of specimens for diagnosis by electron microscopy.

immediately after collection. Once in fixative, the specimen is cut into smaller samples using a scalpel or razor blade. At this point the tissue should be orientated and dissected to optimize exposure of the critical diagnostic features during sectioning and screening. Dissection must also facilitate the penetration of fixatives and processing reagents. The final tissue blocks may be in the form of thin sheets or small cubes (~1 mm³), although the risk of sampling error increases as the sample size decreases. In general, the volume of fixative should be at least 10 times the volume of the tissue. It is also vital to ensure that the tissue remains completely submerged in the fixative – small pieces may adhere to the inside of the lid of the biopsy container; these will be poorly fixed even if they have been exposed to fixative vapor. Gently agitating the vial on a mechanical rotator should help to overcome this problem and improve fixation.

The importance of using small samples cannot be overemphasized. The use of cold fixative assists in minimizing postmortem changes but fixation may be hindered as a consequence. In addition, the penetration rate of most TEM fixatives is quite slow, increasing the risk of artifact formation. It should also be noted that fixatives and processing reagents penetrate different tissues at different rates, and some tissues (such as liver) very poorly. Needle biopsies of liver may need to be cut longitudinally to ensure adequate fixation. If a delay in fixation is unavoidable, damage can be minimized by holding the tissue (for a short time only) in chilled normal saline. However, the tissue must not be frozen at any point.

Fixation

The fixatives used in TEM generally comprise a fixing agent in buffer (to maintain pH) and, if necessary, with various additives to control osmolarity and ionic composition. Other factors that affect fixation include fixative concentration and temperature, and the duration of fixation. The standard protocol involves primary fixation with an aldehyde (usually glutaraldehyde) to stabilize proteins, followed by secondary fixation in osmium tetroxide to retain lipids (Hayat 1981).

Fixative concentration

Glutaraldehyde is effective at a concentration of between 1.5% and 4%, with 2.5% the simplest to prepare from the 25% stock solutions available commercially. Osmium tetroxide is usually used at a concentration of 1% or 2%.

Temperature

Many practitioners prefer to place tissues in cold primary fixative solution but this is not essential.

Fixation at room temperature improves the penetration rate (particularly of aldehyde fixatives) and reduces the time required for fixation although it also increases the risk of autolytic change. Osmium tetroxide is generally used at room temperature.

Duration of fixation

The time required for optimal fixation depends on a range of factors, including the type of tissue, the size of the sample, and the type of fixative and buffer system used. In most circumstances immersion of 0.5–1.0 mm^3 blocks of tissue in 2.5% glutaraldehyde fixative for 2–6 hours is sufficient. It is recommended that punch biopsies of skin taken for cerebral autosomal dominant arteriopathy with subcortical infarcts and leukoencephalopathy (CADASIL) screening should be fixed overnight (to ensure adequate preservation), particularly if they are left whole (i.e., not dissected) and sent to a distant laboratory for processing and screening. Secondary fixation in 1% osmium tetroxide for 60–90 minutes is usually effective; much longer times are required if osmium tetroxide is the primary fixative. The use of microwave irradiation can accelerate fixation times in aldehyde fixative to as little as 5–10 seconds (Leong 1994), after which the sample may be stored in buffer or processed immediately.

Buffers

Fixatives are normally buffered within the range of pH 7.2–7.6 (Robinson & Gray 1996). Ideally the osmolarity and ionic composition of the buffer should mimic that of the tissue being fixed. In general practice this is not a major requirement but, if required, 300–330 mOsm (the osmolarity equivalent to that of plasma or slightly hypertonic) is suitable for most circumstances. Non-ionic molecules such as glucose, sucrose or dextran are used to adjust tonicity as these will not influence the ionic constitution of the buffer. The addition of various salts, particularly calcium and magnesium, is thought to improve tissue preservation, possibly by stabilizing membranes (Hayat 1981). This is unlikely to have a major effect in routine diagnostic applications.

Phosphate buffers

Phosphate buffers (Gomori 1955) have the disadvantage of being good growth media for molds and other microorganisms. Additionally, most metal ions form insoluble phosphates, which restricts the use of this buffer (the phosphates of sodium, potassium and ammonium are soluble). Nevertheless, phosphate buffers are the buffer of choice as they are non-toxic and work well with most tissues.

Phosphate buffer (0.1 M, pH 7.4)	
Stock reagents	
Solution A	
Disodium hydrogen phosphate	14.2 g
(Na$_2$HPO$_4$ anhydrous)	
Distilled water	1000 ml
Solution B	
Sodium dihydrogen phosphate	51.6 g
(NaH$_2$PO$_4$·2H$_2$O)	
Distilled water	1000 ml
Method	
Mix 40.5 ml of solution A with 9.5 ml of solution B. The pH should be checked and adjusted if necessary, using 0.1 M hydrochloric acid or 0.1 M sodium hydroxide.	

Alternative buffers

Other buffers that have been recommended for use in TEM include cacodylate (Plumel 1948; Sabatini et al. 1963), HEPES (N-2-hydroxyethylpiperazine-N´-2-ethanesulfonic acid), MOPS (3-(N-morpholino) propanesulfonic acid) and PIPES (piperazine-N,N´-bis2-ethanesulfonic acid) (Good et al. 1966; Good & Izawa 1972; Massie et al. 1972; Salema & Brandão 1973; Ferguson et al. 1980).

Aldehyde fixatives

Glutaraldehyde

Although glutaraldehyde is the most widely used primary fixative in TEM, its fixation reactions are not well understood. The most important reaction of glutaraldehyde, that of stabilizing proteins, is thought to occur via a cross-linking mechanism involving the amino groups of lysine and other amino acids through the formation of pyridine intermediaries. Lipids and most phospholipids (those that do not contain free amino groups) are not fixed and will be extracted during subsequent processing without secondary fixation (Hayat 2000).

Glutaraldehyde fixative (2.5%, buffered)	
Stock reagents	
25% glutaraldehyde stock solution	10 ml
0.1 M phosphate buffer, pH 7.4	90 ml
Method	
Combine glutaraldehyde and phosphate buffer in the proportions indicated.	

Formaldehyde

Commercially supplied formaldehyde solutions (i.e. formalin) normally contain some level of formic acid and considerable quantities of methanol. As such it is a poor cytological fixative and should not be used for TEM. By contrast, formaldehyde that has been freshly prepared from paraformaldehyde powder is adequate for TEM as it lacks impurities and also has the advantage of a faster penetration rate compared with glutaraldehyde. Paraformaldehyde is often recommended in electron immunocytochemistry as epitopes are less likely to be significantly altered during fixation and, if required, antigen unmasking is more effective.

Aldehyde combinations

The use of an aldehyde mixture has been proposed as a way of offsetting the disadvantages of glutaraldehyde (a slow penetration rate) and formaldehyde (less stable fixation) when applied individually (Karnovsky 1965).

Paraformaldehyde (2%) and glutaraldehyde (2.5%) fixative (buffered) (based on Glauert 1972; Karnovsky 1965)	
Stock reagents	
0.2 M buffer, pH 7.4	50 ml
(phosphate, cacodylate)	
Paraformaldehyde	2.0 g
25% aqueous glutaraldehyde	10 ml
Distilled/deionized water to	100 ml

Method

1. Completely dissolve paraformaldehyde in buffer using heat and with continuous stirring. It may be necessary to add a few drops of 1.0 M sodium hydroxide to clarify the solution.
2. Cool the solution rapidly under running water.
3. Add aqueous glutaraldehyde. Check the pH of the mixture and adjust if necessary to pH 7.4.
4. Add distilled water to make 100 ml.

Note

Adding 0.2 ml of 1.0 M calcium chloride is thought to have a membrane stabilizing effect but this may precipitate if phosphate buffer is used.

Osmium tetroxide

The use of osmium tetroxide fixation to preserve lipids is fundamental to electron microscopy (Palade 1952; Millonig & Marinozzi 1968). While primary fixation in osmium tetroxide is effective, its extremely slow penetration rate can give rise to autolytic changes. For this reason osmium tetroxide is almost always used as a secondary fixative (termed 'post-fixation') after primary fixation in aldehyde. The penetration rate of osmium tetroxide is also higher in stabilized tissue, such that immersion for 60–90 minutes is usually sufficient for most specimens.

Osmium tetroxide is usually supplied in crystalline form sealed in glass ampoules. Extreme care should be exercised when preparing this material and gloves and eye protection should always be worn. It is essential to only handle osmium tetroxide in a fume-hood, as the vapor will also fix tissue.

Specimens fixed in aldehyde solutions should be washed thoroughly in buffer before post-fixation in osmium tetroxide to prevent interaction between the fixatives which can cause precipitation of reduced osmium. Osmium tetroxide can be prepared as an aqueous solution, although it can also be made in the same buffer used to prepare the primary fixative. Osmium tetroxide should be avoided if electron immunogold labeling studies are to be performed, as it has the potential to alter significantly protein structure, rendering antigenic determinants unreactive.

Osmium tetroxide fixative (2% aqueous)

Stock reagent

Osmium tetroxide	1.0 g
Distilled/deionized water	50 ml

Method

1. Clean, then score the glass ampoule with a diamond pencil and place in a dark-glass storage bottle.
2. Break the ampoule with a glass rod and add water. It may take 24 hours or longer for the osmium tetroxide to dissolve completely.
3. Prepared solutions may be stored for short periods at room temperature in the dark in a well-sealed bottle (double wrap the bottle in aluminum foil); for long periods store at 4°C. All osmium solutions should be stored inside a second closed container to prevent the leakage of osmium fumes. Aqueous osmium solutions that are prepared and stored in a clean container should last for ~1 year; solutions in buffer may only last a few days before they deteriorate.
4. For a 1% working solution combine 1:1 with water or buffer.

Note

Osmium is readily reduced by dust and light. Only glassware that has been acid cleaned and thoroughly rinsed in distilled water should be used. Prepared solutions should be monitored during storage and discarded if a pink color develops.

Wash buffer and staining

After primary fixation in glutaraldehyde, tissue may be treated in several ways. Material that is to be retained may be rinsed briefly (in a buffer compatible with the fixative vehicle), then stored in fresh buffer. Tissue that is for immediate processing should be washed in buffer before post-fixation in osmium tetroxide, then washed again in buffer or water to remove excess osmium. This is critical as osmium tetroxide and alcohol react to form a black precipitate. An optional step at this point is to immerse tissues after post-fixation in 2% aqueous uranyl acetate. This *en bloc* staining procedure adds to the contrast of the final sections and improves preservation. However, note that uranyl acetate can extract glycogen.

Dehydration

The most common embedding compounds used in TEM are epoxy resins. These are totally immiscible with water, thus requiring specimens to be dehydrated.

Dehydration is performed by passing the specimen through increasing concentrations of an organic solvent. It is necessary to use a graded series to prevent the damage that would occur with extreme changes in solvent concentration, but it is also important to keep the dehydration times as brief as possible to minimize the risk of extracting cellular constituents. The most frequently used dehydrants are acetone and ethanol. Acetone should be avoided if *en bloc* staining with uranyl acetate has been performed to prevent precipitation of uranium salts. Ethanol overcomes this difficulty but requires the use of propylene oxide (1,2-epoxypropane) as a transition solvent to facilitate resin infiltration. Residual dehydrant can result in soft or patchy blocks.

Commercially available 'absolute' ethanol normally contains a small percentage of water. This will severely restrict infiltration and polymerization of the resin and it is necessary to complete dehydration in anhydrous ethanol (which can be obtained commercially or prepared by using an appropriate molecular sieve). Propylene oxide is highly volatile, flammable and may form explosive peroxides; it should be stored at room temperature in a flammable solvents facility.

Embedding

The standard practice following dehydration and, if required, treatment with a transitional solvent, is to infiltrate the tissue sample with liquid resin. This usually requires gradual introduction of the resin, beginning with a 50:50 mix of transition solvent (propylene oxide) and resin followed by a 25:75

transition solvent resin mix, then, finally, pure resin. An hour in each of the preliminary infiltration steps is usually adequate, although it is preferable to leave samples in pure resin for 24 hours. Gentle agitation using a low-speed, angled rotator during these steps is recommended, as failure to completely infiltrate the tissue will cause major sectioning difficulties.

Once infiltrated, tissue samples are placed in an appropriate mold which is filled with resin and allowed to polymerize using heat. A paper strip bearing the tissue identification code written in pencil or laser-printed is included. Various shaped and sized molds are available. Capsules made from polyethylene are recommended as they do not react with resin, as are flat embedding molds made of silicone rubber. Polymerized blocks can be easily removed from the latter by bending the mold, which can then be reused. Polyethylene capsules can be cut away from the block using a razor or scalpel blade or the block can be extruded from the capsule using large forceps or pliers.

Epoxy resins

Epoxy resins have been the embedding medium of choice in TEM since their introduction in the mid-1950s (Glauert et al. 1956). These resins contain a characteristic chemical group in which an oxygen and two carbon atoms bond to form a three-membered ring ('epoxide'). Cross-linking between these groups creates a three-dimensional polymer of great mechanical strength. The polymerization process generates very little shrinkage (usually less than 2%) and, once complete, is permanent. As well as their properties of uniform polymerization and low shrinkage, epoxy resins also preserve tissue ultrastructure, are stable in the electron beam, section easily and are readily available.

Epoxy resins usually comprise four ingredients: the monomeric resin, a hardener, an accelerator and a plasticizer. Although manufacturers provide advice on the appropriate proportions, the hardness and flexibility of blocks and polymerization times can be manipulated by varying the amount of the individual components. It is the proportion of each component that is important; hence resins can be prepared by volume or weight. The simplest approach is to weigh the components into a disposable paper or plastic cup; as unused resin can be polymerized and discarded in the container. Thorough mixing of the components is absolutely essential. When prepared, the resin is best delivered through a non-reactive plastic syringe or pipette.

Examples of widely used epoxy resin composites include Araldite (Glauert & Glauert 1958), Epon (Luft 1961) and Spurr's resin (Spurr 1969). Although the original product names Araldite and Epon refer to epoxy resins developed by the CIBA Chemical Company and Shell Chemical Company, respectively, these terms are now in general use. Araldite polymers are preferred as these react with a higher degree of cross-linking and are the most stable.

Occupational exposure to epoxy resins is a common cause of allergic contact dermatitis (Kanerva et al. 1989; Jolanki et al. 1990). These agents are also probable carcinogens, primary irritants and systemically toxic (Causton 1981). Spurr's resin in particular is toxic and should be handled with great care (Ringo et al. 1982).

Acrylic resins

Acrylic resins (methacrylates) derive from methacrylic acid [$CH_2=C \cdot (CH_3)COOH$] and acrylic acid [$CH_2=CH \cdot COOH$] and were the original synthetic media developed for use in TEM. Acrylic resins can rapidly infiltrate fixed, dehydrated tissues at room temperature. However, marked, variable shrinkage of tissue components was common due to unreliable polymerization and acrylic resins are relatively unstable in the electron beam. Currently available acrylics are now polymerized using a cross-linking process, thereby overcoming earlier disadvantages. Acrylic monomers are of low viscosity, and both hydrophilic and hydrophobic forms are obtainable. Acrylic resins react by free radical polymerization, which can be initiated using light, heat or a chemical accelerator (catalyst) at room temperature.

The main commercial acrylic resins are LR White and LR Gold and the Lowicryl series (K4M, K11M, HM20 and HM23). Each of these can be used for low-temperature dehydration and embedding to reduce the heat damage from exothermic polymerization and extraction by solvents and resin components (Acetarin et al. 1986; Newman and Hobot 1987, 1993). These characteristics make several forms of acrylic resin ideally suited to electron immunogold labeling (Stirling 1994) and enzyme cytochemical studies.

Tissue processing schedules

Manual tissue processing is best performed by keeping the tissue sample in the same vial throughout, and using a fine pipette to change solutions. When processing multiple samples, take care not to cross-contaminate specimens – use separate pipettes. All vials must be clearly labeled and labels must be 'solvent-proof'. It is advantageous to agitate tissue specimens throughout the processing cycle to enhance reagent permeation. A protocol for the routine processing of solid tissue samples is given in Table 22.1.

Procedures for other tissue samples

Cultured cells

Cell cultures may be fixed *in situ*, then separated from the substrate, centrifuged into a pellet and treated as a solid tissue. Alternatively, cells can be harvested into a centrifuge tube, pelleted lightly, resuspended in fixative and again pelleted by gentle centrifugation. After fixation the tube is inverted to dislodge the pellet, which is then cut into cubes for further processing. Finally cell cultures can be fixed and processed while attached to the substratum, after which inverted embedding capsules are pressed onto the cell layer. Once polymerized, blocks can be separated by force or after being cooled in liquid nitrogen (see 'Pop-off' technique, below).

Table 22.1 Standard processing schedule for solid tissue cut into 1 mm³ blocks (each step is performed at room temperature unless stated otherwise)

Primary fixation	2.5% glutaraldehyde in 0.1 M phosphate buffer	2–24 hours (room temperature or 4°C)
Wash	0.1 M phosphate buffer	2 × 10 minutes on rotator
Wash	Distilled water	2 × 10 minutes
En bloc staining (optional)	2% aqueous uranyl acetate	20 minutes
Dehydration	70% ethanol	10 minutes on rotator*
	90% ethanol	10 minutes on rotator
	95% ethanol	10 minutes on rotator
	100% ethanol	15 minutes on rotator
	Dry absolute ethanol	2 × 20 minutes on rotator
Transition solvent (clearing)	1,2-epoxypropane	2 × 15 minutes on rotator
Infiltration	50:50, clearant:resin[#]	1 hour
	25:75, clearant:resin	1 hour
	Resin only	1–24 hours (with vacuum to remove bubbles)
Embedding	Fresh resin in embedding capsules	12–24 hours at 60–70°C

*Tissues may be stored at this stage.
[#]As batches may vary, resin should be prepared in accordance with manufacturer's instructions.

Cell suspensions or particulate matter

Cell suspensions (such as fine needle biopsy aspirates, bone marrow specimens or cytology samples) or particulate materials (including fluid aspirates, tissue fragments or products and specimens for the assessment of ciliary structures) are best embedded in a protein support medium before processing. Plasma, agar or bovine serum albumen (BSA) can be used. The addition of tannic acid (Hayat 1993) during the preparation of ciliary specimens gives improved visualization of axonemal components (Sturgess & Turner 1984; Glauert & Lewis 1998). The tannic acid is thought to act as a fixative and also a mordant, facilitating the binding of heavy metal stains (Hayat 2000). Double en bloc staining with uranyl acetate and lead aspartate may also improve the visibility of dynein arms (Rippstein et al. 1987).

Preparing particulate specimens

Stock reagents
15% aqueous bovine serum albumen (BSA)
0.1% tannic acid (low molecular weight) in buffer, pH 7.4 (phosphate)

Method
1. Centrifuge the material in buffer in a plastic centrifuge tube to form a loose pellet.
2. Discard supernatant and resuspend the material in glutaraldehyde fixative at room temperature for a minimum of 1 hour.
3. Centrifuge the material and carefully discard the supernatant.
4. Wash the specimen by resuspending it in buffer for 10–15 minutes.
5. Centrifuge the material to form a loose pellet.

6. Discard supernatant and introduce 0.5 ml of 15% aqueous BSA. Resuspend the specimen and allow it to infiltrate for a minimum of 1 hour.

7. Centrifuge the material and discard most of the supernatant, leaving sufficient to cover the pellet to a depth of approximately 1 mm.

8. Introduce an equal volume of glutaraldehyde fixative to form a layer above the BSA. Allow material to solidify for 2–24 hours.

9. Remove the material (this is most easily achieved by cutting away the plastic centrifuge tube) and divide into small portions.

10. Wash in four changes of buffer, each for 5 minutes (for ciliary biopsies only, incubate for 15 minutes in buffered tannic acid solution, then wash in four changes of buffer, each for 5 minutes, before proceeding to step 11).

11. Postfix in 1% aqueous osmium tetroxide and process as normal.

Material embedded in paraffin/cell smears

Occasionally it becomes necessary to examine the ultrastructure of a cell smear or specimen originally embedded in paraffin and intended for light microscopy. As the preservation quality may vary, considerable care must be exercised in the electron microscopic interpretation of such material. Nevertheless it is often possible to obtain information sufficient for diagnostic purposes.

Reprocessing paraffin-embedded material

Method

1. Remove the area of interest from the block, taking care not to damage the tissue.

2. Dewax the specimen by passing through several changes of xylene. The time required depends on the size of the sample but should be at least 1 hour. A minimum of three changes is recommended.

3. Rehydrate the material in a graded ethanol series.

4. Wash in water, postfix in osmium tetroxide and process as routine specimen (see above).

Pop-off technique for slide-mounted sections

(after Bretschneider et al.1981)

Method

1. Remove the coverslip by soaking the slide in xylene. (This may take some time. An alternative is to firstly cool slides to –20°C for up to one hour, then carefully pry off coverslip with a blade.)

If additional fixation is required

2. Rehydrate the tissue in a graded ethanol series.

3. Wash in buffer and fix the tissue in glutaraldehyde fixative for 15–20 minutes.

4. Wash in buffer and postfix in 1% osmium tetroxide for 20–30 minutes.

5. Wash in buffer or distilled water, and then cover with 2% uranyl acetate for 15 minutes.

6. Dehydrate the tissue by passing the slide through 70%, 90%, 95%, 100% and super dry ethanol for 5 minutes in each stage.

7. Dip the slide into propylene oxide for 5 minutes. The tissue should not be allowed to dry.

8. Cover the tissue with a 2 : 1 mixture of propylene oxide and epoxy resin for 5–15 minutes. The tissue should not be allowed to dry.

9. Cover the tissue with a 1 : 2 mixture of propylene oxide and epoxy resin for 5–15 minutes. The tissue should not be allowed to dry.

10. Cover the tissue with neat epoxy resin for 5–15 minutes.

11. Drain off surplus resin mixture. Invert a freshly filled (to overflowing) embedding capsule over the section and press onto the slide.

12. Incubate the slide and capsule at 60°C for 24 hours for polymerization to occur.

13. Remove the slide and, while still warm, separate the capsule and the newly embedded tissue from the glass slide.

If additional fixation is not required

2. Dip the slide in equal parts of propylene oxide and xylene, then into propylene oxide for 5–10 minutes. The tissue should not be allowed to dry.

3. Cover the tissue with a 2 : 1 mixture of propylene oxide and epoxy resin for 5–15 minutes. The tissue should not be allowed to dry.

4. Cover the tissue with a 1 : 2 mixture of propylene oxide and epoxy resin for 5–15 minutes. The tissue should not be allowed to dry.

5. Cover the tissue with neat epoxy resin for 5–15 minutes.

6. Drain off surplus resin mixture. Invert a freshly filled (to overflowing) embedding capsule over the section and press onto the slide.

7. Incubate the slide and capsule at 60°C for 24 hours for polymerization to occur.

8. Remove the slide and, while still warm, separate the capsule and the newly embedded tissue from the glass slide.

Note

Sections (or cell cultures) are easier to prepare using the pop-off method if mounted (or grown) directly on Thermanox coverslips. (Thermanox coverslips are made of a proprietary polystyrene-like compound that is resistant to fixatives and common solvents and which separates easily from the face of resin blocks.)

Ultramicrotomy

Glass knives

Knives are prepared from commercially available plate glass strips manufactured specifically for ultramicrotomy. Before use, the strips should be washed thoroughly with detergent, then rinsed in distilled water and alcohol and dried using lint-free paper. Most knifemakers will allow knives of different cutting edge angles to be produced. Higher angle knives (up to 55°) are best suited to cutting hard materials, while softer blocks respond better to shallower (35°) angle knives. Glass squares and knives should be prepared just before use to avoid contamination and stored in a dust-free, lidded box.

Knives should always be inspected before use. If the knife edge is correctly formed, when it is observed face-on it should be straight and even but with a small glass spur on the top right-hand end (Fig. 22.2).

The edge need not be horizontal, but those that are obviously convex or concave should be discarded. The knife should also display a conchoidal fracture mark that curves across and down from the top left-hand edge of the knife until it meets, and runs parallel to, the right-hand edge of the glass. Each of these characteristics is visible macroscopically. When placed in the ultramicrotome and viewed under the

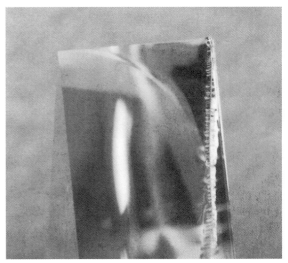

Figure 22.2 Glass knife prepared from 6.4 mm thick glass strip. Note the straight cutting edge and conchoidal fracture mark.

microscope the cutting edge will appear as a bright line against a dark background. The left third of the cutting edge should appear as a smooth line and is the zone recommended for thin sectioning. The middle third is quite frequently also adequate but can show minute imperfections, and is best reserved for trimming blocks prior to sectioning and for cutting semi-thin sections.

In ultramicrotomy, thin sections are floated out for collection as they are cut. This requires a small trough to be attached directly to the knife. Preformed plastic or metal troughs that can be fitted to the back of the knife are commercially available. These must be sealed with molten dental wax or nail varnish after attachment but they are expedient and simple to use. An alternative approach is to prepare a trough using self-adhesive PVC insulating tape. The lower edge of the trough so formed is then sealed with molten dental wax (Fig. 22.3).

Diamond knives

A well-maintained diamond knife is capable of cutting any type of resin block and most biological and many non-biological materials. Knives are priced according to the length of the actual cutting

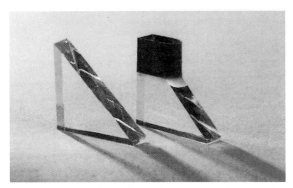

Figure 22.3 Glass knives: left, bare knife used for trimming and semi-thin sectioning; right, knife used for ultra-thin sectioning with trough (prepared from plastic (PVC) tape) fitted.

edge. Manufacturers supply diamond knives already mounted in a metal block (incorporating a section collection trough) designed to fit directly into the knife holder of the ultramicrotome. Diamond knives are brittle but very durable and will continue to cut for quite some time provided they are kept clean and treated carefully. The cutting edge can be cleaned by carefully running a polystyrene cleaning strip (available commercially) along (never across)

the edge. A diamond knife must only be used to cut ultra-thin sections and should never be used 'dry' without a trough fluid.

Trough fluids

The simplest and most suitable fluid routinely used in section collecting troughs is distilled or deionized water; 10–15% solutions of ethanol or acetone can also be used (not with a diamond knife). It is important to ensure that the correct level of fluid is added. If the level is too high, the fluid will be drawn over the cutting edge and down the back of the knife, thereby preventing proper sectioning. If the level is too low, sections will accumulate on the cutting edge and will not float out.

Block trimming

Once polymerized, blocks must be cleared of excess resin to expose the tissue for sectioning. At the completion of this process the trimmed area should resemble a flat-topped pyramid with a square or trapezium-shaped face (Fig. 22.4).

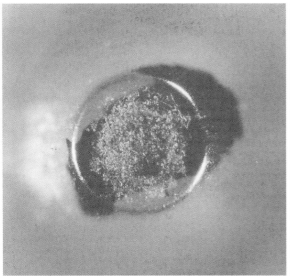
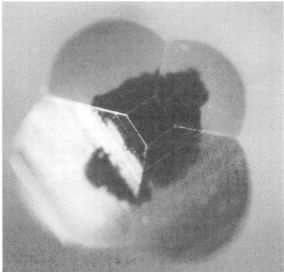

a
b

Figure 22.4 Araldite blocks (a) untrimmed, (b) trimmed of excess resin.

Trimming the block can be achieved manually or by using the ultramicrotome. At its simplest, manual trimming can be performed by mounting the block in a suitable holder under a dissecting microscope and removing the surplus resin with a single-edged razor blade. Although this method is quite speedy, considerable care is required to ensure the ultimate cutting surface is as level as possible to facilitate sectioning. Alternatively, the block is positioned in the ultramicrotome and mechanically trimmed using a glass knife.

Semi-thin sections

Semi-thin (or 'survey') sections allow samples to be screened for specific features and to select areas for thin sectioning. Semi-thin sections are usually cut on a glass knife. However, there are now diamond knives specifically produced for semi-thin section microtomy.

Commonly, semi-thin sections are cut at between 0.5 and 1.0 µm from trimmed or partly trimmed blocks using the ultramicrotome and a glass knife. Sections can be cut dry (using a slow cutting speed) and picked up with forceps or directly into the flotation bath attached to the knife. Sections are transferred to a drop of water on a glass microscope slide and dried on a hot plate at 70–80°C. Semi-thin sections can be examined using phase contrast or be stained and viewed by bright-field microscopy. Various cationic dyes, including methylene blue, azure B (Richardson et al. 1960) and crystal violet, can be used for this purpose, although the most common is toluidine blue (with borax). All are applied at high alkaline pH and with heat to facilitate penetration of the resin.

Toluidine blue stain for semi-thin sections

Stock reagents	
Sodium tetraborate (borax)	1 g
Toluidine blue	1 g
Distilled water	100 ml

Dissolve the borax in the distilled water and then add the toluidine blue. After filtering, the final solution can be stored at room temperature.

Method

1. Cover sections with staining solution and heat on a hot plate at 70–80°C.
2. Allow to stain adequately (the time is not crucial – up to 60 seconds is usually sufficient), then wash thoroughly in running water. Allow section to dry.
3. Sections can be viewed dry or mounted in DPX or epoxy resin.

Note

Borax raises the pH of the final stain to around pH 11.

Collection of sections

Ultra-thin sections are mounted onto specimen grids for viewing. Grids measure 3.05 mm in diameter and are made of conductive material, commonly copper, nickel or gold, although silver, palladium, molybdenum, aluminum, titanium, stainless steel, nylon-carbon and combination varieties are available. A large range of patterns and mesh sizes are available (Fig. 22.5), with 200 square mesh being commonly used, although slotted, parallel bar and hexagonal patterns are also standard. As electrons cannot pass through the metal grid bars, the choice

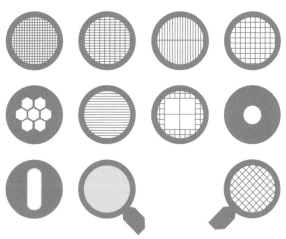

Figure 22.5 Some examples of specimen grids. From top left: mesh (200 size); slotted (200 size); parallel with divider (200 size); mesh (50 size); hexagonal (7 size); parallel (75 size); freeze fracture; single hole; slotted; tabbed mesh (400 size); tabbed mesh (75 size).

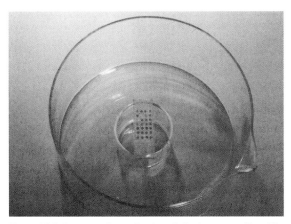

Figure 22.6 Apparatus for application of plastic support films. The water level is raised over the level of the wire mesh, on which grids are then placed. Approximately 0.2 ml of liquid plastic film is dropped onto the water surface over the submerged grids and the solvent allowed to evaporate. The water is then drawn off, allowing the film of plastic to settle onto the grids.

of grid becomes a compromise between support for the sections (better with grids of smaller mesh size) and the relative proportion of exposed section (better with grids of larger mesh size). The latter provides a large area of section for viewing but with less stability.

Support films

The use of support films is generally unnecessary with contemporary, routine embedding media that have been properly prepared. If, however, larger viewing areas are required, it may be necessary to use support films to provide greater section stability.

Electron-transparent plastic films prepared from collodion, Formvar or Butvar are commonly used. There are many methods for applying plastic films, with one of the simpler being illustrated in Figure 22.6. The major problem with using plastic films is that the conductive properties of the grid become compromised. Re-instating the thermal and electrical properties is usually achieved by adding a 5–10 nm layer of carbon in a sputter coater or vacuum-evaporating unit.

Ultra-thin sectioning

The basic principles of ultramicrotomy are similar, regardless of the ultramicrotome used (Reid 1975; Dykstra 1992). Difficulties with sectioning usually relate to tissue that is poorly fixed or inadequately infiltrated, an imperfectly polymerized block or a dull knife (see Table 22.2). Specific instructions on operating particular ultramicrotomes are normally provided by the instrument manufacturer.

A key element in ultramicrotomy is to ensure the sections are cut at a thickness that allows optimal resolution and specimen contrast. The most effective estimate of section thickness is given by viewing the interference color reflected from the section as it is cut; this color is the result of interactions between light waves reflected from the upper and lower surfaces of the section and is directly related to section thickness (Table 22.3).

Silver to gold sections (around 80 nm) are recommended. Thinner sections will give improved resolution but may not provide sufficient contrast for adequate on-screen viewing. Although it is possible to collect and examine individual sections, ribbons are easier to manage and, as the sections are in series, usually offer additional morphological information. Before collection, sections should be flattened (to remove wrinkles) using heat or ether, chloroform, xylene or amyl-acetate vapor. Vapors are applied using a sharpened orange-wood stick which is soaked in the fluid of choice, then held over the sections. Do not allow the stick to come into contact with the flotation fluid as the sections may be spoiled. Heat is best applied using a fine hot wire.

To collect sections, immerse the grid in the flotation fluid, then position it under the ribbon (sections may be maneuvered while they are floating on the knife bath using a fine hair mounted on an orange-wood stick). If the grid is then angled slightly, the ribbon of sections will fall across the diameter of the grid as it is lifted from the fluid. It is important to remove any remaining fluid by gently touching the grid against lint-free absorbent paper to insure the sections become firmly fixed. A pair of very fine-point forceps should always be used to grasp the grid; this requires great care to avoid damaging the

Table 22.2 Causes and remedies for common sectioning faults

Fault	Effect	Potential cause	Remedy
Scoring	Scratches, tears in section running perpendicular to cutting edge	Knife edge damaged or dirty	Use a new section of knife Replace knife
		Hard material in block	Use diamond knife
Sections contaminated	Artifacts, dirt on section	Dirt on knife edge	Replace knife
		Dirty trough fluid	Replace trough fluid
		Trough dirty	Replace with new knife and trough
		Block face dirty	Trim and re-face block
Chatter	Periodic variations in the part (or all) of the section running parallel to the cutting edge	Vibrations in knife, block or block holder on ultramicrotome	Tighten components
		Dull knife	Replace knife
		Block soft or unevenly polymerized	Re-incubate block (60–70°C) for up to 24 hours Modify processing schedule and/or resin formulation
		Cutting speed too fast	Reduce cutting speed
		Clearance angle too great	Reduce clearance angle
Compression	Specimen distortion with compression in the direction parallel to the cutting edge and extension in the direction perpendicular to the cutting edge	Block soft	Re-incubate block (60–70°C) for up to 24 hours Modify processing schedule and/or resin formulation
		Sections too thin	Increase section thickness
		Cutting speed too fast	Reduce cutting speed
		Cutting edge angle too high	Prepare knife with shallower cutting edge angle
Section wrinkling or folding	Electron-dense bands with straight sides but of variable width	Block soft or unevenly polymerized	Re-incubate block (60–70°C) for up to 24 hours Modify processing schedule and/or resin formulation
		Dull knife	Replace knife
		Block face too large	Trim to a smaller block face
		Knife angle too shallow	Increase knife angle
		Section collection technique poor	Improve technique
		Picking up single sections	Use ribbons

Table 22.2 *(continued)*

Fault	Effect	Potential cause	Remedy
Alternating thick and thin sections	Only some sections useful	Block face too large	Trim to a smaller block face
		Incorrect knife angle	Adjust knife angle
		Cutting speed too fast	Reduce cutting speed
		Dull knife	Replace knife
		Block soft or unevenly polymerized	Re-incubate block (60–70°C) for up to 24 hours
		Vibration in ultramicrotome	Modify processing schedule and/or resin formulation
		Air movement over sections during cutting	Tighten components Eliminate air drafts
Failure to cut sections as ribbon	Single sections	Upper and lower block edges not parallel	Re-trim block face
		Upper and lower block edges not straight	Re-trim block face
		Fluid level in trough too high or too low	Adjust fluid level
		Cutting speed too slow	Increase cutting speed
Skipping (sections cut on alternate strokes)	Single sections	Dull knife	Replace knife
		Clearance angle too high	Reduce clearance angle
		Knife angle too high	Reduce knife angle

Table 22.3 Relation between section thickness and interference color

Color	Section thickness (nm)
Gray	<60
Silver	60–90
Gold	90–150
Purple	150–190
Blue	190–240

grid either before or after collecting the sections. After collecting the sections, grids should be placed on filter paper in a lidded container, such as a Petri dish, and allowed to dry completely before staining. The specimens should be clearly labeled (on the filter paper). As they are extremely fragile, it is strongly recommended that grids be kept in suitable storage boxes. These not only afford protection but also provide a means of identifying individual grids.

Staining

The purpose of staining sections in TEM is to increase the capacity of selected structural elements to scatter electrons and thus give the specimen contrast. This is achieved by introducing heavy metal atoms which deposit on the tissue components. It should be noted that image contrast can also be manipulated by changing the size of the objective lens aperture. Thus, image contrast is a function of the interactions between accelerating voltage, size of objective lens aperture, thickness of the section and the staining used.

Tissues are stained at several points during preparation (Glauert & Lewis 1998; Hayat 2000):

1. During secondary fixation (as osmium is deposited in membranes).
2. When uranyl acetate is used during the post-fixation wash.
3. By staining the sections with lead and uranium salts (known as en-section staining).

The standard method for staining sections is to float the grids, section-side-down, on drops of staining solution for the required time. Alternatively, grids may be completely immersed in the solution. The procedure is carried out on a clean surface (such as a Petri dish) to minimize contamination. Normally, sections are stained in uranyl acetate followed by lead citrate (Reynolds 1963). After each staining step, the grid is washed under a gentle stream of distilled water or by dipping in distilled water. Finally, the grids are dried using clean lint-free filter paper. If the level of contrast achieved is not sufficient, a double lead staining method can be used (Daddow 1983).

Uranyl salts

Uranyl acetate is the uranium salt normally used in TEM although uranyl nitrate and magnesium uranyl acetate are also effective. The uranyl ions combine in large quantities with phosphate groups in nucleic acids as well as phosphate and carboxyl groups on the cell surface (Hayat 2000). Aqueous solutions of between 2% and 5%, applied to the section, will give satisfactory contrast but more intense staining can be achieved in less time by using a saturated ethanolic (or methanolic) solution (~7%). Uranyl acetate is radioactive and highly toxic; its effects are cumulative and appropriate precautions should be followed.

Uranyl acetate (2% aqueous)	
Stock reagents	
Uranyl acetate	2.0 g
Distilled water	100 ml

Combine reagents in proportions indicated. Filter, divide into suitable aliquots and store at 4°C in the dark. Centrifuge before use.

Method
1. Place droplets of the staining solution on a clean surface (as in a Petri dish).
2. Place grid section, side down, on the droplets for up to 10 minutes.
3. Rinse grids in three changes of distilled water.

Lead salts

Lead stains increase the contrast of a range of tissue components. Lead stains must be prepared and used carefully as lead ions have the potential to react with atmospheric carbon dioxide, forming a fine precipitate of lead carbonate. The deposit appears as an electron-dense contaminant on sections that cannot be removed easily. The preparation method of Reynolds, which is in common use, addresses this problem by chelating and thus shielding the lead ion from exposure to the carbon dioxide (Reynolds 1963).

Reynolds' lead citrate stain *(Reynolds 1963)*	
Stock reagents	
Lead nitrate	2.66 g
Trisodium citrate	3.52 g
1 M sodium hydroxide (freshly prepared)	16.0 ml
Distilled water (freshly prepared, carbonate-free)	84.0 ml

Mix the reagents in an alkaline-cleaned stoppered flask with approximately 60 ml of the water, inverting continuously for 1 minute. Allow to stand for 30 minutes with occasional mixing. Add sodium hydroxide and mix until the solution becomes clear. Make up to 100 ml with remaining water. Divide into suitable aliquots and store at 4°C. Centrifuge before use.

Method
1. Place droplets of the staining solution in a Petri dish containing a few pellets of sodium hydroxide (for preferential absorption of carbon dioxide).
2. Place grid section, side down, on the droplets for up to 10 minutes.
3. Rinse grids in three changes of distilled water.

Diagnostic applications

Here we describe only the essential features of selected diseases in which TEM plays a major diagnostic role. For in-depth analyses there are a large number of specialist texts that contain a wealth of information on the interpretation of ultrastructural morphology. For example, the ultrastructural pathology of the cell has been covered comprehensively by Ghadially (1997), renal disease by Jennette et al. (1998) and Tisher and Brenner (1994), and non-neoplastic diseases by Papadimitriou et al. (1992b). The ultrastructure of neoplastic diseases has been described in several texts; those by Henderson et al. (1986), Erlandson (1994) and Ghadially (1985) are recommended.

The use of TEM for diagnostics

TEM is used to obtain structural and compositional information that cannot be acquired realistically using an alternative technique. In practice, TEM is rarely used alone and is generally part of an integrated diagnostic protocol. The following criteria can be used to decide if TEM is appropriate (Stirling et al. 1999a):

1. Will TEM give useful additional information in respect to a differential diagnosis?
2. Is TEM time- and cost-effective in respect to alternative techniques?
3. Will the TEM diagnosis result in improved treatment strategies and patient care?

Renal disease

The basic diagnostic features of the major renal diseases are outlined in Tables 22.4–22.8 and Figs 22.7–22.20.

The location and morphology of immune complex deposits

Immune complex deposits are seen as accumulations of electron-dense finely granular material in, or adjacent to, the glomerular basement membrane (GBM) and mesangial matrix (Figs 22.7–22.12). Deposits may also have an 'organized' structure, most commonly fibrils (Figs 22.13 and 22.14) or tubules (Herrera & Turbat-Herrera 2010). The principal forms of deposit are (Stirling et al. 1999b):

- *Subepithelial (epimembranous):* raised dome-shaped deposits that protrude from the outer surface of the GBM (between the GBM and the visceral epithelial cell foot processes). Large well-formed deposits, typical of post-infectious glomerulonephritis (GN), are termed 'humps' (Fig. 22.7). Smaller deposits are typical of membranous GN (Fig. 22.9). In membranous GN the deposits may eventually encroach into the GBM, provoking a GBM reaction. In this case the GBM may become thickened, with 'spikes' of new membrane forming adjacent to the deposits (Fig. 22.9). Such deposits may eventually be completely surrounded by the GBM. Finally, where deposits have been absorbed, only electron-lucent areas surrounded by thickened GBM may remain (Fig. 22.9).
- *Intramembranous:* nodular or, more rarely, linear deposits that are completely incorporated into the GBM, such as in advanced membranous GN. In dense deposit disease (mesangiocapillary GN type II) (Fig. 22.12) the deposit has the appearance of a linear uniform (non-granular) dense 'transformation' that, arguably, may be described as either intramembranous or subendothelial in location.
- *Subendothelial:* linear or plaque-like deposits situated between the inner (luminal) aspect of the GBM and the endothelium (Fig. 22.8). Subendothelial deposits may be massive and visible by LM. The latter are seen typically in systemic lupus erythematosus (SLE) as nodular hyaline 'thrombi' or 'wire-loop' capillary wall thickening (light microscopy description).
- *Mesangial:* deposits that lie completely within the mesangial matrix. Mesangial deposits may be massive and are seen typically in IgA disease (Fig. 22.10).

Table 22.4 Renal diseases with fine granular deposits: the ultrastructural features of post-infectious glomerulonephritis (GN), systemic lupus erythematosus (SLE), membranous GN, and IgA nephropathy

	Diagnostic ultrastructural features			
	Post-infectious GN	Systemic lupus erythematosus (SLE)	Membranous GN	IgA nephropathy
Capillary wall				
GBM morphology: contour, width, texture	Normal	Normal to irregular and thickened depending on the extent and location of membrane deposits	Stage I: minimal irregular thickening Stage II: marked thickening with membrane spikes (argyrophilic by LM) Stage III: thickened membrane surrounding deposits Stage IV and V: much thickened with irregular patchy lucent areas common in stage V (Stages II–V, see Fig. 22.9)	Focal irregular thinning ('etching')
GBM deposit: type, location	Prominent subepithelial dome-shaped deposits (humps) are characteristic (Fig. 22.7): number of humps correlates approximately to intensity of inflammation Intramembranous and subendothelial deposits may also be present	Deposits increase in extent and location with severity of inflammation GBM deposits (subepithelial, intramembranous, and subendothelial) (Fig. 22.8) indicate severe or global inflammation. In well-established disease, deposits may be found throughout the glomerulus SLE can mimic other diseases because of the variety of damage caused	Stage I: subepithelial deposits Stage II: subepithelial deposits with membrane spikes Stage III: intramembranous deposits Stage IV: some deposits resorbed, leaving lucent areas Stage V: many deposits resorbed, leaving poorly defined lucent and rarefied areas	Subendothelial Deposits variable but present in some cases Subepithelial and intramembranous deposits rare

Table 22.4 *(continued)*

	Diagnostic ultrastructural features			
	Post-infectious GN	**Systemic lupus erythematosus (SLE)**	**Membranous GN**	**IgA nephropathy**
Capillary wall				
Visceral epithelium	Foot processes usually effaced over humps so that their outer surface is covered by epithelial cell cytoplasm	Cells may contain tubuloreticular inclusions	Foot process obliteration	Focal foot process obliteration
Endothelium, subendothelial plane	Normal	Tubuloreticular inclusions common in endothelial cells (see Fig. 22.20) (Note that tubuloreticular inclusions may be found in small numbers in other renal diseases)	Normal	Normal
Mesangium				
Matrix	Areas of matrix separated by cellular swelling, proliferation, and infiltration	Diffuse expansion	Normal	Increased
Deposits	Peripheral humps with deposits common within matrix	Minor inflammation has exclusively mesangial deposits only	Deposits absent in primary GN; may be present in secondary membranous GN	Present, sometimes nodular (Fig. 22.10)
Cells	Proliferation (endocapillary) with infiltration by inflammatory cells including macrophages and polymorphs	Diffuse but irregular proliferation with segmental inflammation	No increase	Variable mesangial cell proliferation

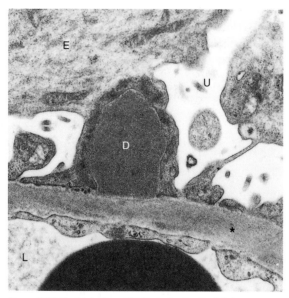

Figure 22.7 Post-infectious GN. Typical subepithelial dome-shaped deposit (hump) (D). GBM (*), epithelial cell cytoplasm (E), urinary space (U), capillary lumen (L) with part of a red blood cell also visible.

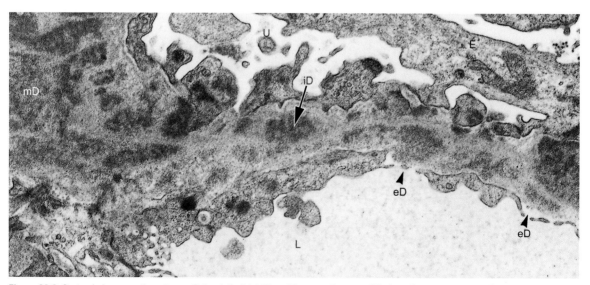

Figure 22.8 Systemic lupus erythematosus. Subendothelial (eD) and intramembranous (iD) deposits are seen in the GBM; mesangial deposits (mD) are also present. Epithelial cell cytoplasm (E), urinary space (U), capillary lumen (L).

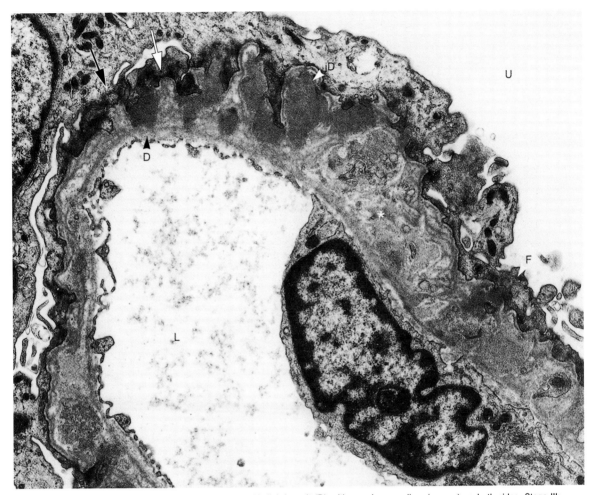

Figure 22.9 Membranous GN Stages II–V. Stage II: subepithelial deposit (D) with membrane spikes (arrows) on both sides. Stage III: intramembranous deposit (iD). Stage IV–V: thickened and disrupted GBM with patches of partially resorbed deposit and lucent areas (*). Epithelial cell foot processes are extensively effaced (F). Urinary space (U), capillary lumen (L).

- *Paramesangial:* deposits within the peripheral mesangial matrix, particularly at the junction of the mesangium and loop GBM (Fig. 22.10).

Variations in the thickness and/or texture of the GBM

The normal GBM has a mean thickness of approximately 390 nm (reported by Coleman et al. 1986 as: mean 394 nm, with a range of 356–432 nm) (Fig. 22.15).

The principal changes in the thickness and/or texture of the GBM are (Stirling et al. 1999b):

- *Thickness:* the GBM may be thickened, thinned or irregular (Figs 22.16–22.19).
- *Texture:* the GBM may be laminated, fragmented or split. Electron-lucent zones may represent areas of resorbed deposits (Fig. 22.9).
- *Surface structure:* the GBM may appear 'etched' (frayed or uneven).
- *Inclusions:* electron-dense granules and debris, microparticles, fibrils, fingerprint-like whorls, small vesicles and virus-like particles, fibrillar collagen and fibrin, all of doubtful or unknown diagnostic significance. Amyloid may also be found occasionally within the GBM (Fig. 22.13).

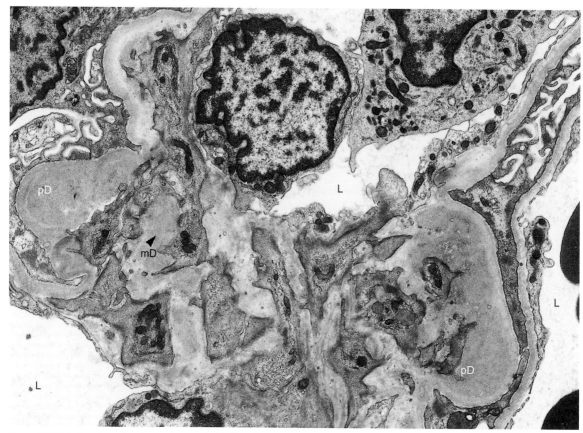

Figure 22.10 IgA nephropathy. Areas of mesangial (mD) and nodular paramesangial (pD) deposit are seen within the mesangium (M). Capillary lumens (L).

Table 22.5 Renal diseases with fine granular deposits: the ultrastructural features of mesangiocapillary GN types I and II

	Diagnostic ultrastructural features	
	Mesangiocapillary GN type I (with subendothelial deposits)	Mesangiocapillary GN type II (dense deposit disease)
Capillary wall		
GBM morphology: contour, width, texture	Double contouring ('tram tracking' by LM) due to mesangial interposition in well-developed disease (Fig. 22.11)	Interposition in some cases
GBM deposit: type, location	Deposits mainly in interposition zone (Fig. 22.11)	Linear dense deposit, typically discontinuous (Fig. 22.12)
Visceral epithelium	Variable foot process obliteration	Normal
Endothelium, subendothelial plane	Interposition of mesangial cells, with deposits and new GBM-like material (Fig. 22.11)	Mesangial interposition
Mesangium		
Matrix	Greatly increased	Increased
Deposits	Present	Present, dense and finely granular
Cells	Endocapillary proliferation	Endocapillary proliferation

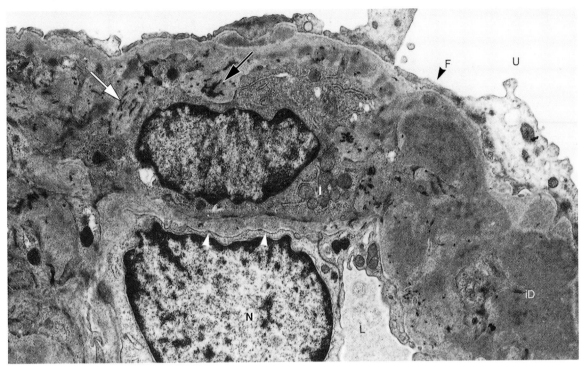

Figure 22.11 Mesangiocapillary GN type I. The capillary wall is considerably thickened due to mesangial cell interposition (I) and the formation of new basement membrane-like material (arrowheads) giving rise to the appearance of double contouring, as seen by LM. Collagen fibers (arrows) and large areas of intramembranous deposit (iD) can also be seen in the capillary wall. Epithelial cell foot processes are extensively effaced (F). Urinary space (U), capillary lumen (L), endothelial cell nucleus (N).

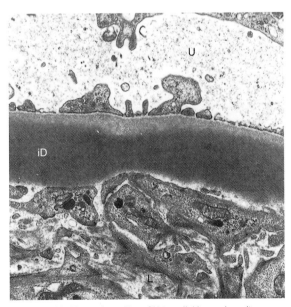

Figure 22.12 Mesangiocapillary GN type II (dense deposit disease). A continuous linear zone of dense intramembranous deposit (iD) is seen along the length of the GBM. Cells of indeterminate type are seen in the capillary lumen (L). Urinary space (U).

- *Folds and wrinkles:* folds and concertina-like wrinkling may result from ischemic collapse. Eventually, folds may consolidate as a thickened and laminated area of GBM; similar changes may also be seen around the periphery of the mesangium.
- *Double contouring (interposition):* the GBM appears duplicated due to the interposition of mesangial cells and matrix between the GBM and the endothelium in the capillary loop (sometimes called 'tram-tracking' when seen by light microscopy) (Fig. 22.11).

- *Subendothelial widening:* the space between the endothelium and the GBM may become widened with an accumulation of flocculent material or, more rarely, cellular elements from the blood (as in hemolytic uremic syndrome).
- *Gaps:* rarely, small discontinuities are seen in the GBM. Such gaps are of unknown diagnostic significance. Although it has been speculated that GBM discontinuities are responsible for hematuria, few are seen, even in cases of macroscopic hematuria.

Table 22.6 Renal diseases with fibrillar deposits: the ultrastructural features of renal amyloid and immunotactoid glomerulopathy (fibrillary glomerulonephritis)

	Diagnostic ultrastructural features	
	Amyloid	Immunotactoid glomerulopathy (fibrillary glomerulonephritis)*
Capillary wall		
GBM morphology: contour, width, texture	Thickened and irregular due to deposition of amyloid fibrils	Diffuse thickening frequent
GBM deposit: type, location	Deposits Congo red positive by LM Typical amyloid deposits: extracellular fine non-branching fibrils ~7–10 nm in diameter; variable in location Fibrils tangled and irregular; not organized (Fig. 22.13)	Deposits Congo red negative by LM Extracellular non-branching fibrils or tubules ~9 to >50 nm in diameter, mostly randomly arranged but sometimes packed into parallel arrays (Fig. 22.14) (Schwartz 1998) Fibrils variable in location: subendothelial, subepithelial, and intramembranous
Visceral epithelium	Often widespread foot process obliteration	Diffuse foot process effacement may be present
Endothelium, subendothelial plane	Normal	Normal
Mesangium		
Matrix	Amyloid deposits	Expansion may be present
Deposits	Amyloid fibrils Fibrils tangled and irregular; not organized (Fig. 22.13)	Mesangial deposits present in most cases Fibrillar/tubular, mostly randomly arranged; 9–50 nm (or greater) in diameter
Cells	Normal	Mild hypercellularity associated with deposits

*Note: some authors use 'fibrillary glomerulonephritis' for disease where the fibril diameter averages ~20 nm, reserving 'immunotactoid glomerulopathy' for cases in which the fibrils are tubular with a diameter of ~30–50 nm; others use the terms synonymously (Alpers 1992; Verani 1993; Jennette et al. 1994; Rostagno et al. 1996; Strom et al. 1996; Schwartz 1998).

Furthermore, some authors restrict a diagnosis of immunotactoid glomerulopathy to situations in which no underlying systemic disease has been identified (Schwartz 1998).

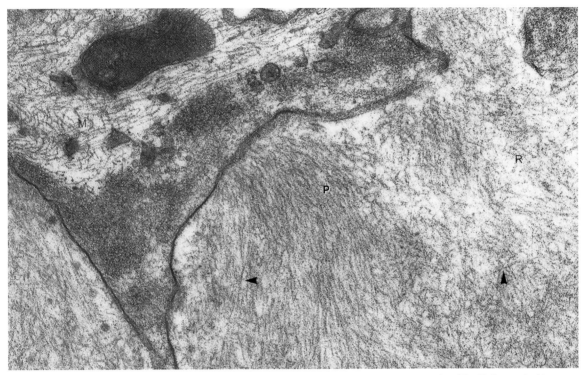

Figure 22.13 Amyloid. Typical fine, non-branching, extracellular amyloid fibrils in the glomerular mesangium. The fibrils seen in this micrograph are arranged randomly (R) and in parallel (P). Individual fibrils (arrowheads) are 8–10 nm in diameter. Mesangial cell cytoplasm (M).

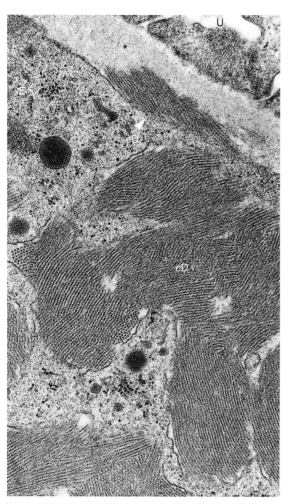

Figure 22.14 Immunotactoid glomerulopathy (fibrillary GN). Fibrillar deposits are seen in the subendothelial zone (eD) and within the capillary lumen (cD). Individual fibrils are ~20 nm in diameter. GBM (*), endothelial cell cytoplasm (En), urinary space (U).

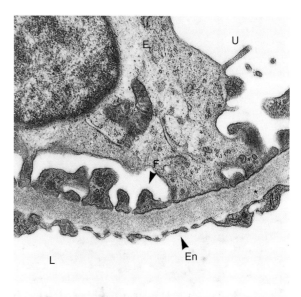

Figure 22.15 Normal GBM. A length of normal GBM (*) with a mean width of ~390 nm. Compare this membrane with Figures 22.16–22.19, which illustrate various types of abnormal GBM at the same magnification. Urinary space (U), epithelial cell (E) and foot processes (F), fenestrated endothelium (En), capillary lumen (L).

	Diagnostic ultrastructural features		
	Diabetic glomerulosclerosis	Minimal change disease	Nephrotic focal/segmental glomerulosclerosis
Capillary wall			
GBM morphology: contour, width, texture	Uniform increase in GBM thickness Thickening may be considerable with GBM greater than 1000 nm in width (Fig. 22.16)	Variable thinning (Coleman & Stirling 1991) Thinning minor but GBM may be less than ~300 nm in width (Fig. 22.17)	Segmental sclerosis; secondary ischemic change (GBM folding and consolidation)
GBM deposit: type, location	Nil	Nil	Nil
Visceral epithelium	Variable foot process obliteration	Diffuse foot process obliteration is the main feature (Fig. 22.17) Microvillous transformation	Diffuse foot process obliteration (Segmental sclerosis and foot process obliteration are essential for the diagnosis)
Endothelium, subendothelial plane	Normal	Normal	Normal
Mesangium			
Matrix	Increased, sometimes into nodular aggregates	Normal	Segmental sclerosis in some cases, especially juxtamedullary glomeruli
Deposits	Nil	Nil	Nil
Cells	Normal	Normal	Proliferation in some cases

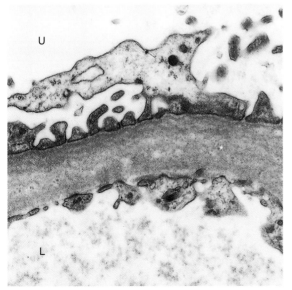

Figure 22.16 Diabetes. In diabetes the GBM (*) typically shows uniform thickening. In this case the GBM is moderately thickened, with a mean width of ~919 nm. Urinary space (U), capillary lumen (L).

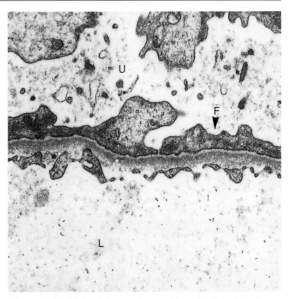

Figure 22.17 Minimal change disease. The epithelial cell foot processes (F) are completely effaced. The GBM (*) is slightly thinned, with a mean width of ~226 nm. Urinary space (U), capillary lumen (L).

Table 22.8 Familial renal diseases with changes in GBM thickness or texture: the ultrastructural features of benign essential hematuria and Alport's disease

	Diagnostic ultrastructural features	
	Benign essential hematuria	Alport's syndrome
Capillary wall		
GBM morphology: contour, width, texture	Variable thinning is the main feature Thinning may be considerable with GBM less than 150 nm in width (Fig. 22.18)	Alternating areas of thinning and thickening with lamellation (basket-weave pattern) Variability in width of GBM may be extreme (reported by Stirling et al. 1999b as 127–886 nm) (Fig. 22.19) Thickness calculations may be misleading, with overall GBM mean near normal value
GBM deposit: type, location	Normal	Normal
Visceral epithelium	May show focal foot process obliteration	May show focal foot process obliteration
Endothelium, subendothelial plane	Normal	Normal
Mesangium		
Matrix	Normal	Normal
Deposits	Normal	Normal
Cells	Normal	Normal

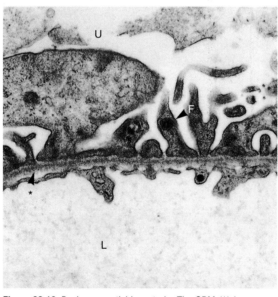

Figure 22.18 Benign essential hematuria. The GBM (*) is extremely thin, with a mean width of ~183 nm. The foot processes (F) are generally intact but show minor areas of effacement ('smudging'). Urinary space (U), capillary lumen (L).

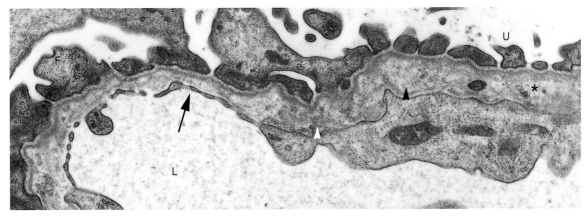

Figure 22.19 Alport's syndrome. In Alport's syndrome the GBM may be extremely irregular, with thickened, thinned and lamellated areas. In this example the membrane is 260–900 nm in width. The thickened section of the GBM (*) is lamellated (arrowheads). Foot processes are 'smudged' (F). Thinned area (arrow), urinary space (U), capillary lumen (L).

Morphological and numerical changes in the cellular components of the glomerulus

Changes of diagnostic significance may also occur in the cellular elements of the glomerulus. The most significant include (Stirling et al. 1999b):

- *Capillary endothelium:* cytoplasmic tubuloreticular inclusions may be found in the endothelial cytoplasm and are most common in SLE (Fig. 22.20).
- *Visceral epithelium:* the epithelial cell foot processes may be effaced to form a continuous (or semi-continuous) layer of cytoplasm (Fig. 22.17).
- *Mesangial cells:* mesangial cells may increase in number; the matrix may also be increased.

Malignant tumors

Mesothelioma

Mesothelioma is morphologically diverse, with three major types generally recognized: epithelial, mixed (biphasic) and sarcomatoid (Ray & Kindler 2009). Unusual variants and subtypes also occur and mesothelioma may mimic other tumor types

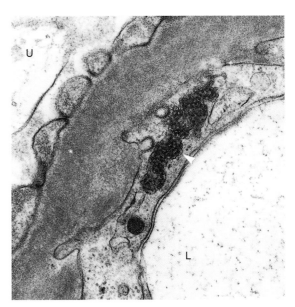

Figure 22.20 Systemic lupus erythematosus. Tubuloreticular inclusion (arrowhead) in the cytoplasm of an endothelial cell. GBM (*), urinary space (U), capillary lumen (L).

(Henderson et al. 1992, 1997) so that diagnosis is problematic (Addis & Roche 2009).

TEM is recommended when (Comin et al. 1997):

- the sample is small (cytological specimens, including cell block preparations)

- the histological appearances are atypical
- the immunohistological findings are atypical

For an unequivocal diagnosis of mesothelioma, mesothelial hyperplasia and metastatic tumor mimicking mesothelioma (especially adenocarcinoma) must be excluded (Henderson 1982; Oury et al. 1998).

Ultrastructural features that can help to distinguish between epithelial mesothelioma and adenocarcinoma include:

- *Microvilli:* mesothelial cells have longer microvilli than those of adenocarcinoma (Fig. 22.21) (Coleman et al. 1989; Henderson et al. 1992), with a mean length-to-diameter ratio (LDR) of 11.9 (standard deviation 5.87, range 4.8–21.3) (Warhol et al. 1982) versus a mean LDR of 5.28 (standard deviation 2.3, range 2.3–10).

- *Contact between stromal collagen fibrils and microvilli:* in mesothelioma, microvilli may be found interdigitating, or in contact, with stromal collagen fibrils (Fig. 22.21) (Carstens 1992). This feature is also found occasionally in adenocarcinoma and is regarded as predictive of mesothelioma rather than an absolute discriminator (Carstens 1992).

- *Cytoplasmic filaments:* intermediate filaments are common in mesothelioma. Filaments are often aggregated into tonofilaments and are characteristically seen near the nucleus (Fig. 22.22) (Henderson et al. 1992).

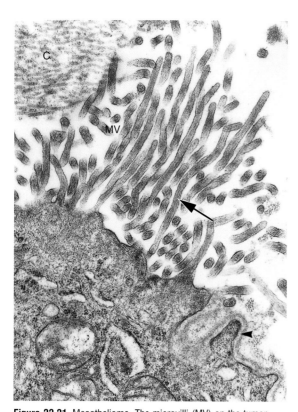

Figure 22.21 Mesothelioma. The microvilli (MV) on the tumor cell shown here project through a discontinuous basal lamina (arrowhead) and are in contact with stromal collagen fibrils (C). In mesothelioma the microvilli are much longer than those of adenocarcinoma and have an LDR greater than 11.9. The microvillus marked (arrow) is ~1900 nm long and 86 nm wide (LDR = 22).

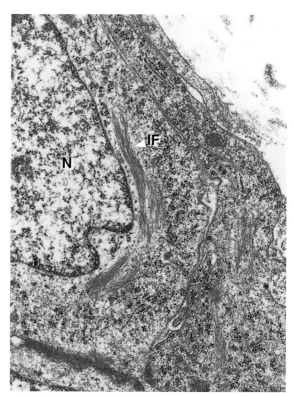

Figure 22.22 Mesothelioma. Cytoplasmic intermediate filaments (IF) are common in mesothelioma, especially near the nucleus (N).

- *Mucin granules:* for a diagnosis of mesothelioma, mucin granules should be absent.

Langerhans' histiocytosis (histiocytosis X)

In Langerhans' histiocytosis (LH) the tumor cells are deviant macrophage-dendritic cells that are structurally similar to the Langerhans' histiocyte (Egeler et al. 2010). LH cells are identified at the ultrastructural level by the presence of Langerhans' cell granules (Birbeck bodies or X bodies) (Fig. 22.23) which are induced by the expression of langerin (Valladeau et al. 2000). TEM has been the gold standard for diagnosing LH for many years. However, although TEM might still be useful, the immunohistochemical detection of langerin expression may now be a better option (Egeler et al. 2010). It should be noted that Birbeck bodies are not specific for LH as they may also be found in other disorders (Henderson et al. 1986; Erlandson 1994).

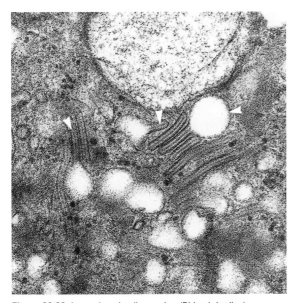

Figure 22.23 Langerhans' cell granules (Birbeck bodies). Langerhans' cell granules (arrowheads) are typical of the Langerhans' histiocyte and the tumor cells of Langerhans' histiocytosis. The granules comprise a short rod-like structure with a clear vesicle at one end.

Primitive neuroectodermal (neuroepithelial) tumor (PNET) and Ewing's tumor

The Ewing's sarcoma family of tumors is a histologically heterogeneous group now considered to consist of three subgroups: PNET (with neuroectodermal phenotype); Ewing's sarcoma (ES); and atypical ES/PNET (Llombart-Bosch et al. 2009). The group have a common translocation, typically t(11;22) *EWSR1-FLI1* (Lessnick et al. 2009). Tumor identification is often problematic and generally requires a combination of immunohistochemical and molecular techniques (Llombart-Bosch et al. 2009).

At the ultrastructural level PNETs typically consist of cells 10–17 µm in size with little intervening stroma. The principal characteristic feature is the presence of variable numbers of cytoplasmic processes which may be elongate (sometimes sinuous and branching) or short and blunt. Within these processes, microtubules and filaments are found in small numbers. Neurosecretory granules vary in number and appearance. Some are lysosomal in appearance, whilst others are similar to typical dense-core neurosecretory granules (Henderson et al. 1989). In comparison, the cells of Ewing's tumor are completely undifferentiated (Henderson et al. 1989).

Non-neoplastic diseases

Skeletal muscle

A wide range of ultrastructural changes are seen in skeletal muscle in primary muscle diseases, as secondary events in neurological diseases and in some systemic diseases. Since it is contractile, skeletal muscle is prone to sampling artifacts and must be biopsied and processed carefully. Practical guidelines are given by Pearl and Ghatak (1995) and Dubowitz and Sewry (2007). Only a small number of the ultrastructural changes that may be found are specific and diagnostically significant (Papadimitriou et al. 1992a; Stirling et al. 1999b); the principal features are summarized in Table 22.9.

Table 22.9 Skeletal muscle – summary of major ultrastructural abnormalities (Schochet & Lampert 1978; Papadimitriou et al. 1992a; Stirling et al. 1999b)

Structural element	Alteration and disease state
Satellite cells	Rare in normal muscle.
	Frequent in regenerating and denervated muscle.
	Increased in polymyositis, Duchenne muscular dystrophy, congenital myotonic dystrophy, Werdnig-Hoffman disease, and Kugelberg-Welander syndrome.
	May display evidence of activation and myogenic differentiation.
	May be confused with invading inflammatory cells.
Nuclei	Large internal nuclei in recently regenerated myofibers.
	Contours convoluted in atrophy and nemaline myopathy.
	Abundant internal nuclei found in various myopathies. Internal nuclei especially numerous, and arranged in chains, in myotonic dystrophy. Chains of internal nuclei a distinctive feature of centronuclear (myotubular) myopathy.
	A variety of vacuoles, inclusions, and pseudoinclusions present in a wide range of diseases.
	Nemaline bodies found in a few cases of polymyositis and some cases of late-onset rod diseases.
	Filamentous intranuclear inclusions resembling myxovirus in polymyositis and chronic distal myopathy. Fibrillar inclusions present in inclusion body myositis and polymyositis.
	Annulate lamellae present in a range of diseases.
Myofibrils	Hypercontracted myofibrils non-specific and often artifactual.
	Aberrant bundles of normal fibrils spiraling, or encircling, the long axis of myofibers are frequent in myotonic dystrophy. This feature is also observed in other diseases.
	Sarcomeres with disorganized myofibrils are non-specific but common in congenital myopathies (multicore and minicore diseases).
	Extensive disorganization of central region of type 1 myofibers is the major lesion in 'target' and 'core-targetoid' fibers.
	Target fibers occur in denervation, re-innervation, polymyositis, and familial periodic paralysis.
	Core-targetoid lesions present in denervating and myopathic conditions and in the aged.
	Peripheral subsarcolemmal aggregates of disorganized myofibrils and sarcoplasm are found in a variety of disorders but are characteristic of myotonic dystrophy.
Z-discs	Z-disc abnormalities are common in many disease states. Streaming of Z-disc material, Z-disc duplication, and zig-zag irregularities are the most common lesions.
	Characteristic rod-shaped electron-dense bodies (nemaline bodies), 6–7 μm long and similar in appearance to Z-discs, are common in nemaline myopathy. These bodies contain actin and α-actinin and are also found sporadically in other diseases.
	Widespread loss of Z-disc material noted in a variety of diseases.
	Discrete osmiophilic cytoplasmic bodies, thought to be related to Z-discs, noted in a wide range of diseased myofibers.

Table 22.9 *(continued)*

Structural element	Alteration and disease state
Mitochondria	Swelling, with deposition of osmiophilic material or formation of myelin figures, common and non-specific. Swelling may result from suboptimal fixation. Changes in numbers common and non-specific. Re-orientation of intermyofibrillar mitochondria (in relation to myofiber) occurs in a range of diseases. Structural abnormalities common (some associated with biochemical deficiencies) and present in a wide range of diseases, including the 'mitochondrial myopathies' and 'mitochondrial encephalomyopathies'. Electron-dense granules and crystalline inclusions present in a wide range of diseases.
Transverse tubular system	Abnormalities in triads common in injured and atrophic fibers. Dilation is a common artifact but may also be present in a variety of diseases. Coalescence of T-system tubules to give a honeycomb pattern may be present in a wide range of diseases.
Sarcoplasmic reticulum	Dilation of cisternae prominent in periodic paralyses and some other diseases. Elongated tubular aggregates (probably derived from sarcoplasmic reticulum) reported in the periodic paralyses and other diseases. Cylindrical structures in a spiral pattern, and with a core of glycogen, observed in a variety of diseases.
Inclusions and deposits	Filamentous bodies; concentric laminated bodies; zebra-striped bodies; fingerprint bodies; reducing bodies; spheroidal bodies; and paracrystalline arrays present in the sarcoplasm in a range of diseases. Excessive lipid accumulation present in a wide range of diseases. Glycogen abundant in fetal muscle and regenerating myofibers. Glycogen moderately increased in a range of diseases; massively increased in various glycogenoses. Autophagic vaculoes and lipopigments present in degenerative diseases and in almost any myopathic state.

Epidermolysis bullosa – mechanobullous dermatoses

Epidermolysis bullosa (EB) is a heterogeneous group of rare, inherited or acquired diseases in which the skin blisters easily under normal levels of mechanical stress. Based on the level of blister formation within the dermal-epidermal junction, EB has traditionally been classified into three major groups: simplex, junctional and dystrophic (Anton-Lamprecht 1992; Mellerio 1999; Pulkkinen and Uitto 1999). A fourth category, the hemidesmosomal group, has also been recognized. In this group, blister formation is at the basal cell/lamina lucida interface at the level of the hemidesmosomes (Pulkkinen & Uitto 1999).

TEM allows the precise level of blister formation to be determined, in combination with a morphological assessment of the basement membrane components (Table 22.10) (Anton-Lamprecht 1992; Jaunzems & Woods 1997; Jaunzems et al. 1997). For best results a fresh blister should be biopsied (Marinkovich 1999).

Cerebral autosomal dominant arteriopathy with subcortical infarcts and leukoencephalopathy (CADASIL)

CADASIL is a familial form of early-onset vascular dementia associated with single missense mutations to chromosome 19 (Notch 3 gene); at least 170

Table 22.10 Basic ultrastructural features of the major groups of congenital epidermolysis bullosa (EB)

EB main category	Plane of cleavage and ultrastructural features
Simplex (epidermolytic EB)	• Split above basal lamina through the cytoplasm of the basal keratinocytes, causing intra-epidermal blister formation • Degenerative cytolytic changes in basal keratinocytes • Tonofilaments are clumped in EB herpetiformis (Dowling-Meara) variant
Hemidesmosomal	• Split at basal keratinocyte/lamina lucida interface at the level of the hemidesmosomes • Hemidesmosomes rudimentary
Junctional (atrophicans)	• Split at level of lamina lucida, causing junctional blister formation • Hemidesmosomes abnormal and reduced in size or number
Dystrophic (dermolytic or scarring EB)	• Split below the lamina densa, causing dermolytic blister formation • Anchoring fibers absent, or few, or rudimentary • Collagen degradation present in some variants

mutations in 20 exons have been described (Ruchoux & Maurage 1997; Kalimo et al. 1999; Tikka et al. 2009). In addition to missense mutations, a pathogenic insertion has been reported by Mazzei et al. (2008) and a duplication of three codons has been described by Tikka et al. (2009). In affected vessels, basophilic, periodic acid Schiff positive deposits accumulate between the smooth muscle cells of the vessel walls. At the ultrastructural level these classic CADASIL-type deposits are often referred to as granular osmiophilic material (GOM) (Kalimo et al. 1999; Tikka et al. 2009).

Genetic screening for such a wide range of mutations is difficult. Strategies for diagnosis will depend on the patient's background and the presence of known mutations that will allow genetic testing to be targeted to a limited number of exons. Although the sensitivity of TEM screening of skin biopsies has been debated, a retrospective study of genetically positive CADASIL cases by Tikka et al. (2009) found typical GOMs in all the patients tested. TEM was therefore regarded as both reliable and practical. TEM also has the added advantage of being able to identify cases in which the mutation present has not been previously described. For TEM screening, a 4 mm punch biopsy of skin is generally adequate. However, the tissue must be well-fixed in glutaraldehyde (tissue fixed in formalin may not be

adequate). GOMs may be patchy in distribution so, to ensure that enough tissue is screened, it is recommended that a minimum of three blocks and 50 vessels are observed. Furthermore, because GOMs are more common adjacent to larger vessels, Tikka et al. (2009) also recommend that the material should include a number of small arterial vessels with well-differentiated pericytes or smooth muscle cells such as those found in the border zone between deep dermis and upper subcutis.

Ultrastructurally, GOMs are seen as extracellular electron-dense granular material that is often in contact with the vascular pericytes and smooth muscle cells and sited in a small indentation (Fig. 22.24). Both GOMs and non-specific granular osmiophilic material may also be found within the intercellular stroma: for an unequivocal diagnosis, GOMs sited in cellular indentations must be identified (Bergmann et al. 1996; Ruchoux & Maurage 1998; Tikka et al. 2009).

Amyloid

Amyloid deposition is associated with a wide range of disorders and can be either hereditary or acquired. Amyloid deposits may also be focal, localized or systemic (Gillmore et al. 1997). By TEM, amyloid is seen as randomly arranged extracellular

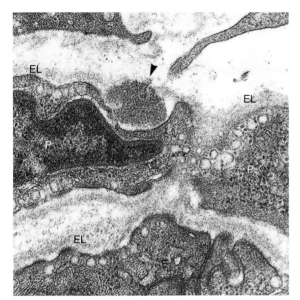

Figure 22.24 CADASIL. In affected vessels electron-dense material (arrowhead) is seen in close proximity to the pericytes or perivascular smooth muscle cells. The material is often sited (as seen here) in an indentation in the cell wall. Pericytes (P), external lamina (EL), capillary endothelial cell (E).

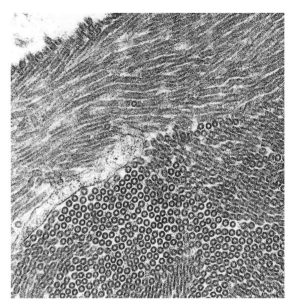

Figure 22.25 Paraproteinemic crystalloidal keratopathy. Extracellular tubular crystalloids are found throughout the corneal stroma in this case. Tubules are thick-walled and of indeterminate length. Overall tubule diameter is 40–45 nm. The crystalloids labeled for κ-light chains in immunogold labeling studies (Henderson et al. 1993).

non-branching fibrils. Individual fibrils are of indeterminate length and approximately 7–10 nm in diameter (Fig. 22.13) (Harvey & Anton-Lamprecht 1992; Gillmore et al. 1997).

Cornea

TEM is useful for identifying corneal deposits and inclusions, particularly amyloid and immunoglobulin deposits in diseases such as paraproteinemic crystalloidal keratopathy (PCK). In PCK, immunoglobulin deposits may be seen in the corneal stroma either as organized or randomly arranged extracellular tubules (Fig. 22.25) (Stirling & Graff 1995; Stirling et al. 1997) or as intracellular crystalloids with a fine fibrillar substructure (Fig. 22.26) (Henderson et al. 1993).

Cilia

Cilia are small motile structures approximately 5–10 μm long and 0.5 μm in diameter. Within the

ciliary shaft there is a core of microtubules (the axoneme) composed of nine outer pairs of microtubules and one inner (central) pair, an arrangement referred to as the '9 + 2' configuration (Fig. 22.27) (Sturgess & Turner 1984; Young & Heath 2000).

A wide range of primary and secondary structural defects may be found in cilia; secondary defects, such as disorganized microtubules, can be ignored (Sturgess & Turner 1984; Carson et al. 1994). Primary defects are caused by a heterogeneous group of genetic abnormalities that result in immotile cilia syndrome (primary ciliary dyskinesia – PCD) and a range of associated diseases (Meeks & Bush 2000; Cardenas-Rodriguez & Badano 2009). In PCD, the ciliary defects are permanent and all cilia in the body are affected (Corrin & Dewar 1992; Mierau et al. 1992). With this fact in mind it is generally said that the finding of a single normal cilium mitigates against a diagnosis of PCD. However, it should also be noted that not all genetic defects result in abnormal ciliary morphology (Santamaria et al. 1999).

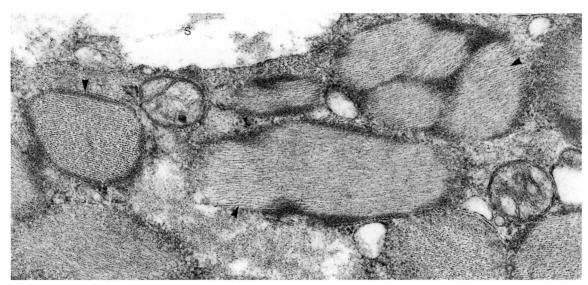

Figure 22.26 Paraproteinemic crystalloidal keratopathy. Intracellular fibrillary crystalloids (arrowheads) in the cytoplasm of a corneal keratinocyte. Filaments are approximately 8–10 nm in diameter. The crystalloids labeled for κ-light chains in immunogold labeling studies (Henderson et al. 1993). Extracellular stroma (S).

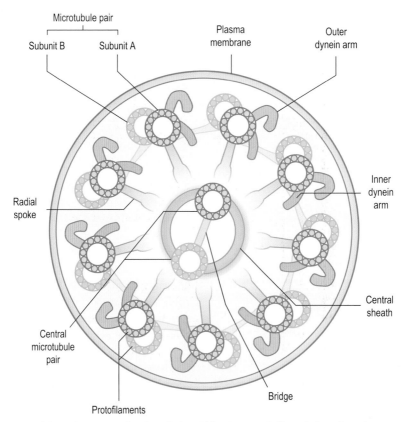

Figure 22.27 Normal cilium. Schematic cross-section through the middle of a normal ciliary shaft to show the structure of the axoneme. The axoneme is formed from an outer ring of nine microtubule pairs with one central pair (the 9 + 2 configuration). The outer microtubule pairs are formed from two subunits (A and B); each subunit is formed from a ring of protofilaments. Projecting from each complete microtubule in the outer microtubule pairs (subunit A) is a pair of inner and outer dynein arms. A variety of structures (the radial spokes, bridge and sheath) appear to link the tubule pairs together.

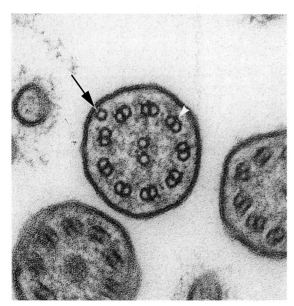

Figure 22.28 Primary ciliary dyskinesia: dynein arm defect. The outer microtubule pairs (arrowhead) lack dynein arms. A single extra displaced microtubule is also present (arrow).

In general it is recommended that screening for PCD should combine an analysis of cilial beat frequency and pattern using high-resolution digital high-speed video (DHSV) with a morphological analysis using TEM (Chilvers et al. 2003; Armengot et al. 2010). The principal morphological defects are (Sturgess & Turner 1984; Corrin & Dewar 1992; Mierau et al. 1992; Carson et al. 1994):

- Outer and/or inner dynein arms absent or short (most cases) (Fig. 22.28)
- Ciliary spokes absent
- Outer microtubular pairs absent, displaced, or discontinuous
- Central microtubular pair with one or both microtubules absent

Observations should be made in the middle of the ciliary shaft, and approximately 50 cilia are recommended as a minimum number for examination. In routinely processed specimens the inner arms are often indistinct. While this is undoubtedly a processing artifact, and such cilia are generally presumed to be normal, care must be taken to identify genuine inner arm defects.

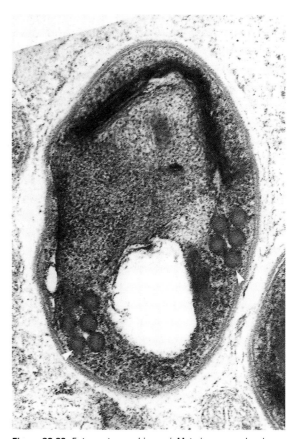

Figure 22.29 *Enterocytozoon bieneusi*. Maturing spore showing the coils of the polar tube. In *E. bieneusi* the polar tube has a range of 4–7 coils which, in cross-section, are seen arranged in two rows on either side of the spore. The spore shown has 5–6 coils on either side (arrowheads). (Electron micrograph courtesy of Dr Alan Curry.)

Microsporidia

The microsporidians are a group of obligate intracellular parasites belonging to the phylum Microspora (Curry 1998; Wasson & Peper 2000; Smith, 2009). Unclassified organisms are conveniently called by the collective name 'microsporidium' but this is not an official genus. Enterocytozoon oganisms are the most common species infecting humans (Figs 22.29 and 22.30) but an increasing number of species are being identified (Table 22.11) (Didier et al. 2009). In some cases the identification of the organism involved is preliminary or tentative. Although,

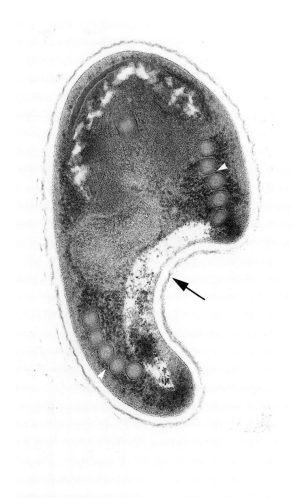

Figure 22.30 *Encephalitozoon hellem*. Spore of *E. hellem* showing the polar tube with five coils arranged in a single row on each side of the spore (arrowheads). The indentation (arrow) is an artifact caused by the collapse of the posterior vacuole. (Electron micrograph courtesy of Dr Alan Curry.)

Table 22.11 Microsporidia found in humans	
Species	**Citation**
Encephalitozoon hellem (Fig. 22.30)	Didier et al. 1991a, 1991b
Encephalitozoon cuniculi	Pakes et al. 1975, Canning et al. 1986
Encephalitozoon (Septata) intestinalis	Cali et al. 1993, Hartskeerl et al. 1995
Pleistophora ronneafiei	Cali & Takvorian 2003, Cali et al. 2005
Pleistophora sp.	Canning et al. 1986, Weber et al. 1994
Trachipleistophora hominis	Hollister et al. 1996
Trachipleistophora anthropophthera	Vavra et al. 1998
Enterocytozoon bieneusi (Fig 22.29)	Desportes et al. 1985, Curry 2000
Nosema ocularum	Cali et al. 1991
Nosema sp.	Curry et al. 2007
Vittaforma corneae (Nosema corneum)	Silveira & Canning 1995
Vittaforma sp.	Sulaiman et al. 2003
*Anncaliia vesicularum**	Cali et al. 1998
Anncaliia connori (Nosema connori)*	Sprague 1974, Cali et al. 1998
Anncaliia algerae (Nosema algerae)*	Visvesvara et al. 1999
Microsporidium ceylonensis[#]	Ashton & Wirasinha 1973, Canning et al. 1998
Microsporidium africanum[#]	Pinnolis et al. 1981

*Anncaliia replaces the genus *Brachiola* (Franzen et al. 2006).

[#]Unclassified organisms are conveniently called by the collective name 'microsporidium': this is not an official genus.

several types of *Nosema* have been found, the diversity of this group means that changes are likely to occur. Microsporidia may be found in almost any human tissue and, while the majority of infections occur in immunocompromised individuals such as HIV-positive persons and organ transplant recipients, healthy individuals may also be infected. The eye is particularly susceptible, especially if the use of topical steroids creates a locally immunocompromised state (Chan et al. 2003; Curry et al. 2007; Badenoch et al. in press). Co-infection by two species may also occur (Didier et al. 2009).

TEM plays an important role in the identification and speciation of microsporidians and is regarded by some as the gold standard for diagnosis (Curry 2000). The organisms can be examined using fecal material or tissue biopsies with standard TEM fixation and processing protocols (Weber et al. 1994). Miller and Simakova (2009) have suggested that staining with oolong tea extract may enhance the visibility of the substructure of the polar filament (Sato et al. 2008; Yamaguchi et al. 2010).

The major ultrastructural features used for typing microsporidia (see Garcia 1993; Bryan 1994; Weber et al. 1994; Curry 1998) are as follows:

- the size and morphology of the various developmental stages

- the configuration of the nuclei in spores and developmental stages

- the host-parasite interface

- the number, arrangement and diameter of coils in the tubular extrusion apparatus (polar tube) in spores (Figs 22.29 and 22.30).

Acknowledgments

We thank Richard Davey (IMVS Pathology) for his assistance in preparing the illustrations for this chapter and Dr Alan Curry (Manchester Royal Infirmary) for his helpful advice on microsporidians.

References

Acetarin, J.-D., Carlemalm, E., Villiger, W., 1986. Developments of new Lowicryl® resins for embedding biological specimens at even lower temperatures. Journal of Microscopy 143, 81–88.

Addis, B., Roche, H., 2009. Problems in mesothelioma diagnosis. Histopathology 54, 55–68.

Allen, D.E., Lawrence, F.A., 1994–96. Tissue preparation for transmission electron microscopy. In: Woods, A.E., Ellis, R.C. (Eds.), Laboratory histopathology: a complete reference. Churchill Livingstone, Edinburgh.

Alpers, C.E., 1992. Immunotactoid (microtubular) glomerulopathy: an entity distinct from fibrillary glomerulonephritis? American Journal of Kidney Disease 2, 185–191.

Anton-Lamprecht, I., 1992. The skin. In: Papadimitriou, J.M., Henderson, D.W., Spagnolo, D.V. (Eds.), Diagnostic ultrastructure of non-neoplastic diseases. Churchill Livingstone, Edinburgh, Ch. 22, pp. 459–550.

Armengot, M., Milara, J., Mata, M., et al., 2010. Cilia motility and structure in primary and secondary ciliary dyskinesia. American Journal of Rhinology & Allergy 24, 175–180.

Ashton, N., Wirasinha, P.A., 1973. Encephalitozoonosis (Nosematosis) of the cornea. British Journal of Ophthalmology 57, 669–674.

Badenoch, P.R., Coster, D.J., Sadlon, T.A., et al., (in press) Deep microsporidial keratitis after keratoconjunctivitis. Clinical and Experimental Ophthalmology.

Bergmann, M., Ebke, M., Yuan, Y., et al., 1996. Cerebral autosomal dominant arteriopathy with subcortical infarcts and leukoencephalopathy (CADASIL): a morphological study of a German family. Acta Neuropathologica (Berlin) 92, 341–350.

Bretschneider, A., Burns, W., Morrison, A., 1981. 'Pop-off' technic. The ultrastructure of paraffin-embedded sections. American Journal of Clinical Pathology 76, 450–453.

Bryan, R.T., 1994. Microsporidia. In: Mandell, G.L. Bennett, J.E., Dolin, R. (Eds.), Principles and practice of infectious diseases, fourth ed. Churchill Livingstone, New York, Part III, Ch. 264, pp. 2513–2524.

Cali, A., Takvorian, P.M., 2003. Ultrastructure and development of *Pleistophora ronneafiei* n. sp., a microsporidium (Protista) in the skeletal muscle of an immune-compromised individual. Journal of Eukaryotic Microbiology 50 (2), 77-85.

Cali, A., Meisler, D., Lowder, C.Y., et al., 1991. Corneal microsporidioses: characterisation and identification. Journal of Eucaryotic Microbiology 38, 215S–217S.

Cali, A., Kotler, D.P., Orenstein, J.M., 1993. *Septata intestinalis* n.g., n.sp., an intestinal microsporidian associated with chronic diarrhea and dissemination in AIDS patients. Journal of Protozoologyy 40, 101–112.

Cali, A., Takvorian, P.M., Lewin, S., et al., 1998. *Brachiola vesicularum*, n.g., n. sp., a new microsporium associated with AIDS and myositis. Journal of Eucaryotic Microbiology 45, 240–251.

Cali, A., Weiss, L.M., Takvorian, L.M., 2005. A review of the development of two types of human skeletal muscle infections from microsporidia associated with pathology in invertebrates and cold-blooded vertebrates. Folia Parasitologica 52, 1–11.

Canning, E.U., Lom, J., Dykova, I., 1986. The microporidia of vertebrates. Academic Press, New York.

Canning, E.U., Curry, A., Vavra, J., Bonshek, R.E., 1998. Some ultrastructural data on *Microsporidium ceylonensis*, a cause of corneal microsporidiosis. Parasite 5 (3), 247–254.

Cardenas-Rodriguez M., Badano J.L., 2009. Ciliary biology: understanding the cellular and genetic basis of human ciliopathies. American Journal of Medical Genetics Part C: Seminars in Medical Genetics 151C, 263–280.

Carson, J.L., Collier, A.M., Fernald, G.W., Hu, S.S., 1994. Microtubular discontinuities as acquired ciliary defects in airway epithelium of patients with chronic respiratory diseases. Ultrastructural Pathology 18, 327–332.

Carstens, P.H.B., 1992. Contact between abluminal microvilli and collagen fibrils in metastatic adenocarcinoma and mesothelioma. Journal of Pathology 166, 179–182.

Causton, B.E., 1981. Resins: toxicity, hazards and safe handling. Proceedings of the Royal Microscopy Society 16, 265–269.

Chan, C.C., Theng, J.T., Li, L., Tan, D.T., 2003. Microsporidial keratoconjunctivitis in healthy individuals. Ophthalmology 110(7), 1420–1425.

Chilvers, M.A., Rutman, A., O'Callaghan, C., 2003. Functional analysis of cilia and ciliated epithelial ultrastructure in healthy children and young adults. Thorax 58, 333–338.

Coleman, M., Stirling, J.W., 1991. Glomerular basement membrane thinning is acquired in minimal change disease. American Journal of Nephrology 11, 437–438.

Coleman, M., Haynes, W.D.G., Dimopoulos, P., et al., 1986. Glomerular basement membrane abnormalities associated with apparently idiopathic hematuria: ultrastructural morphometric analysis. Human Pathology 17, 1022–1030.

Coleman, M., Henderson, D.W., Mukherjee, T.M., 1989. The ultrastructural pathology of malignant pleural mesothelioma. Pathology Annual 24(1), 303–353.

Comin, C.E., de Klerk, N.H., Henderson, D.W., 1997. Malignant mesothelioma: current conundrums over risk estimates and whither electron microscopy for diagnosis? Ultrastructural Pathology 21, 315–320.

Corrin, B., Dewar, A., 1992. Respiratory diseases. In: Papadimitriou, J.M., Henderson, D.W., Spagnolo, D.V. (Eds.), Diagnostic ultrastructure of non-neoplastic diseases. Churchill Livingstone, Edinburgh, Ch. 13, pp. 264–286.

Curry, A., 1998. Microsporidians. In: Cox, F., Kreier, J., Wakelin, D. (Eds.), Topley and Wilson's microbiology and microbial infections, Vol. 5, ninth ed. Arnold, London, Ch. 21, pp. 411–430.

Curry, A., 2000. Electron microscopy as a tool for identifying new pathogens. Journal of Infection 40, 107–115.

Curry, A., Mudhar, H.S., Dewan, S., et al., 2007. A case of bilateral microsporidial keratitis from Bangladesh – infection by an insect parasite from the genus *Nosema*. Journal of Medical Microbiology 56, 1250–1252.

Daddow, L.Y.M., 1983. A double lead stain method for enhancing contrast of ultrathin sections in electron microscopy: a modified multiple staining technique. Journal of Microscopy 129, 147–153.

Desportes, I., Le Charpentier, Y., Galian, A., et al., 1985. Occurrence of a new microsporidian: *Enterozoon bieneusi* n.g., n.sp., in the enterocytes of a human patient with AIDS. Journal of Protozoology 32, 250–254.

Didier, E.S., Didier, P.J., Friedberg, D.N., et al., 1991a. Isolation and characterisation of a new human microsporidian, *Encephalitozoon hellem* (n.sp.), from three AIDS patients with keratoconjunctivitis. Journal of Infectious Diseases 163, 617–621.

Didier, P.J., Didier, E.S., Orenstein, J.M., Shadduck, J.A., 1991b. Fine structure of a new human microsporidian, *Encephalitozoon hellem*, in culture. Journal of Protozoology 38, 502–507.

Didier, E.S., Weiss, L.M., Cali, A., Marciano-Cabral, F., 2009. Overview of presentations on microsporidia and free-living amebae at the 10th International Workshops on Opportunistic Protists. Eukaryotic Cell 8(4), 441–445.

Dubowitz, V., Sewry, C.A., Lane, R., 2007. Muscle biopsy: a practical approach. Saunders Elsevier, London.

Dykstra, M.J., 1992. Biological electron microscopy: theory, techniques and troubleshooting. Plenum Press, New York.

Egeler, R.M., van Halteren, A.G.S., Hogendoorn, P.C.W., et al., 2010. Langerhans cell histiocytosis: fascinating dynamics of the dendritic cell–macrophage lineage. Immunological Reviews 234, 213–232.

Erlandson, R.A., 1994. Diagnostic transmission electron microscopy of tumors. Raven Press, New York.

Ferguson, W.J., Braunschweiger, K.I., Braunschweiger, W.R., et al., 1980. Hydrogen ion buffers for biological research. Analytical Biochemistry 104, 300–310.

Franzen, C., Nassonova, E.S., Schölmerich, J., Issi, I.V., 2006. Transfer of the members of the genus *Brachiola* (Microsporidia) to the genus *Anncaliia* based on ultrastructural and molecular data. Journal of Eukaryotic Microbiology 53, 26–35.

Garcia, L.S., Bruckner, D.A., 1993. Diagnostic medical microbiology, second ed. American Society for Microbiology, Washington DC.

Ghadially, F.N., 1985. Diagnostic electron microscopy of tumors, second ed. Butterworths, London.

Ghadially, F.N., 1997. Ultrastructural pathology of the cell and matrix, fourth ed, Vols 1–2. Butterworth-Heinemann, Boston.

Gillmore, J.D., Hawkins, P.N., Pepys, M.B., 1997. Amyloidosis: a review of recent diagnostic and therapeutic developments. British Journal of Haematology 99, 245–256.

Glauert, A.M., 1972–1998. Practical methods in electron microscopy, Vols 1–17. North Holland, Amsterdam.

Glauert, A.M., Glauert, R.H., 1958. Araldite as an embedding medium for electron microscopy. Journal of Biophysical and Biochemical Cytology 4, 191–194.

Glauert, A.M., Lewis, P.R., 1998. Biological specimen preparation for transmission electron microscopy. Practical methods in electron microscopy, Vol. 17. Portland Press, London.

Glauert, A.M., Rogers, G.E., Glauert, R.H., 1956. A new embedding medium for electron microscopy. Nature 178, 803.

Gomori, G., 1955. Preparation of buffers for use in enzyme studies. Methods in Enzymology 1, 138–146.

Good, N.E., Izawa, S., 1972. Hydrogen ion buffers. Methods in Enzymology 24, 53–68.

Good, N.E., Winget, G.D., Winter, W., et al., 1966. Hydrogen ions for biological research. Biochemistry 5, 467–477.

Hartskeerl, R.A., Van Gool, T., Schuitema, A.R., et al., 1995. Genetic and immunological characterisation of the microsporidian *Septata intestinalis Cali*, Kotler and Orenstein 1993: reclassification to *Encephalitozoon intestinalis*. Parasitology 110, 277–285.

Harvey, J.M., Anton-Lamprecht, I., 1992. Stromal aberrations. In: Papadimitriou, J.M., Henderson, D.W., Spagnolo, D.V. (Eds.), Diagnostic ultrastructure of non-neoplastic diseases. Churchill Livingstone, Edinburgh, Ch. 5, pp. 84–109.

Hayat, M.A., 1981. Fixation for electron microscopy. Academic Press, New York.

Hayat, M.A., 1993. Stains and cytochemical methods. Plenum Press, New York.

Hayat, M.A., 2000. Principles and techniques of electron microscopy, biological applications, fourth ed. Cambridge University Press, Cambridge.

Henderson, D.W., 1982. Asbestos-related pleuropulmonary diseases: asbestosis, mesothelioma and lung cancer. Pathology 14, 239–243.

Henderson, D.W., Papadimitriou, J.M., Coleman, M., 1986. Ultrastructural appearances of tumors. diagnosis and classification of human neoplasia by electron microscopy, second ed. Churchill Livingstone, Edinburgh.

Henderson, D.W., Leppard, P.J., Brennan, J.S., et al., 1989. Primitive neuroepithelial tumors of soft tissues and bone: further ultrastructural and immunocytochemical clarification of 'Ewing's sarcoma', including freeze-fracture analysis. Journal of Submicroscopic Cytology and Pathology 21(1), 35–57.

Henderson, D.W., Shilkin, K.B., Whitaker, D., et al., 1992. The pathology of malignant mesothelioma, including immunohistology and ultrastructure. In: Henderson, D.W., Shilkin, K.B., Langlois, S., Le P., Whitaker, D., (Eds.), Malignant mesothelioma. Hemisphere, New York, Ch. 2, pp. 69–139.

Henderson, D.W., Stirling, J.W., Lipsett, J., et al., 1993. Paraproteinemic crystalloidal keratopathy: an ultrastructural study of two cases, including immunoelectron microscopy. Ultrastructural Pathology 17, 643–668.

Henderson, D.W., Comin, C.E., Hammar, S.P., et al., 1997. Malignant mesothelioma of the pleura: current surgical pathology. In: Corrin, B. (Ed.), Pathology of lung tumors. Churchill Livingstone, New York, Ch. 15, pp. 241–280.

Herrera, G.A., Turbat-Herrera, E.A., 2010. Renal diseases with organized deposits. An algorithmic approach to classification and clinicopathologic diagnosis. Archives of Pathology and Laboratory Medicine 134, 512–531.

Hollister, W.S., Canning, E.U., Weidner, E., et al., 1996. Development and ultrastructure of *Trachipleistophora hominis* n.g., n.sp. after *in vitro* isolation from an AIDS patient and inoculation into athymic mice. Parasitology 112 (1), 143–154.

Jaunzems, A.E., Woods, A.E., 1997. Ultrastructural differentiation of epidermolysis bullosa subtypes and porphyria cutanea tarda. Pathology, Research and Practice 193, 207–217.

Jaunzems, A.E., Woods, A.E., Staples, A., 1997. Electron microscopy and morphometry enhances differentiation of epidermolysis bullosa subtypes with normal values for 24 parameters in skin. Archives of Dermatological Research 289(11), 631–639.

Jennette, J.C., Iskandar, S.S., Falk, R.J., 1994. Fibrillary glomerulonephritis. In: Tisher, C.C., Brenner, B.M. (Eds.), Renal pathology with clinical and functional correlations, second ed. Lippincott, Philadelphia.

Jennette, J.C., Olson, J.L., Schwartz, M.M., Silva, F.G. (Eds.), 1998. Heptinstall's pathology of the kidney, fifth ed, Vols 1–2. Lippincott-Raven, Philadelphia.

Jolanki, R., Kanerva, L., Estlander, T., et al., 1990. Occupational dermatoses from epoxy resin compounds. Contact Dermatitis 23, 172–183.

Kalimo, H., Viitanen, M., Amberla, K., et al., 1999. CADASIL: hereditary disease of arteries causing brain infarcts and dementia. Neuropathology and Applied Neurobiology 25(4), 257–265.

Kanerva, L., Estlander, T., Jolanki, R., 1989. Allergic contact dermatitis from dental composite resins due to aromatic epoxy acrylates and aliphatic acrylates. Contact Dermatitis 20, 201–211.

Karnovsky, M.J., 1965. A formaldehyde-glutaraldehyde fixative of high osmolarity for use in electron microscopy. Journal of Cell Biology 27, 137A.

Leong, A.S.-Y., 1994. Fixation and fixatives. In: Woods, A.E., Ellis, R.C. (Eds.), Laboratory histopathology: a complete reference. Churchill Livingstone, Edinburgh.

Lessnick, S.L., Tos, A.P.D., Sorensen, P.H.B., et al., 2009. Small round cell sarcomas. Seminars in Oncology 36, 338–346.

Llombart-Bosch, A., Machado, L., Navarro, S., et al., 2009. Histological heterogeneity of Ewing's sarcoma/PNET: an immunohistochemical analysis of 415 genetically confirmed cases with clinical support. Virchows Archive 455, 397–411.

Luft, J.H., 1961. Improvements in epoxy resin embedding methods. Journal of Biophysical and Biochemical Cytology 9, 409–414.

Marinkovich, M.P., 1999. Update on inherited bullous dermatoses. Dermatologic Clinics 17(3), 473–485.

Massie, H.R., Samis, H.V., Baird, M.B., 1972. The effects of the buffer HEPES on the division potential of WI-38 cells. In Vitro 7, 191–197.

Mazzei, R., Guidetti, D., Ungaro, C., et al., 2008. First evidence of a pathogenic insertion in the NOTCH3 gene causing CADASIL. Journal of Neurology, Neurosurgery & Psychiatry 79(1), 108–110.

Meeks, M., Bush, A., 2000. Primary ciliary dyskinesia (PCD). Pediatric Pulmonology 29(4), 307–316.

Mellerio, J.E., 1999. Molecular pathology of the cutaneous basement membrane zone. Clinical and Experimental Dermatology 24, 25–32.

Mierau, G.W., Agostini, R., Beals, T.F., et al., 1992. The role of electron microscopy in evaluating ciliary dysfunction: Report of a workshop. Ultrastructural Pathology 16, 245–254.

Miller, A.A., Simakova, A.V., 2009. Use of the OTE-staining method for ultrathin sections on the example of microsporidia. Tsitologiia 51(9), 741–747.

Millonig, G., Marinozzi, V., 1968. Fixation and embedding in electron microscopy. In: Barer, R., Cosslett, V.E. (Eds.), Advances in optical and electron microscopy, Vol. 2. Academic Press, New York, p. 251.

Newman, G.R., Hobot, J.A., 1987. Modern acrylics for post-embedding immunostaining techniques. Journal of Histochemistry and Cytochemistry 35, 971–981.

Newman, G.R., Hobot, J.A., 1993. Resin microscopy and on-section immunocytochemistry. Springer-Verlag, Berlin.

Oury, T.D., Hammar, S.P., Roggli, V.L., 1998. Ultrastructural features of diffuse malignant mesotheliomas. Human Pathology 29(12), 1382–1392.

Pakes, S.P., Shadduck, J.A., Cali, A., 1975. Fine structure of *Encephalitozoon cuniculi* from rabbits, mice and hamsters. Journal of Protozoology 22, 481–488.

Palade, G.E., 1952. A study of fixation for electron microscopy. Journal of Experimental Medicine 95, 285–298.

Papadimitriou, J.M., Henderson, D.W., Spagnolo, D.V., 1992a. Skeletal muscle. In: Papadimitriou, J.M., Henderson, D.W., Spagnolo, D.V. (Eds.), Diagnostic ultrastructure of non-neoplastic diseases. Churchill Livingstone, Edinburgh, Ch. 26, pp. 594–614.

Papadimitriou, J.M., Henderson, D.W., Spagnolo, D.V. (Eds.), 1992b. Diagnostic ultrastructure of non-neoplastic diseases. Churchill Livingstone, Edinburgh.

Pearl, G.S., Ghatak, N.R., 1995. Muscle biopsy. Archives of Pathology and Laboratory Medicine 119, 303–306.

Pinnolis, M., Egbert, P.R., Font, R.L., Winter, F.C., 1981. Nosematosis of the cornea. Archives of Ophthalmology 99, 1044–1047.

Plumel, M., 1948. Sodium cacodylate buffer solutions. Bulletin de la Société de Chimie Biologique 30, 129–130.

Pulkkinen, L., Uitto, J., 1999. Mutation analysis and molecular genetics of epidermolysis bullosa. Matrix Biology 18, 29–42.

Ray, M., Kindler, H.L., 2009. Malignant pleural mesothelioma. An update on biomarkers and treatment. Chest 136, 888–896.

Reid, N., 1975. Ultramicrotomy. In: Glauert, A.M. (Ed.), Practical methods in electron microscopy, Vol. 3 Part 2. North Holland, Amsterdam.

Reynolds, E.S., 1963. The use of lead citrate at high pH as an electron opaque stain based on metal chelation. Journal of Cell Biology 17, 208–212.

Richardson, K.C., Jarett, L., Finke, E.H., 1960. Embedding in epoxy resins for ultrathin sectioning in EM. Stain Technology 35, 313–316.

Ringo, D.L., Brennan, E.F., Costa-Robles, E.H., 1982. Epoxy resins are mutagenic: implications for electron microscopists. Journal of Ultrastructural Research 80, 280–287.

Rippstein, P., Cavell, S., Boivin, M., Dardick, I., 1987. Low magnification transmission electron microscopy in diagnostic pathology. Ultrastructural Pathology 11, 723–729.

Robards, A.W., Wilson, A.J., 1993. Procedures in electron microscopy. Wiley, New York.

Robinson, G., Gray, T., 1996. Electron microscopy 2: practical procedures. In: Bancroft, J.D., Stevens, A. (Eds.), Theory and practice of histological techniques, fourth ed. Churchill Livingstone, Edinburgh.

Rostagno, A., Vidal, R., Kumar, A., et al., 1996. Fibrillary glomerulonephritis related to serum fibrillar immunoglobulin-fibronectin complexes. American Journal of Kidney Disease 28, 676–684.

Ruchoux, M.M., Maurage, C.A., 1997. CADASIL: Cerebral autosomal dominant arteriopathy with subcortical infarcts and leukoencephalopathy. Journal of Neuropathology and Experimental Neurology 56(9), 947–964.

Ruchoux, M.M., Maurage, C.A., 1998. Endothelial changes in muscle and skin biopsies in patients with CADASIL. Neuropathology and Applied Neurobiology 24(1), 60–65.

Sabatini, D.D., Bensch, K., Barrnett, R.J., 1963. Cytochemistry and electron microscopy: the preservation of cellular ultrastructure and enzymic activity by aldehyde fixation. Journal of Cell Biology 17, 19–25.

Salema, R., Brandão, I., 1973. The use of PIPES buffer in the fixation of plant cells for electron microscopy. Journal of Submicroscopic Cytology 5, 79–96.

Santamaria, F., de Santi, M.M., Grillo, G., et al., 1999. Ciliary motility at light microscopy: a screening technique for ciliary defects. Acta Paediatrica 88(8), 853–857.

Sato, S., Adachi, A., Sasaki, Y., Ghazizadeh, M., 2008. Oolong tea extract as a substitute for uranyl acetate in staining for ultrathin sections. Journal of Microscopy 229(1), 17–20.

Schochet, S.S., Lampert, P.W., 1978. Diagnostic electron microscopy of skeletal muscle. In: Trump, B.F., Jones, R.T. (Eds.), Diagnostic electron microscopy, Vol. 1. John Wiley and Sons, New York, pp. 209–251.

Schwartz, M.M., 1998. Glomerular diseases with organised deposits. In: Jennette, J.C., Olson, J.L., Schwartz, M.M., Silva, F.G. (Eds.), Heptinstall's pathology of the kidney, Vol. 1, fifth ed. Lippincott-Raven, Philadelphia, pp. 369–388.

Silveira, H., Canning, E.U., 1995. *Vittaforma corneae* n.comb. for the human microsporidium *Nosema corneum*, Shadduck, Meccoli, Davis & Font, 1990 based on its ultrastructure in the liver of experimentally infected athymic mice. Journal of Eukaryotic Microbiology 42, 158–165.

Smith, J.E., 2009. The ecology and evolution of microsporidian parasites. Parasitology 136, 1901–1914.

Sprague, V., 1974. *Nosema connori* n.sp., microsporidian parasite of man. Transactions of the American Microscopy Society 93, 400–403.

Spurr, A., 1969. A low viscosity epoxy resin embedding medium for electron microscopy. Journal of Ultrastructural Research 26, 31–43.

Stirling, J.W., 1994. Immunogold labelling: resin sections. In: Woods, A.E., Ellis, R.C. (Eds.), Laboratory histopathology: a complete reference. Churchill Livingstone, Edinburgh.

Stirling, J.W., Graff, P.S., 1995. Antigen unmasking for electron microscopy. Journal of Histochemistry and Cytochemistry 43, 115–123.

Stirling, J.W., Henderson, D.W., Rozenbilds, M.A.M., et al., 1997. Crystalloidal paraprotein deposits in the cornea: an ultrastructural study of two new cases with tubular crystalloids that contain IgG κ light chains and IgG δ heavy chains. Ultrastructural Pathology 21, 337–344.

Stirling, J.W., Coleman, M., Thomas, A., Woods, A.E., 1999a. Role of transmission electron microscopy in tissue diagnosis. Journal of Cellular Pathology 4(4), 219–221.

Stirling, J.W., Coleman, M., Thomas, A., Woods, A.E., 1999b. Role of transmission electron microscopy in tissue diagnosis: diseases of the kidney, skeletal muscle and myocardium. Journal of Cellular Pathology 4(4), 223–243.

Strom, E.H., Hurwitz, N., Mayr, A.C., et al., 1996. Immunotactoid-like glomerulopathy with massive fibrillary deposits in liver and bone marrow in monoclonal gammopathy. American Journal of Nephrology 16, 523–528.

Sturgess, J.M., Turner, J.A.P., 1984. Ultrastructural pathology of cilia in the immotile cilia syndrome. Perspectives in Paediatric Pathology 8, 133–161.

Sulaiman, I.M., Matos, O., Lobo, M.L., Xiao, L., 2003. Identification of a new microsporidian parasite related to *Vittaforma corneae* in HIV-positive and HIV-negative patients from Portugal. Journal of Eukaryotic Microbiology 50 (Suppl), 586–590.

Tikka, S., Mykkänen, K., Ruchoux, M.-M., et al., 2009. Congruence between NOTCH3 mutations and GOM in 131 CADASIL patients. Brain 132, 933–939.

Tisher, C.C., Brenner, B.M., 1994. Renal pathology with clinical and functional correlations, second ed. Lippincott, Philadelphia.

Valladeau, J., Ravel, O., Dezutter-Dambuyant, C., et al., 2000. Langerin, a novel C-type lectin specific to Langerhans cells, is an endocytic receptor that induces the formation of Birbeck granules. Immunity 12, 71–81.

Vavra, J., Yachnis, A.T., Shadduck, J.A., Orenstein, J.M., 1998. Microsporidia of the genus Trachipleistophora – causative agents of human microsporidiosis – description of *Trachipleistophora anthropophthera* n.sp. (Protozoa, Microsporidia). Journal of Eukaryotic Microbiology 45, 273–283.

Verani, R.R., 1993. Fibrillary glomerulopathy. Kidney 2, 63–66.

Visvesvara, G.S., Belloso, M., Moura, H., et al., 1999. Isolation of *Nosema algarae* from the cornea of an immunocompetent patient. Journal of Eukaryotic Microbiology 46, 10S.

Warhol, M.J., Hickey, W.F., Corson, J.M., 1982. Malignant mesothelioma. Ultrastructural distinction from adenocarcinoma. American Journal of Surgical Pathology 6(4), 307–314.

Wasson, K., Peper, R.L., 2000. Mammalian microsporidiosis. Veterinary Pathology 37(2), 113–128.

Weber, R., Bryan, R.T., Schwartz, D.A., Owen, R.L., 1994. Human microsporidial infections. Clinical Microbiology Reviews 7(4), 426–461.

Yamaguchi, K., Suzuki K.-I., Tanaka, K., 2010. Examination of electron stains as a substitute for uranyl acetate for the ultrathin sections of bacterial cells. Journal of Microscopy 59(2), 113–118.

Young, B., Heath, J.W., 2000. Wheater's functional histology: a text and colour atlas, fourth ed. Churchill Livingstone, Edinburgh.

Quantitative data from microscopic specimens

23

Alton D. Floyd

Introduction

The practice of histology and histopathology has traditionally relied upon the *subjective* interpretation of microscopic preparations by a highly trained individual. The accuracy with which such interpretations can be made is the foundation of histology and of histopathology. That said, it is important to note that these interpretations are based on *pattern recognition*: that is, overall arrangements of elements within the specimen, a task for which the human visual system is well suited. The human visual system is not well suited for quantitative functions, such as assessment of linear measurements, areas, or density of stain. The human eye is a remarkable sensor, but one that is highly adaptable. It is able to alter its sensitivity depending on the brightness of the object being viewed. The eye is also a non-linear sensor, with a response to brightness that more closely approaches a logarithmic response. These two characteristics preclude accurate assessment of the density of specimens viewed through a microscope.

Human observers do not accurately estimate physical distances and areas of specimens. The eye is reasonably good at comparisons, and most microscopists will 'estimate' sizes based on some internal specimen object, such as the diameter of red blood cells. Even with such comparisons, length and size estimates made by microscopists are neither accurate nor highly repeatable. It is the purpose of image quantitation to eliminate observer-to-observer variation, and produce evaluations that are accurate and repeatable.

In recognition of the problem of accurately describing physical measurements in microscopic specimens, manufacturers of microscopes have included various calibration devices. For spatial measurements within the object, an eyepiece (ocular) reticule is used. These reticules typically consist of either a single line, or crossed lines (like the '+' symbol) that are marked off in even increments. Reticules are also available in the form of a grid. For a reticule to be useful for measurement, it must be calibrated for each magnification at which it is used. This is done by use of a stage micrometer, which is a microscope slide with an accurate scale etched or photographically applied to the slide. Typically, these stage micrometers have divisions of 0.1 and 0.01 millimeters. After calibrating the reticule with a stage micrometer, the reticule can be used directly to measure linear dimensions of microscopic objects.

Microscopes also are calibrated in the 'z' axis, which is the axis that controls stage (or nosepiece) movement. This calibration is found around the focus control knob, and is generally calibrated in microns. The z-axis calibration can be used to estimate the thickness of a microscopic specimen, assuming that one can accurately determine the 'top' and 'bottom' of the focal plane through the object of interest. Accuracy can be improved by using a high numerical aperture, shallow depth of field objective, since this assists in finding the top and bottom focal plane of the object. Modern usage of z-axis movement is more commonly associated with collection of a series of images at various focal planes (an image stack) that can be used subsequently to construct three-dimensional representations of the specimen.

Morphometry is the general term used to describe the measurement of size parameters of a specimen. Size is here defined as length, height, and area of an object of interest. These basic measurements can be combined to provide additional measurements, such as perimeter, smoothness, centers, etc. For some of these additional measurement parameters, it is important to understand the specific mathematical formula (algorithm) used, as there may be more than one definition of a particular parameter, and two different implementations of what appears (by algorithm name) to be an identical measurement may not be the same.

Traditional approaches

The history of development of the microscope is filled with clever devices designed to assist in performing morphometry of specimens. One such device is the camera lucida, which is an optical system that projects an image of the specimen onto a surface adjacent to the microscope. This projected image can be used to draw the specimen, or to measure portions of the image. Accurate measurements within these projected images require calibration of the projection, in a manner identical to that used to calibrate reticules.

Photographic and computer-aided imaging approaches have eliminated the use of the camera lucida in many laboratories, as convenient cameras have become universally available for microscopes. As with projections, a photographic system must be calibrated, using a stage micrometer. In addition to the calibration of the photographic negative, the enlarging process must also be calibrated for accurate measurement. For both camera lucida drawings and photographs, areas are generally determined using a device called a planimeter. This is a mechanical device that is used manually to trace the outline of objects of interest. Using a set of 'x' and 'y' calibrated wheels, the total area of the object is determined. For the planimeter data to be accurate, a standard area at the magnification of the specimen must be determined, and this then becomes a calibration factor used to interpret the planimeter data.

Stereology is a technique developed for analysis of metals and minerals, where generally the properties being measured relate to number, size, and distribution of some particle in the sample. It is based on geometry and probability theory and, using statistical mathematics, stereology makes specific assumptions about the object being analyzed. A general discussion of the theoretical basis of stereology can be found in DeHoff and Rhines (1968), and in Underwood (1970). Stereological techniques have been applied to many biological images, both light and electron microscopical. General principles and applications can be found in Weibel (1979, 1980, 1990), in Elias and Hyde (1983), and in Elias et al. (1978). Although there is a long history of use of stereology in histology and histopathology, the use of this technique makes assumptions about the specimen that may not be applicable. Since the foundation of stereology is statistical, the general nature of the distribution of whatever is being measured should be describable using some statistic. This condition may be met under specific conditions, such as examining the distribution of chromatin 'clumps' within a cell nucleus, where the only object being examined is a single nucleus. For highly ordered structures, such as gland elements within an organ, the organization of the structure implies that there is no statistical distribution. Stereology can make estimates of some parameters of specimens, such as area of a total image occupied by some particular component. Note that this is an estimate. The use of stereology to derive measures of the three-dimensional structure of cell and tissue specimens may provide misleading information, since the probabilities used in the mathematics assume that the entire volume of the specimen is accurately reflected in the portion measured. Due to the polarization of cell organelles, and the arrangement of tissues and organs, this is generally not the case.

While one cannot disagree that stereology has provided many useful insights into microscopic specimens, modern techniques of measurement can provide real measures of the specimen without any assumptions of the distribution pattern. The development of newer forms of microscopy (confocal) has extended this direct measurement capability to the third dimension. With the speed of modern image analysis systems, there is little justification for performing an estimate of a cell or tissue parameter when the actual parameter can be accurately measured, often in less time than is required for the stereological approach. An in-depth review of stereology can be found in the fourth edition of this book.

Electronic light microscopy

An electronic measurement of light transmitted through microscopic specimens has a long history, and roughly parallels the development of photometers, spectrophotometers, and light-detecting devices. Until recently (1980s), these devices simply detected light, and did not produce images. To use these early devices to produce images, the portion of the specimen visible to the light detector had to be restricted, and the specimen or image moved across this restricted area to generate an actual image. Many mechanisms were developed to acquire images using such techniques (Wied 1966; Wied & Bahr 1970). These mechanisms tended to be expensive, since they required high precision, and were also slow, as the image had to be acquired a small area at a time, and then 'put together' or reconstructed into a recognizable image. The majority of literature relating to quantitative light microscopy which utilized electronic measurement of light therefore was actually related to photometric and spectrophotometric studies, rather than analysis of images as currently defined.

Microscope photometry

A detailed theoretical account of microscope photometry can be found in Piller (1977). The hardware systems for obtaining data described in Piller have been superseded by modern devices, but the theoretical foundations are sound. The fundamental requirement for photometry is described by the Beer-Lambert law:

$$A = t \cdot c \cdot \varepsilon$$

where A is the absorbance, t is the path length of the absorbing material, c is the concentration of the absorbing material, and ε is the absorptivity.

In practical terms, for microscopic images, the path length (t) is approximately a constant, and for a given material being measured (usually a dye bound to the specimen) the absorptivity (ε) is also a constant. Therefore, the absorbance of the specimen is directly proportional to the concentration of the absorbing material.

Absorbance is defined as: $A = \log 1/T$, where T is the transmittance. Transmittance is defined as the fraction of light that is transmitted through the specimen (Light through specimen/Light through blank).

A requirement of the Beer-Lambert law is that material being measured is homogeneous (there are a few other restrictions, regarding maximum absorptivities, but these are not ordinarily met in transmitted light microscopy). The requirement of homogeneity is a significant one, as we routinely examine specimens with a microscope to observe structure, and this by definition is non-homogeneous.

The measurement of non-homogeneous materials using photometry gives rise to distributional error. While one can illustrate these errors nicely with mathematical equations, microscopists can grasp the concept intuitively with a simple, classical example. Suppose you have a chamber filled with water, such as an aquarium, and you shine light through the aquarium and measure the light traversing the chamber. Now, place a capped bottle of ink in the water of the aquarium. Depending on the size of the bottle, you may note a small effect on the amount of light that passes through the chamber. If you now uncap the ink bottle, and let the ink diffuse through the aquarium contents, the amount of light that passes through the chamber will be significantly reduced. When you think about this example, note that the amount of ink in the aquarium is identical in the two cases: the capped and the uncapped bottle. The difference is the *distribution* of the ink. For this reason, the error that results from photometry of non-homogeneous materials is referred to as *distributional error* and can be shown to induce error as large as 50% with certain distributions.

Recognition of distributional error was the reason that quantitative microscopes employed various devices to permit restricting the area of the specimen seen by the detector to a small area. This strategy was successful because of the optics of the microscope itself. A given lens resolution is defined as the ability to separate two points (point resolution). If a lens cannot separate two points, then they look like a single object. If a light detector sees an area of the specimen that is smaller than the point resolution of the microscope lens combination in use, then, by definition, that area is homogeneous, since the lens cannot see any structure in that area. For microscope lenses of 40x magnification and above, general 'area examined' sizes for photometry range from 0.25 to 0.5 µm diameter spots. Such spot sizes generally avoid significant distributional error. When such spots are generated by mechanical 'stops' or pinholes in the optical path of the microscope, they may introduce other, significant, sources of error, such as edge diffraction. These sources of error, as well as many others, such as glare within the optical system, are discussed in detail in Piller (1977). The above discussion applies to absorbing images only: that is, microscope images obtained with transmitted light microscopy. Fluorescence emission microscopy and particle reflectance (autoradiography) are based on different physical principles, and require different optics and sensor configurations.

Image acquisition

As mentioned earlier, images can be acquired with systems that examine specimens a small spot at a time. Using mechanical systems such as scanning stages or Nipkow discs, an image similar to that seen through the microscope can be acquired. With a scanning stage device, the time required to acquire such an image may range into hours. In all mechanical scanning systems, the precision and repeatability required for high-quality images translate to slow, expensive, and difficult-to-use systems.

The development of television cameras provided hope for acquiring images through microscopes. Early television cameras were vacuum tube devices, and were not suitable for quantitative microscope image use. Images collected with these devices were of low resolution, and suffered from a variety of geometric and photometric distortions related to

the electronics used to operate the scanning circuits of the tube, and to read out the resulting image signals.

During the decade of the 1980s, a variety of solid-state sensors were developed for television (video) purposes. One technology in particular, the CCD (charge-coupled device) camera, matured into a significantly useful device for microscopic imaging work. CCD cameras continue to evolve, and are the technology of choice for most photometric and imaging microscopic studies. Recently, a new technology has emerged in solid-state cameras: CMOS or complementary metal oxide semiconductor cameras. These devices promise rapid image acquisition, low cost, and the potential for some image manipulation within the camera detector itself. At this time, CMOS cameras still lag behind CCD cameras in suitability for microscope photometry, but this may change in the near future. Solid-state cameras have a number of characteristics that make them ideal for microscope imaging. The detecting element itself consists of individual sensors (pixels) that are arranged in a square or rectangular array. The physical size of individual sensors or pixels in the array is in the order of a few microns, with values of 6 to 10 µm square pixels being common (there are solid-state cameras available with rectangular pixels, but these are not suitable for quantitative image use). The technique used to manufacture solid-state detectors is similar to that used to produce electronic chips such as are used in microcomputers. Therefore, sensor chips can be manufactured that may have one million or more individual sensors (pixels) and each will have similar characteristics, such as response to light (gain and linearity). Most solid-state detectors have a reasonably linear response over a wide range of light intensities, and this implies that each pixel within the sensor is also linear. Within limits, each pixel in the sensor array also generates a similar signal to a given light input (identical gain per pixel).

The camera detector consists of many individual but essentially identical detectors (the pixels): hence, each individual pixel can be considered to be a photometric detector. To use a solid-state camera detector for photometry, the image that the individual detectors (pixels) see must meet the requirements of the Beer-Lambert law; i.e., they must see a homogeneous portion of the specimen. By calibrating the microscope lens system used, and deriving the area of the specimen in square microns seen by each pixel of the solid-state camera chip, an appropriate magnification can be selected which permits accurate photometry. For modern cameras with an array size of 1024×1024 pixels, a microscope objective lens of 20× magnification will achieve approximately 0.50 µm per pixel, and a 40× objective will be in the range of 0.25 µm per pixel. Both of these values are close to the resolving power of the respective lenses, and therefore meet the homogeneity requirement of the Beer-Lambert law. As yet, cameras with high enough pixel density to perform photometry at lower magnifications are not commonly available, and those that do exist are both expensive and slow. With the rapid advancements in camera technology, this is expected to change in the near future.

Solid-state cameras, whether CCD or CMOS, are available in either monochrome or color versions. Color cameras may use two different techniques to generate a color image. In one approach, there are three separate detector arrays, each with a color filter in front of the array. A prism or mirror system is used to split the image coming from the microscope into three separate but identical images, so each detector sees the same image. The color filters are red, green, and blue, since a red image, a green image, and a blue image can be combined to create a full color image. This type of camera is called a three-chip color camera. The second approach to color cameras uses a single detector chip, and places a pattern of color dots over the individual pixels. Again, these color dots are red, blue, and green. The most common pattern for these dots is the Bayer pattern (Fig. 23.1). Note that in the Bayer pattern there are actually four dots per 'repeat', since for each red and each blue dot there are two green dots. This type of camera is called a single-chip color camera.

The three-chip camera has three individual detectors, and a beam-splitting system to divide the image; these cameras are therefore more expensive than a single-chip camera. Essentially, a three-chip camera is three separate cameras in one. The advantage of the three-chip camera is that every pixel is 'real': that is, it is generating a true signal. The disadvantage is that there may be differences in sensitivity of a 'red' pixel and a 'green' pixel that are seeing the exact same spot of an image. Use of a three-chip camera for photometry where various colors are examined requires careful calibration and correction of any variation in output between the separate detector chips.

The single-chip camera can produce excellent color images, but must be used carefully for quantitative work, and is unsuitable for photometry. This is because only one pixel out of four (two in the case of green) is actually seeing the specimen at the point of maximum absorption. The other pixels in the Bayer pattern are being approximated, by assigning their 'red' value to the same value as the one real 'red' pixel in the pattern. In addition to the approximation of true signal for a given color, the Bayer pattern results in a real loss of resolution at the sensor level. Since only one of every four pixels (for red and blue) actually sees a red or blue portion of the specimen, the true resolution of the single-chip camera is one-fourth the total number of pixels in the array. In practical terms this means that if a single pixel sees an area of the specimen that is 0.5 µm square, the true resolution of the Bayer pattern single-chip camera is 2.0 µm per pixel, for color detection. The camera does have true pixel number spatial resolution, but in colored specimens this may be reduced by the distribution of color within the specimen.

The three-chip color camera is essentially three monochrome cameras, with each camera having a different colored filter in front of the camera detector. Software is then used to combine the three separate images into a full-color image. This suggests that it is possible to use a monochrome camera to capture full-color images. A number of cameras provide a mechanism for doing this. Within the camera itself there is either an electronic filter, or a filter wheel carrying glass filters. To capture an image, three sequential images are taken, each through a different colored filter. These images are then combined to produce the full-color image. It is

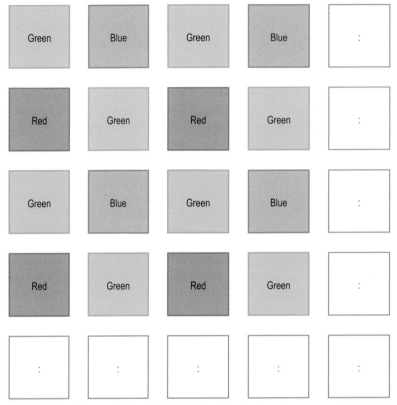

Figure 23.1 The Bayer pattern of color filters applied to individual pixels of single-chip color cameras. Note that this effectively reduces the color resolution of the chip to one-fourth that of the true number of pixels.

possible also to do this using a simple monochrome camera. One would place a red filter in the light path of the microscope, and capture a 'red' image. The same thing would then be done for 'blue' and for 'green'. The result would be three separate images of the same specimen, in different colors, and when these three color planes are combined using software, the result is a full-color image.

Cameras used for imaging are also described in terms of signal resolution per individual pixel. This signal resolution is commonly described as *bit depth* or *gray levels* (for monochrome cameras). The signal resolution is a specification that describes the number of divisions of the signal between zero (no signal) and maximum signal. A common value is 256 levels, and these divisions are often also described as gray levels. They are based on the digital progression by powers of two, and therefore a 256-level

signal corresponds to 8 bits of resolution (2 to the eighth power). Many modern cameras provide 10- or 12-bit signal resolutions. With a 12-bit camera, 4096 gray levels can be obtained. As the signal resolution increases, the susceptibility of the signal to perturbation increases. In particular, sources of electronic noise, such as internally generated heat within the detector itself, may become a problem. With high bit-depth cameras, it is common to find cooling systems which lower the detector temperature, and thereby reduce electronic noise. Such cooling systems also translate to higher prices for cameras so equipped and, if the cooling system contains a fan, may introduce vibration to the microscope.

It is important to note the differences between cameras used to capture images through the microscope, and the same image viewed with the human eye. The human eye is a remarkable detector of light and of color. However, it is a non-linear, highly adaptive sensor. In addition, the resolution of the eye detector (retina) varies across the surface of the retina, being highest in the fovea. Under ideal conditions, most individuals with excellent eyesight can distinguish between 30 and 35 brightness levels (gray levels). This is a far cry from the 256 or higher number of levels seen by a digital camera. A solid-state camera can always detect intensity variations that would be invisible to the human observer. This translates to the ability to detect finer detail within an image than can be resolved by a human observer.

The human eye adapts to light intensity, so the 30 or 35 gray levels that are detected vary, depending on the intensity of the light, and the immediately preceding light exposure of the eye. This is one of the reasons why individuals must 'dark adapt' prior to doing fluorescence microscopy. The same phenomenon occurs in bright-field microscopy, but is seldom recognized. If an individual is asked to assess the density or 'darkness' of a stain, the assessment will vary depending on whether the individual has been in a dim environment or a bright environment just prior to performing the assessment.

Color capture is another area in which a camera differs from the human eye. While there is much that is still unknown as to the way in which the eye-brain combination processes color, the camera provides a fixed model. The construction of the camera itself is based on the RGB (red, green, blue) model of color. There are many other models of color, and those that incorporate intensity and saturation information appear more intuitive to human users of image systems. One common model that employs such a system is the HSI (hue, saturation, intensity) model. Software programs are available that permit images to be converted from one type of color space model to another, and often such conversions are useful when one works with full-color images.

Photographic color film is balanced for the type of light used to illuminate the scene. The type of light is specified by a 'color temperature' number. Film sold for routine color photography is generally balanced for correct color in 'sunlight', which is specified as a color temperature of 5000 K. Specialty films intended for microphotography may be balanced for 'tungsten' illumination, with a color temperature of 3200 K. Because of the narrow limits of intensity for which the film is balanced, photomicrography requires the microscope illuminator to be set to a specified level (generally bright) prior to taking a photograph. The 'color temperature' of a light source is actually a measure of the intensity of the various components of the light source, in the red, green, and blue regions of the spectrum. Photographic film records all of these components simultaneously, and there is little opportunity to 'correct' values, other than limited adjustment during processing. With a solid-state camera and capture software, the situation is different. Each of the image components (red, green and blue) is available as an individual image. They are combined to produce the final image. Since the individual components (color planes) are available, it is possible to 'color correct' the image. This is generally done in the capture software, or the camera itself. The result is that 'white' is a true white (defined as a particular level of R, G, and B), regardless of the 'color temperature' of the microscope illuminator. This eliminates the requirement for presetting the brightness of the microscope prior to taking a picture with a solid-state camera. However, it does mean that each time the microscope is adjusted, in either magnification or illumination intensity, the user may have to calibrate the 'white balance' of the system again. Note that these same software techniques can be used to correct or modify any color image that can be converted into electronic form.

Solid-state cameras used on microscopes are generally coupled to the microscope in a manner to optimize the area of the visible field (to a user looking through the eyepieces of the microscope) that is captured. As is true of photographic cameras, the solid-state camera captures a rectangular (or in a few cases, square) portion of the circular image displayed in the microscope. The camera sensor pixels are, as previously described, quite uniform in response to light intensity. The nature of microscope lens systems, even in those that have been carefully aligned, is a higher intensity along the optical axis (center of the image) than in the periphery of the field. For an adaptive sensor such as the eye, and one with a limited number of intensity step discriminations, the field of view of a carefully aligned microscope appears to be quite uniform. That this is not the case is amply illustrated in many lectures that display photomicrographs, where a common flaw is dark corners. In the case of solid-state cameras, the increased intensity level sensitivity, as compared to the eye, accentuates this problem. Since all solid-state cameras use some type of software, either within the capture system or on the capturing computer to control the camera, this software frequently contains some type of 'field flattening' or 'background subtraction' mechanism to correct this variation in intensity from center to edge of the image. Additional details of requirements for acquiring images through microscopes using electronic cameras can be found in Shotton (1993).

Image analysis

Overview

Image analysis is a broad term that may be defined quite differently by those working in diverse fields. Originally, image analysis was used to describe the extraction of numerical information from pictures. Since the process of placing pictures into a form that could be analyzed digitally was cumbersome, and the computers used to analyze such pictures were slow, image analysis was performed 'off line' and quite often at sites far removed from where the image was originally recorded. As software techniques for image analysis improved, and computers became faster and more affordable, image analysis became more widely used, in many fields and disciplines. Image analysis encompasses many areas: machine vision, graphic arts, pattern matching, photometry, optical character recognition, surveillance, security, and scores of others. While many of the same techniques are used in each of these areas (at the software level), we will restrict the remainder of this discussion to the use of image analytic techniques to extract numerical data from microscopic preparations. The emphasis will be on

transmitted light preparations, although in many cases identical approaches are used for fluorescence preparations.

The minimal requirement for image analysis of microscope preparations is a microscope equipped with a camera that can capture and transmit images to a computer equipped with suitable image analytic tools. The camera requirements have been discussed above. Computers suitable for image analysis range from RISC-based workstations to personal computers, either IBM PCs (or clones) or Apple PCs. A variety of sophisticated image analytic tools (programs) are available for each of these platforms. In addition to commercial offerings, there are a number of freeware or shareware programs available for personal computers. Among the best known of these is the program originally designed for the Apple computers, named NIH Image. There are now versions of this program available for the IBM (Windows) computers as well. A recent addition to the list of available image analytic programs is ImageJ, written by the original author of NIH Image. This program is also freely available, and, because it is written in the JAVA language, can run on any computer which supports JAVA (http://rsb.info.nih.gov/ij/.)

All image analysis programs must provide mechanisms to display images, read images from a source (camera or storage), and ultimately save the image and any derived data to storage. In modern computers, these functions are part of a GUI (graphical user interface) that permits the user actually to see the image and the various alterations to it during and after various image analytic or manipulation steps.

As camera resolutions increase, they often exceed the display capability of many computer displays. As an example, consider a common camera resolution available today, 1024 × 1310. The actual image from such a camera is larger than the common display resolution of many computers, which may be 800 × 600. Another common display resolution is 1024 × 756. In both cases, the larger image is displayed completely on the monitor. This is accomplished within the display program, by simply reducing the image to fit within the monitor resolution. Thus, the displayed image may not accurately represent the 'real' image that has been captured and is available for analysis. Some capture/display programs provide tools to permit the user to display the image at actual resolution, even though only a portion of the image is seen on the screen. Such programs allow the user to scroll over the image in order to see the entire image. Note also that many output devices, such as printers, actually reduce the size of the image, and therefore lose resolution as compared to the original image. This display resolution, which may be different from the actual image resolution, is one reason why high-resolution images may not appear as 'sharp' when viewed on a display device.

It is important to realize that an image, to the computer, is simply an array of values of the individual pixels. For 8-bit monochrome images, this would be a sequence of numbers, with values for each ranging between 0 and 255. Image file storage formats specify the number of pixels per row, and the total number of rows. This information is part of the 'header' information in the file storage, and is required for proper display and analysis of the images. The user ordinarily does not have to worry about this information, since it is taken care of transparently by the image software. Because the computer software considers the image to be an array of x y dimension, any pixel in the image can be individually addressed if its location is known within the array. In the case of color images, the actual image is stored as a sequence of colored pixels, i.e., red, green and blue. To extract the 'green' image, one would read every third pixel from the file. Note that there are a variety of formats for image file storage, and the programmer should be sure to verify the 'bit order' in use prior to attempting to extract specific information.

From the information presented to this point, it should be understood that image analysis of images simply accepts that the image being analyzed contains useful information. This may or may not be true, and is highly dependent on the integrity of the specimen for the parameter being measured. Numerous examples are presented throughout this chapter for specific types of specimens. As a basic tenet, you cannot measure something in a specimen if the preparation methods have not preserved that aspect of the specimen. Not only must the material of interest be preserved but also it must be preserved in a manner that permits extrapolation back to the living state: that is, in the live specimen. Throughout this text, specific methods are presented for demonstration of specific substances in biological specimens. For purely visual assessment, one only needs to selectively identify a material. For image analysis, if one is interested in the amount of material present, then the ability to retain this material during processing and the ability of the staining methods to clearly mark all of the contained material is critically important. Not only must the user of image analysis understand the limitations of the devices used for image acquisition but also a complete understanding of tissue preparation is required. The use of control objects for instrument validation and for specimen preparation are highly encouraged. Without these control objects and studies, it will be impossible to interpret image analytical results.

Image analysis processes

Point processes

Most forms of image analysis of microscope images start with a category of operations classically defined as point processes. These processes are relatively simple, yet are basic to most image operations. A point process acts on an individual pixel within the image, and may modify the value of that pixel depending on the previous value. A common use of a point process is to change the value of each pixel to some other value, depending on the original value. Such an operation may make use of a LUT (look-up table). A common use for such an operation is in a pseudo-color operation, where a gray-scale image is divided into a number of 'levels': i.e., all pixel values between 0 and 20 might be colored 'red', all values between 21 and 50 might be colored 'blue', etc. Since the human eye recognizes color variations much more easily than density variations, such a point operation might well make interpretation of a gray-scale image easier.

Point processes are used to change the overall intensity of an image. Suppose an image is captured, and the background appears too dark. By adding a constant to every pixel, the result is an image that looks brighter. (Note: This depends on the scale being used for display of images. In this case, it is assumed that '0' is black, and '255' is white. There are systems in which this is reversed.) Often, in the process of color balancing the individual color planes of a color image, it is a point process that is used to set the 'clear' or 'background' pixels to 'white'. Point processes can also be used to convert an image to a negative of the original image. In this process, each pixel is mapped to the value it would have if the scale of black to white values were inverted (black = 255, rather than 0). This is quite useful if the image is analyzed with a system different from the one used for capture. It is also a useful function for many intermediate image manipulations, particularly where images may be combined with one another.

Image contrast stretching is another example of a point process. In a contrast stretch (image equalization), the range of gray levels in the image is expanded. In many specimens, the actual image values cover a relatively narrow range of the total available gray values. As an example, in a nuclear preparation stained for DNA with the Feulgen procedure, the total gray levels represented by the stained nuclei occupy only about 30% of the total available levels. By contrast stretching these gray levels to cover the entire range of available values (256 levels), additional details can often be seen and/or measured in such contrast-stretched images. By far the most common point process in image analysis is image thresholding. This is used to segment an image into areas that have some particular interest, such as a particular staining pattern. The action of a threshold is simple. The user selects a particular gray level (generally with some type of interactive tool in the graphical user interface). The point process then sets all pixels with a value lower than this threshold value to '0', and all values above this threshold value to '1'. In other words, the image is converted to a binary image. While this simple threshold is sufficient for some purposes, such as

determining the total area in the image that is above some level (generally, the area of the image that is 'stained' by whatever is being analyzed), the simple binary image is more generally used to combine with the original image to produce some type of 'mask'. A common implementation is to combine the binary image with the original image in such a way that all '0' or background pixels are left '0', while all '1' pixels are left with their original image value. Such an operation leaves the desired portions of the image visible, with the remainder eliminated from the image. A second threshold step is often performed, thresholding from the opposite direction. After this step, a group of objects of 'medium' gray level could be separated or segmented from both lighter and darker objects. Another common implementation of threshold point operations is to combine the two threshold operations with a pseudo-color or LUT operation, and simply place a transparent colored mask over the desired objects, leaving the entire original image visible.

Area processes

Area processes use groups of pixels either to derive information from the image or to alter the image in some specific manner. In general, area processes involve a small portion of the image, in a two-dimensional matrix. The matrix is generally made up of an odd number of 'row' pixels and an odd number of 'column' pixels (a convolution kernel). It is the pixel in the center of this matrix that may be altered after performing the area process. Many of the area processes are often referred to as convolutions. Convolutions commonly are based on matrix sizes of 3, 5, 7, or sometimes larger dimensions. In the area process, a convolution matrix is defined. The convolution matrix is placed over the image, and each pixel over which the convolution mask lies is multiplied by the number contained within the convolution mask. All of these multiplied pixel values are then summed, and the sum is used to replace the central pixel. The mask is then moved one pixel further along, and the process repeated (Fig. 23.2). Note that, in practice, the 'changed' pixel is used to construct a new image, since the process

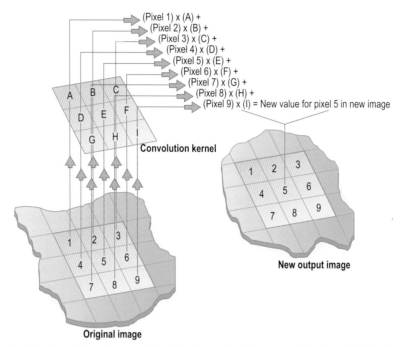

Figure 23.2 The manner of implementation of a convolution. The diagram illustrates a convolution kernel of nine elements.

of convolution would fail if the image being analyzed were being altered during analysis. In other words, the convolution does not change the 'original' image, but creates a new, modified image based on the original (Fig. 23.2).

Area processes in general are often called spatial filtering operations, since they yield information about the rate of change of intensities within the image. In fact, it is these rates of change that are exploited by many common convolution filters. Typical area processes are those used for spatial filtering such as high-pass and low-pass filters. A low-pass filtered image will reduce the contrast of an image. Such an operation is often useful to remove unwanted noise spikes within an image. A high-pass filtered image increases contrast within the image, and is often used to improve the ability to detect edges or other structures within the image.

An important type of spatial filtering is edge detection. A variety of convolution matrices are available to perform it. Often, some type of edge detection is used to perform segmentation within an image, particularly if the area to be segmented is

close in gray value to other structures within the image, and thresholding is difficult.

While area processes are extremely important in image analysis, they are computationally intensive processes. As an example, a point process need only look at each pixel in an image one time. An area process, in the simplest case, must look at each pixel times the size of the convolution matrix. For a convolution matrix of 3 × 3, and an image of 1 million pixels, 9 million operations would have to be performed. For matrices of 7 × 7, 49 million operations would be required. In actuality, the number of operations required is somewhat greater than the figures given here, as impressive as they are. Because of the amount of computer processing required, image analysis requires fast computers, with large amounts of memory. Also, high-resolution, full-color images require a considerable amount of space for storage. A full-color image of 1024 × 1310 pixels will require almost 4 million bytes of storage (4 MB). While there are various methods of making images smaller (image compression), most of these forms of compression are 'lossy': that is, they discard image information, and this information cannot be retrieved from the stored image. Certain image storage formats allow a type of compression that is based on sequences of image data where all the pixels are the same (like large areas of background). This form of compression is called run length encoding, and does not discard any image information. However, for a typical image of a microscope specimen, where there are few or no 'constant value' areas, run length encoding may actually result in a larger image storage size than the original image. As a practical matter, any image intended for future analysis should not be stored in a compressed format, particularly in view of the low cost of large-capacity storage devices.

Frame processes

Both point processes and area processes treat the image as a series of pixels, and address each pixel in a specific manner. Frame processes, in contrast, operate on the entire image. Often frame processes use simple boolean (logic) operations to add, subtract, multiply, divide, or otherwise combine two images to produce a new third 'result' image. A common use of a frame operation is to correct a microscope image for uneven illumination. By collecting and 'temporarily' saving an image of the 'background' (when no specimen is present), the background image can then be subtracted from the specimen image. This will effectively remove any debris or other image-degrading elements that are inherent in the microscope and illuminator. A similar operation is commonly used in security systems, where a 'scene' image is collected at intervals. By subtracting the 'next' image from the previous image, any change in the 'scene' will be immediately recognized. A common biological application for a frame process would be to detect movement in a cell culture being observed at intervals. By tracking these changes over time, a 'trail' can be mapped and applied over the image to follow the movement of cells over time. Frame processes are common in many of the operators employed in image analysis systems, particularly with respect to boolean operations. They are frequently used in the display

portions of image analysis systems, where they can be used to combine the results of various area processes or thresholding operations with the original image, in order to evaluate the effectiveness of a particular operation.

Geometric processes

Geometric processes are quite different from the processes discussed previously, since they are mainly used to reconstruct or correct images. Geometric processes actually move pixels within the image, and can therefore be used to correct defects such as geometric distortion. Geometric processes are used to rotate images, change scale, translate images, and produce mirror images. It is geometric processes that are used to interpolate images from 'real' size to a size that can be displayed on the monitor in use. Geometric distortion would include such image defects as a microscopic section that was attached to the slide in a manner that distorted normal morphology. In such a case, a geometric process could 'transform' the image to straighten or otherwise return it to the shape believed to be correct. Geometric processes are used to make the specimen 'look better', and to prepare the image for display or output to a print device. Until recently, geometric processes were not used extensively in microscope imaging, other than for display and printing. However, with the advent of microscope systems that can collect multiple images from various focal planes of the specimen (confocal microscopes), geometric processes have become much more widely used. These processes can be used to align 'stacks' of images that are used to reconstruct three-dimensional models of specimens.

Geometric processes can also be used to create mosaic images. A mosaic image is an image that is created from several smaller images. Using a motor-driven stage (scanning stage), an image system can travel over a slide, each time moving the exact width of the previous image, and collecting another image. Each collected image can then be 'added' to the previous one to create a large, mosaic image. With appropriate software, the area where these small images join can be a perfect, seamless match. Creation of such mosaic images requires an automatic focusing mechanism, to insure that each image collected is properly focused. While it has been suggested that such mosaic images can be retained in place of the original specimen, the resolution required to prevent loss of data (with current cameras) would mean the minimum objective magnification used to create the mosaic would be 20× and preferably 40–60×, and for large specimens this would create exceptionally large image files. Some 'virtual slide' microscopes produce image sizes that are hundreds of megabytes in size.

Image analysis software

Many commercial image software packages are available, for both the PC and Mac personal computers. All of these offerings include the variety of image analysis processes described above, although there is little standardization of terminology for specific types of process. The user should work with each algorithm of interest, and verify that it is doing the desired function, as the implementation of common algorithms does differ from one software program to another. In general, these software systems are organized as a way to display an image. The image may be either captured from a camera, or retrieved from storage. Once the image is available, the user can select, through menus or tool bars, a variety of image manipulation tools. When the tool is applied to the image, the results can be seen immediately. Most systems also provide a mechanism to back up or undo, in case the result was not satisfactory. Such an image system is an ideal learning tool, and a user should expect to spend some time becoming familiar with any new image analysis system.

In addition to commercial software packages, there are a number of 'freeware' or 'shareware' image analysis packages available. One of the best known of these is NIH Image, written for the Mac platform, and freely available worldwide. There is also a version of this software for the PC platform. Recently, the original author of NIH Image produced a new image software package, ImageJ. This software is written in the Java language, and offers the advantage of running on any computer. ImageJ is available at no cost, and is constantly being upgraded and expanded.

Most vendors of commercial image analysis software packages provide support through user groups, and these groups are a rich source of assistance with image analysis problems. There are also a number of generic image analysis groups that maintain discussions via the Internet, and these groups can provide assistance with specific image analysis problems. The Internet is also a rich source of images, and a number of histology and pathology image archives are available. Note that currently most of these images are available as JPEG images. The JPEG format is a file storage format used for many Internet images, and is a compressed image format (with compression based on a discrete cosine transform). Such compression is a 'lossy' format, which means that image data are lost during compression and cannot be retrieved. This is a critical issue for some types of image analysis, but is not necessarily a problem for simply viewing the image. The newer form of JPEG image is JPEG 2000. This compression uses a wavelet transform, and produces somewhat better visual results. However, it is still a 'lossy' compression format, and therefore not suitable for many types of image analysis.

Specimen analysis

The goal of most image analysis of microscope images is the generation of numerical data that describe some aspect of the specimen. If the specimen is stained for some specific constituent, and the mechanism with which the stain interacts with the constituent is known, then it may be possible to use photometric techniques to produce numbers corresponding to the actual amount of the constituent present in the specimen, or in selected portions of the specimen. Generally, there will be more than one area of interest within the specimen. In the case of a specimen stained for cell nuclei, one could expect several hundred nuclei in a single image. In such a case, the first step of analysis would be to segment the objects of interest (nuclei) from the remainder of the specimen. If only the nuclei are stained, this can most likely be accomplished with a simple thresholding operation. After the nuclei are located by segmentation, it may be found that some nuclei touch each other. In such a case, additional image operations (specific area processes) may be required to separate these touching objects (see Fig. 23.3). In some cases it may be more expedient to use interactive tools, and simply draw a line between the touching objects, to effect a separation.

The above description illustrates an interesting point regarding image analysis. In many cases a particular operation may be performed in a totally automated manner, or the same result may be obtained with manual use of a particular tool. The decision of which approach to use depends on the complexity of the specimen being analyzed, the speed of the hardware and software being used, and the validity of the result. While it is difficult to deny the capability of modern image analysis programs, it is sometimes more time-advantageous simply to perform some manual intervention, thereby saving hours of analysis time. Once objects have been segmented, data can be collected from each. Common measures available include properties such as integrated optical density (absorbance), size (area), length of perimeter, shape, and a variety of other measures of the variation of intensity of pixels within the object. Many image analysis programs provide interactive tools to permit direct measurement of portions of the image. These tools commonly permit simply drawing a line on the displayed image, and having the length of this line displayed in the calibration units of the system (usually microns). Collected data can be saved, analyzed statistically, and displayed in graphs. Many programs permit direct export of data in formats compatible with common analysis tools, such as spreadsheets.

In the case of color images, analysis generally proceeds by selecting a particular color plane, which provides maximal contrast for the object(s) of interest. As an example, consider a specimen stained with an immunostain specific for some feature of cell nuclei. A common example would be a proliferation marker such as Ki-67 (MIB-1). Such a stain ordinarily results in a specimen with some number of positive nuclei, and many that are not stained. These nuclei that do not stain with the specific immunostain are then counterstained with a contrasting color. The object of the analysis of such specimens is to determine the percentage of nuclei within the specimen that are proliferating. To derive this result, we need to determine the total number of nuclei in the specimen, and then the number that stain positively.

After capturing the color image, we select the color plane that has maximal contrast for the positively stained nuclei. For a specimen that has been stained with the chromogen diaminobenzidine (DAB), the positive nuclei will be a brown color. These nuclei will have high contrast in the green or blue color plane, and if the counterstained nuclei are blue, then the blue color plane will see these counterstained nuclei as low contrast. By using a simple threshold operation, the positive nuclei can be segmented from the remainder of the specimen. From this segmented binary image alone, we can derive the total area in the specimen of positive nuclei. By switching to the red color plane, we will see high contrast in the counterstained nuclei. Unfortunately, we will also see that the DAB stain appears in the red color plane and at a density close to that of the blue counterstained nuclei. Since we already know where the DAB-positive nuclei are, from our first analysis, we can simply use a frame process to subtract the positive nuclei from the counterstain image. The result is an image that contains the counterstained nuclei, and 'holes' where the DAB-stained nuclei were. We can then threshold on the counterstained nuclei to derive an area of nuclei that did not stain with the specific proliferation stain. With these two numbers, we can add to obtain the total area of nuclei, and then divide this total into the area of positive stain and thereby obtain the desired measure, the percentage of positive staining for the specimen.

In the above example, a number of manipulations of the image were performed. In fact, most image analysis programs provide a variety of tools which can be used to significantly alter an image. This raises the issue of how much manipulation of an

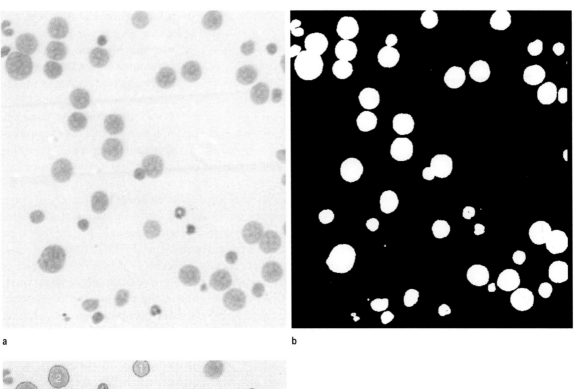

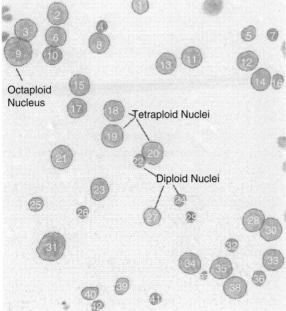

Figure 23.3 An image during analysis. (a) The original image, which is of Feulgen-stained cell nuclei. (b) The image after a threshold operation that converts the image to a binary image. (c) The final image, after isolating objects (nuclei) and separating touching nuclei. Annotations have also been added to this image.

image is permissible in the collection of image data. The answer depends on the purpose of the analysis. When the object of the analysis is to measure some spatial property of the specimen, such as size or shape, then a variety of image tools can be employed to enhance the ability to segment the objects of interest from the remainder of the specimen. The caveat here is that the image manipulations should not alter the property being measured. In the case of photometric measurements, all image enhancement operations must be avoided. Image enhancement operations in this case include any operation that would result in the alteration of any pixel value included in the final measurement result.

It is often assumed, and frequently stated, that image analysis can be used to determine the amount of a particular material present in a specimen (a photometric measurement), assuming a stain that identifies the material of interest. This is in many ways a simplistic statement. A number of specific requirements must be met for this to hold true. First, the stain must have a defined stochiometric relationship with the material of interest. The entirety of the object containing the material must be present in the specimen. In other words, if the material of interest is confined to cell nuclei, then the specimen must contain intact nuclei. In practical terms, this means that one must provide specimens with intact nuclei. Therefore the preparation must be a touch preparation or a cytological preparation, rather than a section. The use of sections complicates photometric measurements. In general, no intact objects (at light microscope resolution) will be present in the section. Essentially all cells, and most cellular constituents, such as nuclei, will be cut. Consequently, there is no way to measure their total content accurately, since part of the content is missing. Another complicating factor is that in the architecture of many tissues every section contains fragments of overlapping cells. With most fixation and staining protocols, cell boundaries are not delineated. One simply cannot tell how much of the thickness through which light is being transmitted is due to the cell on the 'top' of the section or to the one on the 'bottom'.

A sectioned preparation can be used to measure the general concentration per unit volume of a specimen. Assuming an appropriate stain, one can define an area of known size, and sample multiple areas of the specimen with this known area (it is actually a volume, assuming constant section thickness). For this strategy to succeed, one must insure that the areas measured do not contain other, unstained structures such as a fragment of the cell nucleus, if the material being measured is cytoplasmic in location. Although this approach is producing numerical results, it should not be assumed that the results are precise. Such analyses are more properly described as semi-quantitative and, although more accurate and reproducible than subjective visual evaluation of microscope preparations, are not truly quantitative.

Image analysis can be used to provide numerical assessment of many details of microscope specimens. An example is the thickness of an epithelial layer, or the depth of penetration of an epithelial tumor into underlying tissues. Such assessments are simple measurements of distance, but have the advantage of permitting a permanent record to be made of the actual placement of the fiduciary mark used to perform the measurement.

Image analysis can also be used to perform repetitive measurements where many objects must be measured, or where the measurement must be restricted to a particular orientation. An example would be the measurement of the thickness of the myelin sheath around nerve fibers. For areas of cross-sectioned nerve, most myelinated nerve fibers will be cut at a slight angle, rather than a true cross-section. By measuring the long and short axes of the resulting ellipse, the myelin measurement can then be restricted to the short axis of the ellipse, insuring a true measure of the actual myelin thickness.

When many measurements must be performed on a specimen, most image analysis software permits the creation of 'scripts' or 'macros'. These are simply sequences of image analysis steps that can be applied automatically or can be manually invoked for each object of interest. A significant advantage of defined scripts is that they insure that a particular type of measurement is performed in an identical manner each time it is performed. Scripts also insure that data are collected in precisely the same manner, regardless of who performs the analysis. The general examples described here are but a brief introduction to the ways in which an image can be analyzed. Many properties of an image can be documented; with appropriate specimen-preparative methods, the subjective analyses that have been the foundation of histology and cytology may ultimately yield to precise, invariant descriptions of specific features of the cells and tissues in the majority of these microscopy specimens. While many of the tools to provide the framework for such assessments are now available, the actual data on which such descriptions might be based have yet to be collected.

In addition to actual image data, the interpretation and display of data is also an evolving science. As additional parameters are defined for a particular specimen type, one is faced with a significant increase in the number of variables. The complexity of multi-parametric data analysis is beyond the scope of this chapter, but continues to be an area of active research and progress.

Specimen preparation for image analysis

The science of cell and tissue preparation is well developed, as is documented in the contents of this text. The techniques that have been developed and perfected over the course of many years have been designed for the subjective evaluations performed by a skilled microscopist. Stains have been developed that optimize the ability of the human eye to discriminate morphology and colors. Unfortunately, cameras used for image analysis do not mimic the human eye. This means that common staining protocols will not yield optimal results for image analysis. The most common staining protocol for routine pathology is the hematoxylin and eosin (H&E) stain. Interpretation of this stain is straightforward for those trained in microscopic diagnosis. However, this stain is quite difficult to use in image analysis. If we consider the use of a monochrome camera, where all color is converted to shades of gray, the problem becomes apparent. H&E-stained specimens, when viewed as gray-scale objects (like a black-and-white photograph), lack the sharpness and clarity that a human observer would detect when viewing the object in full color through the microscope. Light microscope images depend on absorption of light by the dyes used to stain the specimen. While the eye can readily detect the differences between the blue-purple of hematoxylin and the red of eosin, in a gray-scale image there is little distinction between these two colors. The basis for this lack of differentiation is that the absorption curves of hematoxylin and eosin overlap over a considerable portion of the visible spectrum (Fig. 23.4). This overlap of absorption results in slowly varying shades of gray, rather than abrupt transitions between the blue-purple of hematoxylin and the red

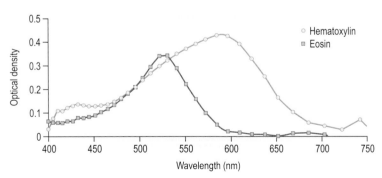

Figure 23.4 The absorbance curves of hematoxylin and eosin, measured from a stained slide. Note the high degree of overlap of the two curves.

of eosin. This problem is not new to image analysis; it has plagued photomicrography for many years. In the case of black-and-white photography, one can improve the appearance of H&E stained specimens by simply substituting some other acid dye for eosin that does not have as great an absorption curve overlap with hematoxylin. Dyes that work well for this are orange G or naphthol yellow S.

The H&E example illustrates the difference between optimum specimen preparation for visual observation versus preparation for image analysis. Recall that the purpose of staining is to permit the observer to detect detail within the cell or tissue specimen. Since the digital cameras used for image analysis respond differently than the eye, specimens intended for image analysis require modifications of traditional staining methods. In the case of specimens intended for analysis with monochrome (black and white) cameras, the staining protocol must be optimized to permit the camera to detect different portions of the specimen. Since essentially all image analysis tasks begin with methods to segregate some portions of the image from other portions, the staining methods should not use dye combinations that produce any absorption overlaps. It is also desirable that the density of the various stained components should be significantly different, so the resulting 'gray levels' are distinct. Remember, in monochrome, color disappears, as far as the camera is concerned. One should always carefully select the specimen preparation method based on the type of analysis to be performed. Careful choice of preparative (staining) method can significantly enhance the speed and accuracy of image analysis of the specimen.

As a common task in image analysis is to determine the size or area of a particular component of the specimen, in many cases the imaging task can be simplified by using single dyes, rather than combinations of dyes. If the dye is specific for a particular component of the specimen, accurate detection is simplified. Many histochemical stains meet this criterion, and are excellent choices for image analysis, if a method is available that specifically detects the cell or tissue component of interest. When it is desired to provide some contrast to the specific stain in order to see the 'non-stained' portions of the specimens, a counterstain may be used. The choice of an appropriate counterstain should include consideration of the spectral overlap and general density of the counterstain. In most cases, the counterstain should be lightly applied, simply to provide contrast. While discussing choices of stains for image analysis, it should be mentioned that for monochrome analysis one can often effectively improve the distinction between components within the specimen by varying the color of the illumination light in the microscope. This is simply done by adding colored filters to the light path. When the desired components are stained with a blue dye, using a red filter will greatly improve the ability to detect the stained components. For objects that are stained red to magenta, a green filter will be found quite useful. Often when the specimen is stained with a method that utilizes a combination of dyes, a filter can be found that will enhance the ability to segment the monochrome image to select the component of interest.

As has been mentioned in the discussion of photometry through the microscope, accurate measurement of the concentration of a material in a stained specimen requires:

- a stoichiometric relationship between the dye and the component of interest
- an absorbing dye
- an intact object, rather than a sectioned object (unless the measurement simply determines concentration per unit volume)

While many staining protocols utilize dyes that are true absorbing chromophores, there are a number of common dyes that are not true absorbing materials. Diaminobenzidine (DAB), which is commonly used as a substrate for peroxidase in immunochemical stains, is a dye that is not a true absorbing dye. DAB staining results in the deposition of a particulate in the specimen, and the concentration of this particulate gives the appearance (when observed visually) of an absorbing stain. However, when observed in reflected or incident illumination, it will be seen that DAB is a true particulate, and an effective scatterer of light. As the concentration of DAB particulate increases (darker stain), the number of particles increases and the amount of light that is scattered increases. As the DAB density increases, the scattered light may not be captured by the objective of the microscope, and the observed (as measured with an image analysis system) density of stain may become non-linear. Light scattering is also influenced by the particle size of the DAB, and this particle size is not necessarily the same for DAB obtained from various sources. Therefore, DAB is not a stain that should be employed when concentrations of a cell or tissue component are desired. Other chromogens for peroxidase in immunostains are true absorbing dyes, and are a more appropriate choice. DAB is useful, however, if the analytical result is simply to measure the areas stained within the specimen.

An important aspect of staining methodologies for quantitative analysis is standardization. Recall that the camera is much more sensitive than the eye. Variations in a particular preparative protocol that might not be detectable to a human observer, who may recognize 30 density levels, may become a significant source of error when these specimens are measured with an image analysis system which identifies 256 levels (8 bit) or 4096 levels (12 bit). In fact, for many types of analysis, every step of the process must be rigidly controlled, beginning with specimen collection and fixation. If the component of interest degrades with time, then the amount of time prior to fixation must be controlled. The length of time in fixative must be precisely defined also, since length of exposure to most fixatives may alter the binding of the final stain to the specimen. If the specimen displays any 'edge effect' – that is, increased or decreased staining at the periphery of the specimen as compared to the center – measurements must always be taken at a specified distance from the periphery. While on the subject of fixation, it should be mentioned that common fixatives may give different results with particular staining protocols. For a quantitative study, it is imperative that all specimens included in the study be fixed in the same fixative.

Staining protocols that are routine for visual examination may prove problematic for quantitative work. As previously, this relates to the increased sensitivity of image detection systems, as compared

to the eye. As the length of time a specimen is exposed to a particular staining step decreases, the percentage of error that can be introduced by the physical time required to insert or remove the slides from the staining solution may become a significant source of error. In other words, if the total time in a particular staining step is only 1 minute, a variation of 10 seconds amounts to almost a 20% variation in staining time. To reduce the potential error introduced by short staining times, staining methods should be modified by decreasing stain concentrations, and then increasing staining times. As a general guide, any staining time that is shorter than 10 minutes should be extended to between 30 minutes and an hour, by reducing stain concentration. This strategy effectively controls errors introduced by the time required to physically introduce or remove specimens from staining solutions. For stains that require differentiation, often this is done with a series of dips, with differentiation controlled by an experienced technician. This type of differentiation should be optimized by changing the concentration of the differentiation solution in order to extend the differentiation steps to a defined time, preferably long enough to eliminate the effect of short times. In addition to times in actual staining solutions, stain results may also be influenced by various dehydration sequences. Standardization of every step of a stain protocol, including deparaffinization, hydration, staining, differentiation, dehydration, clearing and coverslipping, will greatly improve variability of specimens analyzed with image analysis systems.

Quantitation of immunostains is commonly reported in publications. While immunostained specimens do lend themselves to morphometric measurements, photometric techniques can be used only when the chromogen employed is a true absorbing dye, and therefore DAB is not suitable for photometric studies. Standardization of immunostaining is particularly challenging, since most staining protocols involve at least two stages of amplification, and these amplification steps are not controlled to any significant degree. To standardize an immunostaining protocol for photometric analysis, one would have to provide standards that could be used to control the various amplification steps in the staining procedure. Although such standards can be constructed, they are not commercially available, and it is rare to see any use of such controls in published works.

It has been mentioned that, for studies that purport to measure the total amount of a material present, the intact object containing that material must be present in the slide. For many cellular materials, this means that whole cells, such as from tissue cultures, be used. Another strategy is simply to disaggregate tissues and select intact cells for analysis. Sectioned material may be employed for many image analysis tasks, but generally is not suitable for measuring the total amount of material present in a given cell or tissue component. One possible exception to this is the measurement of cell nuclei constituents. However, to measure nuclei, the operator must be certain to include intact nuclei in the section: that is, nuclei which have not been sectioned on either their top or bottom surface. The difficulty with this is that, in most fixed and sectioned material, the average size of cell nuclei is approximately 7 μm in diameter. Since general practice in many laboratories is to section at under 5 μm in thickness, then all nuclei in the specimen will be sectioned. One possible way to address this is to cut thicker sections, and, while this will yield some nuclei that are intact, there is the additional problem of overlap of nuclei from top to bottom of the section.

Morphometry, or the measurement of size and arrangement of cell or tissue constituents, can be done in sections. Such studies must also be carefully controlled, since there will always be a range of 'profiles' of a given object shape in the section. As an example, imagine a perfectly round sphere in a section. If the measurement being done is the total area of the sphere, then one would obtain different values as the section passes through the sphere. The result would be a series of measurements, with only one approaching the true diameter of the sphere. Any measure taken in sections must account for this spread of values that results from the sectioning of spheroidal objects. Obviously, some objects may have shapes other than spheroids, and this particular geometry must be taken into account when establishing a measurement approach.

There are other, subtle sources of error when measuring microscopic preparations. The biological structure should be understood, and the effects of various preparative methods on that structure must be accounted for. In tissues which have oriented, linear structures, one should consider differential shrinkage. In many cases, shrinkage will be more severe at right angles to linear morphology, particularly when that linear morphology is fibrous in nature. A classic example of differential shrinkage occurs in skeletal muscle, where fiber diameter shrinks more than fiber length. The act of sectioning may also induce morphological change, with compression of the section affecting the actual morphology of the specimen. When such compression artifacts are suspected, standards may be included with the specimen to assess the degree of compression. One type of standard that can be used is spherical latex particles, which may be sectioned along with the specimen. One can also use internal standards, and employ elements of the tissue structure that have known shapes to assess the degree of change introduced by the preparative process. Geometry can also provide information on the angle at which tissue elements have been sectioned. Tubular or rod-like elements within a tissue appear perfectly round when sectioned at right angles to the long axis, but appear as ellipses when sectioned at an angle. In such cases, where the diameter of the object is of interest, the minor (shorter) axis of the ellipse will provide the best estimate of the true size of the object.

Standards, or control objects should always be included in quantitative image analysis studies. Many techniques have been developed to construct artificial standard objects, but in many cases a standard biological object can be used. For many studies of nuclear DNA content, populations of cells that contain known amounts of DNA have been used. Common cell types that have been employed in the past are sperm, and the nucleated red blood cells of various amphibian, fish and bird species. For other cellular constituents, a common control object is a defined cell line from tissue culture. Within limits, these types of cell can be accurately characterized and, because of the conditions under which they are grown, can be harvested in such a manner as to provide a reasonably constant control object. It must be appreciated that these control objects are biological in nature and may vary over time. Any analytical procedure using such a biological control should monitor the control itself for any potential change over time.

Multispectral imaging

An emerging technique for image analysis is multispectral imaging. This technique acquires images at many specific wavelengths of light. As an example, one might collect 10 to 30 images over the wavelength range of 400 nm (blue) to 600 nm (red). Each of the selected wavelengths is narrow band, and the approach is similar to that used in chemical spectroscopy. The result is an image stack, made up of images at discrete wavelengths. When the absorbance curves for each compound (stain) within a specimen are known, the multispectral image stack can be used to accurately determine the exact location of each stain within the image. This approach is particularly powerful when the specimen contains areas of mixed stains, and the eye cannot separate the individual stains. An example would be a combination immunohistochemical stain, where one primary antibody is stained with a brown chromogen and the second with a red chromogen. The eye cannot easily separate these two colors, particularly if one is present in small amounts. Using multispectral imaging, one can generate separate images with each individual stain. By then re-coloring, or pseudo-coloring these individual images in some highly contrasting colors, the two images can be recombined into a single, easily evaluated image. Because of the way in which color is produced in display systems, one can also employ a 'trick' and, in the case of two colors, use the pseudo-colors of 'red' and 'green'. When these two pseudo-colored images are then combined for display, any areas that contain both red and green color will appear in yellow. This is obviously quite useful to subjectively evaluate double-stained specimens for label co-localization. Using image logic operations, one can also generate a third image that displays only co-localized staining.

Multispectral imaging requires specific hardware to collect the 'image stack' at specific wavelengths, as well as software to permit extraction of the individual spectral information in the images. There are a variety of devices available to collect multispectral images, ranging from cameras with filter wheels in front of a monochrome sensor, cameras with electronically switchable filters, to systems using switching light sources capable of generating narrow-band light. As the hardware and software for multispectral imaging is rapidly evolving, a search of current literature should be done by those interested in employing this technique.

References

DeHoff, R.T., Rhines, F.N., 1968. Quantitative microscopy. McGraw-Hill, New York.

Elias, H., Hyde, D.M., 1983. A guide to practical stereology. Karger, Basel.

Elias, H., Pauly, J.E., Burns, E.R., 1978. Histology and human microanatomy. John Wiley, New York, Appendix II.

Piller, H., 1977. Microscope photometry. Springer, Berlin.

Shotton, D., 1993. Electronic light microscopy. Wiley-Liss, New York.

Underwood, E.E., 1970. Quantitative stereology. Addison-Wesley, Reading, MA.

Weibel, E.R., 1979. Stereological methods: practical methods for biological morphometry, Vol. 1. Academic Press, New York.

Weibel, E.R., 1980. Stereological methods: theoretical foundations, Vol. 2. Academic Press, New York.

Weibel, E.R., 1990. Morphometry: stereological theory and practical methods. In: Gil, J. (Ed.), Models of lung disease: microscopy and structural methods. Marcel Dekker, New York, pp. 199–247.

Wied, G.L., 1966. Introduction to quantitative cytochemistry. Academic Press, New York.

Wied, G.L., Bahr, G.F., 1970. Introduction to quantitative cytochemistry: II. Academic Press, New York.

Further reading

Baak, J.P.A., 1991. Quantitative pathology in cancer diagnosis and prognosis. Springer, Berlin.

Baxes, G.A., 1994. Digital image processing. John Wiley, New York.

Castleman, K.R., 1995. Digital image processing. Prentice Hall, Englewood Cliffs, NJ.

Crane, R., 1997. A simplified approach to image processing. Prentice Hall, Upper Saddle River, NJ.

Gu, J., 1997. Analytical morphology: theory, applications and protocols. Eaton, Boston.

Jahne, B. 1997. Digital image processing, fourth ed. Springer, Berlin.

Jahne, B., 1997. Image processing for scientific applications. CRC Press, Boca Raton, FL.

Klette, R., Zamperoni, P. 1996. Handbook of image processing operators. John Wiley, New York.

Marchevsky, A.M., Bartels, P.H., 1994. Image analysis: a primer for pathologists. Raven Press, New York.

Parker, J.R., 1997. Algorithms for image processing and computer vision. John Wiley, New York.

Rosenfeld, A., Kak, A.C., 1982. Digital picture processing, Vols 1 and 2. Academic Press, New York.

Russ, J.C., 1995. The image processing handbook. CRC Press, Boca Raton, FL.

Watkins, C., Sadun, A., Marenka, S., 1993. Modern image processing: warping, morphing and classical techniques. Academic Press, New York.

Weeks, A.R., 1996. Fundamentals of electronic image processing. SPIE Press/IEEE Press, New York.

Wootton, R., Springall, D.R., Polak, J.M., 1995. Image analysis in histology. Cambridge University Press, Cambridge.

Diagnostic Appendices

John D. Bancroft

Jennifer H. Stonard

Laura J. Keeling

Sherin Jos Payyappilly

Classical histochemical methods

John D. Bancroft • Jennifer H. Stonard

The aim of this appendix is to include discussion and methodology from the chapters Lipids, Proteins, Nucleic acids and Enzyme Histochemistry which were included in previous editions of this book. These technologies have largely been superseded in the modern laboratory but are still used in teaching courses worldwide.

For a full discussion and omitted methods please refer to the sixth edition of this text.

Lipids

Introduction

These methods have an application in diagnostic pathology for nervous system disorders. The myelin sheath is particularly rich in lipids, being composed of compacted cell membrane, a lamellar structure of cholesterol and phospholipids. The lipid demonstration methods can aid in the diagnosis of demyelination and the lipid storage disorders.

Lipids may be defined as any one of a group of fats or fatlike substances. These fats would include:

- true fats – esters of fatty acids and glycerol
- lipids – phospholipids, cerebrosides and waxes
- sterols – cholesterol and ergosterol
- hydrocarbons – squalene and carotene

Classification

Lipids may be classified as a mixed group of substances with the common characteristics of solubility in organic solvents and insolubility in water. They can be organized as simple lipids, compound lipids or derived lipids.

- Simple lipids: esters of fatty acids with alcohols, including fats, oils and waxes. Fats are neutral esters of glycerol with saturated or unsaturated fatty acids. Oils may be similar to fats but are liquid at room temperature. Waxes are esters of higher alcohols with long-chain fatty acids. Simple lipids are usually found in the body as energy stores in adipose tissue. Waxes are usually found in plant and some animal species.
- Compound lipids: usually consist of a fatty acid, an alcohol and one or more other groups such as phosphorus or nitrogen. These can be found in the brain and central nervous system.
- Derived lipids: fatty acids that can originate from the simple and compound lipids by means of hydrolysis. Cholesterol, bile acids and sex and adrenocortical hormones are examples.

Fixation and microtomy

The common method of demonstrating tissue lipids is with fresh frozen (cryostat) sections. Some degree of fixation may be necessary so that lipids and the sections themselves are able to withstand the potentially destructive or solvent effects of histochemical reagents. The only reagents that truly fix lipids are osmium tetroxide and chromic acid, but both these greatly alter the chemical reactivity of the lipids. Frozen or cryostat sections are required for lipid histochemistry because routine processing for paraffin and resin sections will result in the extraction of all but a few protein-bound lipids from the tissue. Although lipids are not strictly fixed by formaldehyde, they are better retained in a section when the supporting matrix of tissue proteins has been fixed.

Fat stains and the Sudan dyes

Lipids that exist as fats, namely the oily and greasy hydrophobic lipids, have an affinity for the Sudan dyes. For many years a wide range of these compounds has provided almost the sole means of staining lipids.

Oil Red O in dextrin (modified by Churukian (2000)

Fixation

Fresh frozen or NBF, rinse, frozen

Sections

5 μm mount on slides, air dry.

Solutions

Oil Red O solution

Oil Red O	0.5 g
Absolute isopropyl alcohol	100 ml

Allow to stand overnight.

Dextrin solution

Dextrin*	1 g
Distilled water	100 ml

Working solution

Stock Oil Red O	60 ml
Dextrin	40 ml

Allow to stand for a day or more. Stable for months, filter before use.

Method

1. Place slides directly into filtered 0.5% Oil Red O in dextrin. Stain 20 minutes, rinse with running water briefly.
2. Counterstain with Gill II hematoxylin for 20–30 seconds. Rinse with water, blue, coverslip with aqueous mounting media.

Results

Fat	brilliant red
Nuclei	blue.

*Dextrin, bacteriological grade or Type III from Sigma, from corn. Dextrin is hydrolyzed corn starch. VWR (VWR Scientific) also has small quantities, must be most soluble form of dextrin.

Standard Sudan black B method for fats and phospholipids

Fixation and sections

Cryostat sections post-fixed in formal calcium; short fixed frozen sections; unfixed cryostat sections (preferred).

Method

1. Rinse sections in 70% ethanol.
2. Stain for up to 2 hours in saturated Sudan black B in 70% ethanol.
3. Rinse in 70% ethanol to remove excess surface dye, and wash in tap water.
4. Counterstain nuclei with Kernechtrot for 2–5 minutes.
5. Wash well and mount in glycerine jelly.

Results

The standard Sudan black procedure stains unsaturated esters and triglycerides *blue-black*. Some phospholipids appear *gray* and those in myelin exhibit a *bronze* dichroism in polarized light.

Bromination enhances the reaction of these lipids and in addition stains lecithin, free fatty acids and free cholesterol.

Note

The Sudan black solution should not be oversaturated or sections will be covered in a fine deposit. Fixation enhances the staining of phospholipids (present in all tissues) and this is unwanted in general use; thus unfixed sections are preferred.

Cholesterol

Perchloric acid-naphthoquinone (PAN) method for cholesterol (Adams, 1961)

Fixation and sections

Formal calcium fixed frozen section; cryostat sections post-fixed in formal calcium.

Preparation of reagent

1:2 naphthoquinone-4-sulfonic acid	40 mg
Ethanol	20 ml
60% perchloric acid	10 ml
40% formaldehyde	1 ml
Distilled water	9 ml

Mix and use within 24 hours.

Method

1. Air dry sections onto slides.
2. Treat with 1% ferric chloride for 4 hours.
3. Wash well in distilled water.
4. Carefully paint the sections sparingly with the reagent using a soft camel-hair brush. (Note: wash the brush thoroughly with water after each use, and dry.) Heat them on a surface at 70°C for 1 or 2 minutes, until the color develops. The sections are kept moist by gently replenishing the reagent from time to time.
5. Place a drop of perchloric acid on a cover glass and lower section into position.

Results

Cholesterol and related steroids	blue

Sphingomyelin

Sodium hydroxide-ferric hematoxylin/ DAH method

Fixation and sections

Formalin fixed sections, preferably mounted on chrome gelatin subbed slides.

Method

1. Treat sections with 2 M sodium hydroxide for 1 hour at room temperature.
2. Wash gently but thoroughly in a large volume of water.
3. Rinse in 1% acetic acid for 5 seconds.
4. If section has become detached from the slide, remount it and proceed with the ferric hematoxylin method described above.

Results

Sphingomyelin	blue

Cerebrosides

Modified PAS reaction for cerebroside
(Adams & Bayliss 1963)

Fixation and sections

Cryostat sections post-fixed in formal calcium; fixed frozen sections.

Preparation of reagent

Performic acid

98% formic acid	45 ml
100 vol hydrogen peroxide	4.5 ml
Concentrated H_2SO_4	0.5 ml

Prepare an hour before use and stir occasionally with a glass rod, inside a fume hood, to release bubbles of gas from the solution.

Method

1. Mount duplicate sections onto separate slides and extract one of these with chloroform methanol (2 : 1 v/v) for 1 hour at room temperature.
2. Deaminate both sections in 10% aqueous chloramine T for 1 hour at 37°C.
3. Wash slides vigorously and as rapidly as possible, one at a time, in a large volume of water before transferring them immediately to performic acid for 10 minutes. The washing must be swift yet thorough, to avoid swelling and detachment of sections from slides.
4. Wash well in distilled water.
5. Treat with a filtered saturated solution of 2 : 4 dinitrophenyl hydrazine in 1 M HCl at 4°C for 2 hours.
6. Wash well in water.
7. Treat with 0.5% periodic acid for 10 minutes.
8. Wash in distilled water.
9. Stain in Schiff's reagent for 15 minutes.
10. Rinse in distilled water and wash in tap water for 15 minutes to develop color.
11. Counterstain nuclei with Mayer's hematoxylin or Carazzi's hematoxylin if required.
12. Wash in tap water, distilled water and finally mount sections in glycerine jelly.

Results

Cerebroside	magenta

Indicated by the difference in staining intensity between the two sections.

Sulfatides

Toluidine blue-acetone method for sulfatide
(Bodian & Lake 1963)

Fixation and sections

Post-fixed cryostat sections; formal calcium fixed frozen sections.

Reagents

0.01% toluidine blue in phosphate-citrate buffer at pH 4.7.

Buffer solution

0.2 M Na_2HPO_4	96 ml
0.1 M citric acid	104 ml

Method

1. Mount sections onto slides.
2. Stain for 16–18 hours in buffered toluidine blue.
3. Wash in water.
4. Dehydrate with acetone for 5 minutes.
5. Mount in DPX.

Result

Sulfatide deposits appear metachromatic red-brown or yellow.

Gangliosides

Borohydride-periodate-Schiff (BHPS) method

Fixation and sections

Cryostat sections post-fixed in formal calcium; frozen sections of fixed tissue.

Method

1. Destroy existing aldehyde groups (endogenous or from formalin or glutaraldehyde fixation) by reduction with 0.1 M (0.38%) sodium borohydride in 1% disodium hydrogen phosphate for 1 hour at room temperature.
2. Wash thoroughly in distilled water.
3. Oxidize with 1.2 mM (0.03%) sodium periodate for 30 minutes at room temperature.
4. Wash twice for 5 minutes each time in distilled water.
5. Stain with Schiff's reagent for 10 minutes.
6. Rinse in distilled water and wash well in tap water.
7. Counterstain with Mayer's hematoxylin or Carazzi's hematoxylin.
8. Blue in tap water, rinse in distilled, then mount sections in glycerine jelly.

Results

Gangliosides (in Tay-Sachs' disease and GM_1 gangliosidosis)	red
Nuclei	blue

Note

A chloroform methanol-extracted section should be used for comparison to exclude interference from non-lipid sialomucins.

Proteins and nucleic acids

Introduction

Proteins and nucleic acids are major cell and tissue constituents. Proteins are highly organized complex macromolecules that are made up of 20 common amino acids linked together by peptide bonds. They occur in cells and tissues as simple and conjugated proteins. Simple proteins are made up of amino acids only: e.g. albumins, globulins, fibrous structure proteins and enzymes.

Phenyl groups

These can be demonstrated by a modification of the well-known biochemical test, the Millon reaction (Baker, 1956). A red or pinkish color develops at the site of tyrosine-containing proteins when the section is treated with a hot mercuric sulfate-sulfuric acid-sodium nitrite mixture. Tyrosine is the only amino acid which contains the hydroxyphenyl group in a form which can be demonstrated histochemically. The method can therefore be regarded as specific for tyrosine, but since tyrosine is an almost invariable constituent of all tissue proteins, the Millon reaction is a suitable general protein method. The color reaction of the Millon reaction is rarely strong and there may be difficulty encountered in keeping the sections on the slide. A less well-known, but more reliable, technique is the diazotization-coupling method (Glenner & Lillie, 1959).

Millon reaction for tyrosine (Baker 1956)

Fixation

Neutral buffered formalin; formaldehyde vapor (for freeze-dried tissue).

Sections

Paraffin, fixed cryostat, freeze-dried or celloidin.

Solutions

Solution a

10 g of mercuric sulfate is added to a mixture of 90 ml distilled water and 10 ml of concentrated sulfuric acid, and is dissolved by heating. After cooling to room temperature, 100 ml of distilled water is added.

Solution b

250 mg of sodium nitrite is dissolved in 10 ml of distilled water.

Staining solution

5 ml of Solution b is added to 50 ml of Solution a.

Method

1. Take sections to water.
2. Immerse sections in staining solution in a small beaker and gently bring to boil; simmer for 2 minutes.
3. Allow to cool to room temperature.
4. Wash in three changes of distilled water, 2 minutes each.
5. Dehydrate through alcohols, clear in xylene, and mount.

Result

Tyrosine-containing proteins   red or pink

Notes

a. A suitable positive control tissue is pancreas.
b. Mercury-containing reagents must be disposed of according to the law.
c. Caution should be used when diluting sulfuric acid with water.

Performic acid-Alcian blue method *(Adams & Sloper 1955)*

Fixation

Neutral buffered formalin; formaldehyde vapor (for freeze-dried tissue).

Sections

Paraffin, freeze-dried, frozen cryostat sections

Solutions

Performic acid solution

Concentrated formic acid	40 ml
30% hydrogen peroxide	4 ml
Concentrated sulfuric acid	0.5 ml

Alcian blue solution

Alcian blue	1 g
Concentrated sulfuric acid	2.7 ml
Distilled water	47.2 ml

Method

1. Take sections to water; blot to remove surplus water.
2. Immerse sections in performic acid solution (see Note a), 5 minutes.
3. Wash well in tap water (see Note b), 10 minutes.
4. Dry in 60°C oven until just dry.
5. Rinse in tap water.
6. Stain in Alcian blue solution at room temperature, 1 hour.
7. Wash in running tap water.
8. Counterstain (e.g. neutral red) if required.
9. Wash in tap water.
10. Dehydrate through alcohols, clear in xylene and mount.

Result

Disulfides   blue

The intensity of the blue color will depend on the amount of disulfide present.

Note

a. The performic acid solution should be prepared fresh and allowed to stand for 1 hour before use.
b. The section should be washed adequately but carefully; it may lift off if the washing is too vigorous following treatment in performic acid. The drying stage reduces the risk of section loss.

Indole groups

These can be demonstrated by the histochemical reaction of the amino acids tryptamine and tryptophan. The most reliable method is the DMAB-nitrite method of Adams (1957). The best results (i.e. most intense coloration and most precise localization) are obtained with freeze-dried sections, but satisfactory results are obtainable with paraffin sections. The principle of the method is that tryptophan reacts with DMAB (*p*-dimethylaminobenzaldehyde) to produce a substance known as β-carboline, which is then oxidized by the nitrite solution to produce a deep blue pigment.

DMAB-nitrite method for tryptophan *(Adams 1957)*

Fixation

Neutral buffered formalin; formaldehyde vapor (for freeze-dried tissue).

Sections

Paraffin, freeze-dried, frozen cryostat sections.

Solutions

DMAB solution

5 g of *p*-dimethylaminobenzaldehyde is dissolved in 100 ml of concentrated hydrochloric acid.

Nitrite solution

1 g of sodium nitrite is dissolved in 100 ml of concentrated hydrochloric acid.

Method

1. Take sections to absolute ethanol.
2. Celloidinize in 0.5% celloidin.
3. Place sections in DMAB solution for 1 minute.
4. Transfer sections to nitrite solution for 1–2 minutes.
5. Wash gently in tap water for 30 seconds.
6. Rinse in acid alcohol for 15 seconds.
7. Wash in water and optionally counterstain in 1% aqueous neutral red for 5 minutes.
8. Dehydrate through ethanols, clear in xylene and mount.

Results

Tryptophan	dark blue
Nuclei	red

Notes

a. Pancreas is an excellent positive control tissue.
b. This is one of the most satisfactory and rewarding of amino acid histochemical methods.
c. The reagents give off toxic fumes and should be prepared (and used if possible) in a fume hood.

Nucleic acids

Nucleoproteins are combinations of basic proteins (protamines and histones) and nucleic acids. The two nucleic acids are deoxyribonucleic acid (DNA), which is mainly found in the nucleus of the cell, and ribonucleic acid (RNA), which is located in the cytoplasm of cells, mainly in the ribosomes. Both the DNA and RNA molecules consist of alternate sugar and phosphate groups with a nitrogenous base (either a purine or pyrimidine) being attached to each sugar group. The sugar in DNA is the 5-carbon sugar deoxyribose; in RNA it is ribose. Histochemical techniques for the demonstration of nucleic acids in tissue are based on all their constituents. DNA and RNA can be localized in cells by the affinity of their negatively charged phosphate ester groups for almost any basic dye, particularly hematoxylin or methyl green and pyronin (Spicer 1987). RNA is usually only evident in cells whose cytoplasm is particularly rich in this nucleic acid (e.g. plasma cells and serous acinar cells). Hematoxylin is by no means specific for DNA and RNA, and it will also stain glycosaminoglycans and other anionic complexes.

Demonstration of nucleic acids

Fixation

In general terms, the nucleic acids are best preserved in alcoholic and acidic fixatives, a good example being Carnoy's fluid which contains both alcohol and glacial acetic acid. Formalin has only a limited reaction with DNA and RNA, but for routine work gives acceptable results. Low (4°C) temperature fixation in neutral buffered formalin has been shown to prevent DNA degradation by cell nucleases, which is of some importance when carrying out molecular biology studies (Tokuda et al. 1990).

Basophilia

DNA and RNA both stain strongly with most cationic dyes. Selectivity of staining can be achieved by using, for example, methylene blue at a pH range of 3.0–4.0. A distinction has been drawn between the link formed by simple cationic dyes such as neutral red and methylene blue and nucleic acid and the nuclear stain formed by metal complex dyes such as alum hematoxylin (Marshall & Horobin 1973). The former type of staining can be markedly reduced by prior treatment with acids, and is considered to be largely coulombic (electrostatic) in nature. Alum hematoxylin staining of cellular nuclei is much less affected by prior acid treatment. This part acid-fast effect is attributed to the metal-dye complex also forming non-electrostatic bonding interactions, such as hydrophobic bonding and van der Waals' attraction forces, with nucleic acids. Interestingly, whilst nucleic acids exhibit strong basophilia, they do not usually exhibit metachromasia with the standard metachromatic dyes such as toluidine blue or azure A.

Deoxyribonucleic acid (DNA)

The typical demonstration of DNA is ether by the Feulgen technique, which will demonstrate the sugar deoxyribose, or the methyl green-pyronin technique in which the phosphates combine with the basic dye methyl green at an acid pH. DNA can also be demonstrated by fluorescent methods using acridine orange, although the reliability of this type of method is less than the previous methods. Both DNA and RNA can be demonstrated by the gallocyanin chrome alum method; the method does not separate the two nucleic acids and suitable extraction techniques must be used. The definitive, most sensitive technique for identifying DNA is that of *in situ* hybridization.

Feulgen reaction

The method of Feulgen and Rossenbeck (1924) is the standard technique for demonstrating deoxyribose. Mild acid hydrolysis, employing 1 M hydrochloric acid at 60°C, is used to break the purine-deoxyribose bond; the resulting 'exposed' aldehydes are then demonstrated by the use of Schiff's reagent. The hydrolysis is the critical part of the method; an increasingly stronger reaction is obtained as the hydrolysis time is increased until the optimum is reached. Beyond this, the reaction becomes weaker, and if the hydrolysis is continued the reaction may fail completely. An important consideration in selecting the correct hydrolysis time is the fixative used. Bouin's fixative is not suitable as it causes over-hydrolysis of the nucleic acid during fixation. Bauer (1932) discussed the times of hydrolysis for various fixatives; some of these are reproduced in the sixth edition.

Feulgen nuclear reaction for DNA (Feulgen & Rossenbeck 1924)

Fixation

Not critical but not Bouin's.

Solutions

a. 1 M hydrochloric acid

Hydrochloric acid (conc.)	8.5 ml
Distilled water	91.5 ml

b. Schiff's reagent

c. Bisulfite solution

10% potassium metabisulfite	5 ml
1 M hydrochloric acid	5 ml
Distilled water	90 ml

Method

1. Bring all sections to water.
2. Rinse sections in 1 M HCl at room temperature.
3. Place sections in 1 M HCl at 60°C.
4. Rinse in 1 M HCl at room temperature, 1 minute.
5. Transfer sections to Schiff's reagent, 45 minutes.
6. Rinse sections in bisulfite solution, 2 minutes.
7. Repeat wash in bisulfite solution, 2 minutes.
8. Repeat wash in bisulfite solution, 2 minutes.
9. Rinse well in distilled water.
10. Counterstain if required in 1% light green, 2 minutes.
11. Wash in water.
12. Dehydrate through alcohols to xylene and mount.

Results

DNA	red-purple
Cytoplasm	green

Ribonucleic acid (RNA)

The method of choice for demonstrating RNA is the methyl green-pyronin technique. RNA can also be demonstrated by acridine orange and by the gallocyanin-chrome alum technique, along with DNA, given suitable extraction procedures.

Methyl green-pyronin

This will demonstrate both DNA and RNA. Methyl green is an impure dye containing methyl violet. By removing the methyl with chloroform, the pure methyl green (when used at a slightly acid pH) appears to be specific for DNA.

The rationale of the technique is that both dyes are cationic when used in combination: methyl green binds preferentially, and specifically to DNA, leaving the pyronin to bind to RNA. The methyl green-specific reactivity is attributed to the spatial alignment of the NH_2 groups of the dye to phosphate radicals on the DNA double helix. Pyronin staining, on the other hand, does not show this spatial affinity and any negatively charged tissue constituent will stain red. In practice, this means that as well as RNA, acid mucins present in epithelium as well as cartilage also will stain.

Methyl green-pyronin method (Pappenheim 1899; Unna 1902 from Bancroft & Cook 1994)

Fixation

Carnoy preferred, but formalin acceptable.

Solution

Methyl green pyronin Y

2% methyl green in distilled water (chloroform washed)	9 ml
2% pyronin Y in distilled water	4 ml
Acetate buffer, pH 4.8	23 ml
Glycerol	14 ml

Mix well before use.

Method

1. Take sections down to water.
2. Rinse in acetate buffer, pH 4.8.
3. Place in methyl green pyronin Y solution for 25 minutes.
4. Rinse in buffer.
5. Blot dry.
6. Rinse in 93% ethanol, then in absolute ethanol.
7. Rinse in xylene and mount.

Results

DNA	green-blue
RNA	red

Digestion methods for nucleic acids

Specific enzymes can be used to digest DNA and RNA in tissue sections. Pure deoxyribonuclease will remove DNA, while ribonuclease will digest RNA. In a pure state the enzymes will not affect the other nucleic acid.

Enzyme extraction of DNA (Brachet 1940)

Fixation

Potassium dichromate will inhibit digestion, and should be avoided.

Digestion solution

Deoxyribonuclease	10 mg
0.2 M Tris buffer, pH 7.6	10 ml
Distilled water	50 ml

Method

1. Bring both test and control sections to water.
2. Place test section in extraction solution, control in Tris buffer, pH 7.6, incubate both test and control section at 37°C, for 4 hours.
3. Wash in running tap water.
4. Stain both sections by the Feulgen method.

Results

Test section	DNA negative
Control section	DNA red

Enzyme extraction of RNA (Brachet 1940)

Fixation

Potassium dichromate and mercuric chloride should be avoided, as digestion is inhibited.

Digestion solution

Ribonuclease	8 mg
Distilled water	10 ml

Method

1. Bring both test and control slides to water.
2. Place test slide in ribonuclease solution, and control slide in distilled water, incubate both test and control section at 37°C for 1 hour.
3. Wash in distilled water.
4. Apply methyl green-pyronin method.

Results

Test slide	RNA negative, DNA green
Control slide	RNA red, DNA green

Enzyme histochemistry

This subject has been largely replaced by immunocytochemistry. Below are some of the classical methods that are of diagnostic value.

Fixation for enzyme histochemistry

Enzymes are labile and their preservation is important. The mitochondria, in which many of the oxidative enzymes are located, are rapidly damaged when the blood supply is cut. Freezing and subsequent thawing of blocks or sections damages organelles such as lysosomes, which contain many of the hydrolytic enzymes. Hydrolytic enzymes show considerable diffusion if demonstrated on frozen, unfixed sections. Tissues to be used for the demonstration of the majority of hydrolytic enzymes may be subjected to controlled fixation, which, whilst decreasing the amount of demonstrable enzyme within the section, does allow for a considerably sharper localization of the remaining enzyme activity. Fixation will destroy many of the oxidative enzymes; there are a few exceptions to this, and these are indicated in the relevant enzyme methods. For the demonstration of hydrolytic enzymes, histochemical techniques are usually applied to sections that have been prefixed in cold (4°C) formal calcium.

Smears

In enzyme histochemistry, the use of smears for cytochemical identification and evaluation of cells is used. Such smears, whose preparation may be achieved in various ways, include blood, bone marrow and tissue cell suspensions. Three of the most useful enzymes are non-specific esterase, acid phosphatase and chloroacetate esterase. It is usual to fix smears before histochemical staining to preserve cell structure and enzyme localization.

Enzyme types

Oxidoreductases

Oxidases: catalyze oxidation of a substrate in the presence of oxygen
Peroxidases: catalyze oxidation of a substrate by removing hydrogen, which combines with hydrogen peroxide

Dehydrogenases: catalyze oxidation of a substrate by removal of hydrogen
Diaphorases: catalyze oxidation of NADH and NADPH by removal of hydrogen.

Transferases

Catalyze the transfer of the radicals of two compounds without the loss or uptake of water.

Hydrolases

Catalyze the introduction of water or its elements into specific substrate bonds, although in some instances water may be removed. These enzymes include:

- phosphatases (acid, alkaline and specific)
- esterases
- lipases
- glycosidases
- peptidases
- pyrophosphatases

Diagnostic applications

The current common uses of enzyme histochemistry in surgical histopathology laboratories can be summarized:

- skeletal muscle biopsy
- colonic biopsy in cases of suspected Hirschsprung's disease

Skeletal muscle biopsy

The application of enzyme histochemical methods to cryostat sections of unfixed skeletal muscle shows the presence of different fiber types, and changes in the number, size and relative proportions of the different fibers are valuable in establishing the diagnosis.

Methods in common use for muscle biopsy diagnosis:

- Adenosine triphosphatase (ATPase)
- Cytochrome oxidase (COX)
- NADH diaphorase
- Phosphorylase (after Meijer 1968)

Adenosine triphosphatase (ATPase)

Sections

Unfixed cryostat.

Solutions

a. 0.1 M glycine buffer

Glycine	0.75 g
NaCl	0.585 g

Make up to 100 ml with distilled water.

b. 0.1 M glycine buffer with 0.75 M CaCl$_2$

0.1 M glycine buffer (Solution a)	50 ml
0.75 M CaCl$_2$ (11.03 g CaCl$_2$•2H$_2$O in 100 ml distilled water)	10 ml

Mix, then add approx. 22 ml 0.1 M NaOH until pH 9.4.

c. 0.1 M solution veronal-acetate buffer, pH 4.2 and pH 4.6 (see Appendix III)

d. Incubating solution

ATP	5 mg
Solution b	10 ml

Adjust to pH 9.4 with 0.1 M NaOH or 0.1 M HCl if necessary.

Method (at pH 9.4)

1. Incubate freshly cut sections in incubating Solution d at 37°C.
2. Rinse well in distilled water.
3. Immerse in 2% cobalt chloride for 5 minutes.
4. Rinse well in tap water, then in three changes of distilled water.
5. Immerse in dilute (1:10) ammonium sulfide solution for 30 seconds (in fume cupboard).
6. Rinse well in running tap water.
7. Stain lightly in Harris's hematoxylin, blue in tap water (see Note).
8. Mount in glycerine jelly or dehydrate, clear and mount in DPX.

Method (at pH 4.2 and 4.6)

1. Pre-incubate freshly cut sections at 4°C in appropriate 0.1 M veronal-acetate buffer (Solution c above) for 10 minutes.
2. Rinse briefly in distilled water.
3. Proceed as from Step 1 in the pH 9.4 method above.

Results

Differential enzyme staining of skeletal muscle fibers (based on Dubowitz 1985). See table below.

Note

Only the pH 4.2 sections need counterstaining in hematoxylin. Sections must be well washed after the cobalt chloride and ammonium sulfide steps.

Differential enzyme staining of skeletal muscle fibers (based on Dubowitz 1985)

Fiber type	ATPase, pH 4.2	ATPase, pH 4.6	ATPase, pH 9.4	NADH diaphorase, SDH, and LDH	Phosphorylase
Type 1	+++	+++	+	+++	+/–
Type 2A	–	–	+++	++	+++
Type 2B	–	+++	+++	+	+++
Type 2C	+	+++	+++	++	+++

Small regenerating fibers are usually strongly NADH positive, irrespective of fiber type. Type 2C fibers are a very small minority in normal human muscle.

Cytochrome oxidase (COX) *(Seligman et al. 1968)*

Sections

Cryostat sections (fresh).

Incubating solution

Catalase, 20 µg/ml (4 mg in 10 ml; remove 2.5 ml and make up to 50 ml in distilled water)	1 ml
Cytochrome c (type 2)	10 mg
0.1 M phosphate buffer, pH 7.4	9 ml
3,3'-Diaminobenzidine tetrahydrochloride (DAB)	5 mg

Adjust pH to 7.4 before use with 0.1 M NaOH or 0.1 M HCl as required.

Method

1. Incubate sections at room temperature for 2–3 hours.
2. Rinse in distilled water.
3. Fix in formal calcium, 15 minutes.
4. Counterstain in hematoxylin, 15 seconds.
5. Wash and blue.
6. Dehydrate, clear, and mount in DPX.

Results

Brown reaction product at sites of cytochrome oxidase activity.

Notes

Many tissues are rich in this enzyme. It is involved in the main oxidation pathway. The enzyme is also known as cytochrome a_3.

All muscle fibers should demonstrate activity, but type 1 fibers are the most strongly positive. All fibers are negative in congenital cytochrome oxidase deficiency.

Phosphorylase *(after Meijer 1968)*

Sections

Unfixed cryostat.

Incubating solution (add the reagents in the following order)

0.1 M acetate buffer, pH 5.9	100 ml
0.1 M magnesium chloride	10 ml
Glucose-1-phosphate	1 g
Glycogen (oyster/rabbit liver)	20 mg
ATP salt	50 mg
Sodium fluoride	1.8 g
Ethanol	20 ml
Polyvinyl pyrrolidine	9 g

Store at –20°C.

Method

1. Incubate in solution at 37°C for 90 minutes.
2. Wash in 40% ethanol for 5 seconds; air dry.
3. Fix in ethanol for 3 minutes; air dry.
4. Wash in 1 : 30 Lugol's iodine for 5 minutes.
5. Mount in 9 : 1 glycerine jelly/Lugol's iodine.

Results

Phosphorylase activity	blue/black

Notes

The solution is kept in a closed Columbia jar and is frozen after each incubation. Replace when its potency is diminished.

Colonic biopsy in cases of suspected Hirschsprung's disease

In the normal colon and rectum, there are ganglion cells in both the submucosa and the so-called myenteric plexus between the circular and longitudinal muscle of the outer bowel wall. These ganglia, and their associated nerves, are responsible for colonic motility.

In Hirschsprung's disease in children, a variable segment of the rectum and colon is devoid of ganglion cells ('aganglionic segment'). In the affected segment peristalsis is impossible and the large bowel becomes obstructed. The diagnosis may be suspected clinically and radiologically but requires histological confirmation, usually by the examination of one or more suction biopsy specimens of rectal mucosa and submucosa with the aid of the enzyme histochemical method, acetylcholinesterase.

Acetylcholinesterase *(from Filipe & Lake 1983)*

Preparation of tissue

Cryostat sections of snap-frozen tissue cut at 10 µm are air-dried and fixed for 30 seconds in 4% formaldehyde in 0.1 M calcium acetate (formal calcium).

Frozen sections of formal calcium-gum sucrose treated blocks of tissue.

Incubation medium

Acetylthiocholine iodide	5 mg
0.1 M acetate buffer, pH 6.0	6.5 ml
0.1 M sodium citrate	0.5 ml
30 mM copper sulfate	1 ml
Distilled water	1 ml
4 mM iso-octamethyl pyrophosphoramide (iso OMPA)	0.2 ml

Add 1.0 ml 5 mM potassium ferricyanide just before use.

Method

1. Rinse the fixed sections for 10 seconds in tap water.
2. Incubate at 37°C for 1 hour in the above medium.
3. Wash briefly in tap water.
4. Treat with 0.05% *p*-phenylene diamine dihydrochoride in 0.05 M phosphate buffer, pH 6.8 for 45 minutes at room temperature.
5. Wash in tap water.
6. Treat with 1% osmium tetroxide for 10 minutes at room temperature.
7. Wash well in tap water, counterstain lightly (10 seconds) in Carrazzi hematoxylin (or Mayer's hemalum), wash, dehydrate, clear and mount in DPX.

Results

Nerve fibers and cells containing acetylcholinesterase are stained dark brown to black.

References

Adams, C.W.M., 1957. A *p*-dimethylaminoben-zaldehyde-nitrite method for the histochemical demonstration of tryptophane and related compounds. Journal of Clinical Pathology 10, 56.

Adams, C.W.M., 1961. A perchloric acid-naphthoquinone method for the histochemical localization of cholesterol. Nature (London) 193, 331.

Adams, C.W.M., Bayliss, O.B., 1963. Histochemical observations on the localization and origin of sphyingomyelin, cerebroside and cholesterol in normal and atherosclerotic human artery. Journal of Pathology and Bacteriology 85, 113.

Adams, C.W.M., Sloper, J.C., 1955. Technique for demonstrating neurosecretory material in the human hypothalamus. Lancet 1, 651.

Bancroft, J.D., Cook, H.C., 1994. Manual of histological techniques and their diagnostic applications. Churchill Livingstone, Edinburgh.

Baker, J.R., 1956. The histochemical recognition of phenols, especially tyrosine. Quarterly Journal of Microscopical Science 88, 115.

Bauer, H., 1932. Die Feulgensche Nuklealfarbung in ihrer Anwendungaufcytologische Untersuchungen. Zeitschrift für Zellforschung und Mikroskopische Anatomie 15, 225.

Bodian, M., Lake, B.D., 1963. The rectal approach to neuropathology. British Journal of Surgery 50, 702.

Brachet, J., 1940. La detection histochemique des acides pentose-nucleiques. Comptes Rendus des Seances de la Societe de Biologie et des ses Filaiales 133, 88.

Churukian, C.J., 2000. Manual of the special stains laboratory, eighth ed. University of Rochester, Rochester, NY.

Dubowitz, V., 1985. Muscle biopsy: a practical approach. Baillière Tindall, London.

Feulgen, R., Rossenbeck, H., 1924. Mikroskopischchemischer Nachweis einen Nucleinsaure von Typus der Thymonucleinsaure und die darauf berhende elective Farbung von Zellkernen in mikroskopischen Preparaten. Zeitschrift für Physiologische Chemie 135, 203.

Filipe, M.I., Lake, B.D. (Eds.), 1983. Histochemistry in pathology. Churchill Livingstone, Edinburgh.

Marshall, P.N., Horobin, R.W., 1973. The mechanism of action of 'mordant' dyes – using preformed metal complexes. Histochemie 35, 361.

Meijer, A.E.F.H., 1968. Improved histochemical method for the demonstration of the activity of α glucan phosphorylase. Histochemie 12, 244.

Pappenheim, A., 1899. Vergleichende Untersuchungen uber die elementare Zusammensetzung des rothen Knockenmarkes einiger Saugenthiere. Virchows Archiv für

Pathologische Anatomie und Physiologie 157, 19.

Seligman, A.M., Karnovsky, M.J., Wasserkrug, H.L., Honker, J.S., 1968. Non-droplet ultrastructural demonstration of cytochrome oxidase activity with a polymerising osmiophilic reagent, DAB. Journal of Cell Biology 38, 1.

Spicer, S.S., 1987. Histochemistry in pathologic diagnosis. Marcel Dekker, Oxford.

Tokuda, Y., Nakamura, T., Satonaka, K., et al., 1990. Fundamental study on the mechanism of DNA degradation in tissues fixed in formaldehyde. Journal of Clinical Pathology 43, 748.

Unna, P.G., 1902. Eine Modifikation der Pappenheimschen Farbung auf Granoplasma. Monatshefte für Praktische Dermatologie 35, 76.

Applications of immunohistochemistry

Appendix

II

Laura J. Keeling • Sherin Jos Payyappilly

Introduction

The histological diagnosis is often clear from light microscopic examination of tinctorial-stained slides. However, in cases with varying differential diagnoses or where molecular subtleties will add to case interpretation, immunohistochemistry may be employed to reach a conclusion. In certain circumstances, immunohistology also has a role in predicting prognosis and potential response to therapy.

It is beyond the scope of this text to provide a comprehensive list of all possible applications and the hundreds of antibodies currently available. Other excellent texts devoted entirely to that task are available (see Further reading: Taylor & Cote 2006; Dabbs 2010) and there are several excellent Internet-based resources (e.g. Immunohistochemistry vade mecum, Paul Bishop, see below). Therefore, this appendix attempts to provide an overview of the ways in which immunohistochemistry is commonly employed in the diagnostic pathology laboratory, alongside the basic immunohistochemical panels in common usage.

The most frequent application of immunohistology is to consider the nature of neoplasms whose morphology overlaps a range of diagnostic categories. However, other applications include identification of infective agents (e.g. CMV, HSV, *H. pylori*, etc.), deposition of immune complex (renal and skin disease) and typing of active cell populations (Bcl-2, Ki67, etc.), to name but a few.

Classification of neoplasia

A common application of immunohistochemical staining is the classification of neoplasms according to the type of cellular differentiation they display. Previously, electron microscopy was widely used to identify cytoplasmic features that might indicate differentiation toward a particular cell type. However, immunohistochemistry has largely superseded electron microscopy.

Anaplastic tumors

Anaplastic neoplasms are typically composed of relatively large, pleomorphic cells with highly atypical nuclei, which do not resemble any particular normal tissue type (i.e., lack differentiation). The list of differential diagnoses is therefore wide and may include neoplasms of epithelial, hematopoietic, melanocytic, mesenchymal, and in the central nervous system, glial origin. Expense and tissue may be spared by performing stains in a tiered fashion, where the first tier is designed to place a neoplasm into one of the major diagnostic categories, and the second and subsequent tiers are used for subclassification. Using this approach the following table shows a typical panel of stains that would be used in the first tier.

Anaplastic tumors					
	Cytokeratins (AE1/3, MNF116, Cam 5.2)	Lymphoid markers (CD45)	Melan A, S100, HMB45	Vimentin (low specificity)	GFAP[1]
Epithelial origin/carcinoma	+	−	−	Some are positive	−
Hematopoietic/lymphoid	−	+	−	−	−
Melanocytic	−	−	+	−	−
Mesenchymal/sarcoma	+/−	−	+/−	+	−
Central nervous system/glial	−	−	−	+/−	+

1. Glial fibrillary acid protein.

Small round cell tumors

This group of poorly differentiated neoplasms consists of small, immature/somewhat fetal-type cells with relatively round densely stained nuclei and scant cytoplasm. A panel of antibodies that would be useful in distinguishing among these differential diagnostic possibilities is shown in the following table.

Small round cell tumors							
	CD99	CD45	Cytokeratin	Desmin	Neural markers (e.g. CD56)	Muscle markers (e.g. MyoD1)	WT1
Differential diagnosis in children and adults							
Ewing sarcoma/PNET	+	−	+/−	+/−	+	−	−
Neuroblastoma	−	−	−	−	+	−	−
Desmoplastic small round cell tumor	+	−	+	+	+	−	+
Wilms' tumor	−	−	+ (blastema)	+ (blastema)	−	−	+
Rhabdomyosarcoma	+	−	−	+	−	+	−
Lymphoma	+	+	−	−	−	−	−
Differential diagnosis predominantly in adults							
Synovial sarcoma	+	−	+	−	+	−	−
Small cell carcinomas	−	−	+	−	+	−	−

Adenocarcinoma of unknown origin

Some neoplasms can be identified by the presence of specific tumor markers, such as prostate-specific antigen (PSA) in prostate and thyroglobulin in thyroid. However, many neoplasms have no unique markers and require a panel of antibodies for diagnosis (Dennis et al. 2005). One example is the application of a panel of immunohistochemistry to a metastatic tumor with glandular differentiation but no previously diagnosed primary site, or 'adenocarcinoma of unknown origin'. The panel used in this situation will necessarily differ for males and for females; see following table.

Adenocarcinoma of unknown origin									
Primary site (%)	PSA	TTF1	GCDFP15	CDX2	CK20	CK7	ER	Mesothelin	CA 125
Breast	0	0	49	0	0	87	79	4	13
Colon	0	0	6	86	78	3	1	7	1
Lung	0	90	3	1	1	90	6	36	38
Ovary serous	0	0	4	0	0	93	81	96	93
Ovary mucinous	7	0	14	14	21	57	50	36	36
Pancreas	0	4	1	2	15	94	0	49	50
Stomach	2	2	0	21	21	50	0	19	8
Prostate	100	8	4	0	0	0	8	0	0

Spindle cell neoplasms

These neoplasms are composed of thin, elongated cells typically arranged in bundles and may occur at virtually any site in the body, including subcutaneous tissue, deep soft tissues, viscera and nervous systems. Most are mesenchymal or neuroectodermal in type, but lack specific histology clues as to their nature. The differential diagnoses and relevant immunohistochemistry (WHO 2002) are shown in the table below.

Malignant spindle cell neoplasms						
	CD34	ASMA[1]	Desmin	S100	CK	CD99
Synovial sarcoma	−	−	−	−	+	+
MPNST[2]	−	−	−	+	−	−
Leiomyosarcoma	−	+	+	−	Sometimes +	−
Myofibrosarcoma	−	+	−	−	−	−
Fibrosarcoma	−	−	−	−	−	−
Spindle cell carcinoma	−	−	−	−	+	−
Malignant melanoma	−	−	−	+	−	−
GIST[3] (if site appropriate)	+	−	−	Sometimes +	−	−

1. Alpha smooth muscle actin.
2. Malignant peripheral nerve sheath tumor.
3. Gastrointestinal stromal tumor.

Lymphoma

The subclassification of lymphomas often involves molecular tests alongside histology and immunohistology. Several more examples of specific staining combinations for particular neoplasms are given in the table below (Kaufmann et al. 1999; Pileri et al. 2002; WHO 2008; Mitrovic et al. 2009).

Immunohistochemistry in lymphoma diagnosis	
Hodgkin lymphoma	
Classical Hodgkin lymphoma	CD30+, CD15+, MUM1+, CD45–, EMA–
NLPHL[1]	CD20+, CD 30–, CD15–, MUM1–, CD3–, CD57–
Mature B-cell neoplasms	
SLL/CLL[2]	CD20+, CD79a+, CD5+, CD23+, CD10–, cyclin D1–
Follicular lymphoma	CD20+, CD79a+, CD10–/+, Bcl-6+, CD23–, CD5–, cyclin D1–
Mantle cell lymphoma	CD20+, CD79a+, CD5+, cyclin D1+, CD23–, CD10–
Marginal zone lymphoma	CD20+, CD79a+, Bcl2+, CD43 +(50%), Bcl-6–, CD10–, CD5–, cyclin D1–, CD23–
DLBCL[3]	CD20+, CD79a+, CD10+/–, Bcl-6+/–, Bcl-2+/–, CD30+/–. MUM-1+/–, CD5+/–, CD2&3–
Burkitt lymphoma	CD20+, CD79a+, CD10+, Bcl-6+, MIB-1+++, TdT–, Bcl-2–, CD34–, CD2&3–

1. Nodular lymphocyte predominant Hodgkin lymphoma.
2. Small lymphocytic lymphoma/chronic lymphocytic lymphoma.
3. Diffuse large B-cell lymphoma.

Mesothelioma versus adenocarcinoma

Mesothelioma can present with a variety of microscopic phenotypes, the commonest diagnostic conundrum being versus adenocarcinoma, although spindle cell variants of mesothelioma can parallel other spindle cell neoplasia. Immunohistochemistry (Carella et al. 2001; Ordóñez 2005) can be applied to differentiate between these two neoplasms in both surgical and cytological specimens. If proven to be an adenocarcinoma, a second round of antibodies may then be used to identify the primary site.

Epithelial malignant mesothelioma versus lung adenocarcinoma	Mesothelioma	Adenocarcinoma
mesothelin	Usually positive	Usually negative
calretinin	Usually positive	Usually negative
cytokeratin 5/6	Usually positive	Usually negative
Wilms' tumor-1 (WT-1) gene product	Usually positive	Usually negative
D2-40	Usually positive	Usually negative
podoplanin	Usually positive	Usually negative

Epithelial malignant mesothelioma versus lung adenocarcinoma (continued)	Mesothelioma	Adenocarcinoma
BerEP4	Usually negative	Usually positive
AE1/3	Usually negative	Usually positive
CEA[1]	Usually negative	Usually positive
Claudin 4	Usually negative	Usually positive
MOC31	Usually negative	Usually positive
HBME1	Usually negative	Usually positive
TTF1	Usually negative	Usually positive

1. CEA – carcinoembryonic antigen.

Germin cell tumors

Germ cell tumors

There can be significant morphological overlap between the specific types of germ cell tumor, particularly classical seminoma, embryonal carcinoma and yolk sac tumor. Application of an immunohistochemical panel may aid accurate diagnosis and tumor classification (see table below). However, combined forms may exist, complicating interpretation.

Germ cell tumors (excluding teratoma differentiated)	ITGCN[5]	Classical seminoma	Embryonal carcinoma (MTU[6])	Yolk sac tumor	Choriocarcinoma (MTT[7])
CD117 (c-kit)	+	+	−	−	−
PLAP	+	+	+	−	−
CD30	−	−	+	−	−
Epithelial marker (e.g. CK7, EMA[1])	−	−	+	−	+
OCT4	−	−	+	−	−
AFP[2]	−	−	−	+	−
HCG[3]	−	−	−	−	+
HPL[4]	−	−	−	−	+

1. Epithelial membrane antigen.
2. Alpha fetoprotein.
3. Human chorionic gonadotropin.
4. Human placental lactogen.
5. Intratubular germ cell neoplasia.
6. Malignant teratoma undifferentiated.
7. Malignant teratoma trophoblastic.

Renal tumors

The majority of renal tumors can be diagnosed on H&E-stained sections. In cases with morphological uncertainty, the panel in the following table may be useful (Truong & Shen 2011).

Renal tumors				
	Clear cell carcinoma	Papillary carcinoma	Chromophobe carcinoma	Oncocytoma
Vimentin	+	+	−	−
RCC	+	+	−	−
CD10	+	+	−	−
CK7	−	+	+	−
CK19	−	+	+	+
c-kit	−	−	+	+
PAX2	+	+	−	+

Neoplasia versus reactive proliferations

Many reactive proliferations result in masses ('tumors') that may clinically mimic true neoplasms. Immunohistochemistry may play a role in differentiating reactive processes from subtle manifestations of neoplasia, typically by demonstrating the expression of proteins that are not usually expressed at detectable levels in normal tissues (see Further Reading: Fletcher 2007). Several examples are given in the table below.

Reactive versus neoplastic proliferations			
Lymph node	Follicular hyperplasia	Bcl-2 negative in follicles	Ki67 higher in follicles
	Follicular lymphoma	Bcl-2 positive in follicles	Ki67 same as rest of node
Prostate	Benign glands	p63 positive basal myoepithelial layer	P504S negative glands
	Adenocarcinoma	No p63 positive basal layer	P504S positive glands
Bladder	Benign/reactive	CK20 positive only in umbrella cells	
	Carcinoma *in situ*	CK20 positive in full thickness of urothelium	
Brain	Reactive gliosis	p53 and Ki67 are mostly negative	
	Low-grade astrocytoma	p53 positive astrocyte nuclei	
		Ki67 shows high proliferation fraction	

Prediction of prognosis and therapeutic response

Immunohistochemistry can be used to identify biological processes or altered proteins that are related to the prognosis or likely therapeutic response of a given tumor. For example, objective measurement of the proliferative activity by the Ki67 labeling index (MIB-1 antibody) is an important component of the histological grading system for endocrine tumors of the intestines.

Another application is the detection of small metastatic deposits which are difficult to see by routine histological examination ('micrometastases') in sentinel lymph nodes, commonly applied in cases of melanoma and breast carcinoma. The clinical and prognostic significance of identifying such micrometastases is still under investigation (Balch et al. 2009).

Several examples of the application of immunohistochemistry in the selection of patients who would benefit from targeted therapies are given in the table below.

Cell surface receptors	
Neoplasm	**Cell surface receptor**
GIST	C-kit
Breast carcinoma	HER2, ER
Carcinoma colon and lung	EGFR

Examples of immunohistology staining reactions are present in the sixth edition of this book.

References

Balch, C.M., Jeffrey, E., Gerschenwald, J.E., Soond, S., et al., 2009. Final version of the 2009 AJCC Melanoma Staging and Classification. Journal Clinical Oncology 27 (36), 6199–6206.

Carella, R., Deleonardi, G., et al., 2001. Immunohistochemical panels for differentiating epithelial malignant mesothelioma from lung adenocarcinoma: a study with logistic regression analysis. Am J Surg Pathol 25 (1), 43–50.

Dennis, J. L., Hvidsten, T.R., Wit, E. C., et al., 2005. Markers of adenocarcinoma characteristic of the site of origin: development of diagnostic algorithm. Clinical Cancer Research 11 (10), 3766–3772.

Kaufmann, O., Flath, B. Spath-Schwalbe, E.. et al., 1999. Immunohistochemical detection of CD10 with monoclonal antibody 56C6 on paraffin sections. Am J Clin Pathol 111, 117–122.

Mitrovic, Z., Ilic, I., Nola, M., et al., 2009. CD43 expression is an adverse prognostic factor in diffuse large B-cell lymphoma. Clinical Lymphoma Myeloma 9 (2),133–137.

Ordóñez, N.G., 2005. Immunohistochemical diagnosis of epithelioid mesothelioma: an update. Archives of Pathology and Laboratory Medicine 129 (11), 1407–1414.

Pileri, S.A., Dirnhofer, S., Went, P., et al., 2002. Diffuse large B-cell lymphoma: one or more entities? Present controversies and possible tools for its subclassification. Histopathology 41, 482–509.

Truong, L.D., Shen, S.S., 2011. Immunohistochemical diagnosis of renal neoplasms.. Archives of Pathology and Laboratory Medicine. 135 (1), 92–109.

WHO 2002. World Health Organization classification of tumors: pathology and genetics of tumors of soft tissue and bone, third ed. World Health Organization, Geneva.

WHO 2008. World Health Organization classification of tumors of haematopoietic and lymphoid tissues, fourth ed. World Health Organization, Geneva.

Further reading

Dabbs, D.J., 2010. Diagnostic immunohistochemistry, third ed. Elsevier Health, Philadelphia.

Fletcher, C.D.M., 2007. Diagnostic histopathology of tumors, third ed. Elsevier Health, Philadelphia.

Taylor, C.R., Cote, R.J., 2006. Immunomicroscopy: a diagnostic tool for the surgical pathologist, third ed. Elsevier Saunders, Philadelphia.

Internet resource

Immunohistochemistry vade mecum. http://e-immunohistochemistry.info/

Technical Appendices

Stuart Inglut

Danielle Maddocks

Anne Michelle Moon

Paul Samuels

Diane L. Sterchi

Jennifer H. Stonard

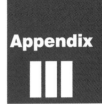

Measurement units

Jennifer H. Stonard

SI Units (Système International d'Unités) are used throughout this text.

Structure of SI units

The SI consists of units of three types: base units, derived units and supplementary units. It also includes a series of prefixes by means of which decimal multiples and submultiples of units can be formed.

Base units

Seven units have been selected to serve as the basis of the system. The four units relevant to the topics included in this book are given in Table Appendix III.1.

Derived units

If a base unit is multiplied by itself or by combining two or more base units, a group of units known as SI derived units are produced. Table Appendix III.2 gives some examples.

Volume

The unit of volume is the cubic meter (m^3) but the liter (litre) (1 liter = 1000 cm^3 = 10^{-3} m^3) is allowed. Squared and cubed are expressed as numerical powers and not by abbreviations. The volume in histology and scientific laboratories is specified either as liters, or more frequently as milliliters (ml) (Table Appendix III.3).

Table Appendix III.2 SI derived units

Quantity	Name of derived unit	Symbol for unit
Area	Square meter	m^2
Volume	Cubic meter	m^3
Substance concentration	Moles per cubic meter	mol/m^3

Table Appendix III.1 SI base units

Quantity	Name of unit	Symbol for unit
Length	Meter (metre)	m
Mass	Kilogram	kg
Amount of substance	Mole	mol
Time	Second	s

Table Appendix III.3 Non-SI units to be retained for general use

Quantity	Unit	Symbol for unit	Value in SI units
Time	Minute	min	60 s
	Hour	h	3,600 s
	Day	d	86,400 s
Volume	Liter	l	1 dm^3 = 10^{-3} m^3
Mass	Tonne	t	1,000 kg

Appendix **III**

© 2013 Elsevier Ltd

Length

The basic unit of length is the meter/metre (m) and all other units of length are expressed as multiples or submultiples of the meter (Table Appendix III.4).

Table Appendix III.4	Length	
Unit	Abbreviation	Size
Meter	m	
Millimeter	mm	10^{-3} m
Micrometer	µm	10^{-6} m
Nanometer	nm	10^{-9} m
Picometer	pm	10^{-12} m

Temperature conversion

Several temperature scales are used, the most common of which are the Fahrenheit scale (°F) and the Celsius scale (°C). To convert from Celsius to Fahrenheit you multiply the Celsius temperature by 9/5 and add 32. Thus, the temperature of boiling water, 100°C, converts to (9/5) (100°C) + 32 = 180 + 32 = 212°F. Similarly, the freezing point of water is 0°C or 9/5 (0°) + 32 = 32°F. To convert from Fahrenheit you first subtract (32°F) and then multiply by 5/9. The 212°F boiling point converts to (212 − 32) × 5/9 = 180 (5/9) = 100°C. Table Appendix III.5 provides some simple conversions.

Mass

The basic unit is the kilogram (kg) and the working unit is the gram (g). The multiples and submultiples of the gram are shown in Table Appendix III.6.

Table Appendix III.5	Conversion of °C to °F
°C	°F
−80	−112
−70	−94
−40	−40
−20	−4
−17.7	0
−10	14
0 (water freezes)	32
10	50
20	68
30	86
40 (hot day)	104
50	122
60	140
70	158
80	176
90	194
100 (water boils)	212

Table Appendix III.6	Mass	
Unit	Abbreviation	Size
Milligram	mg	10^{-3} g
Microgram	µg	10^{-6} g
Nanogram	ng	10^{-9} g
Picogram	pg	10^{-12} g

References

Missel, D.L., 1979. Proceedings of the Royal Microscopical Society 14, 385.

World Health Organization, 1977. The SI for the health professions. WHO, Geneva.

Preparation of solutions

Danielle Maddocks

Introduction

Most solutions in histology are made using water as a solvent. The agent dissolved in water to make an aqueous solution is the solute. Solutions typically are made as volume to volume or weight to volume. Concentrated formaldehyde is a 40% solution of formaldehyde in water. This represents the maximum solubility of the molecule, CH_3CH_2O (solute), in water (the solvent) and the resulting solution is a 40% w/v (weight-to-volume) solution.

The majority of histology laboratories now purchase commercially produced solutions in a prepared form. This is largely to reduce user exposure to a variety of hazardous chemicals and stains, thus minimizing any associated risk. In addition, the use of commercial solutions is beneficial in maintaining quality, as they allow standardization of staining.

Volume-to-volume solution

Making 10% formalin from a concentrated solution of formaldehyde (40% w/v) is an example of preparing a volume-to-volume solution. Add one part of concentrated formaldehyde to nine parts of water and this yields a 10% solution of formalin equivalent to a 4% solution of formaldehyde. Ten percent formalin is buffered to make 10% neutral buffered formalin – the most commonly used fixative in the USA and Europe.

For accuracy in preparing a solution, measure small volumes, unless volume-calibrated pipettes are available. The accuracy of a dilute solution is based more upon the accuracy of the measurement of the solute than of the measurement of the solvent. Thus, if 1.1 ml of solute is added instead of 1 ml, the error is 10% in the concentration of a 1% solution. However, if 1 ml of solute is added to 99.1 ml instead of 99 ml of solvent, the error is of the order of 1%.

A stock solution is generally used to prevent having to measure small amounts of the solute, and also sometimes for molecular stability. For a 1% stock solution, a 0.1% solution is prepared by adding 10 ml of 1% solution to 90 ml of water, and a 0.01% solution is prepared by adding 1 ml of 1% stock solution to 99 ml of water.

Use at least reagent grade chemicals and distilled/deionized water. Note the state of hydration specified on the chemical container, as calibration may be required as the state of hydration must be considered in the molecular weight of the chemical.

In preparing various solutions, the equation: volume of solution 1 × concentration 1 = volume of solution 2 × concentration 2 ($V_1C_1 = V_2C_2$) is very useful in modifying one solution in terms of an original solution. Examples of its use are as follows:

Using 100 ml of a solution of 1% sodium hydroxide, prepare a 0.5% solution of sodium hydroxide:

$$100 \text{ ml} \times 1\% = X \text{ ml} \times 0.5\%$$
$$X \text{ ml} = 200 \text{ ml}$$

Therefore add 100 ml of water to the 100 ml original solution to go from 100 ml of 1% to 200 ml of 0.5% sodium hydroxide.

Using 50 ml of 5% potassium permanganate, prepare a 2% solution of potassium permanganate:

$$50 \text{ ml} \times 5\% = X \text{ ml} \times 2\%$$
$$X \text{ ml} = 125 \text{ ml}$$

Table Appendix IV.1 Volume-to-volume solutions: preparation of 100 ml of a solution		
% aqueous solution	ml of solute	ml of water
1%	1 ml	99 ml
5%	5 ml	95 ml
10%	10 ml	90 ml
50%	50 ml	50 ml

For a 1-liter solution, multiply the solute and water by 10.

Table Appendix IV.2 Preparation of weight-to-volume solutions		
% weight	Solute	Solvent
1	1 g	100 ml
2.5	2.5 g	100 ml
5	5 g	100 ml
7.5	7.5 g	100 ml
10	10 g	100 ml
0.1	10 ml of 1%	90 ml
0.01	1 ml of 1%	99 ml
0.001	1 ml of 0.1%	99 ml

Therefore add 75 ml of water to the 50 ml original solution to go from 50 ml of 5% to 125 ml of 2% potassium permanganate.

See Appendix Table IV.1 for preparation of 100 ml of solution.

Weight-to-volume solutions

Weight-to-volume solutions are typically used when a weight of a solute, typically a solid, is dissolved in an aqueous or other solvent. In such a preparation, takes assume the weight of 100 ml of water to be 100 grams. To make a 1% solution of potassium permanganate, add 1 gram of potassium permanganate to 99 ml of water and make the final solution up to 100 ml. This usually requires a 100-ml volumetric flask. In histology, such accuracy is seldom required and a good approximation is to dissolve the solute in 100 ml of the solvent. Just like volume-to-volume solutions, do not try to measure small quantities of the solute (less than 1 gram). If a dilute solution is to be made, dilute a more concentrated solution, as shown below for solutions of 0.1% or less. As above, be careful to note the state of hydration of the chemical being used. The weight of the complexed water must be calculated and removed from the chemical weight.

To avoid measuring less than 1 g, change the preparation from weight-to-volume to a volume-to-volume solution, as shown in Table Appendix IV.2.

Examples

Prepare a 0.0025% solution of sodium chloride. (Note for a % weight:volume solution the molecular weight of NaCl is not needed). Start by preparing a 2.5% solution or 2.5 g of NaCl in 100 ml of water. Add 1 ml of this 2.5% solution to 1000 ml of water. This would provide a 0.0025% solution without weighing or measuring small quantities.

Again the equation $V_1C_1 = V_2C_2$ is very useful.

How much water do you add to 100 ml of 20% sodium chloride to obtain a 7.5% solution?

$$100 \text{ ml} \times 20\% = X \text{ ml} \times 7.5\%$$
$$X \text{ ml} = 2000/7.5 = 267 \text{ ml}$$

Thus you need to add 167 ml of water to the 100 ml of 20% solution to produce 267 ml of a 7.5% solution.

Molar solutions (M)

These are based upon the molecular weight of the solute. The molecular weight is normally stated on the label of the container of the chemical. It can be looked up in the *Merck Index* or *CRC Handbook of Chemistry*. If water is bound to the solute, the amount of water typically bound at laboratory conditions must be considered in weighing the molecular weight of the solute. A 1 molar solution is the molecular weight in grams of the solute dissolved in 1 liter (1000 ml) of the solvent. A 1 molar solution of sodium chloride (molecular weight = 58.5 g) is prepared by dissolving 58.5 grams of sodium chloride in 1 liter of water. A 0.1 molar solution of sodium chloride is 5.85 grams dissolved in 1 liter. See Appendix Table IV.3.

Normal solutions (N)

The preparation of a normal solution is based upon dissolving an equivalent weight of an equivalent single positive ionic species. Sometimes this is called the equivalent (molecular) weight. For example, if only one positive ion is present in a molecule, such as sodium chloride (NaCl), then the equivalent weight is the same as the molecular weight and a 1 normal solution is the same as a 1 molar solution; thus, one molecular weight of sodium ions is present in the 1 N solution. By contrast, potassium sulfate (K_2SO_4) has two positive ions per molecule; thus, the equivalent weight is the molecular weight divided by 2. In the case of calcium chloride [$Ca(Cl)_2$], the calcium with a positive charge (valence) of 2 is equivalent to two positive ions, so the normal (equivalent) weight is half the molecular weight. Thus, the equivalent weight used to prepare normal solutions depends on the molecular weight and the ionic form of the molecule. The preparation of normal solutions is described in Table Appendix IV.4.

Table Appendix IV.3 Preparation of molar solutions

Solution	Weight of solute	Final volume of solution
1 molar	Molecular weight in grams	1000 ml
0.1 molar	0.1 × molecular weight	1000 ml
0.01 molar	10 ml of 0.1 molar	100 ml (90 ml solvent)
0.001 molar	10 ml of 0.01 molar	100 ml (90 ml solvent)

Table Appendix IV.4 Preparation of normal solutions

Normality	Species	Equivalent weight
1 N	$X^{+1}Y^{-1}$	Molecular weight
1 N	$X^{+2}Y^{-2}$	½ the molecular weight
1 N	$X^{+3}(Y^{-1})_3$	⅓ the molecular weight
0.5 N	$X^{+1}Y^{-1}$	½ the molecular weight
0.5 N	$X^{+2}Y^{-2}$	¼ the molecular weight
0.1 N	Any species	1 part 1 N and 9 parts water
0.01 N	Any species	1 part 0.1 N and 9 parts water
0.001 N	Any species	1 part 0.1 N and 99 parts water

Preparation of useful solutions

Acid alcohol

70% alcohol	99 ml
Concentrated hydrochloric acid	1 ml

Acid permanganate

0.5% aqueous potassium permanganate	50 ml
3% sulfuric acid	2.5 ml

Gram's iodine

Iodine	3 g
Potassium iodide	6 g
Distilled water	900 ml

For hemotoxylin solutions, see Chapter 10.

Lugol's iodine

Iodine	1 g
Potassium iodide	2 g
Distilled water	100 ml

Alcian blue *(varying pH of solution)*

pH 0.2	1 g in 100 ml of 10% sulfuric acid
pH 0.5	1 g in 100 ml of 0.2 M hydrochloric acid
pH 1.0	1 g in 100 ml of 0.1 M hydrochloric acid
pH 2.5	1 g in 100 ml of 3% acetic acid
pH 3.2	1 g in 100 ml of 0.5% acetic acid

Magnesium chloride

(for Alcian blue at different electrolyte concentrations)

0.05 M	1.01 g in 100 ml of distilled water
0.06 M	1.22 g in 100 ml of distilled water
0.3 M	6.09 g in 100 ml of distilled water
0.5 M	10.15 g in 100 ml of distilled water
0.7 M	14.21 g in 100 ml of distilled water
0.9 M	18.27 g in 100 ml of distilled water

Picric acid *(saturated)*

The solubility of picric acid is 1.2 g/100 ml or 1.2%. Due to the hazards of dry picric acid, it is typically sold in a form containing 30–35% water.

Picric acid (hydrated)	1.6 g
Distilled water	100 ml

Note: Solutions of picric acid should not be allowed to evaporate, as dry picric acid is potentially explosive.

Scott's tap water

Potassium bicarbonate	2 g
Magnesium sulfate	20 g
Distilled water	1000 ml

Tris-HCl buffered saline, pH 7.6 *(for immunoperoxidase wash)*

Sodium chloride	8.1 g
Tris(hydroxymethyl)aminomethane	0.6 g
1 M HCl	3.8 ml
Distilled water	to 1000 ml

IMPORTANT

Chemicals should not be used if not in their original container.

Buffer solutions

Paul Samuel

Introduction

The pH of a solution is defined as the logarithm to base 10 of 1 divided by the concentration of the free hydrogen ions in solution (i.e. $pH = \log_{10} 1/[A^+] = -\log_{10}[H^+]$). A neutral solution is defined as $pH = -\log_{10}[10^{-7}] = 7$. The pH may greatly affect many chemical and immunohistochemical reactions, and consequently it is frequently important to minimize large changes in free hydrogen ion content (i.e., in pH).

Buffers are typically solutions in which the addition of small quantities of acids or bases causes little or no change in the pH of the solution. In other words, the solution 'buffers' against a change in pH. This is accomplished by solutions of inorganic and organic acids or bases plus salts which together absorb free hydrogen or free hydroxyl ions to prevent major changes in pH. Several major buffer systems are used in histochemical and/or immunohistochemical staining. Buffer systems include citric acid, sodium citrate, acetic acid-sodium acetate, and mixtures of sodium or potassium phosphates. One frequently used system is based on the use of Tris(hydroxylmethyl)aminomethane, often called 'Tris'. Tris buffer systems include Tris-maleic acid. Tris buffers are susceptible to temperature changes, so pH values specified at multiple temperatures are shown. Usually it is milliliters (ml) or cubic centimeters (ml) but may be in grams (g). The following buffer tables are the primary buffers referred to in this edition. For any buffers required and not listed here, the reader is referred to Pearse (1980) and Lillie and Fullmer (1976), or to suitable biochemical texts.

General notes regarding buffer solutions

The salts and acids used in the preparation of buffers should be of at least laboratory reagent grade. When preparing buffers the molecular weight given on the reagent bottle should be checked, as many chemicals are available in a number of states of hydration.

Acetate buffer

Preparation of stock solutions

Stock A: 0.2 M acetic acid (MW 60.05)
1.2 ml of glacial acetic acid in 100 ml of distilled water.

Stock B: 0.2 M sodium acetate (MW 136)
1.64 g of sodium acetate trihydrate (MW 136) in 100 ml of distilled water.

Composition of buffer
x ml of A + y ml of B made up to 100 ml with distilled water

Acetate buffer

pH	x ml of A	y ml of B
3.6	46.3	3.7
3.8	44.0	6.0
4.0	41.0	9.0
4.2	36.8	13.2
4.4	30.5	19.5
4.6	25.5	24.5
4.8	20.0	30.0
5.0	14.8	35.2
5.2	10.5	39.5
5.4	8.8	41.2
5.6	4.8	45.2

Cacodylate buffer

Preparation of stock solutions

Stock A: 0.2 M sodium cacodylate (MW 214)

4.28 g of sodium cacodylate in 100 ml of distilled water.

Stock B: 0.2 M HCl (MW 36.46)

1.7 ml of hydrochloric acid in 100 ml of distilled water.

Composition of buffer

25 ml of A + y ml of B made up to 100 ml with distilled water

Phosphate buffer

Preparation of stock solutions

Stock A: 0.2 M sodium dihydrogen orthophosphate (MW 156)

3.12 g of sodium dihydrogen orthophosphate in 100 ml of distilled water.

Stock B: 0.2 M disodium hydrogen orthophosphate (MW 142)

2.83 g of disodium hydrogen orthophosphate in 100 ml of distilled water.

Composition of buffer

x ml of A + y ml of B made up to 100 ml with distilled water

Cacodylate buffer	
pH	y ml of B
5.0	23.5
5.2	22.5
5.4	21.5
5.6	19.6
5.8	17.4
6.0	14.8
6.2	11.9
6.4	9.2
6.6	6.7
6.8	4.7
7.0	3.2
7.2	2.1
7.4	1.4

Phosphate buffer		
pH	x ml of A	y ml of B
5.8	46.0	4.0
6.0	43.8	6.2
6.2	40.7	9.3
6.4	36.7	13.3
6.6	31.2	18.8
6.8	25.5	24.5
7.0	19.5	30.5
7.2	14.0	36.0
7.4	9.5	40.5
7.6	6.5	43.5
7.8	4.2	45.8
8.0	2.6	47.4

Phosphate-citrate buffer

Preparation of solutions

Stock A: 0.2 M disodium hydrogen orthophosphate (MW 142.0)

2.83 g of disodium hydrogen orthophosphate in 100 ml of distilled water.

Stock B: 0.1 M citric acid (MW 210.0)

2.1 g of citric acid in 100 ml of distilled water.

Composition of buffer

x ml of A + (100 − x) ml of B

Tris-HCl buffer

Preparation of stock solutions

Stock A: 0.2 M Tris (MW 121.0)

2.42 g of Tris(hydroxymethyl)aminomethane in 100 ml of distilled water.

Stock B: 0.2 M HCl (MW 36.46)

1.7 ml of hydrochloric acid in 100 ml of distilled water.

(Note: Do not add water to acid.)

Composition of buffer

25 ml of A + y ml of B made up to 100 ml with distilled water

Phosphate-citrate buffer		
pH	x ml of A	ml of B
3.6	32.2	67.8
3.8	35.5	64.5
4.0	38.5	61.5
4.2	41.4	58.6
4.4	44.1	55.9
4.6	46.7	53.3
4.8	49.3	50.7
5.0	51.5	48.5
5.2	53.6	46.4
5.4	55.7	44.3
5.6	58.0	42.0
5.8	60.4	59.6
6.0	63.1	36.9
6.2	66.1	33.9
6.4	69.2	30.8
6.6	72.7	27.3
6.8	77.2	22.8
7.0	82.3	17.7
7.2	86.9	13.1
7.4	90.8	9.2
7.6	93.6	6.4
7.8	95.7	4.3

Tris-HCl buffer	
pH	y ml of B
7.2	22.1
7.4	20.7
7.6	19.2
7.8	16.3
8.0	13.4
8.2	11.0
8.4	8.3
8.6	6.1
8.8	4.2
9.0	2.5

References

Lillie, R.D., Fullmer, H.M., 1976. Histopathologic technic and practical histochemistry, fourth ed. McGraw-Hill, New York.

Pearse, A.G.E., 1980. Histochemistry: theoretical and applied, third ed. Churchill Livingstone, Edinburgh, Vol. 1.

Further reading

Bancroft, J.D., 1975. Histochemical techniques, second ed. Butterworths, London. (in appendix)

Gomori, G., 1948. Histochemical demonstration of sites of cholinesterase activity. Proceedings of the Society for Experimental Biology and Medicine 68, 354.

Gomori, G., 1955. Preparation of buffers for use in enzyme studies. Methods in Enzymology 1, 138–146.

McIlvaine, T.C., 1921. A buffer solution for colorimetric comparison. Journal of Biological Chemistry 49, 183.

Plumel, M., 1949. Bulletin de la Société de Chimie Biologique 30, 129.

Solubility of some common reagents and dyes

Stuart Inglut

In the following tables, the weight of solute (in the third column), dissolved in the volume of distilled water (in the right-hand column) will produce 100 ml of a saturated solution at the temperature given in the left-hand column.

Solubility of useful reagents

	Temp (°C)	Weight of solute (g)	Volume of distilled water (ml)
Aluminum ammonium sulfate	25	13.00	92.0
Aluminum potassium sulfate	25	7.02	99.1
Aluminum sulfate	25	63.00	66.0
Ammonium molybdate	25	39.00	88.0
Ammonium nitrate	25	90.20	41.8
Ammonium oxalate	25	5.06	97.0
Calcium chloride	25	67.80	79.2
Chloral hydrate	25	120.00	31.0
Citric acid	25	88.60	42.7
Cobalt nitrate	18	78.20	79.1
Cupric sulfate	25	22.30	98.7
Dextrose	25	59.00	60.0
Ferric ammonium sulfate	16.5	22.40	94.3
Ferric chloride	25	131.10	48.3
Ferric nitrate	25	70.20	79.2
Glycine	25	21.70	86.8
L-Glutamic acid	25	0.86	99.15
Hydroquinone	20	6.78	94.4
Lead nitrate	25	53.60	91.0
Lithium carbonate	15	1.38	100.0
Magnesium chloride	25	79.00	47.5

Solubility of useful reagents *(continued)*			
	Temp (°C)	Weight of solute (g)	Volume of distilled water (ml)
Magnesium nitrate	25	58.60	80.5
Magnesium sulfate	25	72.00	58.5
Oxalic acid	25	10.30	94.2
Phenol crystals	20	6.14	94.5
Phosphomolybdic acid	25	135.00	46.0
Phosphotungstic acid	25	160.00	64.0
Potassium acetate	25	97.10	44.3
Potassium bicarbonate	25	31.60	87.5
Potassium bromide	25	56.00	82.0
Potassium carbonate	25	82.20	73.5
Potassium chloride	25	31.20	86.8
Potassium dichromate	25	14.20	95.0
Potassium ferricyanide	22	38.10	80.8
Potassium ferrocyanide	25	28.20	89.2
Potassium hydroxide	15	79.20	74.2
Potassium iodide	25	103.20	69.1
Potassium nitrate	25	33.40	86.0
Potassium permanganate	25	7.43	97.3
Resorcin	25	67.20	47.2
Silver nitrate	25	164.00	65.5
Sodium acetate	25	40.50	80.0
Sodium bicarbonate	15	8.80	97.6
Sodium carbonate	25	28.10	96.5
Sodium chloride	25	31.70	88.1
Disodium hydrogen orthophosphate	17	4.40	99.9
Sodium hydroxide	25	77.00	74.0
Sodium hypophosphite	16	72.40	66.6
Sodium iodate	25	9.21	98.5
Sodium nitrite	20	62.30	73.8
Sodium periodate	25	13.90	96.2
Sodium sulfate	25	28.50	95.5
Sodium sulfite	25	26.40	94.5
Sodium thiosulfate	25	93.00	46.0
Sucrose	25	90.00	43.0
Trichloroacetic acid	25	149.60	12.41

Solubility of some dyes				
Dye name	**Generic name**	**Colour Index No.***	**Approx. solubility (g/100 ml)**	
			Water	**Alcohol**
Acridine Orange	Basic Orange 14	46005	Sol	Sol
Alcian Blue 8GX	Ingrain Blue 1	74240	5	1.6
Alizarin Red S	Mordant Red 3	58005	7.5	0.15
Aniline Blue (H₂O Sol) (Soluble blue 3 M or 2R, water blue)	Acid Blue 22	42755	Sol	Slight
Auramine O	Basic Yellow 2	41000	0.7	4.5
Azophloxine	Acid Red 1	18050	3	Slight
Azur A (McNeal)		52005	Sol	Sol
Biebrich Scarlet	Acid Red 66	26905	Sol	0.05
Bismark Brown Y (Vesuvian Brown)	Basic Brown 1	21000	1.3	1.1
Carmine	Natural Red 4	75470	Sol	Slight
Carminic acid	Natural Red 4	75470	8.3	–
Chromotrope 2R	Acid Red 29	16570	19	0.15
Congo Red	Direct Red 28	22120	Sol	0.2
Cresyl Fast Violet	–	–	Sol	Slight
Crystal Ponceau 6R (brilliant Crystal Scarlet 6R, Ponceau 6R)	Acid Red 44	16250	3	0.5
Crystal Violet	Basic Violet 3	42555	1.7	13
Eosin Yellowish (H₂O & alcohol Sol, Eosin Y)	Acid Red 87	45380	44	2
Eosin Bluish (Eosin B, Erythrosin B)	Acid Red 51	45430	11	2
Fast Garner GBC salt	Azoic Diazo component 4	37210	5	–
Fast Green FCF	Food Green 3	42053	16	0.35
Fast Red B salt	Azoic Diazo component 5	37125	20	–
Fast Red TR salt	Azoic Diazo component 11	37085	20	–
Fluorescein	Acid Yellow 73	45350	–	2.1
Fuchsin acid	Acid Violet 19	42685	20	0.25
Fuchsin basic	Basic Violet 14	42510	0.4	8
Fuchsin new	Basic Violet 2	42520	1.13	0.41
Gallocyanine	Mordant Blue 10	51030	Insol	Slight
Hematoxylin	Natural Black 1	75290	1.5	>30
Indigo carmine	Food Blue 1	73015	1.1	–

Solubility of some dyes *(continued)*

Dye name	Generic name	Colour Index No.*	Approx. solubility (g/100 ml)	
			Water	Alcohol
Janus Green B	–	11050	5.3	1.1
Light Green SF	Acid Green 5	42095	20	0.8
Luxol Fast Blue	Solvent Blue 38	–	V. Sol	Sol
Malachite Green	Basic Green 4	42000	7.60	7.52
Martius Yellow	Acid Yellow 24	10315	4.5	0.15
Metanil Yellow	Acid Yellow 36	13065	5.36	1.45
Methyl Blue	Acid Blue 93	42780	Sol	Slight
Methyl Green	Basic Blue 20	42585	Sol	Insol
Methyl Violet 2B	Basic Violet 1	42535	3	15
Methylene Blue	Basic Blue 9	52015	3.5	1.5
Neutral Red	Basic Red 5	50040	5.5	2.5
Nile Blue sulfate	Basic Blue 12	51180	1.0	1.0
Oil Red O	Solvent Red 27	26125	Insol	0.5
Orange G	Acid Orange 10	16230	10	0.2
Patent Blue	Acid Blue 1	42045	8.4	5.23
Phloxin	Acid Red 92	45410	50	9
Phosphine	Basic Orange 15	46045	Sol	Sol
Picric acid	–	10305	1.2	8
Ponceau 2R (Ponceau de xylidene)	Acid Red 26	16150	6	0.1
Pyronin Y (Pyronin G)		45005	9	0.6
Rhodamine B	Basic Violet 10	45170	0.8	1.5
Safranin O	Basic Red 2	50240	5.5	3.5
Solochrome cyanine RS (Eriochrome cyanine R)	Mordant Blue 3	43820	Sol	Sol
Scarlet R (Sudan IV)	Solvent Red 24	26105	Insol	0.2
Sudan Black B	Solvent Black 3	26150	Insol	1.13
Tartrazine	Food Yellow 4	19140	11	0.1
Thioflavine T	Basic Yellow 1	49005	Sol	Sol
Thionin	–	52000	0.25	0.25
Toluidine Blue	Basic Blue 17	52040	3.8	0.5
Victoria Blue B	Basic Blue 26	44045	0.5	4

*From Colour Index International, third ed. Society of Dyers and Colourists and American Association of Textile Chemists and Colorists, Bradford, UK. Sol = soluble, Insol = insoluble, V. Sol = very soluble.

Mounting media and slide coatings

Ann Michelle Moon

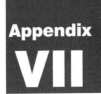

Appendix **VII**

In order to provide the maximum degree of transparency to stained tissue sections, the refractive index of the mounting medium must approximate to that of dried protein, i.e., between 1.53 and 1.54. This is especially important for photographing slides. To visualize detail in unstained tissues, it may be desirable to employ a medium of lower or higher refractive index. The refractive index of a mounting medium may change on drying due to evaporation of solvents. Air bubbles should not be permitted to remain under coverslips since they tend to expand.

Mountants

Most pathology laboratories currently utilize commercial mounting media, usually non-aqueous. From the standpoint of safety and costs, this may be a laboratory's best approach to mounting.

Potassium acetate may be added to mountants, almost to the point of saturation, in order to reduce the 'bleeding' of cationic dyes, at the same time giving a pH of approximately 7.0.

Aqueous mounting media are still important for special stains (e.g. Oil Red O staining), as solvents dissolve the fats to be demonstrated. The aqueous mountant for direct immunofluorescent stained slides should be fluorescence free. Few aqueous mountants have a refractive index higher than 1.5, most being in the range 1.4 to 1.45. Higher refractive indices are usually achieved by the use of high concentrations of sugars.

For other specialized mountants, see the appendices of the sixth edition of this text.

Apathy's mountant *(modified by Lillie & Ashburn 1943)*, refractive index 1.41

Gum arabic crystals	50 g
Cane sugar	50 g
Distilled water	100 ml
Thymol	100 mg

Dissolve with moderate heating.

Apathy's mountant *(Highman's modification, 1946)*, refractive index 1.436

Gum arabic crystals	50 g
Cane sugar	50 g
Potassium acetate	50 g
Distilled water	100 ml

Gentle heat may be used to dissolve the solids.
0.05 g of thymol or merthiolate may be added as a preservative.

Combined coverslip and mountant

Several manufacturers supply a medium of a varnish-like nature which may be used to coat the section surface, by dipping, pouring, or spraying. This type of medium obviates the need for a coverslip.

For low-power microscopy, combined mountant and coverslip may prove quite satisfactory, although little protection of the section to abrasion is given. High-power microscopy demands the use of optically flat slide surfaces with a coverslip of known thickness.

Adhesive slides

Slides may be chemically coated or electronically charged to give them adhesive properties. Microscopic slides may be coated or charged for a variety of reasons:

1. To act as an adhesive to keep difficult tissue specimens attached. For example, fatty tissues such as breast, hard tissues such as bone, synovium, and cartilage, or cellular preparations.

2. To aid in cellular attachment when cells are to be grown on slides or coverslips.

3. To make staining more consistent when staining small structures (e.g. cultured cells) spread across microscope slides.

Slides with adhesive properties are often bought from commercial suppliers. However, if necessary it is possible to create adhesive slides within the laboratory.

Silanized (APES) slides are prepared by cleaning the slides by washing, followed with a rinse in 95% ethanol; 4 ml of 3-aminopropyltriethoxysilane is added to 200 ml of acetone and slides are dipped for 30–60 seconds, followed by 60 seconds in agitated distilled water. The coated slides are then dried for 1 hour, and can be boxed for future use.

Polylysine (PLL) slides are prepared similarly to silanized slides. First wash the slides, followed by a rinse in 95% ethanol. Immerse the non-frosted portion of slides in a 5% solution of polylysine for more than 1 minute. Dry for over 1 hour. The slides can be boxed for future use.

Albumen-coated slides – wash slides, followed by a 95% ethanol wash. Make a 5% aqueous solution of crude egg albumen Grade II and immerse non-frosted portion of slides for over 1 minute. Permit to dry for 1 hour and then fix in a solution of 10% neutral buffered formalin for over 1 hour. Dry and box slides for future use.

References

Highman, B., 1946. Improved methods for demonstrating amyloid in paraffin sections. Archives of Pathology 41, 559–562.

Lillie, R.D., Ashburn, L.L., 1943. A modification of Apathy's mounting medium. Archives of Pathology 36, 432.

Molecular pathology reagents

Diane L. Sterchi

Formulas for the preparation of the reagents used in most ISH methods follow. The majority of these reagents can be purchased pre-mixed or in a kit for easy preparation. Those listed here are for use in a universal no-frills or special equipment ISH procedure (see Chapter 21), but different reagents may be needed for other ISH methods. Purchasing the reagents pre-mixed or in kits is convenient, safer to use and provides some comfort that they are mixed according to manufacturer's specification and guaranteed by them. This may cut down the possibility of human error. Laboratories with limited budgets may find that pre-mixed reagents and kits are not an option as they can be expensive and expire before all the reagents are used.

Diethylpyrocarbonate (DEPC) treated water

Diethylpyrocarbonate	1 ml
Distilled water	1000 ml

Stir while bringing to a boil for 10 minutes (in fume hood). Autoclave to expel DEPC.

2% aminoalkylsilane (positively charged slides)

Aminoalkylsilane (AAS) stored at 4°C	5 ml
Dry acetone	250 ml

Dip clean slides in 2% AAS for 1 minute. Rinse in three changes of deionized water.

Note

These slides may be purchased pre-coated. Make sure they are RNA/DNA free.

Proteinase K

Proteinase K	100 mg
Buffer #1, see below	5 ml

Aliquot and freeze below –20°C.

Hyaluronidase

Hyaluronidase	20 mg
Buffer #1, see below	20 ml

0.1 M triethanolamine (TEA)

Triethanolamine	0.1 ml
DEPC water	100 ml
Acetic anhydride	0.25 ml*

Make fresh.

*Add just prior to use. Stir for 5 minutes, then add an additional 0.25 ml, and stir for another 5 minutes.

1 M Tris (stock)

Trizma base	60.55 g
DEPC water	500 ml
Adjust pH to 8.0 with conc. HCl	20 ml*

*Autoclave.

1 M magnesium chloride (stock)

Magnesium chloride	20.34 g
DEPC water	100 ml*

*Autoclave.

5 M sodium chloride (stock)

Sodium chloride	29.22 g
DEPC water	100 ml*

*Autoclave.

Maleic acid buffer

Maleic acid	100 mM
Sodium chloride	150 mM

Mix 1:10 with water and adjust pH to 7.5 or add Tween 20 (0.3% v/v) for a washing buffer.

Buffer #1: Tris buffered saline, pH 7.5

1 M Tris (stock)	10 ml
5 M sodium chloride (stock)	3.3 ml
1 M magnesium chloride (stock)	0.2 ml
Deionized water	86.7 ml

Adjust pH to 7.5 with HCl.

Buffer #2: Tris buffered saline, pH 9.5

1 M Tris (stock)	10 ml
5 M sodium chloride (stock)	2 ml
1 M magnesium chloride (stock)	5 ml
Deionized water	83 ml

Adjust pH to 9.5 with sodium hydroxide (NaOH).

20x Saline sodium citrate (SSC)

Sodium chloride	348 g
Sodium citrate	167.4 g
DEPC water	1600 ml

Adjust to pH 7.4 with dilute acetic acid, stirring vigorously. Autoclave.

2x SSC

20x SSC	10 ml
DEPC water	100 ml

1x SSC

20x SSC	5 ml
DEPC water	95 ml

Denhart's solution

Ficoll	100 mg*
Polyvinylpyrrolidone	100 mg*
Bovine serum albumin	100 mg
DEPC water	500 ml

*May cause increase in background.

Prehybridization solution

Deionized formamide	5 ml*[1]
20x SSC	2 ml
Denhart's solution	0.10 ml*[2]
50% dextran sulfate	2 ml
Salmon sperm DNA (10 mg/ml)	0.30 ml*[3]
Yeast tRNA (10 mg/ml)	25 ml*[4]

*[1] purified = less non-specific staining
*[2] reduces non-specific probe binding
*[3] denature by boiling for 10 minutes
*[4] blocks non-specific staining

Hybridization solution

Prehybridization solution	1 ml
Labeled probe (500 ng/25 µl)	10 ml

Detection method reagents: choose one

1. Streptavidin-alkaline phosphatase	0.01 ml
Buffer #1	5 ml
2. Anti-digoxigenin	0.01 ml
Buffer #1	2.50 ml
3. Horseradish peroxidase (HRP)	0.01 ml
Buffer #1	5 ml

Colorimetric detection reagents: choose one

1. BCIP-NBT

5 bromo-4-chloro-3-indolyl phosphate (BCIP)	0.5 mg/ml
Nitro-blue tetrazolium salt (NBT)	0.3 mg/ml

2. AEC

3-Amino-9-ethylcarbazole (AEC)	0.08 g
Acetone	10 ml
0.05 M acetate buffer	200 ml
Hydrogen peroxide (30%)	0.10 ml

3. DAB

Diaminobenzidine (DAB)	22 mg
Tris buffer (stock)	50 ml
Hydrogen peroxide (30%)	0.2 ml

Staining methods index

Page numbers followed by 'f' indicate figures, 't' indicate tables, and 'm' indicate methods.

A

acid phosphatase, 319
alcian blue
    amyloid, 284
    carbohydrates, 224–226, 226m
    description of, 166–167, 169
    high iron diamine and, 228, 229m
    low pH technique, 225
    mucins, 225–226
    PAS and, 225–226, 226m, 232
    -performic acid, 567m
    preparation of, 592m
    standard technique for, 224–225, 224m
aldehyde fuchsin
    elastic fibers, 207–208, 208m
    Gomori's
        description of, 168
        lipofuscin staining using, 255f, 256m
    technique for, 208m
alizarin red S method, 257–258, 258m, 259f
alkaline phosphatase, 385, 402–403, 419–421, 419m, 452f, 465
aluminon method, 267m, 345m
alziarin red S, 169
amido black technique, 243
APAAP (alkaline phosphatase-antialkaline phosphatase), 382, 385, 388, 419m
avidin-biotin complex technique
    description of, 389
    immunofluorescence use of, 382
    immunohistochemistry use of, 418
    microorganisms, 293
azodyes, 160
azure A, 230m
azure B, 251

B

BCIP/NBT (5-bromo-4-chloro-3-indoyl phosphate/nitro-blue tetrazolium), 464–465, 604m
BHPS (borohydride-periodate-Schiff) method, 566m
Bielschowsky method for plaques and tangles (modified), 369m–370m
borohydride-periodate-Schiff method, 566m
5-bromo-4-chloro-3-indoyl phosphate/nitro-blue tetrazolium, 464–465
Brown-Brenn method (modified), 295m–296m

C

Celestine blue-alum hematoxylin procedure, 178, 178m, 185
Churukian's method
    chromaffin, 257
    melanin, 249m–250m, 249f
colloidal gold, 388–389
colloidal iron
    carbohydrates, 227, 227m–228m
    technique for, 227m–228m
Congo red
    alkaline, 280m
    amyloid, 271, 279–281, 281f, 286
    chemical structure of, 279f
    description of, 279
    dichroism of, 282
    Highman's technique, 280m
    technique for, 280m
cresyl fast violet, 355m–356m
cresyl violet acetate method, 298m–299m
cresyl violet counterstain, with Luxol fast blue stain, 359m–360m
Crocein scarlet-acid fuchsin, 211

crystal violet
    amyloid, 271, 282
    solubility of, 160
cytochrome oxidase, 573m

D

DAB (diaminobenzidine), 147
    characteristics of, 556–557
    composition of, 604m
    description of, 382, 385, 464–465
    endogenous peroxidase reaction with, 449
    handling of, 28
    immunocytochemical procedures use of, 251
    light scattering, 556–557
    positively stained nuclei, 552
Dako CSAII detection method, 419m
Dako EnVision detection technique, 418m
dehydrogenases, 571
diastase digestion, 231, 231m
diazo methods, 246
DMABR (dimethylaminobenzyidine rhodanine), 259
DMF (dimethylformamide), 28
DMP 30 (dimethylamino methyl phenol), 141
DNA
    cDNA, 487
    counterstain, 481
    definition of, 487, 568
    demonstration methods for, 569
    enzyme extraction of, 570m
    Feulgen reaction for, 569, 569m
    molecular pathology techniques for, 455
    probes for, 460–461, 462t
    recombinant, 488

E

Einarson's gallocyanin method, 355
eosin
  B, 173
  description of, 173–174
  ethyl, 173
  over-differentiation of, 173–174
  Y, 173–174

F

fast red substrate solutions,
  421–422, 421m–422m
fast red TR solution, 421m
Feulgen nuclear technique
  acid hydrolysis-Schiff reagent
    sequence of, 161
  description of, 569, 569m
  problems associated with, 169
Fite method (modified), 298m, 298f
fluorescent methods, for
  mycobacteria, 297m–298m
formaldehyde-induced fluorescence
  biogenic amines, 137
  freeze-dried material used in,
    137
formalin-induced fluorescence, of
  melanins, 253, 253m
Fouchet's technique for liver bile
  pigments (modified), 245,
  245m–246m

G

Gallyas silver technique, 365f,
  367m–368m
Giemsa, 311, 311m–312m
Gimenez method, for *Helicobacter
  pylori*, 299m
GMA
  bone staining, 335–336
  enzyme histochemistry uses of,
    146
Gmelin technique, 246m
Goldner's trichrome method,
  343m–344m
Gomori methenamine silver, 263
Gomori's aldehyde fuchsin
  description of, 168
  lipofuscin staining using, 255f,
    256m
Gomori's hexamine silver
  technique, 260–261
Gomori's method for reticular
  fibers, 210m
Gomori's trichrome, 169

Gordon & Sweets' method,
  209m–210m
Gram
  bacteria in smears, 295m
  description of, 295
  microorganisms, 295, 295m–296m
  modified Brown-Brenn method,
    295m–296m
Gram-Twort stain, 296m
Grocott hexamine silver method
  description of, 169
  fungi, 303, 303m–304m
Grocott methenamine
  (hexamine)-silver
  fungi, 303, 303m–304m
  Histoplasma capsulatum, 306f

H

Harris, 173
HE (hematoxylin and eosin)
  absorbance curves of, 555f
  amyloid, 278
  Aspergillus fumigatus, 305, 305f
  bacteria, 294
  bile pigments, 244–245
  bone sections, 332–333, 333f
  Candida albicans, 305
  Cryptococcus neoformans, 306
  cytoplasm on, 69–70
  decalcified bone sections,
    332–333, 333f
  description of, 555–556
  dysplastic nevus, 252f
  Entamoeba histolytica, 312
  ependymal cells, 361
  fungi, 303, 305
  Giardia duodenalis, 312–313
  Helicobacter pylori, 301
  Histoplasma capsulatum, 306
  Mayer's, 332–333, 333f
  MMA-embedded tissue, 341,
    341m, 341f
  molluscum virus, 310
  neurons, 355
  Nocardia asteroides, 305
  nuclear counterstain use of, 185
  oligodendrocytes, 362
  osteocytes, 334
  paraffin sections, 178m–179m
  Parkinson's disease, 366f
  popularity of, 173
  quality control in, 184–185
  rapid, for urgent frozen
    sections, 179m
  reticular fibers, 190
  Schistosoma sp., 313

technique, 151m, 342m
  Toxoplasma gondii, 312, 312f
  worms, 313
Heidehain's 'Azan' technique,
  203–204
Heidehain's Susa, 263
Heidenhain myelin, 181–182
hematein
  description of, 174
  PTAH staining technique using,
    182m
hematoidin, 244–246
hexazotized new fuchsin, 421m
high iron diamine, 228, 229m
Highman's Congo red technique,
  280m
Holmes' silver impregnation
  method, 334
Hukill and Putt's method for ferric
  and ferrous iron, 241, 242m

I

immunogold techniques
  description of, 420
  indirect, for monoclonal
    antibodies, 420m
  silver staining, 386f, 388–389,
    420m
immunohistochemistry staining
  alkaline phosphatase, 419–421,
    419m
  avidin-biotin, 418
  Dako CSAII detection method,
    419m
  Dako EnVision detection
    technique, 418m
  immunogold, 386f, 388–389,
    420, 420m
  Novolink polymer detection
    technique, 418m–419m
  polymer, 418–419, 418m–419m
  streptavidin/streptavidin-biotin
    complex, 418m
  tyramide signal amplification,
    419, 419m

K

kiton red-almond green technique
  for hemoglobin, 243

L

lead citrate, 508m
Lendrum's phloxine-tartrazine, 307,
  308m

Leuco patent blue V method, for hemoglobin, 243m
Lille's method
    chromaffin, 257
    ferric and ferrous iron, 240–241, 241f, 242m
Lillie's aluminon method, 267m, 267f
Lillie's rhodizonate method, for lead, 265f, 266m
Lindquist's modified rhodanine technique, for copper, 259m–260m, 260f
Long Ziehl-Neelsen method, for lipofuscin, 256m
Lowicryls
    description of, 143–144
    K4M, 152m, 153
    low-temperature embedding procedures used with, 153
    processing and embedding schedule for, 152m
LR Gold, 143–144, 146, 146f, 499
LR White
    acrylic plastic section staining, 151
    processing and embedding schedule for, 150m–151m
    transmission electron microscopy use of, 499
Luxol fast blue
    description of, 359, 359m–360m
    myelin staining, 164–165

M

Macchiavello's, 307, 307m
Mann's methyl blue-eosin, 307
Marchi technique, 360–361
Masson trichrome
    fibrin, 204
    illustration of, 200f
    technique for, 203m
Masson-Fontana method
    chromaffin, 257
    melanin, 249m
    pseudomelanosis pigment, 257
Melan A, 251
Metanil yellow, 227
Methacarn, 88
methenamine, 30
methenamine silver method
    description of, 193, 193m–194m, 257
    senile plaques, 368f, 369m–370m
methyl green, 282

methyl green-pyronin technique, 569–570, 570m
methyl violet
    amyloid, 281–282
    ethyl violet-resorcin and, 207m
    properties of, 281–282
methylene blue
    absorption of, 162
    -azure II-basic fuchsin, 372m
    solubility of, 160
methylene hydrate, 73
methylhippuric acids, 15
microwave ammoniacal silver method, 249m–250m, 249f
Millon reaction for tyrosine, 566, 566m–567m
Movat pentachrome
    illustration of, 210f
    Russell modification of, 210m–212m
MSB (Martius scarlet blue) technique, 204, 204m–205m

N

naphthochrome green, 266
Nile blue method, for melanin, 254m, 254f
nitro-blue tetrazolium for alkaline phosphatase, 420–421, 421m–422m
Novolink polymer detection technique, 418m–419m
nuclear protein-formaldehyde interactions, 73
nuclear stains, for trichrome stains, 201–202

O

oil Red O in dextrin, 564m
oils, 563
Okamoto-Utamura rhodanine method, for silver, 267–268, 268m
Okamoto-Utamura rubeanic acid method, for copper, 259, 259m
osmium tetroxide
    fixation using, 74t–75t, 77–78, 497, 497m
    handling of, 31
    properties of, 77–78
    tissue acidophilia affected by, 163
    transmission electron microscopy uses of, 497, 497m

P

Palmgren technique, 367
Palmgren's method, 357, 357m–358m
PAN (perchloric acid-naphthoquinone) method, 564m–565m
Papanicolaou, 179
    cell overstaining, 164
    formula for, 179m
    Harris's hematoxylin, 179m
    staining method for, 179m–180m
PAS (periodic acid-Schiff)
    alcian blue-PAS technique, 225–226, 226m, 232
    carbohydrates, 221–224, 222t, 224m
    cells that react with, 223t
    cerebrosides, 565m
    colloidal iron technique with, 227
    Cryptococcus neoformans, 306
    description of, 157
    diastase digestion and, 231
    differential diagnosis uses of, 221
    fungal species, 221
    Histoplasma capsulatum, 306
    McManus', for glycogen and fungal cell walls, 304m–305m
    mucopolysaccharides, 334
    mycobacteria, 296–297
    myelin, 359
    rabies virus, 310
    Rhizopus, 306f
    Schiff reagent, 223–224
    starch, 263
    substances oxidized by, 223
    technique for, 221–223, 224m
perchloric acid-naphthoquinone method, 564m–565m
performic acid-alcian blue method, 567m
Perls' Prussian blue reaction for ferric iron, 241m–242m
phloxine B and eosin Y, 173–174
phloxine-tartrazine, 307, 308m
PTAH (phosphotungstic acid hematoxylin) staining
    hematein, 182m
    potassium permanganate, 182m–183m
    technique for, 182, 182m–183m
    uses of, 185t

R

resorcin-fuchsin method
    description of, 191
    elastic fiber staining, 206,
        206m–207m
    Hart's modification of, 207
    modification of, 207
Reynolds' lead citrate, 508m
rhodanine method
    for copper (modified), 259m–
        260m, 260f
    for silver, 268m
rhodizonate method, for lead, 265f,
    266m
Romanowsky, 164
rubeanic acid method, for copper,
    259, 259m
Russell modification of Movat
    pentachrome stain, 210m–212m

S

Schmorl's ferric ferricyanide
    reduction test, 244
Schmorl's picro-thionin, 319f,
    334–335, 335m
Schmorl's reaction, for melanin,
    249, 250m–251m, 250f
Shikata's orcein method for
    hepatitis B surface antigen,
    308m–309m
Sirius red, 281, 281m
sodium hydroxide, 589
sodium hydroxide-ferric
    hematoxylin/DAH method,
    565m
solochrome azurine method
    for aluminum, 266, 266m–267m,
        344, 344m
    for beryllium, 266m–267m
solochrome cyanine
    for mineralized bone sections,
        342, 342m, 342f

for myelin in paraffin sections,
    360m
Steiner for filamentous and
    non-filamentous bacteria
    (modified), 300m–301m, 301f
streptavidin, 389
streptavidin-biotin system, 408,
    418m–419m
Sudan black B, 564m

T

Taenzer-Unna orcein method, 191
Texas Red, 429t
thioflavine S, 283
thioflavine T, 283, 284m, 286
toluidine blue
    absorption of, 162
    amyloid, 284
    cartilage, 334
    Helicobacter sp., 299m
    semi-thin sections, 504m
    in Sorenson's buffer, 299m
toluidine blue-acetone method,
    565m–566m
trichloroacetic acid
    ferric chloride reaction with,
        245, 245f
    fixation using, 72–73
trichrome, 199–202
    applications of, 199t
    decalcified bone sections, 333
    definition of, 199–200
    factors that affect, 200–201
    fixation effects on, 202
    Goldner's, 343m–344m
    heat effects on, 201
    Heidehain's 'Azan' technique,
        203–204
    Masson, 200f, 203m
    nuclear stains for, 201–202
    pH effects on, 201
    phosphomolybdic acid uses in,
        202–204

phosphotungstic acid uses in,
    202–204
tissue permeability effects on,
    200

V

van Gieson
    decalcified bone sections, 333
    picric acid-acid fuchsin mixture
        in, 178, 200, 333
    technique for, 202m
von Kossa silver nitrate method,
    169
    for bone mineral, 342, 343m,
        343f
    for calcium, 258f

W

Warthin-Starry method, for
    spirochetes, 299m–300m
Weigert resorcin-fuchsin method
    description of, 191
    elastic fiber staining, 206,
        206m–207m
    Hart's modification of, 207
    mechanism of, 207
    modification of, 207
Weigert-Pal technique, 184, 185t
Weigert's hematoxylin, 178, 180,
    180m, 185, 185t
Weigert's iron hematoxylin
    solution, 227

Z

Ziehl-Neelsen, 297m

Subject index

Page numbers followed by 'f' indicate figures, 't' indicate tables, and 'm' indicate methods.

A

AA amyloidosis, 276–278
A-bands, 197, 198f
absorbent cloths, 97–98
accreditation, 5–8
  continuous quality
    improvement, 7–8
  description of, 1
  equipment and materials, 7
  examination procedures, 7
  external quality assurance for,
    5–7
  premises, 7
  purpose of, 5–6
  quality control for, 6
  user liaison and organization, 7
acetate buffer, 593m, 593t
acetic acid
  alcoholic formalin and, 89
  eosin Y and, 173
  fixation using, 72–73, 74t–75t,
    466
  handling of, 27
  mechanism of action, 80
  methanol and, 466
  pH affected by, 80
acetone
  dehydration using, 107
  fixation using, 88
  handling of, 27
  properties of, 107
acetylcholinesterase, 573m–574m
achromat, 41
achromatic objectives, 46f, 47
acid alcohol, 592m
acid cabinets, 22
acid dyes, 168
acid permanganate, 592m
acid phosphatase, 319
acid-fast contamination, 297
acrylic acid, 142
acrylic plastics
  development of, 144
  embedding use of, 142–144
  future of, 153

  hydroquinone in, 143
  polymerization of, 144
  processing schedules for,
    148–152, 148m–151m
  sections
    applications of, 144–147
    cutting, 151
    enzyme histochemistry uses
      of, 145–146
    immunohistochemistry uses
      of, 146–147
    in situ hybridization, 148
    staining, 151
    tinctorial staining uses of,
      144–145
acrylic resins, 499
α-actin, 196–197
Actinomyces israelii, 305
additives
  fixation affected by, 82
  paraffin wax, 109
adenocarcinoma of unknown
  origin, 579, 579t
adenosine triphosphatase, 572m
adhesive slides, 602
adhesives
  description of, 127–128
  mineralized bone sections, 336
  paraffin sections, 127–128
adipose tissue, 195
AE1/AE3, 447f–448f, 451f
AEC (aminoethylcarbazole), 147,
  464–465, 604m
aerosol sprays, 132
affinity, 157, 158t, 159–161, 383
agar, 110
agitation, tissue processing rate
  affected by, 106
AIDS, 310
air purification systems, 20
AL amyloidosis, 274–276, 278, 285
albumen-coated slides, 602
alcian blue
  amyloid, 284
  carbohydrates, 224–226, 226m
  description of, 166–167, 169

  high iron diamine and, 228,
    229m
  low pH technique, 225
  mucins, 225–226
  PAS and, 225–226, 226m, 232
  -performic acid, 567m
  preparation of, 592m
  standard technique for, 224–225,
    224m
alcohol
  acid, 592m
  eosin Y solubility in, 173
  protein denaturation by, 72
alcoholic Bouin's solution, 89
alcoholic fixatives
  description of, 107
  uses of, 80
alcoholic formalin
  -acetic acid fixative, 89
  description of, 80
  formula of, 89
  glycogen fixation using, 221
alcoholic hematoxylin, 227
aldehyde fixatives, 496
aldehyde fuchsin
  elastic fibers, 207–208, 208m
  Gomori's
    description of, 168
    lipofuscin staining using, 255f,
      256m
  technique for, 208m
aliphatic hydrocarbon clearing
  agents, 27, 109
alizarin red S method, 257–258,
  258m, 259f
Alkaline Congo red technique, 280m
alkaline phosphatase, 385, 402–403,
  419–421, 419m, 452f, 465
α1-4 glycosidic linkage, 216, 216f
Alport's syndrome, 520t, 521f
alum hematoxylins
  basophilia, 568–569
  Carazzi's hematoxylin, 177m,
    178t, 185t
  Celestine blue and, 178, 178m,
    185

Cole's hematoxylin, 176m, 178t, 185t
  decolorization of, 201–202
  Delafield's hematoxylin, 175m, 178t, 185t
  description of, 174–175
  disadvantages of, 178
  Ehrlich's hematoxylin, 175m, 178t, 185t
  Gill's hematoxylin, 177m, 178t, 185t
  Harris's hematoxylin, 176m, 178t, 179m, 185t
  mordant for, 174–175
  progressive use of, 175
  regressive use of, 175
  staining characteristics of, 174–175
  staining times with, 177–178, 178t
aluminon method, for aluminum, 267m, 345m
aluminum
  aluminon method for, 267m, 345m
  Solochrome azurine method for, 266, 266m–267m, 344, 344m
aluminum ammonium sulfate, 27
aluminum hematoxylin, 166
aluminum potassium sulfate, 27
aluminum sulfate, 27
Alzheimer's disease
  amyloid in, 277
  characteristics of, 364
  description of, 363
  detection of changes in, 365f, 367, 367m–370m
  Gallyas method for tau pathology in, 367m–368m
  neurofibrillary tangles in, 283
  senile plaques in, 368f, 369m–370m
  tau pathology in, 367m–368m
alziarin red S, 169
amalgam tattoo, 264
American Conference of Governmental Industrial Hygienists, 14
amido black technique, 243
amines, 141
aminoalklysilane (2%), 603m
3-aminopropyltriethoxysilane, 127
ammonium hydroxide, 27
amplification, 486–489
α-amylase, 231

amyloid
  β-, 364, 367, 368f
  AA, 285
  acquired fluorescence methods for, 283
  AL, 285
  alcian blue, 284
  in Alzheimer's disease, 277
  birefringence, 282–283
  classification of, 273–274
  composition of, 272–273
  Congo red staining of, 271, 279–281, 280m, 281f, 286
  crystal violet, 271, 282
  definition of, 271
  demonstration of, 278–281
  in diabetes mellitus, 277
  diseases associated with, 277
  dyes for, 278–279
  electron microscopy of, 273, 273f
  fibril extraction, 284–285
  hematoxylin and eosin staining of, 278
  immunohistochemistry for, 285–286, 285f
  laser microdissection-proteomics, 286–287
  metachromatic techniques for, 281–282
  methyl green for, 282
  methyl violet for, 281–282
  polarizing microscopy of, 282–283
  primary, 274
  prior-derived deposits, 286
  proteomics, 286
  renal, 516t, 517f
  SAP scintigraphy of, 278
  secondary, 274
  silver impregnation methods for, 284
  Sirius red technique for, 281, 281m
  structure of, 271–272, 272f
  thioflavine S staining of, 283
  thioflavine T staining of, 283, 284m, 286
  toluidine blue, 284
  transmission electron microscopy of, 516t, 517f, 526–527
  types of, 278
  ultrastructure of, 273
amyloid P, 272–273, 285
amyloid-forming proteins, 274, 275t

amyloidosis
  AA, 276–278
  AL, 274–276, 278, 285
  conformational diseases, 274, 276t
  definition of, 271
  diagnosis of, 277–278
  heavy chain, 276
  hereditary systemic, 276–277
  hereditary transthyretin, 276–277
  LECT2, 277
  pathogenesis of, 274
  systemic, 274
  transthyretin, 274
amyotrophic lateral sclerosis, 366f
analyte-specific reagents, 485–486
analyzer, 57, 60f
anaplastic tumors, 220, 577, 578t
aneuploidy, 474
Angelman syndrome, 475t
angle of incidence, 38, 40f
angle of refraction, 38–39, 40f
aniline, 27
anionic macromolecules, 468
Anncaliia sp., 531t
annealing, 468, 486
anterior horn cells, 355f
anthracosis, 264
antibodies
  clones/dilution chart, 395t–398t, 398f
  concentrated, 438, 449–450
  definition of, 383
  dilution, 440
  immunohistochemistry stain quality affected by, 438
  monoclonal, 384, 419m–420m, 459
  polyclonal, 384, 450, 459
  specificity of, 383, 428–429
  storage temperature of, 438
  tissue microarrays used in production of, 116
  validation of, 439–440
antibody-antigen binding, 383
antigen(s)
  definition of, 383
  deterioration of, 439
  immunofluorescent techniques, 427–428
  low levels of, detection methods for
    amplification, 398–400
    enhancement, 398–400
    multiple labeling techniques, 400–401

proteolytic digestion, 391
  unmasking of, 390–392
antigen retrieval
  autoclave for, 394, 411m
  commercial solutions for,
    394–398, 395t–398t
  heat-mediated, 392–394, 401,
    406m, 409
  microwave
    description of, 392–393, 393f
    technique for, 410m
    trypsin digestion and,
      394–401
  pressure cooker, 393, 393f,
    410m
  proteolytic enzyme methods of,
    408–409, 409m
  steamer for, 393–394, 410m
  water bath for, 394, 410m
anti-roll plate, 134–135
antisense RNA, 486
AP (amyloid P), 272–273, 285
APAAP (alkaline phosphatase-
  antialkaline phosphatase), 382,
  385, 388, 419m
Apathy's mountant, 601m
aperture diaphragm, 48, 48f
apochromat, 41
apochromatic objectives, 46f, 47
apple-green birefringence, 283
aqueous mounting media, 601
arachnoid mater, 355
Araldite, 141
area processes, 548–550, 549f
areolar tissue, 195
argentaffin
  description of, 248
  microwave ammoniacal silver
    method for, 249m–250m, 249f
arrayers
  automated, 119, 120f
  maintenance of, 122–123
  manual, 119–120, 120f
  tissue microarrays, 119–123,
    120f
articular cartilage, 188
artifact(s)
  edge, 448f
  freeze, 132
artifact pigments, 239, 262–263
asbestos, 264–265
Aspergillus fumigatus, 305, 305f
Aspergillus niger, 305
astrocytes, 354, 361–362, 361f
astrocytic gliosis, 361
astrocytomas, 362
ATPase, 572m

audits
  continuous quality
    improvement, 8
  quality management, 5
  risk management, 4–5
autoclave, for antigen retrieval, 394,
  411m
autofluorescence, 63
automated arrayer, 119, 120f
automated incubation methods,
  406–407
autopsies, 363
  central nervous system tissues
    taken at, 375
  medical audit use of, 1
  neurodegenerative diseases, 364
  prion diseases, 375
autoradiography, 137
avidin-biotin complex technique
  description of, 389
  immunofluorescence use of, 382
  immunohistochemistry use of,
    418
  microorganisms, 293
avidity, 383
axons
  description of, 353, 354f
  Palmgren's method for, 357,
    357m–358m
  staining methods for, 357–358,
    357m–358m
'Azan' technique, 203–204
azodyes, 160
azure A, 230m
azure B, 251

B
B cells
  description of, 274
  neoplasms, 580t
B5 fixative, 87
back focal plane, 50, 52
bacteria, 294
  Clostridium difficile, 301–302
  Corynebacterium vaginale, 301
  filamentous and non-
    filamentous bacteria, modified
    Steiner method for, 300m–
    301m, 301f
  Lactobacillus acidophilus, 301
  Legionella pneumophila, 302
  Leptospira interrogans, 302
  Listeria monocytogenes, 302
  mycobacteria, 296–297,
    297m–301m
  Mycobacterium tuberculosis, 302

Neisseria gonorrhoeae, 301
Neisseria meningitidis, 301
Staphylococcus aureus, 301
Treponema pallidum, 302
types of, 294t, 301–302
bacterial-derived ß-D-galactosidase,
  386
barcoding of specimens, 96, 105
barrier filters, 64
basal lamina, 192
base, 486
base pair, 486
base sledge microtome, 125
basement membranes
  description of, 192–193
  glomerular See glomerular
    basement membrane
  methenamine silver
    microwave method for, 193,
      193m–194m
basic dyes, 168
basophilia, 568–569
Batten's disease, 353–354
Bayer pattern of color filters, 543,
  544f
BCIP/NBT (5-bromo-4-chloro-3-
  indoyl phosphate/nitro-blue
  tetrazolium), 464–465, 604m
Bcl-2, 452f
Beer-Lambert law, 541
BEIs (Biological Exposure Indices),
  26–27
benign essential hematuria, 520f,
  520t
benzoyl peroxide, 143
Bertrand lens, 52
beryllium, 266, 266m–267m
BHPS (borohydride-periodate-
  Schiff) method, 566m
Bielschowsky method for plaques
  and tangles (modified),
  369m–370m
bile, 244–246, 245f
bile pigments, 244–246, 245m–
  246m, 245f
bile thrombi, 244
bilirubin, 246
bilirubin-glucuronide, 244
biliverdin, 244, 246
biogenic amines, 137
biohazards, 2
biological exposure indices (BEIs),
  14–15
biological hazards, 25–26
Biological Stain Commission,
  167
biomechanical risk factors, 34

biopsy
  bone, 320–321
  brain, 370–371
  colon, 573, 573m–574m
  core, 99
  muscle, 373–374, 374f, 374t
  peripheral nerve, 371–373,
    372m–373m
  renal, 433f
  skeletal muscle, 571, 572m–573m
  skin, 99–100, 100f
  small
    description of, 99
    rapid processing schedule for,
      113, 114t
  spinal cord, 370–371
  staining procedure for, 431m
biosensors, 168
bioterrorism, 291–292
biotin, 293, 389, 449, 465
biotin-free catalyzed signal
  amplification, 390
biotinylated tyramide signal
  amplification, 389–390
birefringence
  amyloid, 282–283
  anisotropic substances, 282
  apple-green, 283
  signs of, 62
  weak, 62
birefringent crystals, 57, 58f, 61–62
bisphenol A, 141
bit depth, 544
bladder cancer, 479–480, 480m–
  481m, 480f
blocks See tissue blocks
blood smears, 88
blotting, 455
body tube, 47
bone
  amputation specimens of, 321
  biopsy of, 320–321
  cells in, 187, 318–320
  collagen, 317
  compact, 317
  composition of, 317
  cortical, 325–326
  decalcification of See
    decalcification
  development of, 320
  embedding of, 323
  endochondral ossification of,
    320
  fine-detail specimen
    radiography of, 322–323, 327
  fixation of, 321–322
  functions of, 196

growth of, 320
histomorphometric analysis of,
  347
intramembranous ossification
  of, 320
lamellar, 318f
micro computed tomography
  of, 348
morphometry of, 347–348
ossification of, 320
remodeling of, 320, 347
resection/replacement
  specimens of, 321
sawing of, 322, 339
trabecular, 317, 319f, 347
bone marrow, 240
bone mineral
  description of, 318
  staining for, 342, 343f
bone sections
  decalcified
    adhesion, 331–332
    canaliculi, 334–335
    cartilage, 334
    collagen stains, 333
    flattening of, 331–332
    hematoxylin and eosin,
      332–333, 333f
    immunohistochemistry of,
      335–336
    mucopolysaccharides, 334
    Schmorl's picro-thionin stain,
      319f, 334–335, 335m
    staining methods for, 332–335,
      335m
  methacrylate-embedded
    hematoxylin and eosin for,
      341, 341m, 341f
    sectioning, 338
    staining, 339–340
  mineralized
    adhesive tape methods for,
      336
    aluminum demonstration in,
      344, 344m
    description of, 336
    fluorescent labeling of,
      346–347, 346f
    frozen, 337
    grinding and polishing of,
      339
    methacrylate-embedded,
      338–340
    microradiography of, 345–346,
      345f, 346m
    mounting after staining,
      340–341

osteoid demonstration, block
  impregnation for, 336,
  336m–337m
plastic embedding of,
  338–344
preparation of, 336–347,
  336m–337m
sawing of, 339
solochrome cyanine staining
  of, 342, 342m, 342f
undecalcified, 339
bone slabs, 322, 330
bone specimens
  amputation, 321
  fine-detail specimen
    radiography of, 322–323
  resection/replacement, 321
bone volume, 347–348
borohydride-periodate-Schiff
  method, 566m
Bouin's solution
  alcoholic, 89
  decalcifying, 89
  formula of, 87
bovine serum albumin in Tris-
  buffered saline, 420
bovine spongiform encephalopathy,
  277, 311
bowel specimens, 100–101, 100f
Brachyspira aalborgi, 302
brain tissue
  biopsy of, 370–371
  fixation of, 85
  melanin in, 248
  staining of, 452f
breast cancer, 479
breast tissue
  fixation of, 85
  HER2 assessment in, 413f
  processing of, 112–113, 114t
  specimen dissection, 102
bright-field microscope, 50
5-bromo-4-chloro-3-indoyl
  phosphate/nitro-blue
  tetrazolium, 464–465
brown atrophy of the heart, 255
Brown-Brenn method (modified),
  295m–296m
brushes, 127
'bubble' test, for bone
  decalcification, 328
buffer(s)
  definition of, 593
  fixation affected by, 80
  immunohistochemistry stain
    quality affected by, 438
  phosphate, 89, 496, 496m

solutions, 593, 593m–595m, 593t–595t
transmission electron microscopy, 495–496, 496m
buffered saline, 86, 592m
bullous systemic lupus erythematosus, 434t
butyl alcohol
  dehydration using, 107
  properties of, 107
butyl methacrylate, 143

C

cacodylate buffer, 594m, 594t
CADASIL (cerebral autosomal dominant arteriopathy with subcortical infarcts and leukoencephalopathy), 495, 525–526, 527f
calcite, 58f
calcium
  alizarin red S method for, 257–258, 258m, 259f
  staining of, 257–258, 258m, 258f, 340
  von Kossa's silver nitrate method for, 258f
calcium acetate, 86
calcium oxalate
  bone decalcification testing using, 328m
  description of, 258f
calcium pyrophosphate crystals, 260
calcium salts, 257
cameras, 542
canaliculi, 319, 334–335
Candida albicans, 305
CAP *See* College of American Pathologists
CAP (copper-associated protein), 259
Carazzi's hematoxylin, 177m, 178t, 185t
carbohydrates
  alcian blue for, 224–226, 226m
  chemical modification and blocking techniques for, 233–234, 234m–235m
  classification of, 215–220
  colloidal iron technique for, 227, 227m–228m
  enzymatic digestion techniques for, 231–233, 231m
  fixation of, 220–221

GAGs *See* GAGs (glycosaminoglycans)
glycoconjugates, 215, 216t, 218–219, 221
glycoproteins, 216t–217t, 220
high iron diamine technique for, 228, 229m
immunohistochemistry of, 230–231
methylation of, 233, 234m
monosaccharides, 215–216, 216t
mucicarmine technique, 226, 226m–227m
mucins
  alcian blue for, 225–226
  description of, 217t, 219–220
  fixation of, 221
  immunohistochemistry of, 230–231
  methylation of, 233
  mucicarmine technique for, 226
  techniques for demonstrating, 222t
oligosaccharides, 216t
overview of, 215
PAS (periodic acid-Schiff) technique for, 221–224, 222t, 224m
polysaccharides, 216–218
proteoglycans, 217t, 218–219
saponification of, 233–234, 234m–235m
simple, 215
carbon, 264
carbon dioxide, 132
carcinogens, 3
cardiac muscle
  cells of, 255
  description of, 197–198
Carnoy-Lebrun solution, 87
Carnoy's fixative, 88
Carnoy's fluid
  cells affected by, 164
  description of, 107, 568
carousel-type tissue processor, 111
Carson's modified Millonig's phosphate buffered formalin, 86
cartilage
  fibrocartilage, 196
  functions of, 196
  hyaline, 196
  staining of, 334
  structural characteristics of, 195–196

cassette, 34
catalysts, 141
catalyzed signal amplification, 390
cat-scratch disease, 302
CCD cameras, 542
CD3, 407–408
CD15, 399f
CD30, 408f
CD markers, 220
cDNA, 487
CEA, 441–442, 442f
Celestine blue-alum hematoxylin procedure, 178, 178m, 185
cell cultures, 499
cell surface receptors, 583t
cell suspensions, 500, 500m–501m
celloidin
  as embedding agent, 110
  handling of, 27
Celsius, 588, 588t
central lesion, 100, 100f
central nervous system
  description of, 353
  tissues of, from autopsy, 375
cerebral autosomal dominant arteriopathy with subcortical infarcts and leukoencephalopathy (CADASIL), 495, 525–526, 527f
cerebrosides, 565, 565m
ceroid-type lipofuscins, 257, 353–354
charged slides, 127–128
chatter, 164
chelating agents, for bone decalcification, 325
chemical fume hoods, 19–20
chemical hygiene plan, 25
chemical resistance, of gloves, 18
chloroform
  as clearing agent, 108
  handling of, 27–28
  properties of, 108
cholesterol, 564
chondrocalcinosis, 260
chondrocytes, 196
chondroitin sulfate, 195–196, 218, 218t, 219f
Chr17, 459f
chromaffin, 257
chromatic aberration, 41–43, 42f
chromic acid
  fixation using, 78–79
  handling of, 28
  properties of, 78–79
chromic oxide, 263
chromic salts, 79

chromium trioxide, 78–79
chromogens, 385, 445–446, 450–451
chromogranin A, 356–357
chronic lymphocytic lymphoma, 580t
chronic wasting disease, 311
chrysotile, 264–265
Churukian's method
    chromaffin, 257
    melanin, 249m–250m, 249f
chymotrypsin, 409m
cilia, 527–529, 528f
CISH (chromogenic *in situ* hybridization)
    automatic, 458f
    definition of, 457–458
    description of, 413–414, 414f
citrus fruit oils
    as clearing agent, 109
    properties of, 109
CL (ceiling limit), 1
Clarke's solution, 88
clearing agents
    boiling point of, 108
    criteria for, 108
    types of, 108–109
    uses of, 106
CLL (chronic lymphocytic lymphoma), 580t
Clostridium difficile, 301–302
CMOS (complementary metal oxide semiconductor) cameras, 542
coagulant fixatives, 72–73, 164
codon, 487
coherent rays, 54f
Cole's hematoxylin, 176m, 178t, 185t
collagen
    bone, 317
    cross-banding of, 10
    description of, 188
    staining reactions of, 189
    Type I, 188, 189f
    Type II, 188
    Type III, 188–189
    Type IV, 189
    Type V, 189
    Type VI, 189
College of American Pathologists, 6
colloidal gold, 388–389
colloidal iron
    carbohydrates, 227, 227m–228m
    technique for, 227m–228m
colloidal metal labels, 386

colon
    biopsy of, in Hirschsprung's disease, 573, 573m–574m
    description of, 447f, 449f
color cameras, 543
Color Index, 168
color temperature, 37
colorimetric detection regents, 604m
combustibles, 16
compact bone, 317
complementary sequence, 487
compound lipids, 563
computer, ergonomics for, 34
computer-aided imaging, 540
concanavalin A, 230
condensers
    adjusting of, 68
    dark field, 49–50
    description of, 43–45, 43f–44f
    fluorescence microscopy, 64–65
    focal plane of, 53f
    phase contrast, 52
confocal microscope, 66
conformational diseases, 274, 276t
Congo red
    alkaline, 280m
    amyloid, 271, 279–281, 281f, 286
    chemical structure of, 279f
    description of, 279
    dichroism of, 282
    Highman's technique, 280m
    technique for, 280m
conjugate foci, 39
connective tissue, 194–199
    adipose tissue, 195
    anatomy of, 187
    areolar, 195
    bone *See* bone
    cartilage, 195–196
    cells of, 187, 194
    classification of, 187
    collagen *See* collagen
    dense, 195
    elastic fibers, 191–193
    fat cells of, 194
    intercellular substances of, 187–193
    myxoid, 195
    reticular fibers *See* reticular fibers
connective tissue stains
    characteristics of, 199t
    dyes in, 201t
    muscle striations, 205
    phosphotungstic acid, 202–204
    trichrome *See* trichrome stains
    types of, 199t

constructive interference, 50
contact lenses, 18
containers, for hazardous chemical storage, 22
continuous quality improvement, 7–8
Control of Substances Hazardous to Health Regulations, 2–3
control slides, 440–441, 441f
convolutions, 548–549, 549f
copper, 259, 259m
copper-associated protein, 259
corneal deposits and inclusions, 527, 527f
corrosive chemicals, 2
cortical bone, 325–326
cortical Lewy body, 364t
Corynebacterium vaginale, 301
COSHH *See* Control of Substances Hazardous to Health
Coulombic attractions, 158
covalent bonding, 159
coverslip and mountant, 601
Cowdry type A inclusion bodies, 309–310
CPHPC, 287
CQI *See* continuous quality improvement
cresyl fast violet stain, 355m–356m
cresyl violet acetate method, 298m–299m
cresyl violet counterstain, with Luxol fast blue stain, 359m–360m
Creutzfeldt-Jakob disease, 292, 311, 365–366
critical illumination, 48, 48f
cRNA probes, 461
Crocein scarlet-acid fuchsin, 211
crocidolite, 264–265
cross-linking fixatives, 71, 78, 88–89
cryosections, 164
cryostat
    definition of, 132
    fixed tissue and, 133
    frozen sections produced using, 132–133
cryostat sectioning
    anti-roll plate for, 134–135
    blades for, 133–134
    cabinet temperature for, 133–135
    cryoembedding medium for, 133
    equipment for, 135
    knives for, 133–134
    microtome, 133

rapid biopsy for intra-operative
    diagnosis, 135
technique for, 135
ultracryotomy, 135
cryotomy
    description of, 25
    ergonomics of, 35
Cryptococcus neoformans, 306
Cryptosporidium, 313
crystal violet
    amyloid, 271, 282
    solubility of, 160
cultured cells, 499
cyclin D1, 382
cytochrome oxidase, 573m
cytology samples, 1
cytomegalovirus, 309–310, 309t, 457

D

DAB (diaminobenzidine)
    characteristics of, 556–557
    composition of, 604m
    description of, 382, 385, 464–465
    endogenous peroxidase reaction
        with, 449
    handling of, 28
    immunocytochemical
        procedures use of, 251
    light scattering, 556–557
    positively stained nuclei, 552
DAB (3,3'-diaminobenzidine
    tetrahydrochloride), 147
Dako CSAII detection method,
    419m
Dako EnVision detection technique,
    418m
DAPI (4',6-diamidino-2-
    phenylindole), 481
dark-field illumination, 49–50, 49f
data sheets, 11
DDIT3 gene, 478
decalcification
    acid, 324–325, 332
    adhesion, 331–332
    agitation effects on, 326–327
    bone section See decalcified
        bone sections
    'bubble' test for, 328
    calcium oxalate test for, 328m
    chelating agents for, 325
    completion of, 327–328
    decalcified bone, 330–336
    decalcifiers, 324, 326
    definition of, 323
    description of, 323–330
    EDTA for, 325–327

endpoint test for, 327–328
factors that affect, 325–327
FAXITRON X-ray evaluations,
    328, 329f
fixation and, 89
flattening for, 331–332
formic acid for, 324–325
inorganic acids for, 324
knives, 330–331
microtomy, 331
organic acids for, 324–325
radiography evaluations,
    327–328
silver staining of bone before,
    336m–337m
specimen radiography, 327–328
surface, 329–330
suspension effects on, 327
temperature effects on, 326
treatment after, 328–329 See also
    decalcified bone sections
decalcified bone sections
    adhesion, 331–332
    canaliculi, 334–335
    cartilage, 334
    collagen stains, 333
    flattening of, 331–332
    hematoxylin and eosin,
        332–333, 333f
    immunohistochemistry of,
        335–336
    mucopolysaccharides, 334
    Schmorl's picro-thionin stain,
        319f, 334–335, 335m
    staining methods for, 332–335,
        335m
decorin, 190
dehydrant fixatives
    coagulant, 72
    cross-linking, 88–89
    mechanism of action, 88
    types of, 88
dehydration
    description of, 107
    fluids for, 107–108
    transmission electron
        microscopy, 498
dehydrogenases, 571
Delafield's hematoxylin, 175m,
    178t, 185t
dementia
    with Lewy bodies, 364–365
    vascular, 363–364
denaturated alcohol
    composition of, 107
    dehydration using, 107
denature, 487

dendritic tree, 353
Denhart's solution, 604m
dense connective tissue, 195
deparaffinization, 444
DEPC (diethylpyrocarbonate), 469,
    603m
derived lipids, 563
derived units, 587
dermatan sulfate, 218t
dermatitis herpetiformis, 434t
desmoplastic tumors, 578t
destructive interference, 50
diabetes mellitus
    amyloid in, 277
    glomerular basement
        membrane in, 519f
diabetic glomerulosclerosis, 519t
diamond knives, 126, 502–503
diaphorases, 571
diastase digestion, 231, 231m
diazo methods, 246
DIC (differential interference
    contrast), 56
dichroic mirrors, 65–66
dichroism, 57, 61, 62f, 282
dichromate fixation, 78–79, 87
diethyl ether, 28–29
differentiation shrinkage, 558
differentiation staining, 162
diffracted rays, 52
diffuse large B-cell lymphoma,
    580t
DiGeorge syndrome, 475t
digoxigenin, 465–466
diluents, 438
dioxane, 28
direct immunofluorescence, 427
disposal
    biohazardous waste, 26
    hazardous chemical waste,
        23–25
distributional error, 541–542
DLBCL (diffuse large B-cell
    lymphoma), 580t
DMAB-nitrite method for
    tryptophan, 567, 568m
DMABR
    (dimethylaminobenzyidine
    rhodanine), 259
DMF (dimethylformamide), 28
DMP 30 (dimethylamino methyl
    phenol), 141
DNA
    cDNA, 487
    counterstain, 481
    definition of, 487, 568
    demonstration methods for, 569

enzyme extraction of, 570m
Feulgen reaction for, 569, 569m
molecular pathology techniques
for, 455
probes for, 460–461, 462t
recombinant, 488
DNA analysis, 79
DNA polymerase, 487
donor block, tissue microarrays,
117, 119f
DOPA (dihydroxyphenylalanine),
248, 251
dopamine, 248
downstream, 487
dry ice, for frozen sections, 132
drying oven, for paraffin section
cutting, 126–127
dual-color/break-apart probes, 474,
478f
dual-color/dual-fusion probes, 475,
477f
dual-color/single-fusion probes,
474
Dubin-Johnson pigment, 257
Duchenne muscular dystrophy,
374f
dura mater, 355
dye(s) See also specific dye
acid, 168
amyloid, 278–279
basic, 168
chemistry of, staining affected
by, 166–167
classification of, 168, 168t
Color Index numbers for, 168
in connective tissue stains,
201t
dye-dye interactions, 159
glycol methacrylate binding
with, 165
handling of, 28
impurities, 167
molecular size, trichrome stains
affected by, 200
neutral, 168
nomenclature of, 167–168, 168t
non-ionic, 160
properties of, 167
solubility of, 599t–600t
staining affected by, 166–167
suffixes, 167–168
synthetic basic, 168
'dyed in the glass' filters, 64
dysplastic nevi, 251, 252f
dystrophic epidermolysis bullosa,
526t
dystrophin, 374f

E

EAMF (elastin-associated
microfibrils), 191
Echinococcus granulosus, 313
EDAX (electron probe micro
analyzer), 263
edge artifacts, 448f
edge detection, 549
EDTA disodium salt, 325
EDTA (ethylenediaminetetraacetic
acid), 325–327
EFMP (elastic fiber microfibrillar
protein), 191
Ehrlich's hematoxylin, 175m, 178t,
332–333
Einarson's gallocyanin method, 355
elastic fibers
aldehyde fuchsin staining of,
207–208, 208m
description of, 191–193
methyl violet/ethyl violet-
resorcin method for, 207m
orcein staining methods, 206
staining of, 205–208, 206m–208m
Weigert resorcin-fuchsin
staining method for, 206–207,
206m–207m
elaunin fibers, 192
electrical equipment, 26
electrical shock, 26
electrolytes, 82
electromagnetic spectrum, 37, 37f
electron microscopy
amyloid, 273, 273f
cross-linking fixatives for, 78
electronic light microscopy, 541
ELISA (enzyme-linked
immunosorbent assay), 427
embedding
bone, 323
ergonomics for, 34
hard tissues, 139
implants, 139
plastic See plastic embedding
specimen orientation during,
110
embedding reagents
agar, 110
celloidin, 110
gelatin, 110
lipophilic, 165–166
methyl methacrylate, 337–338
paraffin See paraffin
resin, 109
tissue processing use of,
109–110

emission filters, 431–432
emission spectra, 38
empty magnification, 48
Encephalitozoon hellem, 530f, 531t
endochondral ossification, 320
endogenous peroxidase, 449
endomysium, 198–199
endonuclease, 487
endothelial cells, 386f
Entamoeba histolytica, 312
Enterocytozoon sp., 529–531, 529f,
531t
enzymatic digestion techniques
carbohydrates, 231–233, 231m
diastase, 231, 231m
hyaluronidase, 232–233, 233m
sialidase, 232, 232m
enzyme(s)
endogenous, 402–403
as labels, 382, 384–386
enzyme histochemistry
acrylic plastics for, 145–146
enzymes for, 571
fixation for, 571
skeletal muscle biopsy uses of,
571, 572m–573m, 572t
smears, 571
eosin
B, 173
description of, 173–174
ethyl, 173
over-differentiation of, 173–174
Y, 173–174
ependymal cells, 355, 361
epidermolysis bullosa, 525, 526t
epidermolytic epidermolysis
bullosa, 526t
epi-illumination, 432
epimysium, 198–199
epitopes
description of, 382, 391–392
retrieval
heat-induced, 69, 436–437,
445
immunohistochemistry stain
quality affected by, 437,
444–445
incorrect, 447
methods for, 437, 439–440
protein digestion technique
for, 437
requirements for, 437
epoxy plastics
description of, 140–142, 140f
sections, cutting and staining
for light microscopy, 142
epoxy resins, 498–499

Epstein-Barr virus, 309t, 457, 458f
equipment
    epitope retrieval, 437
    physical hazards from, 26
    in situ hybridization, 469
equivalent to aged alcoholic
    Bouin's, 89
ergonomics
    description of, 33–35
    microtome, 128
erythrocyte protein, 200
ethanol
    dehydration using, 107
    fixation using, 72, 466
    handling of, 28
    properties of, 107
    protein denaturation by, 72
ether, 28–29
ethidium bromide, 29
ethylene glycol ethers, 29
Ewing sarcoma, 578t
Ewing's tumor, 523
excitation filters, 431–432
experimental tissue microarrays,
    116
explosive chemicals, 3
exposure control plan, 25
exposure limits, 13–14
extensive dermal melanosis, 251,
    252f
external quality assurance, 5–7
extra-signal probes, 474
eye tissue
    fixation of, 82–85
    melanin in, 248
    processing of, 113, 114t
eyepiece, 47, 67, 539
eyewash bottles, 21
eyewash stations, 21

F

Fab, 383
F(Ab)2 fragments, 429
faceshield, 25
facilities, 7
Fahrenheit, 588, 588t
false-negative staining, 443–446
false-positive staining, 446–451,
    446f–452f
familial amyloid polyneuropathy,
    276–277
fast red substrate solutions,
    421–422, 421m–422m
fast red TR solution, 421m
fat cells, 194
fat clearance, 101

fat stains, 564, 564m
fats, 563
fatty tissue, 90
FAXITRON, 328, 329f, 346m
Fc receptors, 403
fenestrae, 191
ferric ammonium sulfate, 180
ferric chloride
    description of, 182, 206
    trichloroacetic acid reaction,
        245, 245f
ferric hydroxide, 240
ferric iron
    Hukill and Putt's method for,
        241, 242m
    Lille's method for, 240–241,
        241f, 242m
    Perls' Prussian blue reaction
        for, 241m–242m
ferrocyanide, 249
ferrous ion uptake reaction, for
    melanin, 253m
ferrous iron
    Hukill and Putt's method for,
        241, 242m
    Lille's method for, 240–241,
        241f, 242m
'fetal collagen', 188–189
Feulgen nuclear technique
    acid hydrolysis-Schiff reagent
        sequence of, 161
    description of, 569, 569m
    problems associated with, 169
fibril extraction, 284–285
fibrin, 199
    definition of, 199
    Masson trichrome staining of,
        204
    MSB technique for, 204,
        204m–205m
    in paraffin sections, 199
    staining of, 204
fibrinogen, 199
fibrinoid, 199
fibroblasts, 194
fibrocartilage, 196
fibrosarcoma, 579t
filament lamps, 48
film, 545
filters
    barrier, 64
    emission, 431–432
    excitation, 431–432
    fluorescence microscopy, 64
    high-pass, 549
    low-pass, 549
    narrow band, 64

neutral density, 43
    suspension, 64
first aid, 20–21
FISH *See* fluorescence *in situ*
    hybridization
Fite method (modified), 298m, 298f
fixation
    additives that affect, 82
    artifacts caused by, 70
    bone, 321–322
    brain tissue, 85
    breast tissue, 85
    buffers effect on, 80
    carbohydrates, 220–221
    chemical, 71–78
    decalcification and, 89
    duration of, 80–81, 495
    eye tissue, 82–85
    factors affecting quality of,
        80–82
    fatty tissue, 90
    formaldehyde, 73–76, 74t–75t,
        79–80, 466–467
    freeze substitution, 71
    freeze-drying, 71, 136
    heat, 71
    immunohistochemistry stain
        quality affected by, 435–436
    importance of, 69
    in situ hybridization, 466
    lipids, 163
    lung tissue, 85
    lymphoid tissue, 85
    metabolic bone disease, 89
    metallic ions as supplement, 79
    microwave, 71
    mucins, 221
    muscle biopsy, 85
    nucleic acids, 568
    objective of, 69–70
    pH effects on, 80
    physical, 70–71
    post-fixation treatment, 107
    purpose of, 106, 162–163,
        435–436
    quality of, 446
    renal biopsy, 85
    reversal of, 437
    specimen size effects on, 80–81
    staining affected by, 162–163
    temperature of, 81–82
    testes, 85
    for tissue microarrays, 117
    transmission electron
        microscopy, 495–497
    trichrome staining affected by,
        202

types of, 70–71
vapor, 136
fixatives
  aldehyde, 496
  buffering of, 495
  characteristics of, 70
  chromic acid, 78–79
  coagulant, 72–73, 164
  combination, 74t–75t
  compound, 79–80
  concentration of, 82
  cross-linking, 71, 78, 88–89
  dehydrant, 74t–75t, 88
  dichromate-containing, 78–79, 87
  disadvantages of, 69
  DNA analysis, 79
  electrolytes added to, 82
  formaldehyde, 73–76, 74t–75t, 79–80, 466–467, 496
  formulae for, 85–89
  glutaraldehyde, 77
  ideal, 70
  immunohistochemistry stain compatibility with, 436
  interactions, 70
  ionic concentration of, 82
  mechanism of action, 70, 74t–75t
  mercuric, 86–87
  mercuric chloride, 74t–75t, 78
  metallic ions as supplement, 79
  non-coagulant cross-linking, 73
  osmium tetroxide, 74t–75t, 77–78
  osmolality of, 82
  picric acid, 87–88
  protein analysis, 79
  protein inactivation of, 81
  RNA analysis, 79
  selection of, 70
  stains incompatible with, 83t–84t
  tissue penetration depth of, 81
  transmission electron microscopy, 495–497
  vapor, 136
fixed specimens, 25
flammable chemicals, 22
flammable materials, 3
flash point, 16, 22
flotation bath, 126
flow cytometry, 411
fluorescein, 429, 429t
fluorescein isothiocyanate, 381–382, 427

fluorescence *in situ* hybridization
  advantages of, 473
  applications of, 473–480
    bladder cancer, 479–480, 480m–481m, 480f
    breast cancer, 479
    microdeletion syndromes, 474, 475f, 475t
    microduplication syndromes, 474, 475f, 475t
    neuroblastoma, 479
    prenatal chromosome studies, 474, 474f
    solid tumors, 478
  description of, 407, 457, 472
  DNA counterstain, 481
  general technique for, 480m–481m
  HER2, 483, 483m
  HER2 assessment, 412–413, 413f
  interphase scoring criteria, 485
  labeling, 473
  metaphase scoring criteria, 484–485
  methodology of, 472–473
  nomenclature, 486
  PathVysion procedure, 479, 480f, 483, 483m
  probes
    description of, 473
    dual-color/break-apart, 474, 478f
    dual-color/dual-fusion, 475, 477f
    dual-color/single-fusion, 474
    extra-signal, 474
    hematological, 474, 476t
    types of, 476t
    validation of, 485–486
  scoring analysis criteria for, 484–485
  set-up, 481–482, 482m–483m
  steps involved in, 472–473
  tissue types, 473
  troubleshooting, 485, 485t
fluorescence microscopy, 63–67
  condensers, 64–65
  confocal microscope, 66
  filters, 64
  induced light fluorescence, 65–66, 65f
  light sources for, 63–64
  objectives, 65
fluorescent antibody studies, 137
fluorescent dye, 381–382
fluorescent labeling, of mineralized bone sections, 346–347, 346f

fluorescent methods, for mycobacteria, 297m–298m
fluorescent microscope, 431
fluorescent probes
  description of, 168
  vital staining use of, 160
fluorochromes
  description of, 63
  energy output of, 431
  lectin molecule labeling with, 230
  protein conjugation with, 429
  spectral characteristics of, 429t
  types of, 429t
focal length, 39
focal point, 39, 40f
follicular lymphoma, 580t
forceps
  description of, 97–98
  paraffin section cutting, 127
formaldehyde
  biodegradability of, 24
  disadvantages of, 69
  fixation using, 69, 73–76, 74t–75t, 79–80, 202, 466–467, 496
  gelatin and, 135m
  handling of, 29
  macromolecule interactions with
    description of, 73
    reversibility of, 76–77
  nuclear protein interactions with, 73
  nucleic acid interactions with, 73
  peptide-protein bond preservation with, 76–77
  properties of, 73
  recycling of, 23
  trichrome staining affected by, 202
  unbuffered, 80
  ventilation of, 20
formaldehyde dehydrogenase, 24
formaldehyde-induced fluorescence
  biogenic amines, 137
  freeze-dried material used in, 137
formalin
  alcoholic, 80
  alcohols and, 74t–75t
  breast carcinoma, 381f
  buffered saline, 86
  buffered zinc, 86

description of, 436
DNA and, 568
duration of fixation, 440
formation of, 79–80
glycogen loss during fixation
using, 220–221
lymph node tissue fixated
using, 148f, 383f
microwave fixation in, 71
ovarian tissue fixated using,
148f
picric acid and, 74t–75t
pituitary tissue fixated using,
147f
recycling of, 23
reversal of, 437
RNA and, 568
substitutes for, 12
10%, 73, 466, 589
tissue acidophilia affected by,
163
unbuffered, 80
waste disposal, 24
formalin pigment, 262, 262m
formalin-fixed paraffin sections
description of, 402, 411f,
416–417, 458
immunohistochemistry of,
411–412
in situ hybridization of, 459
formalin-induced fluorescence, of
melanins, 253, 253m
formazans, 160
formic acid
bone decalcification using,
324–325
handling of, 29
Fouchet's technique for liver bile
pigments (modified), 245,
245m–246m
FOXO1, 478
fragment binding antigen, 383
frame processes, 550
freeze drying, 136–137
applications of, 136–137
autoradiography, 137
definition of, 136
drying technique, 136
fixation using, 71, 136
fluorescent antibody studies,
137
microspectrofluorimetry of
autofluorescent substances,
137
mucosubstances, 137
protein, 137
quenching, 136

freeze substitution
fixation using, 71
technique for, 137
FRET (fluorescence resonance
energy transfer), 66
frontotemporal lobar degeneration,
365
frozen sections, 129–133
bone, 337
cryostat for, 132–133
freezing of fresh unfixed tissue,
132–133
immunofluorescent techniques,
417, 428, 428m
immunohistochemistry of,
401–402, 417–418
principles of, 131
rapid biopsy for intra-operative
diagnosis, 135
rapid hematoxylin and eosin
stain for, 179m
theoretical considerations for,
131
uses of, 131–133
fuchsin
aldehyde *See* aldehyde
fuchsin
description of, 421m
fume hoods, 19–20
fungi
description of, 302–303
Grocott methenamine
(hexamine)-silver for, 303,
303m–304m
hematoxylin and eosin, 303
identification of, 303,
303m–305m
McManus' PAS method for,
304m–305m
periodic acid-Schiff, 221
types of, 305–307

G

GAGs (glycosaminoglycans)
cell swelling, 164–165
characteristics of, 218t
composition of, 273
definition of, 218
gallstones, 244
Gallyas silver technique, 365f,
367m–368m
gangliosides, 566, 566m
gastrointestinal stromal tumor
(GIST), 579t
G-banding, 473

GBM (glomerular basement
membrane)
in diabetes mellitus, 519f
double contouring, 516
gaps in, 516
inclusions, 513, 517f
methenamine silver microwave
method for, 193, 193m–194m
normal, 518f
renal disease effects on,
510t–511t
subendothelial widening of, 516
surface structure of, 513
texture of, 513–516
thickness of, 192–193, 513–516,
519f–521f, 520t
gelatin
as embedding agent, 110
formaldehyde and, 135m
Gendre's solution, 89
gene, 487
gene cloning, 487
gene library, 487
genome, 487
geometric processes, 550–551
germ cell tumors, 581, 581t
Germann-Straussler-Shienker
disease, 311
GFAP, 361–362, 361f
Giardia duodenalis, 312–313
Giemsa stain, 311, 311m–312m
Gill's hematoxylin, 177m, 178t, 185t
Gimenez method, for *Helicobacter
pylori*, 299m
GIST (gastrointestinal stromal
tumor), 579t
glass knives, 126, 502, 502f–503f
glial cells, 354–355
glial cytoplasmic inclusion, 364t
globin, 242, 244
glomerular basement membrane
in diabetes mellitus, 519f
double contouring, 516
gaps in, 516
inclusions, 513, 517f
normal, 518f
renal disease effects on,
510t–511t
subendothelial widening of, 516
surface structure of, 513
texture of, 513–516
thickness of, 513–516, 519f–521f,
520t
glomerulonephritis, 510t–511t
intramembranous, 509
membranous, 509, 510t–511t,
513f

mesangiocapillary, 514t, 515f
post-infectious, 509, 512f
glomerulosclerosis, 519t
glomerulus, 521
gloves, 18
glucose
chemical structure of, 215, 216f
description of, 215
glucuronyl transferase, 244
glutaraldehyde
cross-linking by, 77
fixation using, 77, 163, 371,
495–496
handling of, 29
limitations of, 163
paraformaldehyde and,
496m–497m
properties of, 77
glycoconjugates, 215, 216t
description of, 215, 216t,
218–219, 221
PAS (periodic acid-Schiff)
technique for, 221–224, 222t,
224m
glycogen
aqueous solubility of, 220–221
characteristics of, 217t
description of, 216
fixation of, 220–221
function of, 217t
McManus' PAS method for,
304m–305m
techniques for demonstrating,
222t
glycogen storage diseases, 216
glycol methacrylate
dye-binding artifacts, 165
methacrylic acid binding, 165
monomer, 29
glycolipids, 216t
glycoproteins, 216t–217t, 220
glycosidic linkages, 216
glycoxal, 29
GMA
bone staining, 335–336
enzyme histochemistry uses of,
146
Gmelin technique, 246m
goggles, 18, 25
Goldner's trichrome method,
343m–344m
Golgi preparation, 358
Gomori methenamine silver, 263
Gomori's aldehyde fuchsin
description of, 168
lipofuscin staining using, 255f,
256m

Gomori's hexamine silver
technique, 260–261
Gomori's method for reticular
fibers, 210m
Gomori's trichrome, 169
Gordon & Sweets' method,
209m–210m
Gram stain
bacteria in smears, 295m
description of, 295
microorganisms, 295, 295m–296m
modified Brown-Brenn method,
295m–296m
Gram's iodine, 592m
Gram-Twort stain, 296m
gray levels, 544
gray matter, 355
grid, tissue microarray, 117, 118f
Grocott hexamine silver method
description of, 169
fungi, 303, 303m–304m
Grocott methenamine
(hexamine)-silver
fungi, 303, 303m–304m
Histoplasma capsulatum, 306f
gross room, 95–96
grossing
description of, 96
tools for, 97f
gum sucrose, 133m
gynecological samples, 101–102

H

H&E (hematoxylin and eosin)
absorbance curves of, 555f
amyloid, 278
Aspergillus fumigatus, 305, 305f
bacteria, 294
bile pigments, 244–245
bone sections, 332–333, 333f
Candida albicans, 305
Cryptococcus neoformans, 306
cytoplasm on, 69–70
decalcified bone sections,
332–333, 333f
description of, 555–556
dysplastic nevus, 252f
Entamoeba histolytica, 312
ependymal cells, 361
fungi, 303, 305
Giardia duodenalis, 312–313
Helicobacter pylori, 301
Histoplasma capsulatum, 306
Mayer's, 332–333, 333f
MMA-embedded tissue, 341,
341m, 341f

molluscum virus, 310
neurons, 355
Nocardia asteroides, 305
nuclear counterstain use of, 185
oligodendrocytes, 362
osteocytes, 334
paraffin sections, 178m–179m
Parkinson's disease, 366f
popularity of, 173
quality control in, 184–185
rapid, for urgent frozen
sections, 179m
reticular fibers, 190
Schistosoma sp., 313
technique, 151m, 342m
Toxoplasma gondii, 312, 312f
worms, 313
Hamazaki-Weisenberg bodies, 257
hapten labeling technique, 389–390
hard tissues, embedding of, 139
Harris stain, 173
Harris's hematoxylin, 174, 176m,
178t, 179m, 185t
Haversian systems, 317–318, 318f
hazardous chemicals
container storage of, 22
containment of, 22–23
control of, 16–25
data sheets for, 11
drain disposal of, 24
elimination of, 12
first aid for, 20–21
flammable, 22
ingestion of, 21
labeling of, 17
occupational exposure limits
for, 13–14
recycling of, 23
reduction of, 12
skin contact of, 21
spill of, 22–23
splashing of, 21
storage of, 21–22
transporting of, 22
types of, 15–16
ventilation of, 19–20
warning signs for, 17–18
waste disposal, 23–25
hazards
biological, 25–26
data sheets for, 11
elimination of, 12
evaluation of, 11–12
identification of, 11–12
occupational exposure limits
for, 13–14
physical, 26

reduction of, 12
standard operating procedures
for working with, 13
types of, 15–16
H-disc, 197, 198f
Health and Safety at Work Act
(1974), 2
Health and Safety Executive, 1–2
Health and Safety Offences Act
(2008), 2
Health Protection Agency, 1–2
heat
tissue processing rate affected
by, 106
trichrome stain affected by, 201
heat fixation, 71
heat-induced epitope retrieval, 69,
436–437, 445
heating and air conditioning, 19
heat-mediated antigen retrieval,
392–394, 401, 406m, 409
heavy chain amyloidosis, 276
Heidehain's 'Azan' technique,
203–204
Heidehain's Susa, 263
Heidenhain myelin stain, 181–182
Heidenhain's hematoxylin,
180–181, 181m, 185t
Helicobacter sp.
cresyl violet acetate method for,
298m–299m
Gimenez method for, 299m
H. pylori, 301
toluidine blue in Sorenson's
buffer for, 299m
Helly's solution, 86–87
HEMA, 143
hematein
description of, 174
PTAH staining technique using,
182m
hematoidin, 244–246
hematoxylin(s)
alcoholic, 227
alum See alum hematoxylins
Carazzi's, 177m, 178t, 185t
chemical oxidation of, 174
Cole's, 176m, 178t, 185t
Delafield's, 175m, 178t, 185t
Ehrlich's, 175m, 178t, 185t,
332–333
Gill's, 177m, 178t, 185t
Harris's, 174, 176m, 178t, 179m,
185t
Heidenhain's, 180–181, 181m,
185t
iron, 180–182, 201–202

lead, 184
Loyez, 181–182, 185t
Mallory, 185t
Mayer's, 174, 175m–176m, 178t,
185t, 333f
molybdenum, 183
mordants for, 174, 184
natural oxidation of, 174
oxidation of, 174
phosphomolybdic acid,
183m–184m
preparation of, 173
Solcia, 185t
sources of, 174
Thomas, 183, 183m–184m, 185t
tungsten, 182, 182m–183m
uses of, 185t
Verhöeff's, 182, 185t, 191–192,
205–206, 206m
Weigert-Pal technique, 184, 185t
Weigert's, 178, 180, 180m, 185,
185t
without mordant, 184
heme, 242–244
hemidesmosomal epidermolysis
bullosa, 526t
hemochromatosis, 240, 241f
hemoglobin, 242–243, 243m, 243f
hemoglobin peroxidase, 243
hemoglobinopathies, 276t
hemoglobinuria, 243f
hemosiderins, 240–241, 241m–242m
hemosiderosis, 240
heparin, 218t
heparin sulfate, 218t, 219
hepatitis B virus, 308, 308m–309m
hepatocytes
bile in, 244
lipofuscins in, 255
HEPES, 496
HER2, 412–414, 413f–414f, 459f, 479
HER2 fluorescence in situ
hybridization procedure, 483,
483m
hereditary systemic amyloidosis,
276–277
herpes simplex, 309t
herpes viruses, 309–310
hexazotized new fuchsin, 421m
high efficiency particulate air
filters, 19–20
high iron diamine, 228, 229m
Highman's Congo red technique,
280m
high-pass filters, 549
high-resolution light microscopy,
139–140

Hirana bodies, 276t
Hirschsprung's disease, 573,
573m–574m
histiocytosis X, 523, 523f
Histology Quality Improvement
Program, 6
Histoplasma capsulatum, 306, 306f
Histo-QIP See Histology Quality
Improvement Program
HMB 45, 251, 252f
H5N1 influenza virus, 310
Hodgkin's disease, 399f, 580t
Hollande's solution, 88
Holmes' silver impregnation
method, 334
HOPE, 79
horseradish peroxidase, 385, 465
hot plate, for paraffin section
cutting, 126–127
HPA See Health Protection Agency
HSE See Health and Safety
Executive
HSI model, 545
Hukill and Putt's method for ferric
and ferrous iron, 241, 242m
human immunodeficiency virus,
309t, 310
human papilloma virus, 309t, 310,
455
human T-cell leukemia virus, 309t
hyaline cartilage, 196
hyaluronic acid
description of, 217t–218t, 219f
techniques for demonstrating,
222t
hyaluronidase
digestion, 232–233, 233m
preparation of, 603m
hybridization
definition of, 487
fluorescence in situ See
fluorescence in situ
hybridization
in situ See in situ hybridization
solution for, 604m
hydrocarbons, 563
hydrochloric acid, 29
hydrogen bonding, 158–159
hydrogen peroxide
handling of, 29
melanin bleaching using,
252m–253m
storage of, 449
hydrogen peroxide-methanol
method, 385
hydrolases, 571
hydrophobic effect, 159

hydroquinone
    in acrylic plastics, 143
    handling of, 29–30
hydroxyapatite, 318
hyperkeratosis, 310
hyphae, 303

I

IDLH, 2
IgA nephropathy, 430, 510t–511t, 514f
illumination
    critical, 48, 48f
    dark-field, 49–50, 49f
    Köhler, 48, 48f
    Rheinberg, 50
    sources of, 63–64
image
    acquisition of, 542–546
    analysis of See image analysis
image analysis
    area processes, 548–550, 549f
    definition of, 546
    frame processes, 550
    geometric processes, 550–551
    illustration of, 553f
    minimal requirement for, 546
    multispectral imaging for, 67, 559
    overview of, 546–547
    point processes, 547–548
    programs, 546
    repetitive measurements using, 554
    scripts for, 554–555
    software for, 551
    specimens
        description of, 551–555
        preparation of, 555–559, 555f
image contrast stretching, 548
image thresholding, 548
immersion objectives, 67
immunocomplexes
    in renal biopsy, 416t
    in skin biopsies, 416t
immunodeficiency, 291
immunofluorescence
    definition of, 427
    direct, 427
    frozen-section, 417
    indirect, 427
immunofluorescent techniques
    advantages of, 427
    applications of, 427
    biopsy staining procedure, 431m
    frozen sections, 428, 428m

microscopy, 431–432
overview of, 427
primary antibodies and conjugates, 428–430
quality control, 432
reagents used in, 428
renal disease, 432–433, 433f
skin diseases, 434, 434t
staining procedure, 430–431, 431m
substrate antigens for, 427–428
immunoglobulins, 383, 407f, 414f, 429
immunogold techniques
    description of, 420
    indirect, for monoclonal antibodies, 420m
    silver staining, 386f, 388–389, 420m
immunohistochemistry
    absorption control, 404, 405f
    acrylic plastic sections for, 146–147
    adenocarcinoma of unknown origin, 579, 579t
    amyloid, 285–286, 285f
    amyotrophic lateral sclerosis, 366f
    anaplastic tumors, 577, 578t
    antibodies
        monoclonal, 384, 419m–420m
        polyclonal, 384
        preparation of, 445
        validation of, 439–440
    antigen sites, 390–392
    avidin-biotin complex technique, 389
    background staining in, blocking of, 403–404
    biotin-free catalyzed signal amplification, 390
    biotinylated tyramide signal amplification, 389–390
    bone, decalcified, 335–336
    carbohydrates, 230–231
    chromogen incompatibility, 445–446
    colloidal metal labels, 386
    controls, 404
    cytological preparations, 402
    decalcified bone sections, 335–336
    definition of, 382–384
    deparaffinization, 444
    description of, 381, 435
    detection system, 450
    direct technique, 386–388, 387f

double, 400f
endogenous enzymes in, blocking of, 402–403
enzyme labels, 384–386
external quality assurance, 442–443
false-negative staining, 443–446
false-positive staining, 446–451, 446f–452f
fast red substrate solutions, 421–422, 421m–422m
frozen sections
    description of, 401–402, 417–418
    immunofluorescence, 417
germ cell tumors, 581, 581t
GFAP, 361–362
hapten labeling technique, 389–390
heat-mediated antigen retrieval, 392–394, 401, 406m, 409
HER2 expression, 412–414, 413f–414f
hydrophobic interactions, 403
immune serum/antibodies, dilution of, 405
immunoglobulin light chains in formalin-fixed paraffin-wax sections, 411–412
immunogold silver staining technique, 386f, 388–389, 420m
immunoperoxidase staining method for formalin-fixed paraffin wax-embedded skin biopsies, 416–417
in situ hybridization versus, 456
incubation methods, 406–407
indirect technique, 387f, 388
influenza virus, 310f
labels, 384–386.
lectins, 230–231, 384
lymph nodes, 447f
lymphoma, 580, 580t
mesothelioma, 580, 580t–581t
microorganisms, 293
MMA sections, 152
monoclonal antibodies, 384, 419m–420m
motor neuron disease, 366f
mucins, 230–231
negative control, 404
neurons, 356–357, 357f
non-gynecological cytology smears, 417–418
non-specific staining, 403
paraffin processing of tissues for, 436–437

paraffin-wax block, 407–408, 408m
polyclonal antibodies, 384
polymer chain two-step indirect technique, 388
positive controls, 404, 441–442, 442f, 444
practical aspects of, 404–406
pretreatment, 152
primary reagents for, 384
proteolytic enzyme digestion, 391–392
quality control
  documentation, 435
  internal, 435
  stain quality, 435–439, 446
radiolabels, 386
reagents for, 384
renal tumors, 582, 582t
rickettsia, 307, 307f
Rocky Mountain spotted fever, 307f
SARS-associated coronavirus, 311f
slides
  control, 440–441, 441f
  daily review of, 442
  preparation of, 443
species cross-reactivity, 451
spindle cell neoplasms, 579, 579t
stain quality in
  block storage conditions effect on, 438–439
  control slides, 440–441, 441f
  daily slide review, 442
  epitope retrieval, 437
  external positive controls for, 441–442
  factors that affect, 435–439
  fixation effects on, 435–437
  internal positive controls for, 441–442, 442f
  monitoring of, 439–443
  processing effects on, 436–437
  reagent effects on, 437–438
  reversal of fixation effects on, 437
  slide storage conditions effect on, 438–439
staining techniques
  alkaline phosphatase, 419–421, 419m
  avidin-biotin, 418
  Dako CSAII detection method, 419m

Dako EnVision detection technique, 418m
immunogold, 386f, 388–389, 420, 420m
Novolink polymer detection technique, 418m–419m
polymer, 418–419, 418m–419m
streptavidin/streptavidin-biotin complex, 418m
tyramide signal amplification, 419, 419m
streptavidin-biotin system, 408
techniques, 386–388, 387f
theory of, 382–386
Toxoplasma gondii, 312f
troubleshooting, 443–451
  false-negative staining, 443–446
  false-positive staining, 446–451, 446f–452f
two-step indirect technique, 388
viral identification using, 457
washes, 405–406
workload, 401
Zygomycetes, 306f
immunolabeling electron microscopy, 459
immunoperoxidase
  for formalin-fixed paraffin wax-embedded skin biopsies, 416–417
  paraffin-wax sections, 417
immunotactoid glomerulopathy, 516t, 518f
implants, 139
impure dyes, 167
in situ hybridization
  acrylic plastics, 148
  advantages of, 456
  applications of, 457–459
  automation of, 470
  chromogenic See CISH (chromogenic in situ hybridization)
  controls, 468–469
  cytological information obtained using, 457
  cytomegalovirus, 457
  definition of, 455, 487
  DEPC-treated solutions, 469
  DEPC-treated water, 469, 603m
  description of, 455
  detection systems, 464–466
  dilution series, 463
  enzymes for detection, 465
  equipment, 469
  fixation for, 466

fluorescence See fluorescence in situ hybridization
glassware preparation, 469
hybridization, 467–468, 487
immunohistochemistry versus, 456
indirect detection systems, 465
microorganisms, 293–294
mRNA detection using, 456, 459, 467
polymerase chain reaction-, 459
positive controls, 468
prehybridization, 467
probes, 460–461
  biotin labeling of, 465
  commercially made, 463–464
  concentration, 464
  definition of, 460
  description of, 460
  DNA, 460–461, 462t
  double-stranded DNA, 461
  5'-end labeling of, 461–462
  labeling of, 461–463
  length of, 464
  oligonucleotide, 460–461, 462t, 464
  preparation of, 461–463
  purification of, 463
  RNA, 461, 462t
  single-stranded DNA, 461
  synthesis methods, 460–461
  testing of, 463, 464f
  3' tailing, 462–463
  3'-end labeling of, 462
  types of, 460–461
radiolabeled probes, 456
reagents for, 459–460, 469, 603m–604m
sample
  fixation of, 466
  proteolytic digestion, 466–467
  slide/section preparation, 466
silver precipitation, 458, 459f
technique of, 455
terminology associated with, 486–489
troubleshooting of, 470–471
universal method for, 469m–470m
in situ zymography, 458–459
incidents
  likelihood values for, 3–4
  severity scoring for, 3–4
incinerator, 24
inclusion body immunostaining, 364t

inclusions
   glomerular basement
      membrane, 513, 517f
   skeletal muscle, 524t–525t
incubation, 406–407
indirect immunofluorescence, 427
indole groups, 567, 568m
induced fluorescence, 63
induced light fluorescence, 65–66,
   65f
industrial methylated spirit
   composition of, 107
   dehydration using, 107
infectious agents, 70
infectious diseases See also specific
   disease
   presentation of, 291–292
   safety issues, 292
infinity corrected objectives, 45, 47
influenza virus, 310
inorganic acids, for bone
   decalcification, 324
intercalated discs, 198
interference microscopy, 52–56, 54f
internal quality control, 5
International Organization for
   Standardization, 5–6
Internet, 551
interpupillary distance, 47
intestinal spirochetosis, 302
intramembranous
   glomerulonephritis, 509
intramembranous ossification, 320
iodine
   Gram's, 592m
   handling of, 30
   Lugol's, 78, 592m
iris diaphragm, 44–45
iron
   absorption of, 240
   demonstration of, 240–241
   dietary, 240
   excess of, 240, 241f
   Lille's method for, 240–241,
      241f, 242m
   metabolism of, 240
   Perls' Prussian blue reaction
      for, 241m–242m
   small intestine absorption of,
      240
iron deficiency, 240
iron hematoxylins, 180–182,
   201–202
iron overload, 239–240
iron salts, 180
irritants, 2
isocitrate dehydrogenase 1, 362

isopentane
   frozen sections produced using,
      132
   handling of, 30
isopropanol, 30
isopropyl alcohol
   dehydration using, 107
   properties of, 107

J

JB4, 149m–150m
JC virus, 309t, 310
JPEG images, 551
junctional epidermolysis bullosa,
   526t

K

Kallmann syndrome, 475t
Kayser-Fleischer ring, 259
keratan sulfate, 218t
Ki-67, 362, 552
kidneys
   diseases of See renal diseases
   glomerular basement
      membrane See glomerular
      basement membrane
   glomerulus changes, 521
kilobase, 487
kiton red-almond green technique
   for hemoglobin, 243
knives
   diamond, 126, 502–503
   glass, 126, 502, 502f–503f
Köhler illumination, 48, 48f
koilocytosis, 310

L

labeling
   fluorescence in situ
      hybridization, 473
   fluorescent, 346–347, 346f
   hapten, 389–390
   hazardous chemicals, 17
labels, for immunohistochemistry,
   384–386.
laboratory
   accreditation of See
      accreditation
   facilities of, 7
   specimen dissection area in, 96
laboratory management
   governance, 1–9
   overview of, 1

   personnel, 8–9
   quality management, 5
   risk management, 1–5
laboratory management team, 2
laboratory manager
   human error prevention by, 2–3
   risk management functions of,
      2
   staff management by, 8–9
laboratory staff
   description of, 7, 95
   laboratory manager's role with,
      8–9
   meeting of, 8–9
Lactobacillus acidophilus, 301
lamellar bone, 318f
lamina densa, 192
lamina lucida, 192
lamina rara, 192
lamina reticularis, 192
Langerhan's histiocytosis, 523, 523f
laser microdissection-proteomics
   amyloid typing using, 286
   future of, 287
latex gloves, 18–19
LCDD (light chain deposition
   disease), 277
lead, 265, 266m
lead citrate stain, 508m
lead hematoxylins, 184
lead salts, 508, 508m
LECT2 amyloidosis, 277
lectins, 230–231, 384
Legionella pneumophila, 302
leiomyosarcoma, 579t
Leishmania tropica, 312
Lendrum's phloxine-tartrazine
   stain, 307, 308m
length measurements, 588, 588t
Leptospira interrogans, 302
leptospirosis, 302
Leuco patent blue V method, for
   hemoglobin, 243m
leukocyte common antigen, 382
levamisole, 385
Lewy body diseases, 276t, 277,
   363–365
light
   birefringent, 57
   energy content of, 38
   image formation, 39–41
   image quality, 41–43, 42f
   interference of, 50–52, 51f, 54f
   monochromatic, 52–56
   polarized, 60–61
   properties of, 37–41, 37f
   refraction of, 38–39, 39f

retardation of, 38–39, 39f
sources of, 37–38
wavelengths of, 37f, 38, 63
white, 37
light microscopy
electronic, 541
high-resolution, 139–140
polarized *See* polarized light
microscopy
light scattering, 556–557
light-emitting diodes, 431
likelihood values, for incidents, 3–4
Lille's method
chromaffin, 257
ferric and ferrous iron, 240–241,
241f, 242m
Lillie's aluminon method, 267m,
267f
Lillie's rhodizonate method, for
lead, 265f, 266m
limonene
as clearing agent, 109
handling of, 30
properties of, 109
Lindquist's modified rhodanine
technique, for copper, 259m–
260m, 260f
lipids
cerebrosides, 565, 565m
cholesterol, 564
classification of, 563
compound, 563
definition of, 563
derived, 563
fixation of, 163, 563–564
gangliosides, 566, 566m
microtomy of, 563–564
simple, 563
sphingomyelin, 565, 565m
stains for, 564, 564m
sulfatides, 565, 565m–566m
lipofuscin
anatomic sites of, 255
bleaching of, 251
ceroid-type, 257
demonstration of, 255, 255f, 256m
description of, 244–245, 353–354
Gomori's aldehyde fuchsin
technique for, 255f
Long Ziehl-Neelsen method for,
256m
in neurons, 353–354
Nile blue method for, 254m,
254f
production of, 255
liposarcoma, 219
liquid nitrogen, 132

Listeria monocytogenes, 302
lithium carbonate extraction-
hexamine silver technique, 261m
Long Ziehl-Neelsen method, for
lipofuscin, 256m
long-chained aliphatics, 109
Lowicryls
description of, 143–144
K4M, 152m, 153
low-temperature embedding
procedures used with, 153
processing and embedding
schedule for, 152m
low-pass filters, 549
Loyez hematoxylin, 181–182, 185t
LR Gold, 143–144, 146, 146f, 499
LR White
acrylic plastic section staining,
151
processing and embedding
schedule for, 150m–151m
transmission electron
microscopy use of, 499
Lugol's iodine, 78, 592m
lung tissue, 85
Luxol fast blue stain
description of, 359, 359m–360m
myelin staining, 164–165
lymph nodes
formalin-fixed tissue, 148f, 383f
identification of, 101
immunohistochemistry of, 447f
lymphoma, 578t, 580, 580t
lyssavirus, 309t

M

Macchiavello's stain, 307, 307m
macromolecules
formaldehyde interactions with
description of, 73
reversibility of, 76–77
solubility of, 72
macroscopic specimen, 97–98, 99f
magnesium chloride, 592m, 603m
magnification
empty, 48
total, 47–48
values, 47–48
major histocompatibility complex
class I, 373
malarial pigment, 262, 262m
maleic acid buffer, 604m
malignant fibrous histiocytoma, 219
malignant melanoma, 247–248, 251,
254f, 579t

malignant peripheral nerve sheath
tumor (MPNST), 579t
malignant tumors
Ewing's tumor, 523
Langerhan's histiocytosis, 523,
523f
mesothelioma, 521–523, 522f
primitive neuroectodermal
tumor, 523
Mann's methyl blue-eosin stain,
307
mantle cell lymphoma, 580t
manual arrayer, 119–120, 120f
manual coverslipping, 35
manual microtomy, 35
manual staining, 35
Marchi technique, 360–361
marginal zone lymphoma, 580t
mass, 588, 588t
Masson trichrome stain
fibrin, 204
illustration of, 200f
technique for, 203m
Masson-Fontana method
chromaffin, 257
melanin, 249m
pseudomelanosis pigment, 257
Mayer's hematoxylin, 174,
175m–176m, 178t, 185t, 333f
measles, 309t
measurement units, 587–588,
587t–588t
Melan A, 251
melanin
anatomic sites of, 247–248
antibodies associated with
activation of, 254–255
argyrophilic nature of, 248
bleaching of, 248, 251,
252m–253m
in brain, 248
Churukian's method for,
249m–250m, 249f
definition of, 247
enzyme methods for, 251
in eyes, 248
ferrous ion uptake reaction for,
253m
fluorescent methods for, 248
formalin-induced fluorescence
of, 253, 253m
hydrogen peroxide bleaching
of, 252m–253m
identification methods for, 248
immunohistochemistry of,
254–255
insolubility of, 248, 251

Masson-Fontana method for, 249m

microwave ammoniacal silver method for, 249m–250m, 249f

Nile blue method for, 254m, 254f

precursor cells, formalin-induced fluorescence of, 253m

protein binding of, 247

reducing methods for, 248–249, 249m–251m, 249f

Schmorl's reaction for, 249, 250m–251m, 250f

in skin, 247–248

solubility methods for, 251

melanin granules, 247

melanocytes, 247–248

melanomas, 248

melanophages, 247–248, 251

melanosis coli, 257

melanosome, 247, 247f

melting temperature, 487

membranous glomerulonephritis, 509, 510t–511t, 513f

meninges, 355

mercuric chloride
  disadvantages of, 78
  fixation using, 74t–75t, 78, 466
  handling of, 30
  reduced use of, 4

mercuric fixatives, 86–87

mercuric oxide, 30, 174

mercury pigment, 263

Merkel cell tumor, 451f

mesangiocapillary glomerulonephritis, 514t, 515f

mesenchymal cells, 197

mesothelioma, 521–523, 522f, 580, 580t–581t

metabolic bone disease, 89

metachromasia, 162
  alcohol fast, 229–230
  alcohol labile, 229–230
  amyloid, 281–282
  azure A technique for, 230m
  definition of, 229
  mechanism of, 229
  staining for, 159, 229–230, 230m

metallic ions as fixative supplement, 79

metallic iron deposits, 240–241

Metanil yellow, 227

meter, 588t

Methacarn, 88

methacrylic acid, 142, 165

methanol
  acetic acid and, 466
  blood smear fixation using, 88

dehydration using, 107

fixation using, 72, 88, 466

handling of, 30

properties of, 107

methenamine, 30

methenamine silver method
  description of, 193, 193m–194m, 257
  senile plaques, 368f, 369m–370m

methyl green, 282

methyl green-pyronin technique, 569–570, 570m

methyl violet
  amyloid, 281–282
  ethyl violet-resorcin and, 207m
  properties of, 281–282

methylation
  carbohydrates, 233, 234m
  saponification and, 234m–235m

methylene blue
  absorption of, 162
  -azure II-basic fuchsin, 372m
  solubility of, 160

methylene hydrate, 73

methylhippuric acids, 15

Michel transport medium, 428

micro computed tomography, 348

microdeletion syndromes, 474, 475f, 475t

microduplication syndromes, 474, 475f, 475t

microglia, 362

microgram, 588t

micrometer, 588t

microorganisms
  adaptive mutations in, 291
  bacteria, 294, 294t
  control secretions for, 294
  definition of, 291
  detection of, 292–294
  Gram stain for, 295, 295m–296m
  Gram-Twort stain for, 296m
  identification of, 292–294
  immunohistochemistry of, 293
  mycobacteria, 296–297
  polymerase chain reaction of, 293–294
  safety of, 292
  in situ hybridization of, 293–294
  size of, 292, 292t

microradiography
  definition of, 345
  of mineralized bone, 345–346, 345f, 346m
  X-ray crystallography for, 346

microscope
  body tube, 47
  bright-field, 50
  calibration devices for, 539
  centering the lamp of, 67–68
  condensers, 43–45, 43f–44f, 52, 68
  confocal, 66
  distributional error, 541–542
  eyepiece, 47, 67, 539
  fluorescent, 431
  image acquisition, 542–546
  iris diaphragm of, 44–45
  light source, 43–47, 431
  morphometry aids, 540–541
  object stage, 45
  objectives, 45, 46f
  phase contrast, 52, 53f
  polarizing, 57
  setting up, 67–68
  slide insertion in, 68
  use of, 67
  'z' axis calibration of, 539

microscope photometry, 541–542

microscopy
  ergonomics of, 35
  fluorescence See fluorescence microscopy
  immunofluorescent, 431–432
  interference, 52–56, 54f
  phase contrast, 50–52, 51f
  polarized light, 56–62, 57f–61f

microspectrofluorimetry, 137

microsporidia, 529–531, 529f–530f, 531t

Microsporidium sp., 531t

microtome
  base sledge, 125
  cryostat sectioning, 133
  ergonomics of, 128
  knives for, 126, 502–503, 502f–503f
  maintenance of, 128
  rotary, 125
  rotary rocking, 125
  setup of, 128
  sliding, 126
  ultra, 126

microtome blades
  description of, 128
  disposable, 126, 133–134
  injuries caused by, 3, 26
  selection of, 330–331

microtomy
  decalcification, 331
  definition of, 125
  instruments used in, 125

lipids, 563–564
  paraffin section cutting, 128
  tissue microarrays, 122
microtubule-associated protein 2, 356
microwave ammoniacal silver method, 249m–250m, 249f
microwave antigen retrieval
  description of, 392–393, 393f
  technique for, 410m
  trypsin digestion and, 394–401
microwave fixation, 71, 81–82
microwave processors, 111, 437
mild methylation technique, 234m
Miller-Dieker syndrome, 475t
Miller's solution, 87
milligram, 588t
millimeter, 588t
Millon reaction for tyrosine, 566, 566m–567m
mineralized bone
  adhesive tape methods for, 336
  aluminum demonstration in, 344, 344m
  description of, 336
  fluorescent labeling of, 346–347, 346f
  frozen, 337
  grinding and polishing of, 339
  methacrylate-embedded, 338–340
  microradiography of, 345–346, 345f, 346m
  mounting after staining, 340–341
  osteoid demonstration, block impregnation for, 336, 336m–337m
  plastic embedding of, 338–344
  preparation of, 336–347, 336m–337m
  sawing of, 339
  solochrome cyanine staining of, 342, 342m, 342f
minerals
  access to, 263
  aluminum, 266, 266m–267m
  asbestos, 264–265
  beryllium, 266, 266m–267m
  calcium, 257–258, 258m, 258f–259f
  carbon, 264
  copper, 259, 259m
  definition of, 239
  exogenous, 239
  lead, 265, 266m

silica, 264
silver, 267–268, 268m
urates, 260–261, 261m, 261f
uric acid, 260–261, 261m, 261f
minimal change disease, 519f, 519t
missense mutation, 488
mission statement, 7
mitochondria, 524t–525t
M-line, 198f
MMA (methyl methacrylate)
  bone, 321–322, 338
  embedding techniques using, 337–338
  embedding uses of, 144–145
  handling of, 30
  hematoxylin and eosin for, 341, 341m, 341f
  processing and embedding schedule for, 150m
  sections, immunohistochemical staining on, 152
MNA (methyl nadic anhydride), 141
molar solutions, 587t, 590–591
'mole', 247–248
molecular cytogenetics, 457
molecular pathology
  applications of, 455, 457–459
  blotting, 455
  description of, 455
  polymerase chain reaction See polymerase chain reaction
  reagents, 603m–604m
  in situ hybridization See in situ hybridization
Möller's solution, 87
molluscum virus, 309t, 310
molybdenum hematoxylins, 183
monochromatic light, 52–56
monoclonal antibodies, 384, 419m–420m, 459
monosaccharides, 215–216, 216t
mordants, 174, 184
morphometry
  bone, 347–348
  definition of, 539–540, 558
mosaic images, 550–551
motor neuron disease, 364t, 366, 366f
motor neurons, 355
mountants, 601, 601m
  coverslip and, 601
Movat pentachrome stain
  illustration of, 210f
  Russell modification of, 210m–212m

MPNST (malignant peripheral nerve sheath tumor), 579t
mRNA, 456, 459, 467, 488
MSB (Martius scarlet blue) technique, 204, 204m–205m
mucicarmine
  carbohydrates, 226, 226m–227m
  mucins, 226
  technique for, 226m–227m
mucins, 217t, 219–221
  alcian blue for, 225–226
  immunohistochemistry of, 230–231
  methylation of, 233
  mucicarmine technique for, 226
  techniques for demonstrating, 222t
mucopolysaccharides, 284, 334
mucopolysaccharidoses, 219
mucosubstances, 137
multispectral imaging, 67, 559
muscle, 196–199
  cardiac, 197–198, 255
  purpose of, 196
  skeletal See skeletal muscle
  smooth, 197
  striated, 197, 198f, 205
  structure of, 198–199
muscle biopsy, 373–374
  description of, 110
  fixation of, 85
  staining methods for, 374t
mutation, 488
mycelium, 303
MYCN oncogene, 479
mycobacteria, 296–297, 297m–301m
Mycobacterium avium/intracellulare, 302
Mycobacterium leprae, 298m, 298f, 302
Mycobacterium tuberculosis, 302
myelin
  description of, 358–359
  loss of, 360–361
  Luxol fast blue stain for, 359, 359m–360m
  Page's solochrome cyanine stain for, 360m
  tinctorial stains for, 359
myelin sheath, 563
myenteric plexus, 573
myofibrils, 197, 524t–525t
myofibrosarcoma, 579t
myosin, 196–197
myxoid chondrosarcomas, 219
myxoid connective tissue, 195

N

NAACLS *See* National Accrediting Agency for Clinical Laboratory Standards
N-acetylneuraminic acid, 220f
nanogram, 588t
nanometer, 588t
naphthochrome green, 266
narrow band filters, 64
National Accrediting Agency for Clinical Laboratory Standards, 9
National External Quality Assurance Scheme, 6
National Institute of Occupational Safety and Health, 13–14
National Society of Histotechnology, 6
NBF (neutral buffered formalin)
  bone fixation, 321
  fixation using, 106, 117, 321
  formulation of, 86
  glycogen fixation using, 221
  lung biopsy fixation in, 85
near field scanning microscopy, 67
necrotising vasculitis, 199
negative birefringence, 260–261
negative staining, 160, 440
Negri bodies, 307
Neisseria gonorrhoeae, 301
Neisseria meningitidis, 301
neoplasia
  adenocarcinoma of unknown origin, 579, 579t
  anaplastic tumors, 577, 578t
  germ cell tumors, 581, 581t
  mesothelioma, 580, 580t–581t
  prognosis for, 583
  reactive proliferations versus, 582
  renal tumors, 582, 582t
  small round cell tumors, 578, 578t
  therapeutic response of, 583
nephrotic focal glomerulosclerosis, 519t
NEQAS *See* National External Quality Assurance Scheme
nerve fibers
  silver binding to, 162
  teased, preparation of, 372m–373m
nervous system
  central
    description of, 353
    tissues of, from autopsy, 375
  components of, 353–355

neuraminidase, 232
neuroblastoma, 479, 578t
neurodegenerative diseases
  Alzheimer's disease *See* Alzheimer's disease
  assessment of, 363
  autopsies, 364
  characteristics of, 363
  description of, 363
  diagnosis of, 363
  frontotemporal lobar degeneration, 365
  motor neuron disease, 366, 366f
  Parkinson's disease, 366f
  pathological characteristics of, 363
  vascular dementia, 363–364
neurofibrillary tangles, 283, 364, 364t, 369m–370m
neurofilaments, 356
neuroglia
  astrocytes, 361–362, 361f
  definition of, 361
  ependymal cells, 361
  microglia, 362
  oligodendrocytes, 358–359, 362
neuromelanin, 353–354
neuron(s)
  anatomy of, 353, 354f
  axons, 353, 354f, 357–358, 357m–358m
  immunohistochemistry of, 356–357, 357f
  lipofuscin in, 353–354
  motor, 355
  Nissl substance, 355, 355m–356m
  tinctorial stains for, 355, 355m–356m
neuronal inclusion bodies, 276t
neuronal nuclear proteins, 356
neuron-specific enolase, 356
neuropil, 355
neurosecretory granules, 356–357
neutral density filters, 43
neutral dyes, 168
nevus, 247–248
Newcastle disease, 459
nickel chloride, 31
Nicol prisms, 57, 58f
Nile blue method, for melanin, 254m, 254f
NIOSH *See* National Institute of Occupational Safety and Health
Nissl substance, 355, 355m–356m
nitric acid, 31
nitrile gloves, 19

nitro-blue tetrazolium for alkaline phosphatase, 420–421, 421m–422m
nitrogen, liquid, 31
Nocardia sp.
  modified Fite method for, 298m
  N. asteroides, 305
non-coagulant cross-linking fixatives, 73
normal solutions, 588t, 591
Nosema sp., 529–531, 531t
Novolink polymer detection technique, 418m–419m
NSH *See* National Society of Histotechnology
nuclear protein-formaldehyde interactions, 73
nuclear stains, for trichrome stains, 201–202
nuclease digestion, 467
nucleic acid sequences, 455–456
nucleic acids
  basophilia, 568–569
  description of, 568
  digestion methods for, 570, 570m
  DNA *See* DNA
  fixation of, 568
  formaldehyde interactions with, 73
  RNA *See* RNA
nucleoproteins, 568
nucleotides, 456f, 488
numerical aperture, 45, 50

O

objectives
  cleaning of, 67
  description of, 45, 46f
  fluorescence microscopy, 65
  immersion, 67
object-to-image ratio, 45
occupational exposure limits, 13–14
Occupational Safety and Health Administration
  flash point, 16
  Permissible Exposure Limits, 13–14
  purpose of, 1–2
odong tea extract, 531
oil Red O in dextrin, 564m
oils, 563
Okamoto-Utamura rhodanine method, for silver, 267–268, 268m

Okamoto-Utamura rubeanic
   acid method, for copper, 259,
   259m
Olig2, 362
oligodendrocytes, 358–359, 362
oligodendroglia, 355
oligodendrogliomas, 362
oligonucleotide, 488
oligonucleotide 3′-end labeling
   with DIG-ddUTP, 472m
oligonucleotide probes, 460–461,
   462t, 464
oligosaccharides, 216t
Olmacher's solution, 87
1p36 deletion syndrome, 475t
orcein
   description of, 206
   Shikata's method for
      hepatitis B surface antigen,
      308m–309m
organic acids, for bone
   decalcification, 324–325
Orth's solution, 87
OSHA See Occupational Safety and
   Health Administration
osmium tetroxide
   fixation using, 74t–75t, 77–78,
      497, 497m
   handling of, 31
   properties of, 77–78
   tissue acidophilia affected by,
      163
   transmission electron
      microscopy uses of, 497,
      497m
ossification of bone, 320
osteoblasts, 319–320
osteoclasts, 319–320, 319f
osteocytes, 319, 319f, 334
osteoid
   block impregnation for
      demonstration of, 336,
      336m–337m
   description of, 318, 333
   volume of, 347
osteomalacia, 266
osteons, 317–318, 318f
ovarian tissue, formalin-fixed,
   148f
ovaries, lipofuscins in, 255
overnight tissue processing, 112,
   113t
oxalic acid, 31
oxidases, 571
oxidizers, 3
oxidoreductases, 571
oxytalan fibers, 191–192

P

Palmgren's method, 357, 357m–
   358m, 367
PAN (perchloric acid-
   naphthoquinone) method,
   564m–565m
PAP (peroxidase-antiperoxidase
   complex), 388
Papanicolaou stain, 179
   cell overstaining, 164
   formula for, 179m
   Harris's hematoxylin, 179m
   staining method for, 179m–180m
papilloma viruses, 309t, 310
paraffin
   additives, 109
   contraindications, 139
   as embedding reagent, 109–110,
      139
   immunohistochemistry, 407–408
   melting point of, 109
   properties of, 109
   reprocessing of tissues
      embedded in, 501, 501m
   tissues embedded in, 501, 501m
   viscosity of, 106
paraffin section cutting
   brushes for, 127
   drying oven for, 126–127
   equipment required for,
      126–127
   flotation bath for, 126
   forceps, 127
   hard tissues, cutting of, 129
   hot plate for, 126–127
   practical microtomy for, 128
   problems and solutions, 129,
      130t–131t
   sections
      adhesives, 127–128
      cutting of, 128–129
      drying, 129
      floating out, 129
      problems and solutions, 129,
         130t–131t
   slides, 127
   surface decalcification, 129
   tissue block trimming, 128
   water bath for, 126, 129
paraffin sections
   cutting of See paraffin section
      cutting
   fibrin in, 199
   formalin-fixed, 402
   hematoxylin and eosin stain for,
      178m–179m
immunohistochemistry, 408m
immunoperoxidase, 417
paraformaldehyde
   glutaraldehyde and, 496–497m
   handling of, 29
paraproteinemic crystalloidal
   keratopathy, 527, 527f–528f
parasites
   Giemsa stain for, 311,
      311m–312m
   microsporidia, 529–531,
      529f–530f, 531t
par-central lenses, 47
par-focal lenses, 47
Parkinsonism, 366
Parkinson's disease, 366f
partially polymerized resins, 373
PAS (periodic acid-Schiff)
   alcian blue-PAS technique,
      225–226, 226m, 232
   carbohydrates, 221–224, 222t,
      224m
   cells that react with, 223t
   cerebrosides, 565m
   colloidal iron technique with,
      227
   Cryptococcus neoformans, 306
   description of, 157
   diastase digestion and, 231
   differential diagnosis uses of,
      221
   fungal species, 221
   Histoplasma capsulatum, 306
   McManus', for glycogen and
      fungal cell walls, 304m–305m
   mucopolysaccharides, 334
   mycobacteria, 296–297
   myelin, 359
   rabies virus, 310
   Rhizopus, 306f
   Schiff reagent, 223–224
   starch, 263
   substances oxidized by, 223
   technique for, 221–223, 224m
pathology service, 1
pattern recognition, 539
peanut agglutinin, 230
PELs (Permissible Exposure
   Limits), 13–14, 26–27
pemphigoid, 434t
pemphigus, 434t
pepsin, 409m, 467
peracetic acid, 251
perchloric acid-naphthoquinone
   method, 564m–565m
performic acid-alcian blue method,
   567m

perimysium, 198–199
periodic acid
    handling of, 31
    -methenamine silver microwave
        method, 193m–194m
periodic reviews, 13
peripheral nerve biopsies, 371–373,
    372m–373m
Perls' Prussian blue reaction for
    ferric iron, 241m–242m
peroxidases, 571
personal hygiene, 16–17
personal protective equipment
    description of, 18
    risk minimization using, 12
personnel
    management of, 8–9
    personal hygiene practices for,
        16–17
    safety training for, 13
PGP9.5, 356
pH
    acetic acid effects on, 80
    alcian blue, 225
    fixation affected by, 80
    solution, 593
    trichrome stain affected by, 201
phase contrast microscope, 52, 53f
phase contrast microscopy, 50–52,
    51f
phenol
    dehydration using, 108
    handling of, 31
    as softening agent, 108
phenyl groups, 566, 566m–567m
phloxine B and eosin Y, 173–174
phloxine-tartrazine stain, 307, 308m
phosphate buffers, 89, 496, 496m,
    594m, 594t
phosphate-citrate buffer, 595m, 595t
phospholipids, 564m
phosphomolybdic acid
    handling of, 31
    hematoxylin stain, 183m–184m
    practical uses of, 203
    trichrome staining and, 202–204
phosphorylase, 573m
phosphotungstic acid
    handling of, 31
    practical uses of, 203
    trichrome staining and,
        202–204
photographs, 98, 99f, 540
physical hazards, 26
pia mater, 355
picogram, 588t
picometer, 588t

picric acid
    fixation using, 72–73, 74t–75t,
        87–88, 402
    formalin and, 74t–75t
    handling of, 31
    picrates formed by, 107
    preparation of, 592m
    solubility of, 592m
pigments
    amalgam tattoo, 264
    artifact, 239, 262–263
    bile, 244–246, 245m–246m, 245f
    chromaffin, 257
    chromic oxide, 263
    definition of, 239
    Dubin-Johnson, 257
    endogenous, 239
        bile pigments, 244–246,
            245m–246m, 245f
        chromaffin, 257
        hemoglobin, 242–243, 243m,
            243f
        hemosiderins, 240–241,
            241m–242m
        melanins See melanin
        porphyrin, 246
    exogenous, 239, 263–268
    formalin, 262, 262m
    hemoglobin, 242–243, 243m,
        243f
    hemosiderins, 240–241,
        241m–242m
    insoluble, 160
    malarial, 262
    melanin See melanin
    mercury, 263
    porphyrin, 246
    pseudomelanosis, 257
    schistosome, 262–263
    starch, 263
    tattoo, 263–268, 264f
pipetting, 35
pituitary tissue, formalin-fixed,
    147f
plan-apochromats, 47
plane of vibration, 57
plasma cells, 274
Plasmodium sp., 262
plastic embedding
    acrylic plastics, 142–144
    description of, 140
    epoxy plastics, 140–142, 140f
    mineralized bone, 338–344
    polyester plastics, 142
Pleistophora sp., 531t
pleochroic, 57
plus slides, 127–128

PMA (phosphomolybdic acid)
    practical uses of, 203
    trichrome staining uses of,
        202–204
PNET (primitive neuroectodermal
    tumor), 523
Pneumocystis jiroveci, 294, 306–307
point processes, 547–548
Poison Control Center, 21
polarized light, 60–61
polarized light microscopy
    amyloid, 282–283
    collagen, 333
    description of, 56–62, 57f–61f
polarizers, 57, 59f, 60–61
poliovirus, 309t
polyclonal antibodies, 384, 450, 459
polyester plastics, 142
Polyglycol methacrylate, 143
poly-L-lysine, 127, 331–332
poly-L-lysine slides, 602
polymerase chain reaction
    description of, 455
    -in situ hybridization, 459
    microorganisms, 293–294
polymerization, 140
polysaccharides
    description of, 163, 216–218
    techniques for, 222t
polyvinyl alcohol, 337
pop-off technique, for slide-
    mounted sections, 501m–502m
porphyrin pigments, 246
positive controls
    immunohistochemistry, 404,
        441–442, 442f, 444
    in situ hybridization, 468
post-infectious glomerulonephritis,
    509, 512f
potassium dichromate, 32
potassium ferricyanide, 32
potassium ferrocyanide, 32
potassium hydroxide, 32
potassium permanganate, 589
    handling of, 32
    PTAH solution chemically
        oxidized with, 182m–183m
Prader-Willi syndrome, 475t
prehybridization solution, 604m
prenatal chromosome studies, 474,
    474f
pressure cooker antigen retrieval,
    393, 393f, 410m
prevalence tissue microarrays, 116
primary ciliary dyskinesia, 527,
    529f
primary fluorescence, 63

primitive neuroectodermal tumor, 523
prion diseases
    autopsy issues, 375
    Creutzfeldt-Jakob disease, 292, 311, 365–366
    description of, 276t, 311, 365
prions
    biological risks associated with, 25
    function of, 365
prior-derived amyloid deposits, 286
probes
    definition of, 488
    fluorescence *in situ* hybridization
        description of, 473
        dual-color/break-apart, 474, 478f
        dual-color/dual-fusion, 475, 477f
        dual-color/single-fusion, 474
        extra-signal, 474
        hematological, 474, 476t
        types of, 476t
        validation of, 485–486
    in situ hybridization, 460–461
        biotin labeling of, 465
        commercially made, 463–464
        concentration, 464
        definition of, 460
        description of, 460
        DNA, 460–461, 462t
        double-stranded DNA, 461
        5'-end labeling of, 461–462
        labeling of, 461–463
        length of, 464
        oligonucleotide, 460–461, 462t, 464
        preparation of, 461–463
        purification of, 463
        RNA, 461, 462t
        single-stranded DNA, 461
        synthesis methods, 460–461
        testing of, 463, 464f
        3' tailing, 462–463
        3'-end labeling of, 462
        types of, 460–461
processors
    carousel-type, 111
    changing solutions on, 34
    closed, 81–82
    continuous input rapid, 111–112
    maintenance of, 112
    microwave, 111
    tissue, 111–112
    vacuum, 111

prognosis tissue microarrays, 116
progression tissue microarrays, 116
propan-2-ol
    dehydration using, 107
    properties of, 107
propidium iodide, 32
propylene glycol ethers, 32
protease, 409m, 458–459
protective equipment, 18–19
protein
    alcohol denaturation of, 72
    description of, 566
    erythrocyte, 200
    ethanol denaturation of, 72
    fixative inactivation by, 81
    fixatives for analysis of, 79
    freeze-dried sections of, 137
    indole groups, 567, 568m
    phenyl groups, 566, 566m–567m
    tertiary structure of, 72
protein digestion technique, 437
proteinase K, 467, 603m
proteoglycans
    description of, 217t, 218–219
    techniques for demonstrating, 222t
proteolytic digestion
    antigens, 391
    immunohistochemistry, 391–392
    in situ hybridization sample, 466–467
    troubleshooting of, 471
proteolytic enzymes
    antigen retrieval, 408–409, 409m
    digestion, 391–392
proteomics, 286
protoplasmic astrocytes, 361
protoporphyrin, 243
protozoa
    Giemsa stain for, 311, 311m–312m
    types of, 312–313
provision, 47
pseudogout, 260, 261f
pseudomelanosis pigment, 257
PTA (phosphotungstic acid)
    practical uses of, 203
    trichrome staining uses of, 202–204
PTAH (phosphotungstic acid hematoxylin) staining
    hematein, 182m
    potassium permanganate, 182m–183m
    technique for, 182, 182m–183m
    uses of, 185t
pyridine, 32

Q
Q-bands, 197, 198f
quality, 5
quality assurance, external, 5–7
quality control
    accreditation use of, 6
    immunofluorescent, 432
    tissue processing, 115
quality management, 5
quenching, 136

R
rabies virus, 310
radioactive chemicals
    description of, 21
    storage of, 22
radiolabels, 386
random priming, 488
reactive proliferations, 582
reagents
    analyte-specific, 485–486
    embedding *See* embedding reagents
    immunohistochemistry, 384, 437–438
    issues associated with, 169
    molecular pathology, 603m–604m
    reactive, 162
    recycling of, 115
    in situ hybridization, 459–460, 469
    solubility of, 597t–598t
    tissue interactions with, 158–159
    uptake rates of, 162
real image, 39, 41f
recombinant DNA, 488
record keeping, 13
recycling of reagents, 115
red blood cells, 244
Regaud's solution, 87
regressive staining, 162
renal amyloid, 516t, 517f
renal biopsy
    fixation of, 85
    high-resolution light microscopy for, 139–140
    immunocomplexes in, 416t
renal diseases
    glomerular basement membrane *See* glomerular basement membrane
    glomerulonephritis *See* glomerulonephritis

immunofluorescent techniques for, 432–433, 433f
systemic lupus erythematosus, 510t–511t
types of, 510t–511t
renal tumors, 582, 582t
replication, 488
reproductive toxins, 16
resin(s)
  acrylic, 499
  epoxy, 498–499
  partially polymerized, 373
  as stain binders, 165
  as stain excluders, 165
  staining patterns affected by chemistry of, 166
resin embedding
  description of, 109
  staining affected by, 165–166
resolution, 45
resolving power, 45–47
resorcin-fuchsin method
  description of, 191
  elastic fiber staining, 206, 206m–207m
  Hart's modification of, 207
  modification of, 207
respirator cartridges, 19
respiratory protection, 19
reticular fibers, 190
  argyrophilia of, 188–189
  definition of, 190
  description of, 188–189
  Gomori's method for, 210m
  Gordon & Sweets' method for, 209m–210m
  metal impregnation techniques for, 208–209
  pattern of, 190f
  Russell modification of Movat pentachrome stain for, 210m–212m
  sections, 209
  staining of, 208–209, 209m–210m
reticules, 539
reticulin staining, 334
reticuloendothelial system, 240, 244
reverse transcriptase, 488
reverse transcription-polymerase chain reaction, 458–459
Reynolds' lead citrate stain, 508m
rhabdomyosarcoma, 578t
Rheinberg illumination, 50
Rhizopus, 305, 306f
rhodamine, 429–430, 429t
rhodanine method

for copper (modified), 259m–260m, 260f
for silver, 268m
rhodizonate method, for lead, 265f, 266m
RI (refractive index), 38–39, 46f, 50, 57, 282
riboprobes, 461
rickettsia, 307
risk analysis/evaluation, 3
risk identification, 3
risk management
  audits, 4–5
  elements of, 2
  funding of, 5
  hazards, 11–12
  in laboratories, 1–5
  methods of, 4
  objective of, 4
  occupational exposure limits, 13–14
  periodic reviews, 13
  personnel training, 13
  plan for, 12
  record keeping, 13
  standard operating procedures, 13
risk minimization, 12
RNA
  analysis, fixatives for, 79
  definition of, 488, 568
  demonstration methods for, 569–570, 570m
  enzyme extraction of, 570m
  methyl green-pyronin technique for, 569–570, 570m
  molecular pathology techniques for, 455
  mRNA, 456, 459, 467, 488
  probes, 461, 462t
  rRNA, 488
  tRNA, 489
RNA polymerase, 488
Rocky Mountain spotted fever, 307, 307f
Romanowsky stain, 164
Rossman's solution
  description of, 89
  glycogen fixation using, 221
rotary microtome, 125
rotary rocking microtome, 125
round cell tumors, 578, 578t
R-Phycoerythrin, 429t
rRNA, 488
rubeanic acid method, for copper, 259, 259m

Russell modification of Movat pentachrome stain, 210m–212m

S

S100 protein, 254–255, 360
SAA (serum amyloid A protein), 276
safety
  personnel training in, 13, 20–21
  specimens, 95
  tissue processing, 115
safranin O-fast green, 334, 342
saline, 86
  buffered, 86, 592m
saline sodium citrate, 604m
SAP (serum amyloid P component), 272–273, 278, 285
saponification, 233–234, 234m–235m
sarcoidosis, 266
sarcoma, 219, 578t
sarcoplasmic reticulum, 524t–525t
SARS (severe acute respiratory syndrome), 310
SARS-associated coronavirus, 310, 311f
satellite cells, 524t–525t
sawing, of bone, 322, 339
scanning electron microscopy, 137
Schaudinn's solution, 87
Schiff reagent, 223–224
Schistosoma sp., 313
schistosome pigment, 262–263
Schmorl's ferric ferricyanide reduction test, 244
Schmorl's picro-thionin stain, 319f, 334–335, 335m
Schmorl's reaction, for melanin, 249, 250m–251m, 250f
Schwann cells, 358–359
Scott's tap water, 592m
secondary fluorescence, 63
sections
  adhesives for, 127–128
  frozen See frozen sections
  paraffin See paraffin sections
  semi-thin, 504
segmental glomerulosclerosis, 519t
self-adhesive labels, 17
semi-automated incubation, 406
semi-thin sections, 503
senile plaques, 368f, 369m–370m
sense strand, 488
sensitivity, 384
serpinopathies, 276t
serum amyloid P component, 272–273

severity scoring, for incidents, 3–4
Shikata's orcein method for
    hepatitis B surface antigen,
    308m–309m
short-chained aliphatics, 109
SI units, 587–588, 587t–588t
sialic acids, 220, 220f
sialidase digestion, 232, 232m
sialomucin, 221
silanized slides, 602
silica, 264
silver, 267–268, 268m
silver precipitation *in situ*
    hybridization, 458, 459f
silver salts and solutions
    amyloid, 284
    bone, before decalcification,
        336m–337m
    handling of, 32
    preparation of, 209
    reduction of, to metallic silver,
        248
    reticular fiber staining using,
        208–209
simple carbohydrates, 215
simple lipids, 563
simplex epidermolysis bullosa, 526t
single-chip camera, 543
Sirius red, 281, 281m
skeletal muscle
    biopsies, enzyme
        histochemistry of, 571,
        572m–573m, 572t
    transmission electron
        microscopy of, 523, 524t–525t,
        558, 572t
skin
    melanin in, 247–248
    staining of, 447f
skin biopsy
    formalin-fixed paraffin
        wax-embedded,
        immunoperoxidase staining
        method for, 416–417
    immunofluorescence of,
        430–431
    specimen dissection, 99–100,
        100f
    specimen orientation, 110
    staining procedure for, 431m
skin diseases, 434, 434t
slide
    adhesive, 602
    albumen-coated, 602
    charged, 127–128
    coating on, 602
    drying temperature for, 439

insertion of, in microscope, 68
paraffin section cutting, 127
plus, 127–128
poly-L-lysine, 602
silanized, 602
storage of, 438–439
slide labeling
    automated systems for, 105
    ergonomics for, 34
slide-mounted sections, pop-off
    technique for, 501m–502m
sliding microtome, 126
small cell carcinoma, 578t
small intestine, iron absorption in,
    240
small lymphocytic lymphoma, 580t
small round cell tumors, 578, 578t
smears
    brain, 370–371
    enzyme histochemistry, 571
    specimen geometry in, 164
    spinal cord, 370–371
Smith-Magenis syndrome, 475t
smooth muscle, 197
sodium azide, 32
sodium bisulfite, 32
sodium chloride, 603m
sodium dibasic, 32
sodium hydroxide, 589
sodium hydroxide-ferric
    hematoxylin/DAH method,
    565m
sodium hypochlorite, 32
sodium iodate, 32, 174
sodium methoxide, 141
sodium monobasic, 32
sodium phosphate, 32
sodium thiosulfate, 32
soft tissue resections, 102
solid tumors, 478
solid-state cameras, 542–543,
    545–546
solochrome azurine method
    for aluminum, 266m–267m, 344,
        344m
    for beryllium, 266m–267m
solochrome cyanine stain
    for mineralized bone sections,
        342, 342m, 342f
    for myelin in paraffin sections,
        360m
solubility, 160, 597t–600t
solutions *See also specific solution*
    buffer, 593, 593m–595m,
        593t–595t
    molar, 587t, 590–591
    neutral, 593

normal, 588t, 591
pH, 593
preparation of, 592
volume-to-volume, 587t,
    589–590
weight-to-volume, 587t, 590
soma, 353
SOPs *See* standard operating
    procedures
Sorenson's buffer, toluidine blue in,
    299m
Sotos syndrome, 475t
spatial filtering, 549
specimen(s)
    analysis of, 98, 551–555
    barcoding of, 96, 105
    bone *See* bone specimens
    bowel, 100–101, 100f
    definition of, 163–164
    fixation affected by size of, 106
    identification of, 96, 105
    image analysis preparations,
        555–559, 555f
    large, 98
    macroscopic, 97–98, 99f
    medium, 98, 98f
    multiple, 96
    particulate, 500, 500m–501m
    reception of, 95–96
    safety considerations, 95
    size of, fixation affected by,
        80–81
    small, 99
    staining affected by geometry
        of, 163–165
    thin, 164
    transmission electron
        microscopy, 493–495, 494f
    two-person rule for, 96
specimen dissection
    breast resections, 102
    core biopsy, 99
    fat clearance, 101
    gynecological samples,
        101–102
    laboratory area for, 96
    lung tissues, 101
    residual tissue storage after, 99
    room for, 96
    skin biopsy, 99–100, 100f
    small samples, 99
    soft tissue resections, 102
specimen identifier, 95
spherical aberration, 42f, 43
sphingomyelin, 565, 565m
spill, of hazardous chemicals,
    22–23

spinal cord
  anterior horn cells in, 355f
  biopsy of, 370–371
spindle cell neoplasms, 579, 579t
spindle-shaped fibroblast, 194
spirochetes, 302
  Warthin-Starry method for,
    299m–300m
Splendore-Hoeppli protein, 305
stain(s) *See also specific stain*
  affinity of, 157, 158t, 159–161
  definition of, 157
  fixatives incompatible with,
    83t–84t
  lipophilic, 166
  quantitation of, 557–558
  reagent-tissue interactions,
    158–159
  resin binding with, 165
  selectivity of, 161–162
  solubility of, 160
  staining patterns affected by
    chemistry of, 165–166
  stain-stain interactions, 159
  tissue retention of, 160–161,
    161f
  uptake mechanisms, 157–160
  vital, 168
staining
  collagen fibers, 189
  definition of, 157
  differentiation, 162
  dye impurity effects on, 167
  errors in, 169
  fixation effects on, 162–163
  histochemical blocking and
    extraction effects on, 163
  introduction to, 157
  metachromasia, 162
  metachromatic, 159
  negative, 160
  problems associated with,
    168–169
  PTAH, 182, 182m–183m
  rate of reaction effects on, 162
  rate of reagent uptake and loss
    effects on, 162
  reagents *See* reagents
  regressive, 162
  resin chemistry effects on, 166
  resin embedding effects on,
    165–166
  solvent-solvent interactions, 159
  specimen geometry effects on,
    163–165
  stain chemistry effects on,
    165–166

stain-stain interactions, 159
standardization of, 557
theory of, 157–166
tissue modification effects on,
  162–163
vital, 160
standard operating procedures
  accreditation standards for, 7
  description of, 2–3
  hazardous substances, 13
  methodology of tests
    documented in, 7
Staphylococcus aureus, 301
starch, 263, 271
steamer, for antigen retrieval,
  393–394, 410m
Steiner for filamentous and
  non-filamentous bacteria
  (modified), 300m–301m, 301f
STEL (short-term exposure limit),
  14
stereology, 540–541
steroid sulfatase deficiency, 475t
sterols, 563
stock solution, 589
storage
  hazardous chemicals, 21–22
  hydrogen peroxide, 449
  radioactive chemicals, 22
  slides, 438–439
streptavidin, 389
streptavidin-biotin system, 408,
  418m–419m
Streptomyces avidin, 389
striated muscle, 197, 198f
stringency, 488
structural glycoproteins, 191
subepithelial immune complex
  deposits, 509
substantia nigra, 248
Sudan dyes
  affinity of, 161
  black B method, 564m
  lipids, 564, 564m
  solvents used with, 159
sulfanilic acid, 246
sulfatides, 565, 565m–566m
sulfomucin, 221
sulfur dioxide, 223–224
sulfuric acid, 32–33
support films, 505, 505f
surface decalcification, 329–330
surgical cut-up, 96, 97f
suspension filters, 64
synapses, 353
synaptophysin, 356–357, 357f
synovial sarcoma, 578t–579t

synthetic basic dye, 168
α-Synuclein, 364–365
systemic amyloidosis, 274
systemic lupus erythematosus,
  434t, 510t–511t, 512f, 521f

T

Taenzer-Unna orcein method, 191
target organ effects, 16
tattoo pigment, 263–268, 264f
Tau pathology, Gallyas method for,
  367m–368m
TDP-43, 365
TdT (terminal deoxynucleotidyl
  transferase), 462
temperature conversions, 588, 588t
template, 488
terminal deoxynucleotidyl
  transferase, 462
testes
  fixation of, 85
  lipofuscins in, 255
tetracycline labeling, 346–347, 346f
tetrahydrofuran, 33
Texas Red, 429t
thioflavine S, 283
thioflavine T staining, 283, 284m,
  286
three-chip camera, 543–544
threshold limit values, 13–14
tinctorial stains
  description of, 144–145
  myelin, 359
  neurons, 355, 355m–356m
tissue
  connective *See* connective tissue
  drying of, 449
  freezing of, 132–133, 134t
  permeability of, trichrome
    stains affected by, 200
  reagent interactions with,
    158–159
  stain affinity for, 157, 158t,
    159–161
tissue blocks
  description of, 97–98, 98f
  storage of, 438–439
tissue microarrays
  advantages of, 116
  antibody production using, 116
  arrayers, 119–123, 120f
  database for, 117–119
  development of, 115–116
  donor block preparation, 117,
    119f, 121
  experimental, 116

fixation of tissues for, 117
grid design for, 117, 118f
illustration of, 116f
microtomy, 122
needle sizes, 117
portable quick ray, 120–121
prevalence, 116
prognosis, 116
progression, 116
punch size for, 117, 122–123
purpose of, 116
recipient block preparation, 121, 121f
smoothing and sectioning, 122
staining procedures used with, 116
tips for, 122
troubleshooting for, 122
types of, 116
tissue processing
  agitation effects on, 106
  automated, 110–113
  breast specimens, 112–113, 114t
  clearing agents for, 108–109
  dehydration stage of, 106–108
  description of, 105
  embedding reagents for, 109–110
  eyes, 113, 114t
  fixation stage of, 106–107
  heat effects on, 106
  immunohistochemistry stain quality affected by, 436–437
  labeling of tissues for, 105
  manual, 114–115
  microwave, 437
  overnight, 112, 113t
  paraffin, 436–437
  post-fixation treatment, 107
  principles of, 105–107, 110
  processors for See processors, tissue
  quality control in, 115
  rate of, factors that affect, 105–106
  safety considerations, 115
  schedules for, 112–113, 500t
  small biopsies, 113, 114t
  stages of, 106–110
  tissue dried in, restoration of, 115
  transmission electron microscopy, 499, 500t
  vacuum effects on, 106
  viscosity effects on, 106
TLV See threshold limit values
TMAs See tissue microarrays

toluene
  as clearing agent, 108
  handling of, 33
  properties of, 108
toluidine blue
  absorption of, 162
  amyloid, 284
  cartilage, 334
  Helicobacter sp., 299m
  semi-thin sections, 504m
  in Sorenson's buffer, 299m
toluidine blue-acetone method, 565m–566m
tonsil, 411, 411f, 452f
tools, grossing, 97f
total internal reflection, 39, 40f
toxic materials, 16
Toxoplasma gondii, 312, 312f
trabecular bone, 317, 319f, 347
traceability, 17
Trachipleistophora sp., 531t
'tram-tracking', 515f, 516
transcription, 488
transferases, 571
transillumination, 101
transmissible spongiform encephalopathy, 277
transmission electron microscopy
  advantages of, 493
  aldehyde fixatives for, 496
  amyloid, 516t, 517f, 526–527
  buffers for, 495–496, 496m
  CADASIL, 495, 525–526, 527f
  cilia, 527–529, 528f
  corneal deposits and inclusions, 527, 527f
  dehydration, 498
  diagnostic uses of, 509
  embedding
    acrylic resins for, 499
    description of, 498
    epoxy resins for, 498–499
  epidermolysis bullosa, 525, 526t
  epoxy resins, 498–499
  fixation for, 495–497
  light microscopy versus, 493
  malignant tumors
    Ewing's tumor, 523
    Langerhan's histiocytosis, 523, 523f
    mesothelioma, 521–523, 522f
    primitive neuroectodermal tumor, 523
  microsporidia, 529–531, 529f–530f, 531t
  non-neoplastic diseases, 523–531

osmium tetroxide fixation for, 497, 497m
paraproteinemic crystalloidal keratopathy, 527, 527f–528f
pop-off technique for slide-mounted sections, 501, 501m
primary ciliary dyskinesia, 527, 529f
principle of, 493
renal diseases
  Alport's syndrome, 520t, 521f
  benign essential hematuria, 520f, 520t
  glomerulonephritis, 510t–511t
  glomerulosclerosis, 519t
  immune complex deposits, 509–513, 512f–515f
  immunotactoid glomerulopathy, 516t, 518f
  minimal change disease, 519f, 519t
  systemic lupus erythematosus, 510t–511t, 512f, 521f
  types of, 510t–511t
sectioning, 506t–507t
sections
  collection of, 504–505
  semi-thin, 503
  silver to gold, 505
  thickness of, 507t
  ultra-thin, 505–507
skeletal muscle, 523, 524t–525t, 558
specimen handling, 493–495, 494f
staining, 497–498
  lead salts for, 508, 508m
  purpose of, 507
  timing of, 507–508
  uranyl salts for, 508, 508m
tissue samples
  cell suspensions, 500, 500m–501m
  cultured cells, 499
  paraffin-embedded material, 501, 501m
  particulate matter, 500
  preparation of, 493
  processing of, 499, 500t
  wash buffer of, 497–498
ultramicrotomy
  diamond knives, 502–503
  glass knives, 502, 502f–503f
  semi-thin sections, 503
  support films, 505, 505f

trough fluids, 503
  ultra-thin sections, 505–507
  wash buffer, 497–498
transmitted light fluorescence
  filters, 64
  light sources, 63–64, 64f
transthyretin amyloidosis, 274, 285
transverse tubular system,
  524t–525t
Treponema pallidum, 302
trichloroacetic acid
  ferric chloride reaction with,
    245, 245f
  fixation using, 72–73
trichloroethane, 33
trichloroethylene, 202
Trichomonas vaginalis, 313
trichrome stain/staining, 199–202
  applications of, 199t
  decalcified bone sections, 333
  definition of, 199–200
  factors that affect, 200–201
  fixation effects on, 202
  Goldner's, 343m–344m
  heat effects on, 201
  Heidehain's 'Azan' technique,
    203–204
  Masson, 200f, 203m
  nuclear stains for, 201–202
  pH effects on, 201
  phosphomolybdic acid uses in,
    202–204
  phosphotungstic acid uses in,
    202–204
  tissue permeability effects on,
    200
triethanolamine (0.1), 603m
trinitrophenol, 72–73
Tris (stock), 603m
Tris-HCl buffer, 593, 595m, 595t
Tris-HCl buffered saline, 592m, 604m
tRNA, 489
tropoelastin, 191
trough fluids, 503
trypsin
  -chymotrypsin, 409m
  description of, 152
  digestion, 394–401
tryptophan, DMAB-nitrite method
  for, 567, 568m
TTR (transthyretin), 274, 276–277
tumors
  anaplastic, 577, 578t
  Ewing's, 523
  primitive neuroectodermal,
    523
  renal, 582, 582t

small round cell, 578, 578t
solid, 478
tungsten hematoxylins, 182,
  182m–183m
TWA (time-weighted average), 1,
  14
two-person rule, for specimens, 96
tyramide
  description of, 152
  signal amplification using, 419,
    419m
  streptavidin biotin method,
    419m
tyrosinase, 247–248, 251, 254–255
tyrosine, Millon reaction for, 566,
  566m–567m
Tzanck smears, 309–310

U

ubiquitin, 363–364
UKNEQAS, 442
Ulex europaeus, 230
ultra microtome, 126
ultracryotomy, 135
ultramicrotomy
  block trimming, 503–504, 503f
  diamond knives, 126, 502–503
  glass knives, 502, 502f–503f
  semi-thin sections, 503
  support films, 505, 505f
  trough fluids, 503
  ultra-thin sections, 505–507
ultrastructural studies
  description of, 139
  epoxy plastics as embedding
    media for, 140
ultra-thin sectioning, 135
unfixed tissue, freezing of, 132–133
universal solvents
  dehydration using, 108
  properties of, 108
uranyl acetate, 508m
uranyl nitrate, 33
uranyl salts, 508, 508m
urates, 260–261, 261m, 261f
uric acid, 260–261, 261m, 261f
users
  liaison with, 7
  organization with, 7
uterine samples, 101–102

V

vacuum, tissue processing rate
  affected by, 106

vacuum tissue processor, 111
van den Burgh test, 246
van der Waals' forces, 158
van Gieson stain
  decalcified bone sections,
    333
  picric acid-acid fuchsin mixture
    in, 178, 200, 333
  technique for, 202m
vaneometer, 19–20
vapor fixation, 136
variant Creutzfeldt-Jakob disease,
  311, 375
varicella-zoster, 309t
vascular dementia, 363–364
VCD (vinylcyclohexande dioxide),
  141–142
Velocardiofacial syndrome, 475t
ventilation, 19–20
Verhöeff's hematoxylin
  description of, 182, 185t,
    191–192
  elastic fiber staining, 205–206,
    206m
vibration direction, 57, 57f
Vibrio cholerae, 232
viral hepatitis, 309
viral inclusion bodies, 307
virtual image, 39–41
viruses
  description of, 307
  immunohistochemistry of,
    457
  infections caused by, 309–310,
    309t
viscosity, tissue processing rate
  affected by, 106
vital stains/staining, 160, 168
Vittaforma sp., 531t
Volkmann's canals, 317–318, 318f
volume, 587, 587t
volume-to-volume solutions, 587t,
  589–590
von Kossa silver nitrate method,
  169
  for bone mineral, 342, 343m,
    343f
  for calcium, 258f

W

Warthin-Starry method, for
  spirochetes, 299m–300m
waste
  biohazardous, 26
  hazardous chemical, 23–25

water bath
    antigen retrieval, 394, 410m
    paraffin section cutting, 126,
       129
Weigert resorcin-fuchsin method
    description of, 191
    elastic fiber staining, 206,
       206m–207m
    Hart's modification of, 207
    mechanism of, 207
    modification of, 207
Weigert-Pal technique, 184, 185t
Weigert's hematoxylin, 178, 180,
    180m, 185, 185t
Weigert's iron hematoxylin
    solution, 227
weight-to-volume solutions, 587t,
    590

Weil's disease, 302
white asbestos, 264–265
white light, 37
white matter, 355
Williams syndrome, 475t
Wilms' tumor, 578t
Wilson's disease, 259
Wollaston prism, 56f
work practice controls, 12
workstation ergonomics, 34
worms, 313

X

xylene
    as clearing agent, 108
    handling of, 33

    isomers of, 15
    properties of, 108
xylene substitutes
    as clearing agent, 109
    properties of, 109

Z

Z7, 79
Z-discs, 524t–525t
Zenker's solution, 86
Ziehl-Neelsen stain, 297m
zinc, 86
    buffered, 86
zinc chloride, 33
zinc formalin, 33
zinc sulfate, 33
zygomycosis, 305